RYAN'S OCCUPATIONAL THERAPY ASSISTANT:
Principles, Practice Issues, and Techniques

FOURTH EDITION

Editor

Karen Sladyk, PhD, OTR, FAOTA

Bay Path College

Longmeadow, Massachusetts

Editor Emeritus

Sally E. Ryan, COTA, ROH, Retired

Mounds View, Minnesota

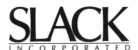

SLACK
INCORPORATED

An innovative information, education, and management company
6900 Grove Road • Thorofare, NJ 08086

www.slackbooks.com

ISBN-13: 978-1-55642-740-4

Ryan's Occupational Therapy Assistant: Principles, Practice Issues, and Techniques, Fourth Edition Instructor's Manual is also available from SLACK Incorporated. Don't miss this important companion to *Ryan's Occupational Therapy Assistant: Principles, Practice Issues, and Techniques, Fourth Edition*. To obtain the Instructor's Manual, please visit http://www.efacultylounge.com.

The following are adapted or reprinted from Ryan, S. E. (1993). *The certified occupational therapy assistant: Principles, concepts, and techniques* (2nd ed.). Thorofare, NJ: SLACK Incorporated: Figures 1-1, 1-2, 1-3, 2-1, 2-2, 2-3, 2-4, 3-1, 8-1, 14-1, 14-2, 14-3, 14-4, 32-2, 32-3, 33-1, 33-2, 33-3, 33-4, 33-5, 33-6, 33-7, 33-8, 33-9, 33-10, 33-11, 33-12, 33-13, 33-14, 33-15, 33-16, 33-17, 36-2, 36-3, 42-1, 42-4, 42-5, Appendix A and Tables 2-1, 3-1.

The work SLACK Incorporated publishes is peer reviewed. Prior to publication, recognized leaders in the field, educators, and clinicians provide important feedback on the concept and content that we publish. We welcome feedback on this work.

Printed in the United States of America.

Ryan's occupational therapy assistant : principles, practice issues, and techniques / [edited by] Sally E. Ryan, Karen Sladyk.-- 4th ed.
    p. ; cm.
  Includes bibliographical references and index.
  ISBN 1-55642-740-9 (alk. paper)
  1. Occupational therapy assistants.
  [DNLM: 1. Occupational Therapy--methods. 2. Allied Health Personnel. 3. Disabled Persons--rehabilitation. 4. Professional Practice. WB 555 R9893 2005] I. Title: Occupational therapy assistant. II. Ryan, Sally E. III. Sladyk, Karen, 1958- IV. Title.

  RM735.4.R95 2005
  615.8'515--dc22

                        2005001026

Published by: SLACK Incorporated
                 6900 Grove Road
                 Thorofare, NJ 08086 USA
                 Telephone: 856-848-1000
                 Fax: 856-853-5991
                 www.slackbooks.com

Contact SLACK Incorporated for more information about other books in this field or about the availability of our books from distributors outside the United States.

Last digit is print number: 10   9   8   7

CONTENTS

About the Editors ix
Current Contributors xi
Introduction xiii

Section I   **Historical, Philosophical, and Theoretical Principles** 1
Chapter 1   Looking Back, Living Forward: Occupational Therapy History 2
             Robert K. Bing, EdD, OTR, FAOTA

Chapter 2   The Occupational Therapy Assistant Heritage: Proud and Dynamic 14
             Shirley Holland Carr, MS, LOTR, FAOTA

Chapter 3   Philosophy and Core Values in Occupational Therapy 24
             Phillip D. Shannon, MA, MPA

Chapter 4   Human Development 34
             Carol Winters-Smith, PhD

Chapter 5   *Occupational Therapy Practice Framework: Domain and Process—Our Language* 44
             Ben Atchison, PhD, OTR, FAOTA

Chapter 6   Activity Analysis: Our Tool 52
             Sally E. Ryan, COTA, ROH, Retired and Karen Sladyk, PhD, OTR, FAOTA

Chapter 7   Theory That Guides Practice: Our Map 66
             Diane K. Dirette, PhD, OT

Chapter 8   Therapeutic Intervention Process 80
             Sally E. Ryan, COTA, ROH, Retired

Chapter 9   Occupation: An Individual's Choice 86
             Bonnie Brooks, MEd, OTR, FAOTA

Chapter 10   Teaching and Learning 96
             Karen Sladyk, PhD, OTR, FAOTA

Section II   **Occupations and Disabilities** 103
Chapter 11   A Young Child With Visual Impairments 104
             Angela E. Scoggin, PhD, OTR, FAOTA; Dickson Rodriguez, MA-CVRT, OTR;
             Mary Kathryn Cowan, MA, OTR, FAOTA; and Patricia K. Benham, MPH, OTR

Chapter 12   A Toddler With Autism Spectrum Disorder 122
             Tara J. Glennon, EdD, OTR, FAOTA

Chapter 13   A Kindergartner With Sensory Integration Dysfunction 138
             Heather Miller Kuhaneck, MS, OTR, BCP and Susanne Smith Roley, MS, OTR, FAOTA

Chapter 14   Two Children With Cerebral Palsy 156
             Tara J. Glennon, EdD, OTR, FAOTA

Chapter 15   A Second-Grader With Oppositional Defiant Disorder 172
             Linda Florey, PhD, OTR, FAOTA

Chapter 16   A Third-Grader With Attention Deficit Hyperactivity Disorder 184
             Sue Gallagher, MA, OTR

Chapter 17 A Teenager With Depression.. 202
Linda Florey, PhD, OTR, FAOTA

Chapter 18 A Car Mechanic With Traumatic Brain Injury............................... 212
Deanna Proulz-Sepelak, OTR and Paula Jo Belice, MS, OTR

Chapter 19 A Telephone Repairman With Spinal Cord Injury........................... 230
M. Laurita (Lita) Fike, MA, OTR; Karen Pendleton, MA, OTR; and Liane Hewitt, MPH, OTR

Chapter 20 A Teacher's Aide With Schizophrenia...................................... 250
Margaret Drake, PhD, OTR, FAOTA and Tonia Taylor, BS, COTA

Chapter 21 A Mother and Caterer With Multiple Sclerosis............................ 258
Lori T. Andersen, EdD, OTR, FAOTA and Barbara L. Kornblau, JD, OT/L, FAOTA

Chapter 22 A Self-Help Group Leader With Anxiety.................................... 272
Margaret Drake, PhD, OTR, FAOTA and Tonia Taylor, BS, COTA

Chapter 23 Three People Across the Age Span With Arthritis......................... 282
Lynda Bishop, MS, OTR

Chapter 24 A Plumber and Golfer With Total Hip Arthroplasty........................ 292
Dairlyn Gower, BAS, COTA/L and Marcia Bowker, OTR, CHT

Chapter 25 A Senior Homemaker With Substance Abuse................................. 304
Frank E. Gainer, MHS, OTR, FAOTA and Denise Rotert, MA, OTR

Chapter 26 A Businessman With a Stroke.. 318
Martha Logigian, MS, OTR

Chapter 27 A Homemaker and Volunteer With Parkinson's Disease...................... 334
Kathryn Melin Eberhardt, MAEd, COTA/L, ROH

Chapter 28 A Retired Librarian With Sensory Deficits............................... 348
Paula W. Jamison, PhD, OTR

Chapter 29 A Married Couple Dealing With Alzheimer's Disease........................ 366
Carolyn M. Baum, PhD, OTR/C, FAOTA

Section III Treatment Techniques, Procedures, and Concepts 381
Chapter 30 Group Intervention.. 382
Roseanna Tufano, LMFT, OTR

Chapter 31 Arts and Crafts as Meaningful Occupation................................ 398
Margaret Drake, PhD, OTR, FAOTA

Chapter 32 Assistive Technology and Adaptive Equipment............................. 406
Mary Kathryn Cowan, MA, OTR, FAOTA and Beth O'Sullivan, MPH, OTR

Chapter 33 Basic Splinting... 416
Jaclyn West-Frasier, MA, OTR

Chapter 34 Wellness and Health Promotion... 428
Karen Sladyk, PhD, OTR, FAOTA

Chapter 35 Life Skills... 432
Denise Rotert, MA, OTR and Frank E. Gainer, MHS, OTR, FAOTA

Chapter 36   Activities of Daily Living 442
              Corina Hall, MS, OTR

Chapter 37   Work Injury Activities 462
              Barbara Larson, MA, OTR, FAOTA

Section IV   Management and Practice Issues **471**
Chapter 38   Evidence-Based Practice 472
              Paula Wright, MS, OTR

Chapter 39   Understanding Research 484
              Sandy Bell, PhD, PT

Chapter 40   Documentation 498
              Karen Sladyk, PhD, OTR, FAOTA

Chapter 41   Occupational Therapy Assistant Supervision 510
              Sally E. Ryan, COTA, ROH, Retired and Karen Sladyk, PhD, OTR, FAOTA

Chapter 42   The Occupational Therapy Assistant as Activity Director 516
              Sally E. Ryan, COTA, ROH, Retired and Karen Sladyk, PhD, OTR, FAOTA

Chapter 43   Functional Ethics 528
              S. Maggie Reitz, PhD, OTR, FAOTA

Chapter 44   Teamwork and Team Building 538
              Ellen Berger Rainville, MS, OTR, FAOTA; Tone Blechert, MA, COTA, ROH;
              Marianne Christiansen, MA, OTR; and Nancy Kari, MPH, OTR

Chapter 45   Management Issues 550
              Claudine Bogosian, MHA, OTR

Chapter 46   Professional Development 560
              Anne Birge James, MS, OTR and Marijke Thamm Kehrhahn, PhD

Appendix A   Human Developmental Chart 573
Appendix B   Standards of Practice for Occupational Therapy 583
Appendix C   Occupational Therapy Code of Ethics—2000 587
Appendix D   Internet Resources 591
              Karen Sladyk, PhD, OTR, FAOTA

Index 595

ABOUT THE EDITORS

Sally E. Ryan, COTA, ROH, *Retired* is a graduate of the first occupational therapy assistant (OTA) program at Duluth, MN in 1964. She has taken extensive coursework at the University of Minnesota as a James Wright Hunt Scholar, and at the College of St. Catherine, St. Paul. Her background includes experience in practice, clinical education supervision, management in long-term care, consultation, and teaching in the professional occupational therapy (OT) program at the College of St. Catherine. In the past, Sally has served in a variety of leadership positions at the local, state, and national levels, including the AOTA Executive Board and on-site evaluator of the AOTA Accreditation Committee. Sally is the recipient of numerous state and national awards. She was the first COTA to receive the AOTA Award of Excellence and was among the first recipients of the AOTA Roster of Honor. Sally has recently retired and is enjoying interior decorating, photography, needlework, and gardening.

Karen Sladyk, PhD, OTR, FAOTA is professor and chair of OT at Bay Path College in Longmeadow, MA. Karen received her Bachelor's degree in OT from Eastern Michigan University and a Master's degree in Community Health Education from Southern Connecticut State University. Her practice interests in mental health and cognitive rehabilitation led to her pursuit of a Doctorate in Adult and Vocational Education at the University of Connecticut. An educator for 15 years, Karen is very interested in how students learn to become clinical reasoners. She has edited several OT texts with a focus on helping OT and OTA students master the content of OT education. In her free time she quilts, antiques for vintage jewelry, and volunteers for the local animal shelter, taking in too many strays.

CURRENT CONTRIBUTORS

Lori T. Andersen, EdD, OTR, FAOTA
Nova Southeastern University
Fort Lauderdale, Florida

Ben Atchison, PhD, OTR, FAOTA
Western Michigan University
Kalamazoo, Michigan

Paula Jo Belice, MS, OTR
Rush University
Chicago, Illinois

Sandy Bell, PhD, PT
University of Connecticut
Storrs, Connecticut

Lynda Bishop, MS, OTR
Bay Path College
Longmeadow, Massachusetts

Claudine Bogosian, MHA, OTR
Burke Rehabilitation Hospital
White Plains, New York

Marcia Bowker, OTR, CHT
Cloquet Community Memorial Hospital
Cloquet, Minnesota

Diane K. Dirette, PhD, OT
Western Michigan University
Kalamazoo, Michigan

Margaret Drake, PhD, OTR, FAOTA
University of Mississippi Medical Center
Jackson, Mississippi

Kathryn Melin Eberhardt, MAEd, COTA/L, ROH
South Suburban College of Cook County
South Holland, Illinois

Linda Florey, PhD, OTR, FAOTA
Neuropsychiatric Institute
Los Angeles, California

Frank E. Gainer, MHS, OTR, FAOTA
American Occupational Therapy Association
Bethesda, Maryland

Sue Gallagher, MA, OTR
Quinnipiac University
Hamden, Connecticut

Tara J. Glennon, EdD, OTR, FAOTA
Quinnipiac University
Hamden, Connecticut

Dairlyn Gower, BAS, COTA/L
Lake Superior College
Duluth, Minnesota

Corina Hall, MS, OTR
Burke Rehabilitation Hospital
White Plains, New York

Liane Hewitt, MPH, OTR
Loma Linda University
Loma Linda, California

Anne Birge James, MS, OTR
Mercy College
Dobbs Ferry, New York

Paula W. Jamison, PhD, OTR
Western Michigan University
Kalamazoo, Michigan

Marijke Thamm Kehrhahn, PhD
University of Connecticut
Storrs, Connecticut

Barbara L. Kornblau, JD, OT/L, FAOTA
Nova Southeastern University
Fort Lauderdale, Florida

Heather Miller Kuhaneck, MS, OTR, BCP
Sacred Heart University
Fairfield, Connecticut

Barbara Larson, MA, OTR, FAOTA
WorkWell Systems, Inc.
Duluth, Minnesota

Martha Logigian, MS, OTR
Keuka College
Keuka Park, New York

Beth O'Sullivan, MPH, OTR
Quinnipiac University
Hamden, Connecticut

Karen Pendleton, MA, OTR
Loma Linda University
Loma Linda, California

Ellen Berger Rainville, MS, OTR, FAOTA
Springfield College
Springfield, Massachusetts

S. Maggie Reitz, PhD, OTR, FAOTA
Towson University
Towson, Maryland

Dickson Rodriguez, MA-CVRT, OTR
Milestones Therapeutic Associates
McAllen, Texas

Susanne Smith Roley, MS, OTR, FAOTA
University of Southern California
Los Angeles, California

Denise Rotert, MA, OTR
American Occupational Therapy Association
Bethesda, Maryland

Angela E. Scoggin, PhD, OTR, FAOTA
University of Texas-Pan American
Edinburg, Texas

Tonia Taylor, BS, COTA
University of Mississippi Medical Center
Jackson, Mississippi

Roseanna Tufano, LMFT, OTR
Quinnipiac University
Hamden, Connecticut

Jaclyn West-Frasier, MA, OTR
Western Michigan University
Kalamazoo, Michigan

Carol Winters-Smith, PhD
Bay Path College
Longmeadow, Massachusetts

Paula Wright, MS, OTR
Southcoast Hospitals Group
New Bedford, Massachusetts

INTRODUCTION

This is now the fourth edition of *Ryan's Occupational Therapy Assistant*. Hundreds of OTs and OTAs have contributed to its success because they cared about the growth and development of the OTA. The reader should know that as he or she begins his or her new career, the proud OTA history stands behind him or her. Best wishes!

How to Use The Real Records

As you will see as you thumb through this new edition, several new sections have been added, including clinical summaries, evidence-based practice reviews, and real records. The real records are just that, client records copied from clinics across the country. You will notice these records are not perfect examples of proper documentation but instead accurate examples of real clinical issues. Each chapter links the real records to cases in the chapter or clinical problem-solving questions posed by the authors. However, using the real records just to support the reading would limit the potential learning. Educators and students should review the records for ethical issues, legal issues, professionalism, communication effectiveness, and as starting points for assessment or treatment planning. The editors and authors hope you find the real records a great starting point for many interesting discussions in the classroom.

Karen Sladyk, PhD, OTR, FAOTA

HISTORICAL, PHILOSOPHICAL, AND THEORETICAL PRINCIPLES

Key Concepts

- Moral treatment: A change from prison-like conditions to more human treatment of people with mental illness.
- Early OT leaders: Dunton and Meyer, psychiatrists; Tracy, a nurse; Slagle, a social worker; Barton, an architect with a disability.

Essential Vocabulary

habit training: Developed by Slagle to provide routine and occupation to severely ill patients.

invalid occupations: Coined by Tracy as activities for the disabled.

moral treatment: Change from jail-like conditions to treatment focus for people with mental illness.

National Society for the Promotion of Occupational Therapy: The forerunner of the American Occupational Therapy Association (AOTA).

occupational nurse: First training of nurses in the use of occupation in treatment.

Looking Back, Living Forward: Occupational Therapy History

Robert K. Bing, EdD, OTR, FAOTA

Introduction

Today, occupational therapy (OT) personnel face numerous predicaments. Educational preparation for practice is based predominantly on knowledge and skills that are marketable in a very competitive health care environment. The *what* of our art, science, and technology is emphasized, often at the expense of the *why*. What is missing is the sense of what has come before, of those recurring patterns that offer legitimacy and uniqueness in the health care profession.

History is an invaluable tool to assess the present and determine future courses of action. The recording of an occupational life or medical history is a testament to the past's influence on current conditions and its ability to offer approaches to alleviate problems. Fundamentally, history is experience, rather than the mere telling of quaint stories or reminiscing about past feats or failures. It is knowing enough about what has come before to know what to consider or what to rule out in evaluating the present on our way to the future. As Neustadt and May (1986) point out, we must learn how to use experience, whether remote or recent, in the process of deciding what to do today about the opportunities for tomorrow.

In the late 1700s, Western Europe was astir with a new view of life. Social, political, economic, and religious theories promoted a general sense of human progress and perfectibility (DeGrazia, 1962). Notions about intolerance, censorship, and economic and social restraints were being abandoned and replaced by a strong faith in rational behavior. Universally valid principles governing humanity, nature, and society directed people's lives and interpersonal relationships.

The changing ethic of work added a rich ingredient to this new, heady brew. Fundamental was Martin Luther's viewpoint, which declared that everyone who could work should do so. Illness and begging were unnatural. Charity should be extended only to those who could not work because of mental or physical infirmities or old age.

Moral Treatment

Near the center of all of this invigorating change was the treatment of sick people, particularly the mentally ill. Whereas long-term survivors of physical disease with physical disabilities were still rare because treatment was so inadequate, the mentally ill were a significant portion of the population.

Up to this time, the insane had been housed and handled no differently than criminals and paupers and were often chained in dungeons. Moral treatment of the insane was one product of the Age of Enlightenment. It sprang from the fundamental attitudes of the day:

- A set of principles that govern humanity and society.
- Faith in the ability of the human to reason.
- Purposeful work as a moral obligation.
- The supreme belief in the individual.

Fast disappearing were the centuries-old notions that the insane were possessed of demons; that they were no better than paupers or criminals; and that crime, sin, vice, and inactivity were the core of insanity.

Two men of the 18th century working in different countries, and unknown to each other, initiated the moral treatment movement. These two could not have been more dissimilar. Phillippe Pinel was of the French Revolution, a physician, a scholar, and a natural philosopher. William Tuke was an English merchant, wealthy, a deeply religious Quaker, and a philanthropist.

Father of Moral Treatment—Phillippe Pinel

According to Pinel, moral treatment meant treating the emotions. He believed the emotionally disturbed individual was out of balance and the patient's own emotions could be used to restore equilibrium. The compassionate Pinel believed the loss of reason was the most calamitous of all human afflictions. The ability to reason, he claimed, principally separates the human from other living forms. As Pinel wrote in his famous treatise in 1806, because of mental illness, the human character is always perverted. His thoughts and actions are diverted, his personal liberty is at length taken from him (Pinel, 1806).

Occupation figured prominently in Pinel's scheme, primarily to take patients' minds away from emotional distress and to develop their abilities. Music and various forms of literature were used. Physical exercise and work were parts of institutional living. Pinel advocated patient farms on the hospital grounds. This period was largely an agricultural era in which one's life revolved around producing products necessary for survival and one's emotional content was elaborately interwoven. The care of animals and the necessary routines of growing crops provided patients with a respect for the authority of nature as well as the most liberty that could be tolerated. The unvarying routine to maintain farming as part of the institution made a strong appeal to moral concepts, such as respect, self-esteem, and dignity for the patient.

The York Retreat—William Tuke

Part of this new humane concern was influenced by the beliefs and work of the Society of Friends, derisively known as the Quakers. They emerged in 17th century England and became one of the most distinctive movements of Puritanism. In the last decades of the 18th century, William Tuke and various members of his family established The York Retreat, primarily because of their religious-based concerns about the deplorable conditions in public insane asylums. Until this time, the term *retreat* had never been applied to an asylum. Tuke's daughter-in-law suggested the term to convey the Quaker belief that such an institution may be a quiet haven, a place in which the unhappy might obtain refuge (Tuke, 1813).

Several fundamental principles became evident within a short time. The approach was primarily one of kindness and consideration. The patients were not thought to be devoid of reason, feelings, or honor. The social environment was to be as nearly like that of a family with an atmosphere of religious sentiment and moral feeling. Tuke and Thomas Fowler, the visiting physician, believed that most insane people retain a considerable amount of self-command. The staff endeavored to gain the patient's confidence, to reinforce self-esteem, and to arrest the attention and fix it on objects that were opposite to the illusions the patient might possess. Employment in various occupations was expected as a way for the patient to maintain control over his or her disorder (Tuke, 1813).

Pinel's major work on moral treatment was published in 1801, and Tuke's description of The York Retreat appeared in 1813. These brought on a rush of reforms in institutions in Europe and, ultimately, the United States.

Sir William and Lady Ellis

Sir William Charles Ellis and his wife were in charge of newly founded county asylums in England during the first half of the 19th century. They regarded the hospital as a community—"a family"—as Sir Ellis called it. He paid little attention to medical remedies and concentrated on moral treatment principles, which he believed to be difficult but most likely to result in the gradual return to reason and happiness.

A remarkable innovation of Sir and Lady Ellis was the establishment of aftercare houses and night hospitals. Keenly aware of environmental and social influences on insanity, they envisioned these halfway houses as steppingstones from the asylum to the world (Hunter & Macalpine, 1963).

Moral Treatment in the United States

The Quakers brought the roots of moral care and occupation as treatment to the United States. They established asylums and immediately implemented Tuke's programs. The programs were popular because they helped maintain relatively low costs by having patients perform most of the necessary work of the asylum: growing crops and vegetables, maintaining herds, and manufacturing clothing and other goods. The typical institution was a beehive of activity largely designed to help it remain as self-sufficient as possible.

Reformers were in abundance. Borrowing heavily from The York Retreat, Thomas Eddy, a member of the board of governors of the Society of the New York Hospital, proposed in 1815 the construction of a building for exclusive use by mental patients. He envisioned a balanced program of exercise, entertainment, and occupations (Hass, 1924).

In the mid 1800s, just when it seemed that the moral movement was expected to be fully realized, unanticipated trouble came from all directions. A reform-minded humanitarian, Dorthea Lynde Dix, had been campaigning vigorously for better care of the mentally ill, including moral principles. State legislatures were responding positively by establishing public mental hospitals. By 1848, Dix decided to approach the federal government. Her vision was the establishment of a federal system of hospitals. After 6 years of wearying work, Dix was rewarded when Congress passed her bill. President Franklin Pierce, however, vetoed it, claiming states' rights would be endangered if the federal government took on the care of mentally ill patients.

State hospitals were experiencing great difficulties with a new type of patient: immigrants from Europe who were unable to adjust to the new conditions. They became public wards, often unable to use the language, and were considered unemployable. Several hospitals attempted to introduce moral principles, even establishing English instruction. The Bloomingdale, a New York Asylum, made such an attempt in 1845. Classes were also held in chemistry, geometry, and the physical sciences. These classes were coupled with manual labor suitable for men and women. This approach eventually failed for many reasons. Patients often were unaccustomed to the American forms of labor. Bilingual instructors could not be found. Foreign-born mechanics and artisans could not find familiar labor. Finally, large numbers of patients were too ill to participate in the available occupations (Hass, 1924).

By the mid 1800s, the American agenda largely consisted of expansionism and slavery issues. These did not bode well for improving or increasing public care of the insane. Moral treatment, including occupations, rapidly began to disappear. By the onset of the Civil War, virtually none existed in state or public-supported institutions. Custodial care continued well into the 20th century (Bockhoven, 1972).

20th Century Progressivism

The 20th century brought with it unparalleled exuberance. The United States had largely recovered from the Civil War and acquired considerable overseas possessions as a result of the Spanish-American War. For a few years before 1900 and for some years after, nearly all Americans had become ardent believers in progress, although they did not always agree about what the word meant. Prosperity was fueled by science and technology and with a flurry of industrial inventions. Cities grew rapidly, particularly in the East and Midwest. Railroads punched their way through all kinds of barriers and in all directions, linking the country's population. The newly invented automobile served important economic purposes and became useful in leisure pursuits (Bates, 1976).

There was more than a modest amount of zaniness during this era. Many physicians regarded increased female education as the primary cause of decreased women's health. These men felt the woman's brain simply could not assimilate a great deal of academic instruction beyond high school. Some physicians went further and claimed that women who worked were in danger of acquiring predominantly male afflictions—alcoholism, paralysis, and insanity. Women were thought to have an inborn immunity to such ills.

Drug therapy was also unusual by today's standards. The pharmaceutical firm that helped to usher in the aspirin craze introduced a new medication for bad coughs—heroin. Other over-the-counter products included cocaine tablets for the throat and general nervousness. Baby syrups were spiked with morphine, and miscarriage-producing pills were, according to the ads, a sure and great remedy for women.

The Progressive Era was not always progressive. Poverty, racial injustice, ethnic unrest, sterilization of mental defectives (as they were known) and possible sterilization of social misfits, repression of women's rights because of leftover Victorian ideals, a marked increase in industrial accidents resulting in chronic disabilities, and a continued lack of concern about the institutionalized insane were all part of the times.

Chicago's Hull House

Social experiments abounded during this period, particularly in urban areas. One such experiment was Hull House, opened by Jane Addams in 1889. Hull House was intended to serve the immigrants and the poor through a variety of educational, social, and investigative programs. Along with Julia Lathrop and Florence Kelley, Addams created an environment that helped bring OT to the forefront, as part of the restorative process of individual freedom. Eleanor Clarke Slagle, a pioneer in OT, spent 2 years as a staff member at Hull House and established the first training program for occupation workers (the forerunner of OT personnel).

Invalid Occupations—Susan Tracy

The first individual in the 20th century to use occupations with acutely ill patients was Susan Tracy, a nurse. She initiated instruction in activities to student nurses as early as 1902. She coined the term *occupational nurse* to signify a specialization. By 1912, she was working full-time to apply moral treatment principles to acute medical conditions. She was convinced that remedial activities should be classified by their physiological effects as stimulants or sedatives (Tracy, 1914). Tracy was also interested in experimentation and observation to enhance her practice. In 1918, she published a research paper on 25 mental tests derived from occupations (Tracy, 1918a) (e.g., instructing a patient in using a piece of leather and a pencil, and asking him or her to make a line of dots at equal distances around the margin and at uniform distances from the edge). This constitutes a test of judgment in estimating distances (Tracy, 1918a). Continuing with the same piece of leather, the patient is instructed to punch a hole at each dot. To do this, the patient must consider the two sides of leather and the two parts of the tool and must bring these together, thus making a simple construction test (Tracy, 1918a).

Tracy (1923) determined that high-quality work was therapeutic, worth doing well, and that practical, well-made articles have a greater therapeutic value than useless, poorly made articles. Tracy's major work, *Studies in Invalid Occupations*, published in 1918, is a revealing compendium of her observations and experiences with different kinds of patients (Tracy, 1918b). Among her many lasting principles, one stands out: the patient is the product, not the article he or she makes.

Re-Education of Convalescents— George Barton

The Progressive Era spawned a number of reformers who, although dissimilar in background, character, and temperament, strove to work together on common goals. George Edward Barton and William Rush Dunton, Jr. were 2 individuals significant to OT. Barton, by profession an architect, contracted tuberculosis during adulthood. His constant struggle led him into a life of service to physically disabled persons.

Barton founded Consolation House in Clifton Springs, NY, in 1914, an early prototype of a rehabilitation center. Today he would be considered an entrepreneur. He was an effective speaker and writer, although often given to exaggeration. Barton's main themes were hospitals and their responsibilities to the discharged patient, the conditions the discharged patient faces, the need to return to employment after an illness, and occupations and education of convalescents.

Barton's first published article in 1914 was based on a speech given to a group of nurses, in which he described a weakness in hospitals—hospitals discharge not efficients, but inefficients. An individual leaves almost any of our institutions only to become a burden upon his family, his friends, the associated charities, or upon another institution. Later in the article he warns to his subject, discharge a patient from the hospital with his fracture healed, to be sure, but to a devastated home, to an empty desk, and to no obvious sustaining employment is to send him out to a world cold. His solution was occupation to shorten convalescence and improve the condition of many patients. He ended his oration with a rallying cry: "...It is time for humanity to cease regarding the hospital as a door closing upon a life which is past and to regard it henceforth as a door opening upon a life which is to come" (Barton, 1914, p. 336).

At Consolation House, physically impaired individuals underwent a thorough review, including a social and medical history, and a consideration of their education, training, experience, successes, and failures. Barton (1922) believed that by "considering these in relation to the condition [the patient] must presumably or inevitably be in for the remainder of his life, we can find some form of occupation for which he will be fitted" (p. 320). Barton's major contribution to the re-emergence of moral treatment principles was an awakening of physical reconstruction and re-education through employment. Convalescence, to him, was a critical time for the inclusion of something to do.

Judicious Regimen of Activity— William Dunton

A medical school graduate of the University of Pennsylvania and a psychiatrist, William Rush Dunton, Jr., devoted his entire life to OT. A prolific writer, he published in excess of 120 books and articles related to OT and rehabilitation. He also served as treasurer and president of the National Society for the Promotion of Occupational Therapy (the forerunner of the AOTA), and for 21 years he was editor of their official journal. As a physician, he spent his professional career treating psychiatric patients in an institutional setting. Key to his treatment methods was what he called a judicious regimen of activity. He read the works of Tuke and Pinel, as well as the efforts of significant alienists (an early term for psychiatrists) of the 19th century.

In 1895, Dunton joined the medical staff at Sheppard and Enoch Pratt Asylum in Towson, MD. From his readings and observations of patients there, he concluded that acutely ill patients generally were not amenable to occupations because their weakened attention span would make involvement in activity fatiguing and harmful. Later, activities might be prescribed that use energies not needed for physical restoration. Stimulating attention and directing the thoughts of the patient in regular and healthful paths would ensure an early discharge from the hospital. Dunton developed a wide variety of activities from knitting and crocheting to printing, the repair of dynamos, and farm work to gain the attention and interest, as well as to meet the needs, of all patients. He stated that a patient makes more rapid progress if his attention is concentrated upon what he is making and he derives stimulating pleasure in its performance (Dunton, 1935). Interest in the activity was paramount in Dunton's thinking.

At the second annual meeting of the National Society for the Promotion of Occupational Therapy in 1918, Dunton unveiled his 9 cardinal principles to guide the emerging practice of OT and to ensure that the new discipline would gain acceptance as a medical entity. These principles were the following:

1. Any activity should have as its objective a cure.

2. The activity should be interesting.
3. There should be a useful purpose other than to merely gain the patient's attention and interest.
4. The activity should preferably lead to an increase in knowledge on the patient's part.
5. Activity should be carried on with others, such as a group.
6. The OT should make a careful study of the patient and attempt to meet as many needs as possible through activity.
7. Activity should cease before the onset of fatigue.
8. Genuine encouragement should be given whenever indicated.
9. Work is much to be preferred over idleness, even when the end product of the patient's labor is of poor quality or is useless (Dunton, 1918).

The major purposes of occupation in the case of the mentally ill were outlined in Dunton's first book, *Occupation Therapy: A Manual for Nurses*, published in 1915. The primary objective is to divert attention from unpleasant subjects, as is true with the depressed patient; or from daydreaming or mental ruminations, as in the case of dementia praecox (schizophrenia), to divert the attention to one main subject.

Another purpose of occupation is to re-educate, to train the patient in developing mental processes through educating the hands, eyes, and muscles, just as is done in the developing child (Dunton, 1915). Fostering an interest in hobbies is a third purpose. Hobbies serve as both present and future safety valves and render a recurrence of mental illness less likely. A final purpose may be to instruct the patient in a craft until he or she has gained enough proficiency to take pride in the work. However, Dunton worried that specialization would limit interest in the world in general (1915).

The Origin of the Term *Occupational Therapy*

There is a continuing controversy about who was initially responsible for the term *occupational therapy*—Dunton or Barton. At Sheppard and Enoch Pratt Asylum, Dunton directed the therapeutic occupations program. A special building was completed in 1902 and named The Casino. It was a dedicated space for a wide variety of occupations and amusements. In 1911, Dunton initiated a training program for nurses in patient occupations, and here he first used the term *occupation therapy*. This term appeared in his handwritten lecture notes, dated October 10, 1911. This is the earliest known record of the use of this term. In later years, Dunton indicated that Adolph Meyer, a renowned psychiatrist and personal and professional friend, was the first to use the terms *therapy* and *therapeutic* in connection with occupations, but that he was the first person to put occupation and therapy together as one phrase (AOTA, 1914-1917).

Barton's claim to the first use of the term appeared initially in March 1915, in the *Trained Nurse and Hospital Review*. The article was based on a speech given in Massachusetts on December 28, 1914. Before then, Barton had preferred the term *occupation re-education*, which accurately described his efforts at

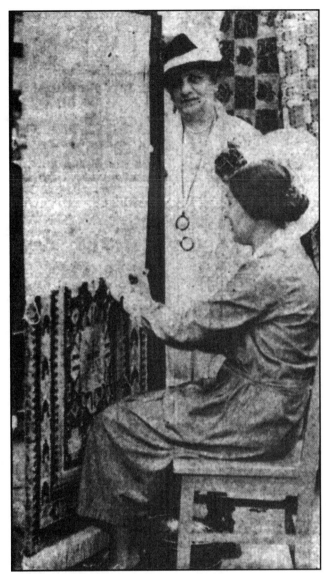

Figure 1-1. Eleanor Clarke Slagle (standing) and Margaret Kransee (1933).

Consolation House. During preliminary discussions between Barton and Dunton about a national organization during 1915 to 1916, a series of squabbles took place, mostly through correspondence. Terminology figured heavily in these differences of opinion. Barton preferred his occupational re-education and Dunton held tenaciously to occupation therapy. Barton finally countered with occupational therapy, preferring the adjectival form. They did agree on the term *occupational workers*, since the word therapist was considered the sole property of the psychiatrist. Dunton did not change his mind until well into the 1920s (Barton, 1915; Bing, 1987).

Habit Training—Eleanor Clarke Slagle

Eleanor Clarke Slagle is considered the most distinguished 20th century OT. One of 5 founders of the national professional organization, she served in every major elective office. She was also executive secretary for 14 years. In the first decade of this century, she was partially trained as a social worker and completed one of the early special courses in curative occupations and recreation at the Chicago School of Civics and Philanthropy, which was associated with Hull House. She worked subsequently in a number of institutions, most notably the new Henry Phipps Clinic, Johns Hopkins Hospital, Baltimore, MD. There she served under the direction of the renowned psychiatrist Adolph Meyer. At this time, she became a devoted friend of William Dunton's family. Later, she moved to New York, where she pioneered in developing OT in the State Department of Mental Hygiene.

Slagle (1934) was knowledgeable about moral treatment principles and embraced them as the core of her thinking and practice. She emphasized that OT must be a purposely planned progressive program of rest, play, occupation, and exercise. She often spoke of the need for the mentally ill person to have a fairly well-balanced day.

Her most long-lasting contribution to the care of the mentally ill was what she entitled *habit training*. This plan was first attempted at the Rochester, New York State Hospital in 1901, but it was Slagle who developed and refined the basic principles for those patients who had been hospitalized for 5 to 20 years and whose behavior had steadily regressed. Habit training was 24 hours long and involved the entire ward staff. It was a re-education program designed to overcome disorganized habits, to modify other habits, and to construct new ones, with the goal of restoring and maintaining of health (Slagle, 1922).

A typical habit-training schedule called for patients to wake at 6:00 a.m., then wash, toilet, brush teeth, and air beds. After breakfast, they returned to the ward and made beds and swept. Classwork followed and lasted for 2 hours. It consisted of a variety of simple crafts and marching exercises. After lunch, there was a rest period, continued classwork, outdoor exercises, folk dancing, and lawn games. After supper, there was music and dancing on the ward, followed by toileting, washing, teeth brushing, and preparing for bed (Slagle & Robeson, 1933).

After maximum benefit was achieved from habit training, the patient progressed through 3 phases of OT. The first was what Slagle called the kindergarten group. Occupations such as music, coloring, and games were graded from simple to complex. The next phase was ward classes in OT. When able to tolerate it, the patient joined in group activities. The third phase was the occupational center. "This promotes opportunities for more advanced projects... a complete change in environment; ...comparative freedom; ...actual responsibilities placed upon patients; the stimulation of seeing work produced; ...all these carry forward the readjustment of patients" (Slagle & Robeson, 1933, p. 29).

Figure 1-1 shows Eleanor Clarke Slagle (standing) when she was the director of OT at the New York Department of Mental Hygiene. She is inspecting the weaving of a woolen rug by Mrs. Margaret Kransee, instructor at the Manhattan State Hospital, Wards Island, NY in 1933.

THE PHILOSOPHY OF OCCUPATIONAL THERAPY—ADOLPH MEYER

A history of this type would not be complete without at least a brief mention of Adolph Meyer, a Swiss physician who immigrated to this country in 1892. By the end of 1910, he became professor of psychiatry at Johns Hopkins University and the first director of the Henry Phipps Clinic. Meyer "borrowed" Eleanor Clarke Slagle from Hull House for 2 years, during which time she founded the therapeutic occupations program in the clinic. Meyer's lasting contribution to psychiatry is the psychobiologic approach to mental illness and health. He coined this term to indicate that the human is an indivisible unit of study, rather than a composite of symptoms (Meyer, 1975).

Because of his friendship with Slagle and Dunton, Meyer agreed to deliver a major address at the fifth annual meeting of the National Society for the Promotion of Occupational Therapy in Baltimore, October 1921. This address has become a classic in OT literature. Meyer emphasized occupation, time, and the productive use of energy. He stated that the whole of human organization has its shape in a kind of rhythm; there are many rhythms to which we must be attuned: the larger rhythms of night, day, sleep, and waking hours; and finally the big four: work, play, rest, and sleep. The only way to attain balance in all this is actual doing, actual practice, a program of wholesome living is the basis of wholesome feeling and thinking and fancy and interests (Meyer, 1922).

In this address, Meyer successfully brought the fundamental moral treatment principles of more than a century before into contemporary OT practice and established the foundation of what is now known as occupational behavior, the model of human occupation and occupational performance.

FOUNDING OF THE AMERICAN OCCUPATIONAL THERAPY ASSOCIATION

The AOTA (1914-1917) archives hold all of the correspondence between George Barton, William Dunton, and Eleanor Clarke Slagle during the era when discussions were held about creating a national organization to be a mechanism for exchanging views and extending information about the fledgling new line of medicine. The first letter in the series was from Dunton to Barton on October 15, 1915, wherein he suggested that Barton take the lead in organizing a central bureau for occupation workers. Barton wrote back, agreed, and suggested a title, Society for the Promotion of Occupation for Re-Education. A series of false starts ensued, and Dunton became exasperated with the lack of progress. Local groups of occupation workers were forming to exchange views, and he felt they needed support and guidance from a national group. On December 7, 1916, Dunton wrote Barton again, proposing a 5-member national executive committee. Disagreements between them arose about who should be invited. They were settled on December 20, 1916, when Barton wrote Dunton with a new

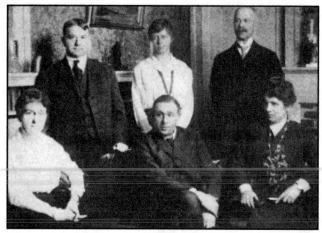

Figure 1-2. The founders of the National Society for the Promotion of Occupational Therapy. Front row, left to right: Susan Cox Johnson, George E. Barton, Eleanor Clarke Slagle. Back row, left to right: William R. Dunton, Isabel Newton, Thomas Kidner.

title, National Society for the Promotion of Occupational Therapy.

After some juggling of dates, March 15 through 17 were set for the organizational meeting and incorporation of the society. Barton invited the "big five," as he called the executive committee, to use his Consolation House for the event, as he wished to be host. The invitees, other than Dunton, included Eleanor Clarke Slagle, then the general superintendent of OT at Hull House; Susan Cox Johnson, the director of occupations, New York State Department of Public Charities; and Thomas B. Kidner, the vocational secretary, Canadian Military Hospital Commission. Susan E. Tracy, instructor in invalid occupations, Presbyterian Hospital, Chicago, was also invited but declined because of her work schedule. Isabelle Newton, Barton's secretary at Consolation House, was invited to attend in that capacity (Figure 1-2). Barton was elected president, a position he nominated himself for a few weeks before the meeting.

The next 6 months proved critical. Barton became increasingly annoyed at Dunton and Slagle, who was vice president. He suspected they were trying to overshadow his presidency. He also became involved in a heated debate about finances with Dunton, the treasurer. Subsequently, Barton refused to attend the first annual meeting on Labor Day weekend, September 1917, in New York City. He cited poor health as the reason. Dunton was elected the new president. There is no record that Barton attended any meetings of the national organization for the remainder of his life; however, he did remain a member (Licht, 1967).

The 1925 Principles

An AOTA committee, made up of physicians and chaired by William Rush Dunton, Jr., compiled an outline of lectures on OT for medical students and physicians (Adams, 1925). The members developed a definition, objectives, statements of the use of a variety of activities with different kinds of patients, therapeutic approaches, and the qualities and qualifications of practitioners. This was the first such effort since Dunton had created his principles in 1918 (Adams, 1925).

The first principle states that OT is a method of training the sick or injured by means of instruction and employment in productive occupation (Adams, 1925). One is struck by the importance of the connection between learning by doing and purposeful activity. This was the dominant theme in several of the principles. The act of doing should be seen from the patient's point of view. For example, the treatment objectives stated that activities sought are to arouse interest, courage, and confidence; to exercise mind and body; to overcome disability; and to re-establish capacity for industrial and social usefulness (Adams, 1925).

Rules were established about the extent of activities, and attention was given to their qualities and effect on the patient. The use of crafts and work-related occupations was emphasized. Games, music, and physical exercise were not to be overlooked. A warning was offered: whereas quality, quantity, and salability may serve some objectives, these must not override the main purpose of the activity. Belief in the various properties of occupation is evident as the patient's strength and capability increase, the type and extent of occupation should be regulated and graded accordingly (Adams, 1925).

The committee made a statement about the quality of work to be expected as a therapeutic approach that inferior workmanship in an occupation that would be trivial for the healthy may be used with the sick or injured, but standards worthy of normal persons must be maintained for proper mental stimulation (Adams, 1925).

The relationship between purposeful activity and the connections between the mind and body is found in the principle, the production of a well-made article, or the accomplishment of a useful task, requires healthy exercise of mind and body. Involvement in group activity is advised because it provides exercise in social adaptation (Adams, 1925). Evaluation rests with measuring the effect of the occupation on the patient, the extent to which objectives are being realized.

Adams (1925) believed one final principle addressed the qualifications of the practitioner as good craftsman, ability to teach, understanding, interest in the patient, and an optimistic, cheerful outlook. Elsewhere in the lecture outline, the committee recommended that therapists and aides should have a therapeutic sense, the teaching instinct, and good mental balance. Personality constitutes 50% of the value of these workers (Adams, 1925).

During this period, a number of issues were combined, including the following:
- Purposeful work and leisure.
- The intricate involvement of the mind and body (interdependence of mental and physical aspects, also known as holism).
- OT as a learning process.
- The therapeutic use of one's personal qualities.

The literature of the next several decades, which was a period of remarkable development in the profession, gives evidence of how these principles became operational.

Purposeful Work and Leisure

In her early endeavors as a practitioner, Clare Spackman (1936) explored the perplexing problem of engaging the patient's interests. Her recommendation was to approach the patient through his or her interests. She noted that there are few people who have not an interest and for the therapist to make the right suggestion at the right time takes both experience and imagination.

Martha Gilbert (1936), an OT at the Choctaw-Chickasaw Sanitarium in Oklahoma, built her entire treatment program around purposeful work and leisure for children. The sanitarium was a federal institution with 75 beds for Native American children with tuberculosis and related diseases. In 1929, times were difficult, not only because of the Great Depression, but also because Native American children were not highly valued, except by those who cared for them on a daily basis. Supplies meager, she used native material to make items of interests, including clay in summer and leaves in fall. The children loved to draw, garden, and march to music. Culture was a focus of activities, especially at holidays. Gilbert's approach may be seen today, as therapists and assistants carry out innovative and imaginative programs in impoverished areas of the United States and, indeed, throughout the world.

Involvement of the Mind and Body

The interaction of mind and body has remained a basic principle throughout our historical evolution. Ida Sands addressed the annual AOTA conference in 1927 with the importance of spiritual rehabilitation (Sands, 1938). Beatrice Wade, a renowned clinician, educator, and administrator, spoke of the treatment of the total patient in an address in 1967. She stated that this approach is unique to OT among the health disciplines. There has always existed a strong component concerned with the ill or disabled, with the entirety of man, and his functioning as a patient (Wade, 1967). This OT concept, she added, prevented an undesired separation of the psychiatric therapist from the physical disabled therapist.

Occupational Therapy as a Learning Process

Throughout the formative years, OT and education held much in common, not so much in how patients were instructed, but in the outcome of that instruction through changes in behavior and performance of a more complex nature. Harriet Robeson, a distinguished therapist, addressed a group of social workers in 1926 and affirmed some longstanding principles that OT is a re-education. She added that many think of OT as only handwork. It is far more; it is a program of work, play, and medicine to meet the mental, physical, and social needs of each patient (Robeson, 1926).

The re-education process follows the same pathway as normal education, a gradual growth through progressive development. The therapist must teach the patient to creep and to creep in the right direction (Robeson, 1926).

Irene O'Brock (1932), director of OT at the University of Oklahoma Hospitals, indicated that her program for children had an extra value, a deeper more intangible significance: the natural tendencies of life, play, and companionship. She based her treatment program on 5 lines of readiness:

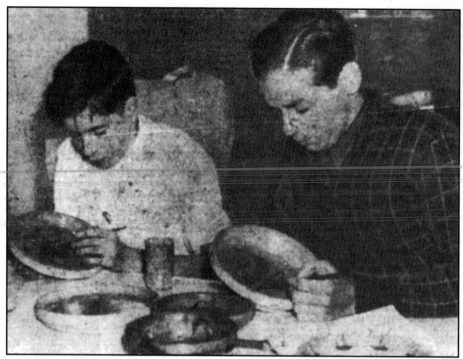

Figure 1-3. Patients in the OT Department at the Jewish Sanitarium and Hospital for Chronic Diseases, Brooklyn, NY.

1. To construct things
2. To communicate things
3. To find out things
4. To compete in things
5. To excel in things

Figure 1-3 shows two men engaged in activities that were typical of the times. These patients were receiving OT treatment at the Jewish Sanitarium and Hospital for Chronic Diseases in Brooklyn, NY. They were painting colorful designs on wooden plates that were sold at a bazaar. The proceeds were used to augment the hospital fund, which provided care for more than 500 disabled men, women, and children.

The Practitioner's Personal Qualities

One of the first student papers published in *Occupational Therapy and Rehabilitation*, the official journal of the AOTA, appeared in 1930. Nelda McKee (1930) of the University of Minnesota wrote *Ethics for the Occupational Therapist*. She discussed the ideals, customs, and habits that members of the profession are accumulating around the name and character of the trained therapist. Essential attributes in dealing with patients include honesty, frankness, and wisdom. She showed her insight when she stated:

> A therapist should endeavor to develop a symmetrical life. We all have a physical, mental, spiritual, and social side to our make-up which needs care and cultivation. The [therapist] is under personal obligation to keep herself from growing narrow...
> Above all, [she] must keep the quality of being "teachable." Then she will never stop developing the possibilities which she possesses. The ideal therapist never forgets that our ambitions are all directed

toward one common end. We are working for the advancement of understanding and the enlargement of human life. (pp. 357, 360)

Joseph C. Doane, MD (1929), who later became president of AOTA, gave an impromptu address to conference attendees at the 1928 AOTA annual meeting. He distinguished between two kinds of workers—the occupationalist and the therapist:

> I regret to say that the occupationalists include not a few physicians and many laymen. [They believe] that OT is a very interesting and very useful plaything which begins and stops there; they see the product, rather than the patient; they comment on the beautiful colors and difficult weaves... They see nothing beyond the mere physical thing which has resulted from the activity.
> Then there is the other party—the therapist. The therapist looks at yarn and raffia, not as materials to be used... but as the implements or tools to be employed in the handling of much more difficult material, the disposition of the persons who are ill, a most varying and a most uncertain commodity. (pp. 13-14)

For Doane (1929), the critical importance is for the therapist to know what sick people do, think, and why they behave as they do, which is much more important than to know how to make something.

WE LIVE FORWARD

Contemporary occupational theorists and visionaries, such as Mary Reilly, Phillip Shannon, Gary Kielhofner, Janice Burke, and Elizabeth Yerxa, find ample support for their concepts in the founding, time-honored principles. For nearly 2 decades, between 1958 and 1977, Reilly wrote extensively about OT principles and the profession's changing role in medicine and health care. As Madigan and Parent (1985) point out:

> Reilly stated that the medical model is designed to prevent and reduce illness and does not address the reduction of incapacity that results from illness. It is the OT's [and assistant's] responsibility to activate residual adaptation of patients and to help deficit humans achieve life satisfaction through work and social involvement. (pp. 25-26)

Reilly (1962) repeatedly called for a renewed conceptualization of OT as reflected in the ideals of Dunton, Slagle, and Tracy. In addition, Reilly argued that OT needed to be concerned about the difficulties people have with their occupations all along the developmental continuum, including play and work. This she called *occupational behavior*.

By 1977, much of OT practice had markedly shifted away from its foundation in the original principles. Shannon (1977) viewed with alarm what was taking place. He called it a derailment:

> ...a new hypothesis has emerged that views man not as a creative being capable of making choices and directing his own future, but as a mechanistic creature susceptible to manipulation and control via the application of techniques... is a derailment from those... values and beliefs that legitimized the practice of OT. If OT persists in this direction, what was once and still is one of the great ideas of 20th century medicine will be swept away by the tide of technique philosophy. Should this happen the legitimacy of OT may be revoked and... its services absorbed by other health care professions. (p. 233)

Shannon was one of many graduate students under Reilly who advanced occupational behavior theory.

Six years later, Kielhofner and Burke (1983) completed an exhaustive review of the early literature and were left with a deep respect for the ideas and accomplishments of the first generation of therapists. Both a science of occupation and the art of using occupation as a medical therapy were conceived, clearly articulated, and applied. Yet, our confidence and willingness to embrace clinical problems was missing, something had been dropped out in the intervening years between the development of the principles and the time of their review.

Kielhofner (1985) and his associates proceeded with the development of what they term a *model of human occupation*, using the concepts of occupational behavior theory. The latest addition to this evolution, starting with the original principles, is called *occupational science* and is viewed by many as a foundation for OT well into the 21st century. Occupational science is believed to be an emerging basic science that supports occupational practice (Yerxa, 1989).

SUMMARY

OT beginnings reach back more than 200 years, to the Age of Enlightenment when human beings were emerging with a new, expanded view of "why on earth they were on Earth."

There was a sense of economic, political, social, and religious progress. Ideas were forming about the importance of each human being, about the human ability to think and learn, about labor as the central focus of life, and about human existence being governed by a prevailing set of principles directed toward everyday living. These same ideals became significant in caring about and for the mentally ill.

In Europe, the birthplace of this new age, men and women such as Phillippe Pinel, William Tuke, and Sir William and Lady Ellis engaged their mental patients in a variety of occupations and amusements for a number of purposes:

- To restore reason.
- To provide feelings of security and self-worth.
- To allow as much freedom of choice and movement as possible, regardless of mental conditions.
- To arrest delusional attention and fix it on objects that would help restore reason.

From their experience, the caregivers established certain principles that were handed down to the present day. For more than 50 years, during the latter decades of the 19th century and the early 20th century, these principles all but disappeared because of social, economic, and political upheavals. They reemerged in the second decade of the 20th century as OT.

In the United States during the Progressive Era, a diverse collection of men and women restated and added to the inherited principles. Among these people were William Rush Dunton, Jr., a psychiatrist; Eleanor Clarke Slagle, a partially trained social worker; Susan Tracy, a nurse; George Edward Barton, a disabled architect; and Adolph Meyer, a psychiatrist. Their contributions remain today as the cornerstone of the 7 OT principles:

1. Activity contains ingredients by which an ill or disabled individual may gain understanding of and control over one's own feelings, thoughts, and actions; habits of attention and interest; usefulness of occupation; creative expression; the process of learning by doing; skill; and concrete evidence of personal accomplishment.

2. Variations of activity provide opportunities to balance the larger rhythms of life: work, play, rest, and sleep, which must remain balanced if health is to be regained, maintained, or attained.

3. Purposeful occupation involves the intricate interplay of the mind and body, which cannot be separated if the human being is to engage in activity.

4. Involvement in remedial activity has as a major purpose the acquiring or restoring of usefulness to one's self and others as a happy, productive human being.

5. The patient is the product of his or her own efforts, not the article made nor the activity accomplished.

6. One's approach to the patient is as significant to treatment and rehabilitation as is the selection and use of an activity.

7. A knowledge of the patient's needs, an appreciation of the pain that accompanies an illness or disability, a strong desire to reduce or remove it, and a gentle firmness are among the major characteristics of the provider of therapeutic occupations.

These principles remain intact, although often restated and reworded. There is considerable evidence they will remain a part of our practice through the efforts of such individuals as Mary Reilly, Phillip Shannon, Gary Kielhofner, Janice Burke, and Elizabeth Yerxa and her associates. Occupational behavior, the model of human occupation, and occupational science offer assurances that these principles will still be with us well into the next century.

LEARNING ACTIVITIES

1. Construct a historical timeline identifying the important people and events that shaped the profession's history.

2. Much of the impetus for the development of the profession grew out of the principles of moral treatment, yet adherence to moral treatment "died out." What implications does this have for the OT profession today?

3. Review the summary of principles and compare and contrast them with those you see in OT literature and practice environments today. Discuss the similarities and differences.

4. If you could have spent time talking with Barton and Dunton, what would you have discussed?

5. Identify ways in which the early beliefs about habit training are reflected in OT practice today.

6. Set up an annual conference for practitioners from 1949 when OTAs were first discussed.

ACKNOWLEDGMENTS

The author wishes to express his profound gratitude to those people who so generously assisted in the search for materials and in the preparation of this chapter: Lillian Hoyle Parent, OTR, FAOTA; James L. Cantwell, OTR; Gary A. Wade, OTR; Florence S. Cromwell, OTR, FAOTA; and Inci Bowman, PhD, director, Truman Blocker History of Medicine Collection (AOTA Archives), Moody Medical Library, The University of Texas Medical Branch at Galveston.

Thanks also to the staff of the *American Journal of Occupational Therapy* for permission to use excerpts from previously published articles: *Occupational Therapy Revisited: A Paraphratic Journey* [1981, Vol. 35(6)] and *Living Forward, Understanding Backwards, Part 1 and 2* [1984, Vol. 38(6 and 7)].

Robert Kendall Bing died in 2003. Described as a gentleman, scholar, and outstanding leader in occupational therapy, he was known for his compassion (Christiansen, Gordon, & Parent, 2004). The chapter was updated by the editors.

REFERENCES

Adams, I. D. (1925). An outline of lectures on OT to medical students and physicians. *OT Rehabilitation, 4,* 277-292.

American Occupational Therapy Association. (1914-1917). Unpublished correspondence in AOTA Archives 1914-1917, Series 1. Truman Blocker History of Medicine Collection, Moody Medical Library, The University of Texas Medical Branch at Galveston.

Barton, G. E. (1914). A view of invalid occupation. *Trained Nurse and Hospital Review, 52,* 328-330.

Barton, G. E. (1915). Occupational nursing. *Trained Nurse and Hospital Review, 54,* 328-336.

Barton, G. E. (1922). The existing hospital system and reconstruction. *Trained Nurse and Hospital Review, 69,* 309,320.

Bates, J. L. (1976). *The United States, 1898-1928: Progressivism and a society in transition.* New York, NY: McGraw-Hill.

Bing, R. K. (1987). Who originated the term OT? *American Journal of Occupational Therapy, 3.* Letter to the editor.

Bockhoven, I. S. (1972). *Moral treatment in community mental health.* New York, NY: Springer Publishing.

Christiansen, C., Gordon, D., & Parent, L. (2004). In memoriam, Robert Kendall Bing, 1929-2003. *American Journal of Occupational Therapy, 58*(3), 258-260.

DeGrazia, S. (1962). *Of time, work, and leisure.* New York, NY: Twentieth Century Fund.

Doane, J. C. (1929). OT. *OT Rehabilitation, 8*(1), 13-14.

Dunton, W. R. (1915). *Occupation therapy: A manual for nurses.* Philadelphia, PA: W. B. Saunders.

Dunton, W. R. (1918). The principles of OT. In *Proceedings of the National Society for the Promotion of OT, Second Annual Meeting.* Catonsville, MD: Spring Grove State Hospital Press.

Dunton, W. R. (1935). The relationship of OT and physical therapy. *Archives of Physical Therapy, 16*(1), 19.

Gilbert, M. E. (1936). OT program at Choctaw-Chickasaw Sanitarium. *OT Rehabilitation, 11,* 113.

Hass, L. J. (1924). One hundred years of OT. *Archives of OT, 3*(2), 83-100.

Hunter, R., & Macalpine, I. (1963). *Three hundred years of psychiatry: 1535-1860* (pp. 871-872). London: Oxford University Press.

Kielhofner, G. (Ed.). (1985). *A model of human occupation: Theory and application.* Baltimore, MD: Williams & Wilkins.

Kielhofner, G., & Burke, J. P. (1983). The evolution of knowledge and practice in OT: Past, present, and future. In G. Kielhofner (Ed.), *Health through occupation: Theory and practice in OT.* Philadelphia, PA: F. A. Davis.

Licht, S. (1967). The founding and founders of the AOTA. *American Journal of Occupational Therapy, 21,* 269-271.

Madigan, M. J., & Parent, L. H. (1985). Preface. In G. Kielhofner (Ed.), *A model of human occupation: Theory and application.* Baltimore, MD: Williams & Wilkins.

McKee, N. (1930). Ethics for the OT. *OT Rehabilitation, 9*(6), 357-360.

Meyer, A. (1922). The philosophy of OT. *Archives in OT, 1*(6). Reprinted in *American Journal of Occupational Therapy* in 1977, 31(10).

Meyer, A. (1975). The psychobiological point of view. In J. B. Brady (Ed.), *Classics in American psychiatry.* St. Louis, MO: Warren H. Green.

Neustadt, R. E., & May, E. R. (1986). *Thinking in time: The uses of history for decision-makers.* New York, NY: The Free Press.

O'Brock, I. (1932). Occupational treatment for crippled children. *OT Rehabilitation, 11*(3), 204-205.

Pinel, P. (1806). *A treatise on insanity in which are contained the principles of a new and more practical nosology of maniacal disorders*. Translated by D. D. Davis. London: Cadell and Davis.

Reilly, M. (1962). OT can be one of the great ideas of 20th century medicine. *American Journal of Occupational Therapy, 26*, 1-2.

Robeson, H. A. (1926). How can occupational therapists help the social service worker? *OT Rehabilitation, 5*, 379-381.

Sands, I. F. (1938). When is occupation curative? *OT Rehabilitation, 17*, 117-119.

Shannon, P. D. (1977). The derailment of OT. *American Journal of Occupational Therapy, 31*, 233.

Slagle, E. C. (1922). Training aides for mental patients. *Archives of OT, 1*, 13-14.

Slagle, E. C. (1934). OT: Recent methods and advances in the United States. *OT Rehabilitation, 13*, 289.

Slagle, E. C., & Robeson, H. A. (1933). *Syllabus for training nurses in occupational therapy*. Utica, NY: State Hospital Press.

Spackman, C. S. (1936). The approach to the patient in a general hospital. Unpublished paper delivered at Tri-Stab Institute on OT, Farnhurst, NJ, March 9, 3-5.

Tracy, S. E. (1914). The place of invalid occupations in the general hospital. *Modern Hospital, 2*(5), 386.

Tracy, S. E. (1918a). Twenty-five suggested mental tests derived from invalid occupations. *Maryland Psychiatric Quarterly, 8*, 15-16.

Tracy, S. E. (1918b). *Studies in invalid occupations*. Boston, MA: Witcomb and Barrows.

Tracy, S. E. (1923). Treatment of disease by employment at St. Elizabeth's Hospital. *Modern Hospital, 20*(2), 198.

Tuke, W. (1813). *Description of the retreat: An institution near York for insane persons of the Society of Friends*. London: Dawson of Pall Mall.

Wade, B. D. (1967). OT: A history of its practice in the psychiatric field. Unpublished paper delivered at the AOTA 51st annual conference, October 1967.

Yerxa, E. (1989). An introduction to occupational science: A foundation for OT in the 21st century. *OT Health Care, 6*(4), 3.

Key Concepts

- Early leaders in OTA history: Ruth A. Robinson, Marion W. Crampton, Ruth Brunyate Wiemer, and Mildred Schwagmeyer.
- Roster of Honor (ROH): AOTA national award for occupational therapy assistants (OTAs) for leadership in OT.

Essential Vocabulary

grandfather clause: Ruling or law that allows OTAs not formally trained to earn credentials once formal training began for all OTAs.

supportive personnel: Aides and technicians other than OTAs.

Chapter 2

THE OCCUPATIONAL THERAPY ASSISTANT HERITAGE: PROUD AND DYNAMIC

Shirley Holland Carr, MS, LOTR, FAOTA

INTRODUCTION

This chapter is about the birth of the certified occupational therapy assistant (COTA). The story begins in the post-World War II era with Ruth A. Robinson and Marion W. Crampton, and later Ruth Brunyate Wiemer and Mildred Schwagmeyer. Described here are the circumstances that led to the creation of the COTA, the roles of some individuals who were instrumental in the development of the concept, educational training, and practice of the OTA, and OTA accomplishments.

You are carried from the "beginnings" to your own entry into our profession, with emphasis on the early years. If you discern more anecdotes than usual, consider that while you are reading contemporary history the writer was reminiscing.

USE OF PERSONNEL BEFORE 1960

Before World War II, many OTs worked in psychiatric institutions. After 1945 and influenced by military experience, increasing numbers of therapists practiced in medical and rehabilitation settings (see Chapter 1). This added to the already severe shortage of OTs in psychiatric settings during and after World War II. Psychiatric hospitals often had patient populations of between 1,000 and 6,000. With a shortage of therapists, OT services were provided by a number of aides, assistants, or technicians who were supervised by one or two OTs.

Supportive personnel (OT aides and technicians) working in psychiatric facilities were valuable and valued employees, having learned the "tricks of the trade" by modeling therapist behaviors or by trial and error. In contrast to the mobility of OTs, the employment stability of aides and technicians often made them the most knowledgeable personnel about individual patient behavior and the availability of activities and equipment in a given setting. Supportive personnel knew how to do things, but lacked goal-oriented intervention methods necessary to work without immediate supervision. This deficit motivated supervisory personnel to organize courses for OTAs (Crampton, 1989).

EARLY TRAINING NEEDS AND SHORT COURSES

Several states and the military recognized the need for in-service training (on-the-job educational opportunities) for OT personnel and developed courses of varying lengths. As early as 1944, the U.S. Army developed a 1-month course. Crampton, employed by the state of Massachusetts, developed and conducted 4- and 6-week courses before approval by the AOTA. Other states with early short courses were New York, Wisconsin, and Pennsylvania (for activity aides) (Crampton, 1989).

AMERICAN OCCUPATIONAL THERAPY'S ROLE IN THE DEVELOPMENT OF THE OCCUPATIONAL THERAPY ASSISTANT

The overlapping employment and association roles of Col. Ruth A. Robinson, Marion W. Crampton, Mildred Schwagmeyer, and Ruth Brunyate Wiemer were fortuitous to the development of the COTA. Each of these women had a long-standing interest in the use of supportive OT personnel, and all but Wiemer were members of the Committee on Occupational Therapy Assistants (AOTA, 1964). This committee was delegated responsibility for all developmental aspects of the OTA, including needs assessment, educational program standards, new program proposal and on-site review, and program approval (Schwagmeyer, 1989).

In addition, members of the Committee on Occupational Therapy Assistants reviewed applications for certification under the grandfather clauses. Of 460 applications, 336 individuals became COTAs. The committee also undertook the continuing education of OTs by preparing documents and acquiring grant funds to sponsor national workshops (Schwagmeyer, 1989). The focus was two-fold: appropriate supervision and use of OTAs.

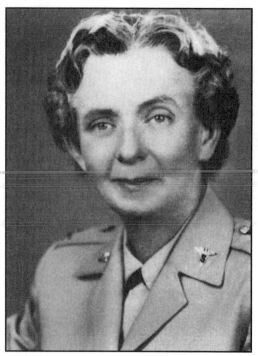

Figure 2-1. Ruth A. Robinson.

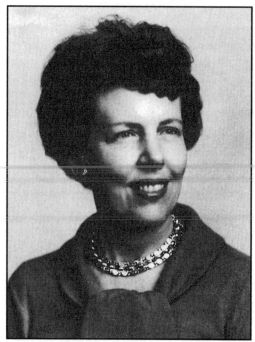

Figure 2-2. Marion W. Crampton, OTR.

Ruth A. Robinson

Col. Ruth A. Robinson was the president of AOTA from 1955 to 1958 (Figure 2-1). About the same time, she became Chief of the Occupational Therapy Section of the Women's (later Army) Medical Specialist Corps, and then the first Chief of the Women's (later Army) Medical Specialist Corps. Both her military and association roles involved advocacy for the training of supportive OT personnel. She served on the Committee on Occupational Therapy Assistants from its inception as a member, chair, and consultant (AOTA, 1967).

In a video interview (Cox, 1977) taped a few years before her death in 1989, Robinson stated that she thought her greatest contribution to the OT profession was the development of the program and curriculum to train OTAs. She also stated:

> We may not realize how far advanced the OT profession was. We set a standard for other professions to follow. At first our program concentrated on the care of the psychiatric patient, just as in the early days of OT. It was frightening to some of us who felt we were not far enough advanced ourselves or secure in our own identities to be able to accept the responsibility of supervising others. We still have a long way to go. I thought the COTA ultimately would be what we thought of then as the OT, and that the COTA would be the best job in OT, leaving the OTR to do the intake work and program planning for individual patients. Recognition of the COTA through certification made me the proudest. (Cox, 1977)

Marion W. Crampton

Marion W. Crampton was a member of the House of Delegates, a delegate member of AOTA's Board of Management, and finally a member of the board itself (Figure 2-2). She was employed by the Massachusetts Department of Mental Health to work with the state psychiatric facilities as well as the state schools under the Division of Mental Retardation. Crampton's employment involved meeting the need for OT services in her state's institutions at a time of OTR shortages. She understood the problems and needs of personnel with less than optimal preparation because that was her daily work. The OTA education program in Massachusetts was an in-service program for employed individuals with experience in OT. Crampton noted (1989):

> The first group of students thought long and hard before applying to the course, which required leaving families for a month and returning to school after many years. Exams were especially threatening, since some students had only a 10th grade education, and had school-aged children who questioned their grades.

She was already involved in Massachusetts when the Committee on Occupational Therapy Assistants was formed and she was appointed chair. Crampton included "members of the loyal opposition" as she made appointments to the committee, so all sides were heard (Crampton, 1989).

As noted earlier, implementation of the OTA program brought a deluge of applications from OT personnel seeking credentialing under the grandfather clause. She recalled, "During the 2-year period, applications were reviewed in a 'round robin' composed of all committee members, who worked evenings, weekends, holidays, and even vacations to process these forms" (Crampton, 1989).

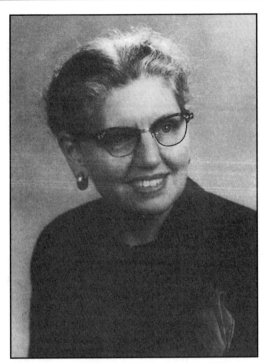

Figure 2-3. Mildred Schwagmeyer, OTR.

Mildred Schwagmeyer

Mildred Schwagmeyer worked in tuberculosis hospitals until recruited as assistant director of education at the AOTA national office in 1958 (Figure 2-3). Nine years later, she became director of technical education, remaining in this position until 1974 (M. Schwagmeyer, personal communication, January 4, 1990). She became the most knowledgeable person on the subject of OTAs at the national office and in the United States. She continued to work in OTA educational services through several title changes until her retirement.

In recalling those years, Schwagmeyer commented:

> I knew in a general way about what was going on, but not that the COTA would have a real impact on my working life. After only 4 months as assistant director of the education, the division became responsible for OTA education. I became liaison to the Committee on Occupational Therapy Assistants, which reported directly to the Board of Management. At first, OTAs were only part of my job, but the work became increasingly time-consuming, demanding, and absorbing. By the 1960s, being technical education director and working with the Committee on Occupational Therapy Assistants was a full-time position. (Schwagmeyer, 1989)

She went on to recount:

> As educational programs moved from hospital-based to academic-based training, concern and discussion increased on topics such as career mobility, entry-level skills, laddering, behavioral objectives, lack of appropriate textbooks and teaching aids, shortage of faculty, and overeducation by some programs leading to disappointment in graduates' work experience. (Schwagmeyer, 1989)

Five federally funded invitational workshops were held at yearly intervals between 1963 and 1968. Four were attended primarily by academic and clinical faculty, and the last included an equal mix of OTRs and COTAs. Topics included role and function, COTA/OTR relationships, and supervision. Excellent teaching materials developed from these workshops, including the present *Guide for Supervision of OT Personnel* (AOTA, 1994).

Schwagmeyer brought a precise use of language to her work. Among other things, she taught us that the term COTA *program* was a non sequitur. Programs are approved, but students cannot seek certification until they graduate. Even today you may sometimes hear the incorrect terminology.

After the 1964 restructuring of AOTA (1964), the functions of the Committee on Occupational Therapy Assistants were slowly integrated into the council structure (Schwagmeyer, 1989), and the committee was dissolved. Seldom have so few accomplished so much.

Ruth Brunyate Wiemer

Ruth Brunyate Wiemer was employed as an OT consultant for the Maryland Department of Health and in 1964 became president of the AOTA (Figure 2-4) (AOTA, 1967). Wiemer guided the association through the difficult period of reorganization (Wiemer, 1966). Of that period she said:

> Communication was slow and labored, with few secretaries in the national office or in OT departments. Flying was not common; one usually traveled by car or train. Expense accounts were unheard of, either at AOTA or on the job. Little money was available for phone calls, retreats, or any type of face-to-face confrontation. (Wiemer, 1989)

She continued:

> Our world changed rapidly in the 1960s after Medicare, with an explosion in the number of proprietary nursing homes and home health agencies. OT was a small, unrecognized profession without precedent for adopting such a concept [as the OTA]. Nursing had supportive personnel, but were protected by licensure; we were not. (Wiemer, 1989)

For professional OTs, OTAs became an added issue because of the following:

- OTs feared the unknown, especially those with no experience working with or supervising supportive personnel.
- OTs feared the AOTA was imposing the OTA on the profession.
- OTs feared giving representation to the OTA and the consequences of OTAs voting.
- Abilities of the OTA highlighted weaknesses in OT skills such as deficits in supervisory techniques and current clinical practice, contentment in their own comfortable niche, naively, and insufficient business acumen.
- There was a lack of country-wide consensus on the appropriate role of OT itself (Wiemer, 1989).

In such an environment, how then were OTAs nurtured? My belief is that the leadership came from those therapists used to hierarchical order, chain of command, and discipline, such as in the military, veterans administration, or health departments. Therapists from psychiatric settings were also familiar with working with supportive personnel (Wiemer, 1989).

While others argued, Wiemer often seemed to be collecting her thoughts. Her responses were graceful, direct, organized, and reasoned, and they did not hide her advocacy for OTAs. She used a convincing metaphor in referring to the OT/OTA problem: "Able seamen far outnumber captains and commodores, yet ships do not sink, and new ship forms, from sail to nuclear power, evolved to meet man's need. So too the varied levels of our profession can be coordinated to achieve efficiency and growth" (Wiemer, 1964).

Therapists who had not stayed abreast of current clinical practice had reason to be concerned about the role of the OTA (AOTA, 1982a). According to a 1967 "Nationally Speaking" column in the *American Journal of Occupational Therapy*, therapists must know that what was taught 15 years ago as functional treatment is taught to OTAs today as maintenance and supportive therapy (Carr, 1971). This writer's attempt to motivate other therapists may sound harsh, but the basic premise about current practice was true.

According to Wiemer (1989):

Change eventually came about in the profession, brought about by the advent of the COTA; these included the sharpening of the roles and functions which opened up part-time positions, increased legislative efforts, and increased state licensure. A physician once asked how the OT profession had the vision to establish a subprofessional group. The profession did not; a few within it did and urged that we follow, and we did.

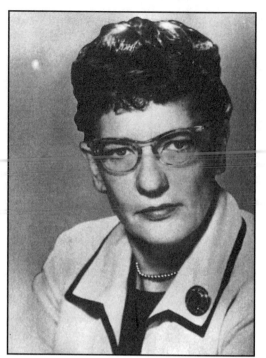

Figure 2-4. Ruth Brunyate Wiemer, OTR.

As the first OTAs practiced and practiced well at the technical level (Wiemer, 1989), OTs and OTAs began building on each other's strengths, learning to identify and complement each other's skills to the betterment of the profession. As you read further in this and in subsequent chapters, you will see how the OT/OTA relationship continues to mature.

FEELINGS OF DISTRUST

Feelings of distrust among some OTs periodically ran high for a number of years, reigning each time new OTA rights and privileges were initiated. The following anecdote is an example of such an emotional response in the early 1970s, when the AOTA Delegate Assembly considered career mobility to allow OTAs to become OTs by fulfilling certain fieldwork requirements and passing the national certification examination for OTs (AOTA, 1982a).

One evening, two AOTA national office staff members spoke on the subject at a district OT meeting. Heated discussion followed the presentations as a few vocal therapists expressed concern that such legislation would directly threaten their jobs. Others disagreed, and still others sat quietly, because the hour was late and the response had become familiar. A stenotypist took notes throughout the meeting so the proceedings could be distributed to therapists statewide. Apparently to prevent such dissemination, the stenotypist's tapes were "lost," but later were retrieved from a lavatory trash can. The proceedings were published (Texas Occupational Therapy Association [TOTA], 1973), the Delegate Assembly voted OTA's career mobility rights terminated in 1982 (AOTA, 1982a), and OTs' employment was unaffected as a consequence of this or any other action pertaining to OTA rights.

OCCUPATIONAL THERAPY ASSISTANT EDUCATION

The initial short-term courses, such as those conducted under the auspices of the state hospital systems in Massachusetts, Wisconsin, and New York, were in-service programs (Crampton, 1989). In 1961, a program in Montgomery County, MD, was approved in general practice to train students to practice in nursing homes (Caskey, 1961). The first approved program combining psychiatric and general practice was at the Duluth Vocational-Technical School in Minnesota; it also targeted student training for nursing homes. Another Minnesota program at St. Mary's Junior College became the first approved 2-year college program (AOTA, 1965). By 1966, the original single-concept programs were being eliminated (AOTA, 1966), and soon all students were enrolled in programs that prepared them to work in general areas of OT practice, rather than in a specialized setting.

Within the parameters set by AOTA guidelines for the number of program hours, program length remained variable depending on the academic setting, length of school day, length of fieldwork, and student backgrounds. One interesting program consolidated all of the academic work into a summer. The program used the college campus and employed faculty members when the campus would otherwise be closed. All students had prior experience in OT or associated departments, or at least 2 years of college and experience working in a health facility. Such students had fewer professional socialization needs than typical junior college students but received the same OT education in an 8-hour classroom day. Fieldwork was arranged when the other college students returned to campus.

PRACTICE SETTINGS

As we have seen, OTAs were trained initially to work in psychiatric hospital practice settings and then in nursing homes and other general medical settings. Many still work in those facilities. The dispersion of OTAs into nontraditional settings came about not because of training, but because of federal legislation (Carr, 1971). Initially, Titles XVIII and XIX of P. L.89-97 (1965), more commonly known as Medicare and Medicaid, opened employment in nursing homes, related facilities, and home health agencies. Other funding opened opportunities in community health and mental health centers, day care centers, and centers for the well aging. Numbers of OTAs increased at the same time some OTs began moving from hospitals to less traditional community practice settings (Carr, 1971). OTAs joined the move to community settings, sometimes in larger numbers than OTs. Carr commented, "It may be either COTA or OTR who meanders away from traditional to new settings, but whichever goes first the other will accompany or soon follow" (TOTA, 1973). NBCOT (2004) surveyed OTAs as part of their practice review and showed the following workplace settings for OTAs:

- Skilled nursing: 40%
- School system: 16%
- Rehabilitation hospital: 12%
- Other long-term care: 8%
- Outpatient/community: 6%
- Acute care hospital: 5%
- Home health: 2%
- Other: 9%

With the passage of P. L. 94-142, the Education for All Handicapped Children Act of 1975, OT personnel were recruited as a related service by public schools to assist children 3 through 21 years old in learning skills necessary to participate in their individualized special education programs. P. L. 99-457, the Handicapped Amendments of 1986, gave a direct OT role in early intervention with children from birth through 2 years, and OTAs and OTs again modified their roles as they moved into schools.

As you read later in this chapter about some individual OTAs who have been singled out for honors, be aware how many have moved to nontraditional roles, some requiring OT supervision and some not. Even in roles requiring no OT supervision, it is observed that OTAs continue their relationships informally with their counterparts.

PRIDE IN RIGHTS AND PRIVILEGES HARD WON

The chronology of OTA developmental milestones, shown in Table 2-1, chronicles hard-won rights and privileges, as well as a few not yet won. In 1980, the AOTA Executive Board formed the OTA Task Force to identify OTA concerns and formulate suggestions (AOTA, 1980, 1981). A year later, the Task Force reported the following recommendations (AOTA, 1981; Barnett, 1981):

- Submit a resolution to the Representative Assembly to establish OTA representation. This was to include a proposal for a nationwide communication network.
- Increase OTAs' participation on key committees and commissions and national office advisory committees.
- Maintain a roster of OTAs qualified and interested in serving on committees at state, regional, and national levels.
- Establish "OTA Share" column in the OT newspaper.
- Design OTA workshops to improve technical skills.
- Encourage utilization of OTAs as educators in professional and technical education programs.
- Appoint a OTA liaison in the national office.

The OTA Task Force was funded for several years (AOTA, 1983) and then replaced by a OTA Advisory Committee in 1986 (Brittell, 1986). All of the original objectives were accomplished, along with many others identified by the networking of the OTA Advisory Committee. Although a proposal to elect a OTA member-at-large in the Representative Assembly was defeated in 1982 (AOTA, 1982b), a similar measure in 1983 (AOTA, 1983) created a OTA representative with voice and vote elected by the membership. It is anticipated that when OTAs are routinely elected to the Representative Assembly from their states, such a special at-large position will be unnecessary. Two OTAs have been elected to the Representative Assembly from their states in the past. Theresa Letois is currently the president of her state association and Terry Olivas De La O is the first elected representative to the Executive Board (AOTA, 1999a).

OTAs describe the 1980s as having had 2 phases. In the early part, they expended their energy, claiming a fair share of responsibility in the Association. Their effort paid off, and in the latter part of the decade, increasing numbers of OTAs were involved in local, state, and national professional activities. The maturity of the OTA group was especially obvious when the OTA Advisory Committee voluntarily withdrew the proposal to change the title of OTAs and discouraged any further action on that long-held dream because the legal and economic implications outweighed the benefits (AOTA, 1980).

In 1989, 21 full-time and 20 part-time OTAs were employed as faculty in technical education programs, and 6 full-time and 20 part-time OTAs were on faculties of professional curricula. Nine OTAs were members of state regulatory (licensure or reg-

---

Table 2-1

Chronology of Occupational Therapy Assistant Developmental Milestones

Year	Milestone
1949	AOTA Board of Management discussed a proposal to the AMA for a 1-year training program for "assistants" by Guy Morrow, OTR, of Ohio.
1956	AOTA Board of Management approved a task force to investigate OT aides and supportive personnel.
1956	AOTA Board of Management changed name of Committee on Recognition of Nonprofessional Personnel to Committee on Recognition of OT Aides to avoid use of term *nonprofessional* in all correspondence. In October of the same year, the name was changed to Committee on Recognition of Occupational Therapy Assistants.
1957	AOTA Board of Management accepted the committee's plan and agreed to implement plan in October, 1958.
1958	First Essentials and Guidelines of an Approved Educational Program for Occupational Therapy Assistants adopted.
1958	Plan implemented.
1958	Grandfather clause established.
1959	First OT assistant education program approved at Westborough State Hospital in Massachusetts.
1960	336 COTAs certified through grandfather clause.
1961	First general practice program approved at Montgomery County, MD.
1962	First OTA directory published.
1963	Board of Management established OTA membership category.
1965	First paper authored by a OTA published in the *American Journal of Occupational Therapy*.
1966	All future educational programs must prepare OTA students as generalists, including both psychosocial and general practice input.
1967	First OTA meeting held at AOTA Annual Conference.
1968	Eight OTAs served on various AOTA committees.
1969	Tenth anniversary of OTAs noted in Schwagmeyer paper.
1970	Effort to change name of OTA to "associate" or "technician" failed in Delegate Assembly.
1971	Military OT technicians eligible for certification as OTAs.
1972	Fifth Annual OTA Workshop held in Baltimore on subject of OT/OTA relationship.
1972	First book review written by OTA published in the *American Journal of Occupational Therapy*.
1973	Career mobility plan endorsed by Executive Board.
1974	First OTAs take certification examination as part of career mobility plan to become OTs.
1974	OTAs get *American Journal of Occupational Therapy* as a membership benefit.
1975	Award of Excellence created for OTA.
1975	OTAs became eligible to receive the Eleanor Clarke Slagle Lectureship Award and the Award of Merit.
1976	First OTA elected member-at-large of the Executive Board.
1977	First national certification examination administered to OTAs.
1978	Roster of Honor (ROH) award established.
1979	Policy adopted that the acronym "OTA" can be used only by assistants currently certified by AOTA.
1980	Funding for 2 year (later refunded) OTA advocacy position for AOTA office.
1981	OTA Task Force established.
1981	Eight OTAs are faculty members of professional OT curricula
1981	Entry-level OT and OTA role delineations adopted.
1982	Career mobility plan terminated.
1982	"OTA Share" column introduced in OT newspaper.
1983	Representative Assembly agreed a OTA member-at-large elected to the assembly would have voice and vote.
1985	First OTA representative and alternate to serve in the Representative Assembly elected.
1987	AOTA Bylaws Revision allowed no distinction between OTA and OT in running for or holding office, including president of the Association.
1989	Twenty-one full-time and 20 part-time OTAs employed in OTA education programs.
1989	Six full-time and 20 part-time OTAs employed in professional OT curricula.
1989	Nine OTAs are members of state regulatory boards.
1990	New guidelines for supervision of OTAs adopted by the Representative Assembly.
1991	Treatment in Groups: A OTA Workshop was sponsored by the AOTA as the association's first continuing education program specifically for OTAs.

(continued)

Table 2-1

Chronology of Occupational Therapy Assistant Developmental Milestones
(continued)

1991	First AOTA OTA/OT Partnership Award received by Ilenna Brown and Cynthia Epstein.
1991	AOTA's Executive Board invites OTA participation.
1992	17,000 COTAs certified by AOTCB.
1998	AOTA establishes Advanced Practitioner (AP) credential and awards first 26 APs.
1998	Theresa Letois is elected first OTA as state president for Indiana. Terry Olivas De La O became the first voting OTA representative member on AOTA's Executive Board.
1999	Teri Black is secretary of AOTA Executive Board.
1999	Robin Jones is secretary of AOTA Executive Board.
2003	Teri Black fights for changes in official documents to support OTAs.
2004	RA votes and confirms changes suggested by Teri Black.

---

istration) boards. Can the day be far off when OTAs with advanced training are directors of educational programs (Jones, 1989)? Only the visionaries among us would even have dreamed that in 1987 the AOTA would change its bylaws (AOTA, 1987), allowing no distinction between OTAs and OTs running for elected national office, including the office of president. Jones (1989) commented that with the labor shortage (where this chapter began), OTAs are becoming administrators, hiring OTs as consultants and clinicians.

ROSTER OF HONOR

The Roster of Honor (ROH) recognizes OTAs with at least 5 years of experience who, with their knowledge and expertise, have made a significant contribution to the continuing education and professional development of members of the association and provide an incentive to contribute to the advancement of the profession (AOTA, 1999b). Become familiar with their names so you will recognize them when you meet them (and you will). Many of the recipients also received the Award of Excellence (AOTA, 1999a), which recognizes the contributions of OTAs to the advancement of OT and provides an incentive to contribute to the development and growth of the profession.

The following people are a select group of early recipients of these honors, which the AOTA bestows on OTAs. Each year other distinguished OTAs join the ranks of these leaders, presented here with our pride in their accomplishments.

- Sally E. Ryan of Mounds View, MN, received the ROH (1979) and the Award of Excellence (1976) for outstanding achievements and contributions in education, committee work in professional organizations at affiliate and national levels, and for identifying the needs of the OTA as a membership group. She is a retired member of a professional OT curriculum faculty and is both an editor and author of textbooks for OTA students.
- Betty Cox of Baltimore, MD, received the ROH (1979) and the Award of Excellence (1977) for leadership in

increasing the involvement of OTAs both in the practice arena and in the Association. Her own business offers professional seminars in health-related subjects, both nationally and internationally. She is president of a publishing company that produces books on OT.

- Terry Brittell of New Hartford, NY, received the ROH (1999) and the Award of Excellence (1979) for outstanding contributions to OT in the areas of practice and clinical education and for service to the profession and for services to the community. At the same psychiatric facility where he was a traditional OTA, he was the coordinator of a stress management program for employees, and of the Mental Health Players, a community prevention program based on role playing.
- Charlotte Gale Seltser of Chevy Chase, MD, received the ROH (1981) in recognition of her program development for the visually handicapped. Once retired, Seltser enjoyed volunteering at the National Eye Institute of the National Institutes of Health, teaching patients appropriate independence and coping skills and referring them to community agencies.
- Toné Frank Blechert of Excelsior, MN, received the ROH (1981) and the Award of Excellence (1981) in recognition of her outstanding contributions to OT in the area of OT technical education. As a master degree faculty member of a junior college, she taught mental health concepts and group dynamics to OTA students and coordinated academic advisement for all students.
- Ilenna Brown of Plainfield, NJ, received the ROH (1984) for fostering pride and pursuit of excellence for OTA practitioners. In a 550-bed nursing facility, Brown was the supervising OTA and rehabilitation coordinator for programs carried on cooperatively by OT, physical therapy, and rehabilitation nursing.
- Barbara Larson of Mahtomedi, MN, received the ROH (1985) for exemplary leadership and promotion of the profession. Larson returned to school to become an OT

and now has a master's degree. She was the coordinator of an industrial rehabilitation clinic and currently consults in occupational health and industrial rehabilitation. She was the past president of her state association at the time of her award.

- Patty Lynn Barnett of Birmingham, AL, received the ROH (1986) for dynamic leadership in the promotion of OTAs. At the time, Barnett was a faculty member of a university OT curriculum where she taught activity classes and coordinated clinical education for assistant students.

- Margaret S. Coffey of Russiaville, IN, received the ROH and Award of Excellence (1986) for excellence in role expansion and commitment to OTAs. With a master's degree, she enjoys a diverse life with the care of two children, a weaver's group, and co-authored Activity Analysis: Application to Occupation (5th ed.) with 2 OTs.

- Barbara Forte of Palm Springs, CA, received the ROH and the Award of Excellence (1986) because through exemplary qualities of dedication and commitment, she provides outstanding leadership in local, state, and national organizations. She articulates the emerging role of OTAs and serves as a role model. Forte has broad experience in delivering community-based clinical services and private mental health programs.

- Robin Jones of Chicago, IL, received the ROH (1987) and the Award of Excellence (1987) because she exemplified excellence and professionalism and is recognized as a strong OTA role model by her peers. She is recognized as an outstanding practitioner, teacher, and advocate for OT. Jones has experience as the director of an independent living center, master's degree student, and vice chair of her state's licensure board.

- Teri Black of Madison, WI, received the ROH (1989) and Award of Excellence (1989) for leadership modeling for OTA/OT professional development. She has experience teaching in an area technical college and practices in a nursing home. Black served 2 terms as chair of her state's licensure board.

- Sue Byers of Gresham, OR, received the ROH (1989) for exemplary role modeling for OTAs and students. As a member of the faculty of an OTA education program, Byers taught and practiced in home health.

- Diane S. Hawkins of Baltimore, MD, received the ROH (1991) in recognition of her significant contributions in staff development and communications. Diane was a faculty consultant for the AOTA workshop "Treatment in Groups: A Workshop for COTAs" and an associate faculty member for the Sheppard and Enoch Pratt National Center for Human Development.

- Kathryn Melin Eberhardt, an author in this book, received the ROH (2000) for her contribution to the education of occupational therapy practitioners such as you, the reader.

In addition, the AOTA (2004) awards OTA and OT partnerships who through collaborative efforts doing outstanding work to benefit consumers and the profession. The Terry Brittell OTA/OT Partnership Award has only been given 6 times, first to Ilenna Leni Brown and Cynthia Epstein in 1991 and most recently to Jacalyn Mardirossian and David Leary in 2004.

ELEANOR CLARKE SLAGLE AWARD

As of yet, no OTA has received the Eleanor Clarke Slagle Award, the highest honor given by the AOTA to any OTA or OT. This honor may be waiting for you or one of your peers.

SUMMARY

To summarize in allegory, picture a young fruit tree growing well, but having the potential of producing a limited amount of fruit. On advice of well-experienced practitioners, a graft of another tree is applied to increase productivity and quality of fruit. Although traumatic to the tree and to the graft bud at first, the surgery is successful. The graft takes well, and the whole tree develops and becomes stronger than before, even stronger than it could have been if left alone to grow naturally. Now after more than 40 years, the subtle difference in a part of the tree is indistinguishable, unless you are up close or know fruit trees very well.

LEARNING ACTIVITIES

1. Identify some of the barriers to acceptance of the OTA in the profession, both historically and currently.

2. Interview at least 3 OTAs and 3 OTs and determine what the current issues are relative to supervision. What efforts are being made to resolve the issues?

3. Write a short paper discussing how OTAs will be viewed by the profession in the next decade. What challenges will assistants face? What new roles will be assumed?

4. List some of the characteristics that contribute to a positive OT and OTA team relationship.

5. If you had the opportunity to talk to Wiemer, Schwagmeyer, or Crampton, what questions would you ask? What advice would you seek?

EDITOR'S NOTE

At the request of the author, the writing style has not been modified to third person, to conform with other chapters. Rather, the terms you and your have been retained where appropriate to assist in engaging the reader in the story as it unfolds.

ACKNOWLEDGMENTS

Marion Crampton, Mildred Schwagmeyer, and Ruth Wiemer shared their early COTA stories and allowed me to use their materials; I avow my appreciation. I also thank those who helped me document memories and flesh out the intervening years. These individuals include Patty Barnett and Sally Ryan, Robert Bing, Bonnie Brooks, Marie Moore, Dottie Renoe, Lauren Rivet, Ira Silvergleit, and the ROH award winners. Lisa Dickey was a patient co-proofreader, and Joel G. Swetnam has generously shared his computer graphic skills. This chapter was updated by the editors in 2004.

REFERENCES

American Occupational Therapy Association. (1964). Annual report, committee on OTAs. *American Journal of Occupational Therapy, 18*, 45-46.

American Occupational Therapy Association. (1965). Board of management report. *American Journal of Occupational Therapy, 19*, 100.

American Occupational Therapy Association. (1966). AOTA: Delegate assembly minutes. *American Journal of Occupational Therapy, 20*, 49-53.

American Occupational Therapy Association. (1967). Presidents of the AOTA (1917-1967). *American Journal of Occupational Therapy, 21*, 290-298.

American Occupational Therapy Association. (1980). Representative assembly minutes. *American Journal of Occupational Therapy, 43*, 844-870.

American Occupational Therapy Association. (1981). COTA task force chart of concerns. *OT News, 35*(8).

American Occupational Therapy Association. (1982a). Representative assembly report. *American Journal of Occupational Therapy, 36*, 808-826.

American Occupational Therapy Association. (1982b). 52nd annual conference, annual business meeting. *American Journal of Occupational Therapy, 36*, 808-826.

American Occupational Therapy Association. (1983). Representative assembly minutes. *American Journal of Occupational Therapy, 37*, 92.

American Occupational Therapy Association. (1987). Member data survey. *OT News,* September.

American Occupational Therapy Association. (1994). Guide for supervision of OT personnel. *American Journal of Occupational Therapy, 48*, 1054-1056.

American Occupational Therapy Association. (1999a). *Award nomination form, ROH.* Bethesda, MD: Author.

American Occupational Therapy Association. (1999b). Fortieth anniversary timeline: OTA history. *OT Practice, 21,* July/August.

American Occupational Therapy Association. (2004). AOTA honors 45 years of OTAs. *OT Practice, October 4,* 2004, 21.

Barnett, P. (1981). COTA task force report. *OT News, 35,* August.

Brittell, T. (1986). *AOTA COTA advisory committee final report.* Bethesda, MD: Author.

Carr, S. H. (1971). Models of manpower utilization. *American Journal of Occupational Therapy, 25,* 259-262.

Caskey, V. (1961). A training program for OTAs. *American Journal of Occupational Therapy, 15,* 157-159.

Cox, B. (1977). *AOTA's visual taped history: Ruth A. Robinson.* AOTA Archives, Moody Medical Library, University of Texas Medical Branch, Galveston, Texas.

Crampton, M. (1989). *Presentation at 30th anniversary COTA forum.* Baltimore, MD.

Jones, R. (1989). *Presentation at 30th anniversary COTA forum.* Baltimore, MD.

National Board of Certification in Occupational Therapy. (2004). A practice analysis study of entry-level occupational therapist registered and certified occupational therapy assistant practice. *OTJR: Occupation, Participation, and Health, 24,* supplement 1.

Schwagmeyer, M. (1989). *Presentation at 30th anniversary COTA forum.* Baltimore, MD.

Texas Occupational Therapy Association, Southeast District (1973). Proceedings of meeting. October 15.

Wiemer, R. (1964). *Unpublished report of workshop summary: Workshop on the training of the OTA.* Detroit, MI.

Wiemer, R. (1966). AOTA conference keynote address. *American Journal of Occupational Therapy, 20,* 9-11.

Wiemer, R. (1989). *Presentation at 30th anniversary COTA forum.* Baltimore, MD.

Key Concepts

- Importance of philosophy: Profession's views guide action, explain practice, appreciation.
- Metaphysics: The ultimate nature of man and life.
- Epistemology: The study of truth.
- Axiology: The study of values.
- Philosophy of Adolph Meyers: Founding beliefs of OT.

Essential Vocabulary

philosophy of life: Personalized view of one's self and the world.
quality of life: Satisfaction in the occupations of living.

Philosophy and Core Values in Occupational Therapy

Phillip D. Shannon, MA, MPA

Introduction

A vital aspect of the educational preparation of the OTA is an appreciation of the philosophy on which the practice of OT is based. Why is this so vital? There are at least 4 reasons that provide a rationale.

First, the philosophy of any profession represents the profession's views on the nature of existence. These views reflect the reasons for its own existence in responding to the needs of the population served. For example, a somewhat complex question addressed in philosophy is, "What is man?" Is man a physical being, a psychological being, a social being, or all of these? If man is perceived by a profession as a physical being only, then in responding to the needs of "man the patient" the action is quite clear: the practitioner deals only with the body, not with the mind. As inconceivable as this particular belief might appear, the practices of some professions reflect a narrow perspective of man. Sometimes, as it will be discussed later, a profession does not practice what it believes.

Guided by its philosophical beliefs, a grand design evolves to specify the purposes or goals of the profession. Lacking an understanding of the philosophical basis for this grand design, the practitioner cannot be sure that the goals he or she is pursuing are worth pursuing or that the services provided are worth providing.

A second reason for understanding the philosophy of the profession is that philosophy guides action. Indeed, it is only within the context of a profession's philosophy that actions have meaning. Attending to the leisure needs of the patient, for instance, is one of the major concerns of OT, because its practitioners believe that man seeks a sense of quality to life. One aspect of a quality life, like a satisfying work life, is a satisfying leisure life. Consequently, using arts and crafts to promote the leisure interests and skills of the patient and, therefore, the quality of life of the patient, is an action that makes sense because the action has philosophical meaning.

One of the primary reasons for studying philosophy, according to Thomas (1983), is to clarify beliefs so that the action that

comes from those beliefs is sound and consistent. Clarifying the beliefs of the profession should be regarded as a critical component of the OTA's education to ensure that his or her actions are sound and consistent (i.e., that the OTA's entry-level behaviors are based on and consistent with a set of guiding philosophical beliefs).

A third rationale for understanding the philosophy of OT is the direct relationship between the growth of the profession and the ability of its practitioners to explain their reasons for existence. In the present era of accountability, where the justification for programs and the competition for resources to support these programs is greater than in previous years, one cannot assume that those external to the profession, such as physicians, will perceive OT as an intrinsically good or essential service. Claims of goodness must be substantiated with evidence. That evidence must be supported philosophically, otherwise it will lack a context for its interpretation. For example, documented evidence that a patient's range of motion in the left elbow was increased by 5 degrees as a result of OT intervention is important. What strengthens this evidence, however, are the reasons for intervening in the first place. These reasons are linked to the philosophical beliefs of the profession.

Finally, it is not sufficient for the OTA to be skilled in applying the techniques of the profession. On the contrary, he or she must have some appreciation, philosophical and theoretical, of the reasons why these techniques are applied. Lacking this appreciation, the OTA will apply these techniques without being able to communicate their value to the patient, thereby failing to motivate the patient's active involvement in treatment.

Certainly from the initial stage of patient referral to the last stage of discontinuing the patient's treatment, the philosophical beliefs of the profession must remain in the foreground. For the OTA, who has major responsibilities along the entire continuum of health care, these beliefs and the actions that stem from them must be understood and practiced. Indeed, this is the first duty of the OTA.

WHAT IS PHILOSOPHY?

To appreciate fully the philosophy of OT, one must appreciate and understand philosophy in general. Basically, philosophy is concerned with the "meaning of human life, and the significance of the world in which man finds himself" (Randall & Buchler, 1960, p. 5). Man is, by nature, a philosophical creature. Questions such as "Who am I?", "What is my destiny?", and "What do I want from life?" are questions of meaning and purpose that concern all human beings. Each individual, in responding to questions such as these, develops a personalized view of one's self and the world, commonly referred to as a philosophy of life. This philosophy represents a fundamental set of values, beliefs, truths, and principles that guide the person's behavior from day to day and from year to year.

The philosophy of a profession also represents a set of values, beliefs, truths, and principles that guides the actions of the profession's practitioners. Typically, as with individuals, the philosophy evolves over time and sometimes changes as a profession matures. Each profession, in shaping and reshaping its philosophy, has choices to make in 3 philosophical dimensions. These include metaphysics, epistemology, and axiology.

Metaphysics

Metaphysics is concerned with questions about the ultimate nature of things, including the nature of man. With regard to the nature of man in particular, the mind/body relationship is of special interest to the philosopher. Are mind and body two separate entities, one superior to the other, or are mind and body a single entity representative of the "whole"—the whole person? The first position, that of mind/body separation, is the dualistic position. The second position, that of mind/body as one entity, is the position of holism.

While most (if not all) professions claim to be holistic, the truth in this claim is seen to the extent to which the actions of the profession are consistent with its beliefs. Assume, for example, that the actions of "profession X" are directed toward exercise as the means for promoting a healthy body (i.e., a healthy "physical" body). Assume also that profession X claims to be holistic, asserting a concern for the whole person. In actuality, it is dualistic because the body is viewed as superior to the mind; the goal of exercise, in this case, is a healthy body, not a healthy body and a healthy mind. There is a contradiction, therefore, in what profession X believes and what it does. Its actions do not follow from its beliefs, and the claim of holism is illegitimate. When exercise is seen as promoting the health of the "whole," a more holistic approach is demonstrated.

Epistemology

The second dimension pertinent to shaping and reshaping the philosophy of a profession is the dimension of epistemology, which is concerned with questions of truth. What is truth? How do we come to know things? How do we know that we know? One way of knowing is by experience. One knows, for example, that the flame of a fire brings pleasure in terms of the warmth it provides, but also that it produces pain if it is touched by the bare hand. Usually, one only needs to experience this pain once to "know that he or she knows." Is experience the only route to truth or knowing? From a holistic perspective, there are many routes to truth and knowing. Intuition, for instance, is considered to be as truthful as experiential learning or the logic reasoned by the powers of the intellect. For the dualist, on the other hand, the subjective realities of intuition and experience cannot be accepted as truths. On the contrary, only the objective reality of rational thought can be admitted as truth; truth is logic.

Axiology

The third dimension of philosophy is axiology, which is concerned with the study of values. Two types of questions are addressed by axiology: questions of value with regard to what is desirable or beautiful in the world (aesthetics) and questions of value with regard to the standards or rules for right conduct (ethics). Most people would agree that a long life is a desirable thing—something that is valued. Some people might argue that a long life without a sense of quality to one's life is a life that is not worth living. Almost everyone would maintain that it is wrong to take a life, yet there are those who believe that "a life for a life" might be justified in some instances.

Conflicting values and standards often produce dilemmas that are difficult to resolve. If life is valued, for example, is it right or moral to disconnect the support systems maintaining the life of the person who has been certified as "brain dead?" Is it right or moral to prolong a life that may not be a life worth living? These are difficult questions of value about what is desirable or beautiful in the world and about the standards that will be applied in pursuing that which is valued.

Each profession has choices to make about what it considers beautiful and desirable in the world and the ethical principles that it will follow in achieving its goals. For medicine, the preservation of life is the first priority, and perhaps this is as it should be, for medicine. But, is this the highest priority of the other health care professions? Should it be the highest priority? A profession that claims to be holistic cannot be satisfied with saving lives. Instead, a holistic profession would maintain that a life worth saving must be a life worth living.

Given this brief glimpse of metaphysics, epistemology, and axiology, dimension can be discussed as it relates to the philosophy of OT. Specifically, 4 questions will be addressed:

1. The metaphysical question of "What is man?"
2. The epistemological question of "How does man know that he knows?"
3. The aesthetic question of "What is beautiful or desirable in the world?"
4. The ethical question of "What are the rules of right conduct?"

Two approaches will be taken in responding to these questions. First, the philosophy of Adolph Meyer (1977), who was primarily responsible for providing OT with a philosophical foundation for practice, will be examined. Second, the extent to which this philosophical base has survived the test of time will be explored.

Home before this
  4 to get inthen 14 up
the stairs to bathroom
  12 down to do laundry
Son lives w/ you 47 y/o
does Meals + laundry

  went to WCA w/ severe flu
constipated for a couple wks.
  turned into pneumonia
afraid of falling b/c
aides almost dropped her
  sent here for OT + PT
to Heritage
  way given 400 units instead
of 48 → could have died
  fell out of ~~bedside~~
~~OOO~~
          harness left

scared of sit to stand

Strength, Endurance, ROM, NMR/Balance training, therapeutic (dynamic) activity, self care/home light training

NMR (Neuromuscular Rehab) 1 hr / 6x week

Energy conservation
Adaptive equip.

what I need to do:
1 stand & tolerate standing
2 walking
3 toileting
4 wiping
5 stand pivot transfer

What I want to do:
1 reading
2 going to casino
3 word finds
4 watch TV
5 clean bedroom

What I'm expected to do:
1 care for dog / chair pushup to start
2 vaccum
3 get up stairs   preparing for sit
4 drove months ago   to sta trans
5 be transposed in car
6 Have O2 @ all times

Loves Disney Movies

NCIS + Law & order

Jeopardy

---

73 y/o

O_2 dep. COPD

pneumonia

IDDM

Morbid Obesity

CAD

HTN

Afib

CHF

Referred to Nursing from WCA resp. pneumonia failure d/t

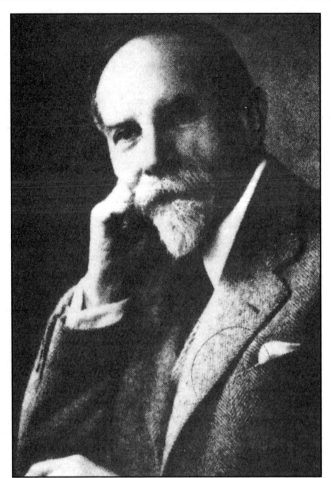

Figure 3-1. Dr. Adolph Meyer, psychiatrist and early occupational therapy proponent and philosopher (Fabian Bachrach photo).

THE EVOLUTION OF OCCUPATIONAL THERAPY

OT evolved from the moral treatment movement that began in the early 19th century (Bockhoven, 1971). If there was a single purpose to which the champions of this movement were committed, it was to humanize and to provide more humane forms of treatment for the mentally ill incarcerated in the large asylums in this country and abroad. Marching under the banner of humanism, the leaders of this movement sought to defend and preserve the dignity of all human beings, particularly the sick and the disabled.

Among these humanists who carried the movement into the 20th century was the psychiatrist Adolph Meyer (Figure 3-1), whose paper *The Philosophy of Occupation Therapy* (1977) laid the foundation for the practice and promotion of OT. Meyer's philosophy was based on his observations of everyday living. From his beliefs about the nature of man, about life, and about a life worth living, the pioneers of the profession emerged to chart its course. Although Meyer has been quoted frequently in the literature of recent years, a more extensive discussion of his philosophy is provided here because, to date, his thoughts have not been examined within the context of metaphysics, epistemology, and axiology.

A Retrospective Glance at the Philosophy of Adolph Meyer

What is Man?

Meyer's perspective of man was holistic: Our body is not merely so many pounds of flesh and bone figuring as a machine, with an abstract mind or soul added to it. Rather it is a live organism acting in harmony with its own nature and the nature about it.

For Meyer, 3 characteristics distinguished man from all other organisms: sense of time, capacity for imagination, and need for occupation.

A sense of time, past, present, and future, was the central theme of Meyer's philosophy. He believed that a sense of time, and particularly time past (experience), provides man with an advantage over other living organisms in terms of adapting in the present and manipulating the future. This capacity to learn from experience, when blended with the capacity for imagination or creativity, allows man to alter his environment. The squirrel, for example, is totally dependent on its environment for food and shelter during the winter months. Man, on the other hand, through experience and imagination, has been able to alter his environment to ensure survival from hunger through food preservation techniques and protection from the cold via heat-producing systems.

The need for occupation was regarded by Meyer (1977) as a distinctly human characteristic. He defined occupation as a form of helpful enjoyment, which clearly transcends the notion of occupation as being limited to work. On the contrary, the meaning of occupation was extended by Meyer to include all of those activities that comprise a normal day, particularly work and play. He considered occupation important to all, the sick as well as the healthy. Each individual must achieve a balance among his occupations, a balanced life of not only work and play, but also of rest and sleep (Meyer, 1977).

How Does Man Know That He Knows?

Man learns not only by experience, but also by "doing": engaging mind and body in occupation. By doing, man is able to achieve. Fidler and Fidler (1978), in reiterating this theme in the 1970s, maintained that doing is linked to becoming, to realizing one's potential. Fundamental to achieving and becoming is doing. In doing, man comes to know about himself and the world. In doing, man knows that he knows.

What Is Beautiful or Desirable in the World?

For Meyer (1977), man is not content simply existing in the world. Instead, man seeks a sense of quality to life that comes from the pleasure in achievement. It is in engaging the total self that man comes to experience the pleasure in achievement, which Reilly (1962), in her Eleanor Clarke Slagle lectureship, articulated so beautifully: "That man, through the use of his hands as they are energized by mind and will, can influence the state of his own health." Again, it is in doing that man achieves and is able to acquire a sense of quality in his life.

What Are the Rules of Right Conduct?

Meyer (1977), in outlining the guiding principles for the practice of OT, maintained that the occupation worker should provide opportunities, not prescriptions. Prescriptions tend to constrain the development of one's potential, whereas opportunities nourish it. To apply prescriptions is to treat the patient as an object; to offer opportunities is to regard the patient as a person. Inherent in this principle of right conduct is a belief in the type of relationship that the occupation worker should maintain with the patient—a helping relationship, a caring relationship, a relationship in which patients are indeed treated as persons and not as objects.

To summarize, Meyer's perspective of man was holistic. He emphasized doing as the primary route to truth and to achieving a sense of quality in one's life. Prerequisite to doing, however, is opportunity. Lacking the opportunity to do, man, like the squirrel, cannot control his own destiny. On the contrary, man becomes the squirrel, controlled and manipulated by his environment.

The Test of Time

Has the philosophy of Adolph Meyer, which provided the direction for the practice and promotion of OT, survived the test of time, or has the profession, as it matured, changed its direction, based on a different set of values, beliefs, truths, and principles? The answer is reflected in the *Report on the AOTA Project to Identify the Philosophical Base of Occupational Therapy* (Shannon, 1983), which was submitted to the Executive Board of the representative assembly. This report did not represent "an official position" of the AOTA with regard to the philosophy of OT, but it is the documentation of a 6.5-year project designed to trace the philosophical beliefs of the profession historically and to interpret those beliefs within the context of more modern times. In reviewing the degree to which the beliefs of Adolph Meyer have withstood the test of time, the 4 philosophical questions addressed earlier are once again discussed in the following sections.

What is Man?

The belief in holism has persisted in the profession (Shannon, 1983). Indeed, one of the unique aspects of OT is its integrating function, where mind and body are activated to promote the patient's total involvement in the treatment process. To lose sight of this function is to lose sight of one of the major contributions of OT—attending to the "whole person."

One might speculate that it is the profession's commitment to holism that has attracted people to OT rather than to some of the other health professions that appear less holistic. Even in OT, however, the concept of holism, although universally professed, is not uniformly applied in practice. Action is not always consistent with belief. When practice takes the form of dealing only with the mind, only with the body, or worse yet, with only parts of the body, the commitment to holism has been compromised, and there is a contradiction between what one believes and what one does.

For example, hand rehabilitation has become a highly specialized area of practice. Unquestionably, there is a significant contribution to be made to health care in this area. However, when some of the practitioners in rehabilitation begin to refer to themselves as "hand therapists" vs. "OTs," there is an implicit shift away from holism. The belief in holism may remain, but the explicit actions that follow are sometimes not holistic. Only when hand rehabilitation focuses on the whole person does it retain its holistic function.

Another contradiction between belief and action is in mental health practice. Probably one of the first signs indicating the shift away from holism in mental health is when the practitioner uses the title "psychiatric occupational therapist" or "psychiatric occupational therapy assistant." "Psychiatric occupational therapy" personnel tend to focus only on the mind of the patient to the exclusion of the patient's body. Furthermore, when the practitioner's actions are directed primarily toward the unconscious mind, as in providing activities for the sublimation of innate drives, attention is not even focused on the whole mind, much less the mind and body. Again, the belief in holism may be contradicted by the practitioner's actions.

Surely these examples are not characteristic of most practitioners in mental health; nor is "hand therapy" necessarily limited to the treatment of the hand. However, when the broad concerns of OT are narrowed, the patient is somehow cheated in the process.

Also surviving the test of time is the belief in Meyer's distinguishing characteristics of man. Indeed, in responding to the needs of "man the patient," OT has placed a high priority on time as a continuum in the life of a patient, designing programs of treatment within the context of the patient's past, present, and future. In implementing these programs, the patient's capacity for imagination or creativity is challenged in the interest of serving the need for occupation.

Occupation, as defined in the *Report on the AOTA Project to Identify the Philosophical Base of Occupational Therapy*, is goal-directed behavior aimed at the development of play, work, and life skills (Shannon, 1983). If, as Reilly (1962) proposed, man's need for occupation is that vital need of man served by OT, then to reduce the concept of occupation to the level of exercising bodily parts with weights and pulleys or to the level of occupying the patient's mind with activities that bear little or no relationship to the nature of his or her occupation, is to deny this vital need. In addition, another unique aspect of the profession is somehow lost in the transformation of belief into action.

In contrast, by drawing on the patient's past experiences in work and play and in exploring the patient's values, capacities, and interests, the therapist should provide experiences that will serve the patient's need for occupation. In addition, in tapping the creative potential of the patient in areas such as problem solving and decision making, the therapist can expand the patient's capacities for altering the environment, thereby, expanding the potential for adapting in the present and for controlling his or her own destiny into the future.

How Does Man Know That He Knows?

From the beginning, OT has believed in the active vs. the passive involvement of the patient in treatment (i.e., in doing). As Meyer believed, however, doing is but one way of knowing. There are multiple routes to truth—experience, thinking, feeling, and doing—which the modern day practitioner also accepts as reality (Shannon, 1983). One knows, for example, what happiness means because it has been experienced and because it can be felt. Happiness cannot be measured, but this does not make it any less real.

Among the many ways of knowing, doing is emphasized in the profession as the means for acquiring the skills for daily living and knowing one's capabilities in the present and one's potential for the future. Here again, the opportunities for doing must be framed within the context of the whole person. Consider, for example, the active engagement of the patient in sensory integration activities. One of the major reasons for involving a patient in this type of activity is that the ability to receive and process sensory information is one way of knowing. For example, one knows that it is cold, and, therefore, that the body should be protected with warm clothing because one is able to feel cold, process this input, and take the appropriate steps to protect one's self.

Lacking the ability to process sensory information, the person is denied an important, if not critical, source of information. In this case, doing, in the form of involving the individual in sensory integration activities, is an important step in the process of knowing. On the other hand, if the patient benefits from involvement in OT are limited to those derived by applying the techniques of sensory integration, then OT has not served its holistic function, nor has it served the patient's need for occupation.

The practitioner takes a step away from this belief in doing when the action of "having the patient do" is replaced with the action of "doing to the patient." Another unique aspect of OT is obscured when the patient is denied the opportunity for doing.

What Is Beautiful or Desirable in the World?

To subsist, according to Meyer, is not enough for man. Man seeks something beyond subsistence or survival: the "good life," a life of quality. In maintaining this position over the years, OT has focused its attention in 2 directions: minimizing the deficits and maximizing the strengths of the patient (Shannon, 1983). Attending to one without attending to the other is incomplete and insufficient if the goals go beyond mere survival.

Traditionally, OT has minimized its contribution to the survival aspects of care and maximized its role in promoting a life of quality for its patients. Perhaps this is as it should be, perhaps not. Perhaps it is a matter of interpretation (i.e., how one defines survival in terms of whether or not this position is legitimate). Consider, for example, the patient who has not learned the techniques of wheelchair mobility. This individual will not survive, at least not as a self-sufficient being. Consider also the patient who cannot dress him- or herself and is unable to organize time to meet the demands of daily living. This patient will not survive with any degree of autonomy or self-respect.

Furthermore, as Shannon (1983) summarized, bodies and minds not active will die. Also, people who lack quality in their lives sometimes engage in self-destructive behaviors, such as alcoholism, that lead to deterioration and death (Shannon, 1985). Does OT contribute to the preservation of life? Surely, as these examples suggest, OT contributes to the survival of the patient directly, if survival is interpreted to mean the ability to care for self, and indirectly, by adding a sense of quality to the lives of those served by the profession.

Reilly (1962) stated that the first duty of an organism is to be alive; the second duty is to grow and be productive. If survival is the first priority of the organism, then perhaps the position of the profession can be strengthened by developing an argument for the practice and promotion of OT that includes a commitment to the survival of the patient, as well as to the quality of his or her life (Shannon, 1985). In developing this argument, it must be made clear that the first priority of the profession is to teach the patient skills that will ensure survival. The second priority is to guide the patient toward the realization of his or her potential and social worth as a member of society, as evidenced, according to Heard (1977), by the ability to perform an occupational role. Indeed, it is for these reasons that man engages in occupation; it is also for these reasons that OT exists.

OT has expressed its commitment to the second priority, but its actions are often directed to the first. As Heard maintained, it is in addressing the second priority, and particularly the social worth of the patient, that OT has been most negligent (Heard, 1977). Yet, in attending to the social worth of the patient, the profession is making a major contribution to a more healthy society. Certainly, in making this contribution, as Yerxa (1979) argued that it must, the profession's value is increased and its survival guaranteed.

What Are the Rules of Right Conduct?

Meyer's principle of providing opportunities, not prescriptions, for patients has been one of the distinguishing characteristics of the profession. In applying the rule of nonprescription, the patient becomes an active partner in treatment. Why is this important?

First, the skills and habits necessary for the performance of occupational roles cannot be administered to the patient, but must be acquired by the patient. Second, prescriptions tend to foster externally controlled behaviors (pawn), whereas opportunities encourage internally controlled behaviors (origin) as defined by Burke (1977). In applying prescriptions, the patient is treated as a pawn, externally controlled by those responsible for his or her care; in offering opportunities, the patient is treated as origin, drawing upon the strengths within him or her to assume control for his or her own life. If taking charge of one's own life is important and assuming control for one's own destiny is valued, providing opportunities and not prescriptions is a necessary first step.

In offering opportunities for patients to take charge of their own lives, two major ethical principles guide the actions of the practitioner (Beauchamp & Childress, 1983). The first of these is the principle of nonmaleficence, which states that not only should one do no harm, but also that one should promote the good. The second is the principle of beneficence, or the rule that one should show kindness and caring. Perhaps no profession can lay greater claim to applying these principles than OT. The principle of showing kindness and caring, however, raises the issue of patient vs. client. Which is more legitimate: a therapist/patient relationship or a therapist/consumer relationship?

In a therapist/patient relationship, the client is perceived as an object, an "it," because only one aspect of the client becomes the focus of attention. The therapist/patient relationship is similar to that of a used car salesperson who has only one goal: to sell the client a used car regardless of whether the client can afford gasoline to operate the car or whether the client has the financial resources to insure and maintain it.

In a therapist/consumer relationship, the patient is perceived not as an object, but as a person. Patients expect that their total well-being will be improved when seeking health care (Reilly, 1984).

Over the years, OT has prided itself on the fact that it cares. In caring about its patients, clients, or consumers, the profession has demonstrated that it is holistic and humanistic. If a different type of caring evolves, then any future claim of being a holistic, humanistic enterprise will have to be denied.

CURRENT PHILOSOPHY OF OCCUPATION

The philosophical beliefs guiding the contemporary practice of OT can be traced to Adolph Meyer, whose philosophy of occupation therapy was framed within the context of metaphysics, epistemology, and axiology. Meyer's philosophy was both holistic and humanistic. As it persists in the present to guide the actions of the OT practitioner, so will it persist in the future to provide direction for the profession as it continues to mature.

The current philosophy statement from AOTA has not changed since 1978, holding proud and steady through many changes in practice, forming a solid foundation for the profession (AOTA, 1979). The statement, available to student members on AOTA's Web site (www.aota.org), states firmly that man is an active being who participates in purposeful activity for life satisfaction. Occupational therapy's use of purposeful activity and occupation can improve man's well-being and health. Essential to providing occupational therapy services is a belief in our core values and attitudes (AOTA, 1993). These include altruism, equality, freedom, justice, dignity, truth, and prudence. Understanding the general concepts of philosophy and the specific strengths of occupational therapy's philosophy will guide the occupational therapy practitioner throughout his or her career.

The philosophical beliefs identified in this chapter and the principles for practice that evolved from these philosophical beliefs are summarized in Table 3-1, which also contains descriptions of situations when these beliefs and principles are compromised. The OTA owes allegiance to these beliefs and principles when responding to the needs of those served by the profession.

LEARNING ACTIVITIES

1. The author cited several ways in which OT practitioners fail to retain a holistic approach to rehabilitation. Outline how OT personnel in a physical dysfunction setting and in a psychosocial dysfunction setting would proceed with evaluation and treatment applying a holistic approach.

2. Reilly, Heard, and Yerxa were cited regarding whether the profession of OT should be concerned with survival or with quality of life. What are the pros and cons of each position? What are the implications of each course of action?

3. Make a list of your basic beliefs about OT. Compare and discuss your list with a classmate or peer.

4. List at least 4 reasons why it is important for OTAs to be able to communicate the philosophy on which the profession of OT is based.

5. Discuss the following questions with a peer: According to Meyer, what 3 characteristics distinguish man from all other organisms? What are the implications for OT practice?

6. Using the fax-on-demand services of AOTA, request the current *Philosophy of Occupational Therapy* from AOTA or use a search engine to find a current copy.

EDITOR'S NOTE

In the context of this chapter, the term "man," in the philosophical sense, refers to the generic term "mankind," which is considered standard and gender inclusive.

REFERENCES

American Occupational Therapy Association. (1979). The philosophical base of occupational therapy. *American Journal of Occupational Therapy, 33,* 785.

American Occupational Therapy Association. (1993). Core values and attitudes of occupational therapy practice. *American Journal of Occupational Therapy, 47,* 1085-1086.

Beauchamp, T. L., & Childress, J. F. (1983). *Principles of biomedical ethics.* New York, NY: Oxford University Press.

Bockhoven, J. S. (1971). Legacy of moral treatment 1800s to 1910. *American Journal of Occupational Therapy, 25,* 223-225.

Burke, J. P. (1977). A clinical perspective on motivation: Pawn versus origin. *American Journal of Occupational Therapy, 31,* 254-258.

Fidler, G. S., & Fidler, J. W. (1978). Doing and becoming: Purposeful action and self-actualization. *American Journal of Occupational Therapy, 32,* 305-310.

Heard, C. (1977). Occupational role acquisition: A perspective on the chronically disabled. *American Journal of Occupational Therapy, 31,* 243-247.

Meyer, A. (1977). The philosophy of occupation therapy. *American Journal of Occupational Therapy, 31,* 639-642.

Randall, J. H., & Buchler, J. (1960). *Philosophy: An introduction.* New York, NY: Barnes and Noble, Inc.

Table 3-1

Summary of Philosophical Beliefs, Principles, and Contradictory Practices

Philosophical Beliefs	Principles for Practice	Beliefs/Principles Compromised
Metaphysical Position		
The belief in holism, in mind and body as one entity	Attending to the whole person	Attending only to the mind or only to the body or parts of the body
The belief in the uniqueness of or in man's distinctly human qualities, that include an appreciation of time, past, present, and future	Designing intervention programs within the context of the patient's past, present, and future	Attending to the present needs of the patient without considering the patient's past experiences and future goals
The capacity for imagination	Challenging the patient's capacity for imagination or creativity	Providing prescriptions vs. opportunities
The need for occupation	Promoting a balanced life of work, play, rest, and sleep	Placing an emphasis on the treatment of pathology to the extent that the acquisition of skills that will support occupational role is minimized or ignored
Epistemological Position		
The belief that there is not just one, but many routes to knowing or learning	Valuing experience, thinking, and feeling in the process of doing en route to knowing or learning	Treating the patient as a passive vs. active participant during the process of intervention
Axiological Position— The Aesthetic Component		
The belief that man seeks a life beyond subsistence, a life of quality	The first principle: teaching survival skills by minimizing deficits and maximizing strengths	Teaching survival skills without attending to the patient's potential beyond survival or his or her social worth
	The second principle: providing opportunities for achievement, for the realization of one's potential and one's social worth	
Axiological Position— The Ethical Component		
The humanistic belief that patients should be treated as persons, not objects	Protecting the patient from harm; promoting good	Neglecting the patient's safety or security needs and/or failing to protect the patient's rights as a patient and as a human being
	Demonstrating kindness and caring	Promoting a therapist/client vs. therapist/patient relationship
	Providing opportunities vs. prescriptions	Applying remedies that discourage individual initiative

Reilly, M. (1962). OT can be one of the great ideas of 20th century medicine. *American Journal of Occupational Therapy, 16,* 1-9.

Reilly, M. (1984). The importance of the patient versus client issue for OT. *American Journal of Occupational Therapy, 6,* 404-406.

Shannon, P. D. (1983). Report on the AOTA project to identify the philosophical base of OT. January, 1983. Condensed under the title: Toward a Philosophy of OT. August, 1983.

Shannon, P. D. (1985). From another perspective: An overview of the issue on the roles of OTs in continuity of care. *OT Health Care, 2,* 3-11.

Thomas, C. E. (1983). *Sport in a philosophic context.* Philadelphia, PA: Lea and Febiger.

Yerxa, E. (1979). The philosophical base of OT. In *OT: 2001 AD.* Rockville, MD: American Occupational Therapy Association.

Key Concepts

- Nature vs. nurture debate: The ongoing controversy over whether the environment or genetics is a more powerful influence on an individual's development.
- Freud's psychosexual stages of development: Steps through which Freud believed each child progressed, emphasizing the focus of libidinal energy and the importance of early experiences.
- Erikson's 8 stages of psychosocial development: Steps that Erikson believed each child must progress through in order to develop personality and the ability to meet the demands of society.
- Piaget's cognitive stages of development: Four stages that Piaget believed explain the acquisition of new information and mental skills.
- Bandura's Social Learning Theory: A theory that emphasizes the importance of learning by observation and imitation.

Essential Vocabulary

cognitive development: Progressive changes in thinking, memory, processing, and problem-solving skills.
physical development: Growth of the body, brain, and motor skills.
social-emotional development: Changes in how one relates to others and responds to life circumstances that develop with time and experience. Includes temperament or the innate personality of a child as well as identity formation during the adolescent years.

HUMAN DEVELOPMENT

Carol Winters-Smith, PhD

OTAs, like all people in helping professions, must observe human behavior carefully and in doing so, maintain an awareness of the multiple influences on typical human development. With scientists now charting the human genome, the age-old issue of nature vs. nurture takes on a new light. As more and more children survive premature births or illnesses that would have been fatal in the past, as treatments are discovered for progressively more illnesses and disorders, as families change their dynamics and constellations, how one develops into an adult becomes progressively more complex.

Despite the rapid changes taking place both in science and society, however, there are certain aspects of the human experience that remain constant. While there are exceptions to every theory, the standard developmental theories seem to hold firm, forming the foundation for the current direction of developmental exploration. From Sigmund Freud to Jean Piaget to Albert Bandura, the early contributors to the study of human nature remain dominant influences on modern thinking. As this chapter explores the main features of human development from prenatal stages to late adulthood and even death, the observations and findings of these early theorists will serve as explanations for experiences at every stage of life.

One factor remains constant: not all theorists agree on the nature of human development. Some, like Freud, Erikson, and Piaget, believed development is discontinuous or occurs in stages (i.e., that each person proceeds in an orderly fashion through predetermined milestones that all experience in the same sequence). Others believe development is continuous or an ongoing but gradual process (Berk, 2002).

Some believe that human development, from physical to cognitive, is determined by a genetic predisposition. This is the nature side of the nature vs. nurture controversy. Those who argue for the influence of "nurture" believe that it is experience or one's environment that determines how the individual grows.

Rather than argue either side of this debate, most current scientists agree that there are a variety of influences on all aspects of development. Research has demonstrated that conditions or traits that once were considered the result of experience, and in some cases parenting, are actually the result of genetic predispositions. Schizophrenia and autism are both examples of disorders that have a strong genetic influence but at one time were attributed to poor parenting. It is important, therefore, to study both the biological and experiential aspects of development. This chapter will begin with a general overview of the theorists most influential in the study of human development. The physical, cognitive, and social changes at each stage of life will be reviewed.

DEVELOPMENTAL THEORISTS

Sigmund Freud (1856-1939) continues to be one of the most influential theorists in all of psychology and in the study of human development. Born in Moravia, Freud spent most of his life in Vienna, Austria, and moved to London late in life to avoid Nazi terrorism.

Freud believed there were 3 parts to the personality: the id, the ego, and the superego. Through tools like psychoanalysis as well as hypnosis and dream interpretation, Freud concluded there are 5 psychosexual stages through which a child must pass on the path to adulthood. If an individual's needs are satisfied at one stage, then he or she moves on successfully. If his or her needs are not satisfied, he or she may well become fixated at that stage, resulting in behavioral or personality traits that strive to fulfill this need indefinitely. Freud's theory on the psychosexual stages of development is based on the recollections of patients, many of who were referred to him for their unexplainable neurological disorders. His observations led to an emphasis on the unconscious mind where threatening or unacceptable memories or impulses are stored (Hall, 1954).

Although Freud's theories are controversial, it is worth understanding these concepts because they form the foundation of all further developmental theories. Most of the later theorists either used Freud's theory as a foundation or, in contrast, rejected his theory all together. One theorist who originally worked as an art teacher for the children at the Vienna Psychoanalytic Institute and who underwent psychoanalysis by Freud's daughter, Anna, was Erik Erikson (1902-1990).

Erikson's theory is unique because he continued to add to it throughout his own lifespan and addressed the fact that indi-

Table 4-1

Comparison of Developmental Stage Theories

Life Cycle	Freud	Erikson	Piaget
	Psychosexual	Psychosocial	Cognitive
Infancy (0 to 3 years)	Oral Anal	Trust vs. mistrust Autonomy vs. shame and doubt	Sensorimotor
Early Childhood (3 to 6 years)	Phallic	Initiative vs. guilt	Preoperational
Middle Childhood (6 to 12 years)	Latency	Industry vs. inferiority	Concrete operational
Adolescence (12 to 21 years)	Genital	Identity vs. identity confusion	Formal operational
Early Adulthood (21 to 30 years)		Intimacy vs. isolation	
Middle Adulthood (30 to 60 years)		Generativity vs. stagnation	
Late Adulthood (60+ years)		Ego integrity vs. despair	

Adapted from Rice, F. P. (1996). *The adolescent: Development, relationships and culture* (8th ed.). Needham Heights, MA: Allyn and Bacon.

viduals continue to grow and change throughout life. Unlike Freud, who focused on the influence of sexual energy on development, Erikson focused on the social relationships in a child's life. Each of Erikson's psychosocial stages, called "crises," represents a time when the individual faces a conflict that must be resolved, hopefully favorably, at each phase. If successful, the individual acquires a "virtue" that enables him or her to move forward.

Rather than look at the development of personality, Jean Piaget (1896-1980) was more interested in how a child's cognitive development changes with age. In fact, Piaget was more interested in what children did not know at each particular age, rather than what they did know (Papert, 1999). Piaget's cognitive theory is also a stage theory based on the belief that the individual seeks equilibrium between his or her units of knowledge, or schemas, and his or her experience. A lack of equilibrium results in the need to change or add to one's knowledge called *adaptation*. Piaget used the terms *assimilation* and *accommodation* to refer to the two types of adaptation. Assimilation refers to the use of schemas that one already possesses, and accommodation refers to the formation of new schemas.

Piaget's work has met with criticism in recent years. Many feel that he underestimated the appropriate ages to develop certain capabilities (Feldman, 2003), and it has even been shown recently that infants possess a comprehension of object permanence fairly earlier than first suggested.

Table 4-1 compares the 3 major stage theories.

Finally, behavioral theorists have influenced the way we view learning in childhood as well as throughout the lifespan. Ivan Pavlov (1849-1936) was a physiologist conducting research directly after World War I in what would become the Soviet Union. He discovered what is now known as classical conditioning. In classical conditioning, the individual (or dog in his case) learns to respond to a neutral stimulus that is paired with a stimulus that normally would not bring about a response. (Feldman, 2003). Not only do dogs learn to salivate to the sound of a caretaker's keys as he or she approaches with food, but humans learn to make associations as well. The founder of American classical conditioning, John B. Watson (1878-1958), conditioned a child known as "Little Albert" to fear a white rat, an animal he naturally did not fear until it was paired with a loud noise. Many theorists believe that humans learn fears, phobias, and other behaviors through classical conditioning.

B. F. Skinner (1904-1990) discovered how the principles of operant conditioning also influence human behavior. In operant conditioning, what happens immediately after a response will strengthen or weaken the behavior that took place immediately prior. Thus, reinforcement will encourage the person to display that behavior again. Punishment is the opposite experience wherein something negative occurs due to one's behavior, thus decreasing the chances of it happening again.

Finally, Albert Bandura took the concept of operant conditioning a step further and developed social learning theory, which suggests that humans learn not only by reinforcement but

Table 4-2
Other Theorists Relevant to the Study of Development

Ivan Pavlov and John B. Watson	Classical conditioning
B. F. Skinner	Operant conditioning
Albert Bandura	Social learning theory
Abraham Maslow	Hierarchy of needs
Lawrence Kohlberg	Moral development
Noam Chomsky	Language acquisition device

via vicarious reinforcement as well. If a child witnesses another child being rewarded for a behavior (e.g., giving the teacher an apple), that child will be more likely to display behaviors similar to that of the model. Bandura's work is relevant today in that he showed through his "Bobo Doll" and other experiments that children imitate what they see in person, on television, and even on cartoons.

Numerous theorists have contributed to our current knowledge of human development and a very incomplete list appears in Table 4-2.

HUMAN DEVELOPMENT

Research into the importance of the early environment in the womb, as well as growing knowledge about the role of genes, suggests that the prenatal environment is a crucial determinant of how the individual develops and experiences life. Many people agree that human life begins at conception. When the sperm successfully penetrates the ovum, the bundle of cells soon forms the zygote. For the first 10 to 14 days after conception, the still undifferentiated cells of the zygote multiply. By the beginning of the third week, the cells start to differentiate by function and the zygote becomes the embryo. At approximately the 21st day after conception, the ball of cells folds over to form the neural tube. The neural tube forms the foundation of the brain and central nervous system of the embryo. Thereafter, the embryo undergoes what is considered a critical period of development. As the organs and limbs develop, this is also a time when the environment, stress, or other factors may interfere with successful development. This period lasts until about the eighth week after conception. During this time, teratogens, or substances that can damage the embryo after they cross the placenta, are most likely to cause harm. Some known teratogens include mercury, nicotine, alcohol, cocaine, and diseases like measles. Once differentiation has occurred, the embryo is called a fetus, bones start to form, and the period from 8 to 40 weeks after conception is spent growing in size (Feldman, 2003).

A full-term baby is one born any time after 36 to 38 weeks of conception. The average full term baby weights 7.5 lbs and is 20 inches long at birth. A baby born prior to this is considered preterm or premature. Babies classified as having low birth weight are less than 5 lbs at birth. Those with very low birth weight are born less than 2.5 lbs. These babies may present with many problems or complications, including anoxia, respiratory distress syndrome, and jaundice (Feldman, 2003).

At birth, the APGAR scale, administered at 1, 5, and 10 minutes after birth, is used to assess the infant's health (Apgar, 1953). This measure evaluates appearance, pulse, grimace, activity, and respiration, rating each on a scale of 0 to 2 with a total possible score of 10.

During the early months of life, infants should receive regular examinations by a pediatrician. At these well-child checkups, the pediatrician will perform an evaluation of the infant's reflexes. A reflex is an innate involuntary behavior (Myers, 2005) and the presence or absence of certain reflexes indicates the proper functioning of the central nervous system (Feldman, 2003). With age, some reflexes are expected to drop out, indicating that the cerebral cortex or higher-order abilities are taking over and that the infant is no longer dominated by reflexive actions. Some of the reflexes and the age at which they should drop out are listed in Table 4-3.

At these regular visits to the pediatrician, the typical infant receives a series of vaccinations that provide immunization to numerous illnesses. Table 4-4 displays the vaccines and when administration normally takes place.

Sometimes it is necessary to continue to evaluate an infant's developmental progress after birth. The measures used include the Brazelton Neonatal Behavioral Assessment Scale (Brazelton, 1973), the Bayley Scales of Infant Development (Bayley, 1949), and the Denver Developmental Screening Test (Frankenburg, Dodds, Archer, Shapiro, & Bresnick, 1992). While each of these has a specific focus, all of them evaluate the infant's motor, perceptual, or language development when appropriate. One flaw in infant tests is that most of them do not predict performance on later developmental tests, which tend to focus on verbal skills.

Other researchers claim that the best predictor of a child's intelligence is the mother's intelligence and level of education. In some circumstances, the Home Observation for Measurement of the Environment (HOME) is used to evaluate the home environment in which the child is living to determine levels of stimulation and available activities (Caldwell & Bradley, 1994).

Table 4-3

Reflexes of Infancy and Ages When Reflexes Should Drop Out of Behaviors

Rooting	Turning face when cheek is stroked	Drops out by 3 weeks
Moro	Startle response when head drops below spine	Drops out 6 months
Palmar	Firmly grasps items placed in hand	Drops out by 3 to 4 months
Babinski	Spreading toes when stroked	Drops by 8 to 12 months
Plantar	Curling down of toes when ball of foot is pressed	Drops by 8 to 12 months
Tonic neck reflex	Fencer position when looks at dominant hand	Drops by 4 months

Adapted from Berk, L. A. (2002). *Infants and children: Prenatal through middle childhood*. Boston: Allyn & Bacon.

Table 4-4

Vaccination Schedule

2 months	4 months	6 months	15 months	18 months	24 months	4 to 6 years.	14 to 16 years.
DTP-1 OPV-1	DTP-2 OPV-2	DTP-3	MMR	DTP-4 OPV-3	Hib	DTP-5 OPV-4	Td

DTP = diphtheria, pertussis, tetanus; Hib = Hemophilias influenza b vaccine; MMR = measles, mumps, and rubella; OPV = oral polio vaccine; Td = adult tetanus, diphtheria

Adapted from Winters-Smith, C. (2003). Normal human development. In K. Sladyk (Ed.), *OT study cards in a box* (2nd ed.). Thorofare, NJ: SLACK Incorporated.

STAGES OF DEVELOPMENT

Infancy/Toddler

Infancy, normally ranging from birth to 18 months more or less, is a time of rapid growth and change. While at birth the average infant weighs just over 7 pounds and is 20 inches long, within the first 5 months of life, his or her weight has doubled. By the first birthday, it has tripled. As the child becomes a toddler (i.e., the second birthday), the weight is four times the birth weight (Feldman, 2003). As shown in Table 4-5, by the infant's second birthday, the average child is 3 feet tall.

Growth and coordination develop in the same sequence for all people. According to the principle of cephalocaudal development, maturation occurs from the head down. In proximodistal development, maturation occurs from the center of the body outward.

One's ability to use parts of the body also develops according to these principles. For example, the infant will be able to lift its head before it can coordinate movement of its arms. Notice how development progresses downward and outward when studying Table 4-6. In general, gross motor skills mature before fine motor skills.

The study of human development involves a variety of other areas beyond physical development. Personality and cognitive development are also important to understand. There are numerous and diverse explanations for personality development. Freud's psychosexual stages begin with the oral stage (0 to 18 months) wherein the infant focuses its libido or sexual energy on oral gratification. Freud was certainly correct in his observation that all children tend to put any and everything in their mouths during this age although his explanation has come under great debate. As will be discussed later, other theorists, like Piaget, had very different explanations for the same observations. During the anal stage (18 months to 3 years), the child's energy is focused on the part of the body around the anus. Coincidentally, during this time the child is experiencing potty training as well as the conflicts that accompany the imposition of such rules. An individual who was potty trained too strictly may either become anal retentive or anal expulsive.

In Erikson's psychosocial theory, the infant experiences a conflict between basic trust and mistrust during the early months of life. If the caregiver is attentive, predictably meeting the needs of the infant, the infant learns positive things about the world and resolves this conflict in favor of trust. This influences his or her entire outlook as he or she marches into the next stage of development. Note that no child will ever experi-

Table 4-5

Average Height and Weight Statistics

	Birth	5 months	12 months	24 months	36 months
Weight	7.5 lbs.	15 lbs.	22 lbs.	28 lbs.	32 lbs.
Height	20 inches	25 inches	30 inches	35 inches	39 inches

Adapted from Feldman, R. S. (2003). *Child development*. New Jersey: Prentice Hall/Pearson Education.

Table 4-6

Milestones of Motor Development

Rolling over	3.2 months
Grasping rattle	3.3 months
Sitting without support	5.9 months
Standing while holding on	7.2 months
Grasping with thumb and finger	8.2 months
Standing alone	11.5 months
Walking	12.3 months
Building a tower of two blocks	14.8 months
Walking up steps	16.6 months
Jumping in place	23.8 months

Adapted from Feldman, R. S. (2003). *Child development*. New Jersey: Prentice Hall/Pearson Education.

ence a perfect environment, and to do so is almost impossible, because the child must learn to mistrust to a healthy degree in order to stay safe.

Erikson believed that the first crisis, basic trust vs. mistrust, (0 to 18 months) formed the foundation for the child's later experiences. During infancy, the infant learns whether the world is a place that is welcoming and safe or one that is cold and untrustworthy. If the mother or caregiver responds to the infant's needs by providing comfort, nutrition, warmth, and attention, the infant will undoubtedly find the world to be a reasonably happy place. Unfortunately, not all mothers are equipped to respond to the infant and are unable or unwilling to satisfy its needs. There are many reasons why this may be so, including the demands of other children; disinterest in an unwanted child; the mother's emotional or mental state; or the mother's dependence on drugs, alcohol, or other substances that distract her from the child's well-being. While all children will experience some unmet needs, and in fact, this is to be not only expected but desired, ideally most of the needs will be met on a timely and appropriate basis. Learning that one isn't the center of mom's world is also important considering not all mothers can be present and available at all times.

The second crisis encountered is that of autonomy vs. shame and doubt (18 months to 3 years). During this time, which coincides with potty training, as did Freud's anal stage, the toddler is experiencing a conflict between the socialization efforts of society and his or her own needs to become independent. Therefore, efforts to prove one's self may result in discipline

from a disproving caregiver. This is also the time commonly known as "the terrible twos" when children are expected to express their individuality by getting into great mischief and possibly throwing frequent temper tantrums. When viewed as expressions of autonomy and self-awareness, the astute caregiver can more easily manage these disruptions with brief time-outs or redirections of behavior rather than allowing the child to dominate the tranquility of the home or public setting.

Another area of interest to researchers related to personality is that of infant temperament. Temperament is inborn and is the infant precursor to personality. In 1968, Thomas, Chess, and Birch determined in the New York Longitudinal Study that temperament differs among individual children based on the components of activity level, rhythmicity, approach/withdrawal, adaptability, intensity of reactions, responsiveness, quality of mood, distractibility, and attention span (Thomas, Chess, & Birch, 1968). By applying these components to children's behavior, Thomas et al. categorized children as easy babies, difficult babies, or slow-to-warm-up babies. As can be expected, easy babies are predictable, generally happy, have a moderate intensity of reactions, and adapt easily to new situations or people. Difficult babies are generally cranky, have very intense reactions, are unpredictable, and have trouble adapting to new situations or people. Slow-to-warm-up babies are a mix of traits but generally are more reserved than the easy babies but are easier to handle than difficult babies. They may well be the future "shy" children who warm up to a situation once they have had time to evaluate it (Feldman, 2003).

Table 4-7

Timeline for Development of Early Communication

1.5 to 3 months	Coos, gurgles
6 to 10 months	Babbles consonants and vowels
9 months	Use of gestures
9 to 10 months	Begins to understand words, imitates adult words
10 to 14 months	First word or holophrases
13 months	Deliberate gestures like pointing or waving
18 to 24 months	First sentence
30 months	Combines three or more words, makes common grammatical mistakes like mouses for mice
36 months	1,000 words in vocabulary

Adapted from Winters-Smith., C. (2003). Normal human development. In K. Sladyk (Ed.), *OT study cards in a box* (2nd ed.). Thorofare, NJ: SLACK Incorporated.

As infants approach 8 to 10 months, the departure of the mother or the appearance of a stranger may cause separation anxiety or stranger anxiety.

Ainsworth studied attachment in infants by creating the "strange situation." This experimental paradigm identifies whether infants are securely attached, using their mother as a source of comfort, or have insecure types of attachment, which she labeled avoidant, ambivalent, or disorganized-disoriented (Feldman, 2003).

Beyond physical and personality development, cognitive development is also of interest. One frequently studied element of cognitive development is the use of language. Learning theory suggests that infants are reinforced for the use of language through attention and imitation. Whether an infant babbles, smiles, coos, or vocalizes a holophrase (i.e., single word with multiple meanings) like "ma" or "da," it is likely that he or she will be reinforced by a response by the caregiver who will smile or vocalize in return. In contrast, Chomsky proposed the existence of an internal language acquisition device that drives infants to learn language. Other researchers believe that the use of motherese, or child-directed speech, teaches conversational skills (Feldman, 2003).

In Piaget's theory, there are 4 stages of cognitive development. For the first 18 to 24 months, the child is in the sensorimotor stage of development. During this stage, the infant begins by experiencing the world through his or her reflexes but at age 2 is demonstrating the presence of mental representations for objects and events that they have experienced in the past. The infant develops object permanence, begins to understand cause-and-effect reactions, and starts to use language.

According to Piaget, the infant in the sensorimotor stage explores the world by combining both sensory and motor modalities. Development progresses from innate or reflexive behaviors to more complex behaviors (primary circular reactions), followed by comprehension that the infant can control objects external to the self (secondary circular reactions). As behavior becomes more intentional, the infant develops object permanence, becomes more actively engaged in experimentation (tertiary circular reactions), and finally the infant displays deferred imitation of previously experienced events and begins to use symbolic thought. Between the ages of 2 and 3 years, the child uses language more extensively and has a more advanced memory for events that occurred in the past.

Prelinguistic speech or communication involves gestures or verbalizations that are not words, and linguistic speech progresses by the approximate timetable shown in Table 4-7.

Early Childhood

Early childhood refers to the preschool ages of 3 to 6. Physical development in early childhood slows compared to infancy, with the average 6 year old weighing 46 lbs and standing 46 inches. There is more variability in height, weight, and shape, with boys being taller and heavier than girls. Much of the baby fat of infancy burns off and their physique becomes more adult-like in proportion (Feldman, 2003). Significant changes in both fine motor and gross motor skills take place as the child passes through the preschool years. Running, hopping, and stopping abilities all improve as do fine motor skills like drawing, cutting, and folding (Feldman, 2003).

During this stage, Freud postulates that the child experiences the Oedipus complex wherein the young child directs his or her sexual energy or libido toward the opposite gendered parent. If this conflict is resolved satisfactorily, the child will not only develop identification with the same gendered parent, but he or she will also successfully form a superego, the part of personality containing the conscience.

The early childhood years involve a crisis Erikson identified as a conflict between initiative and guilt. Children of this age want more independence in planning their own activities, selecting their own wardrobe, or making other decisions that might sometimes come in conflict with what the parents consider safe or appropriate behavior. When punished for trying to take initiative, especially when it has resulted either in safety risks or making messes, the child may experience guilt. Ideally, the child will be given the opportunity to make his or her own decisions on some matters, which will result in a sense of purpose and the ability to carry out plans and organizational tasks in the future.

According to Piaget, the preschooler enters the preoperational stage. During this time, the child improves his or her use of symbolic function and begins to use reasoning. This is one of the more interesting stages because of the limitations still existing in the child's thinking. Piaget believed their thinking is limited by the characteristics of centration, egocentrism, and the lack of conservation. Anyone who has poured drinks for two 4 year olds experiences these limitations first hand.

Middle Childhood

Middle childhood typically refers to the elementary school years or ages 6 through 12. During this time, children grow an average of 2 to 3 inches and gain 5 to 7 pounds per year. For the first time, and in many cases the only time, girls are slightly taller than boys (Feldman, 2003).

Fine motor skills become more refined with pencils gripped at the tip, rather than palmed, and children of this age in general have a more relaxed grasp of pencils, brushes, or other instruments. Gross motor skills continuously improve with skipping possible at age 6 and jumping jacks at age 7 although some awkwardness may appear between the ages of 10 and 12 due to their accelerated rate of growth (Winters-Smith, 2003).

The years of middle childhood include what Freud identified as the latency stage. He believed that during this stage, sexual energy is directed inward and not toward any external source. As will be seen, not all theorists agree with Freud's view.

The school years are a time when the child's curiosity about the world exposes him or her to diverse influences, including peers, television, the educational system, and even competitive sports. Many children begin to experience difficulties in school or in their social relationships, resulting in a diagnosis of learning disabilities or attention deficit disorder (with or without hyperactivity). They may also experience social rejection or bullying (Feldman, 2003).

Bandura's research has demonstrated the effects of television watching on children's behavior and shows that aggressive behavior displayed on the playground or in the classroom may be the result of observational learning. Many schools have adapted the concept of multiple intelligences as espoused by Howard Gardner (1993). Gardner proposes that intelligence includes not just verbal and math skills but also musical, spatial, bodily-kinesthetic, personal, and naturalistic types of intelligence. By trying to challenge all types of intelligence, the emphasis in many classrooms has moved beyond basic math, reading, and writing skills, and students are encouraged to explore music, nature, and other areas of interest.

Another emphasis in some schools is emotional intelligence (called EQ or EI), a quality that has been found to be more predictive of success in later years than traditional concepts of intelligence. Four year olds who were able to regulate their behavior in a test that involved their resisting the temptation to eat marshmallows actually scored 200 points higher on the Standardized Achievement Test (SAT) when they were 18 years old (Goleman, 1995). This study suggests that traditional intelligence as measured by verbal and math ability may not be all that is necessary to succeed in life. One's interpersonal skills may do much to carry one through the challenges of childhood and the complexities to follow during adolescence.

While Freud suggested that the retreat of libidinal interests in middle childhood resulted in little change or growth, Erikson's theory suggests this is a time of dramatic growth. According to Erikson, during the school years, the child experiences a crisis of industry vs. inferiority. The child wants to prove him- or herself as productive and competent while also being accepted by a peer group. At this age, hands-on projects, both at school and home, facilitate a sense of industry. This is when forts are constructed, sand castles built, and tree houses desired. Having one friend is as desirable as having a large group of friends. What is more important is that the child feel accepted by someone. Joining activities at school, church, in the neighborhood, or through sports teams often satisfies this need.

In Piaget's theory, this stage of cognitive development is that of concrete operations. The child becomes less egocentric in his or her thinking and begins to perform mental operations. There is still a preference to hands-on activities and the child cannot think abstractly but begins to use logic in problem solving. The limitations of the previous stage decrease as the child begins to comprehend conservation and can de-center or take multiple points of view (Feldman, 2003).

Adolescence

The term *adolescence* refers to the stage of life between childhood and adulthood. It is a time of growth, change, independence, and often the onset of various emotional problems, including anorexia, depression, and schizophrenia. Drug and alcohol abuse are rampant among both high school and college campuses (Myers, 2005).

Typically, the onset of puberty determines one's entrance into adolescence. The average age is 12 years with females beginning puberty between 10 to 12 and males 13 to 14. Typically, females first experience a growth spurt with a sudden increase in height, followed by development of breasts, followed lastly by the onset of menstrual cycles. The attainment of about 102 pounds in an otherwise average-sized female may predict the onset of the menstrual cycle. Eating disorders are common among adolescent females. Extreme weight loss may indicate anorexia nervosa or hint at bulimia (Feldman, 2003).

Males will experience a growth spurt accompanied by acquisition of secondary sexual characteristics like growth of facial and body hair, expansion of shoulders, and deepening of the voice.

Due to immaturity of the prefrontal lobe, teenagers are unable to understand the dangers of drugs or alcohol and therefore may engage in dangerous behaviors, including driving carelessly or practicing unprotected sex (Grubin, 2002).

According to Freud, with the onset of adolescence the individual enters the genital stage, when adult sexual orientation is established. One area often considered a flaw in Freud's theory is that development concludes at the onset of puberty and there is no consideration for growth at later ages.

In Piaget's theory, the individual enters into the formal operational stage of cognitive development at about age 12 and begins to demonstrate the ability to think abstractly. Both hypothetical thinking and deductive reasoning become possible. When this happens, it becomes possible to consider abstract issues like those encountered in solving an algebra problem or contemplating the universe. Not all people enter formal operations this early, however, and many never really develop this quality of thinking (Feldman, 2003).

Adolescence involves what Erikson called the conflict between identity achievement vs. identity diffusion. This focus on identity causes the adolescent to be overly self-conscious and is expressed both by experimentation with styles of hair or clothing as well as participating in a variety of activities. The adolescent who fails to establish a firm sense of identity will experience self-doubt, may practice self-destructive behaviors, and is more likely to become involved with drugs or alcohol. Fortunately, one's identity can reformulate at later points in life.

Based on an analysis of Erikson's theory, researcher James Marcia (Marcia, 1996) suggested other options for identity formation. These include moratorium, which means the individual puts identity formation on hold, or foreclosure, when one's identity formation is based on the expectations of others or the individual makes a commitment to a career or relationship but has not really experienced a crisis.

The most important developmental tasks are achieved by early adulthood with a great deal of variety in experiences thereafter and the changes being more qualitative rather than quantitative. Some will have married, others not. Some may still be searching for a career; others are on the fast track toward success in a particular field. Therefore, the ever-changing options currently acceptable in society should be taken into account when studying the stages experienced by adults.

Early Adulthood

Although motor functioning and physical well-being peak in the early adult years (ages 18 to 30), many factors determine how well the individual lives. Accidents are the leading cause of death, and unhealthy practices like smoking or drinking will begin to take a toll on the future quality of life. Obesity is a growing problem among young Americans and may result in increased risk of later diseases like diabetes, heart disease, and cancer.

During the years of 18 to 30, the typical individual begins to make decisions or commitments that may last his or her entire life. During this time, the ability to commit to relationships as well as the establishment of career goals are major concerns in one's life. According to Erikson, this is when the individual confronts the crisis of intimacy vs. social isolation. If the identity formed properly during adolescence, the individual is ready for commitment. If not, then the individual may flounder and have trouble finding a career as well as committing to a long-term relationship. Part of identity formation includes the accumulation of the trappings of adulthood: a house, car, furniture, and nowadays a 401K.

With age, the individual becomes more flexible in his or her thinking, expressing transformal thought. Personal experience or tacit knowledge begins to be an important factor in career success, sometimes being a better predictor of success than traditional intelligence. This is consistent with the studies mentioned earlier that attribute adult success to emotional intelligence displayed at an early age (Winters-Smith, 2003).

Middle Adulthood

In the middle adult years (ages 30 to 60), many individuals experience a decline in sensory abilities, especially vision. Reaction time decreases, as do strength and coordination, but endurance may continue, especially if the individual has maintained an exercise regime. Currently, many adults participate in exercise programs or belong to gyms, which will undoubtedly result in healthier experiences as they age.

Later in adulthood, shifts in hormones are experienced by both males and females. Menopause, a term that refers to the changes that women experience during the climacteric, means a woman can no longer reproduce. For some women this experience represents the end of her productive years but to others it represents the beginning of a new and exciting phase of life. In the male, testosterone levels drop but men are able to father children well into old age.

According to Erikson, middle-aged adults experience a crisis of generativity vs. stagnation. Up to age 40, adults are concerned with the formation of families and careers but once established in these areas, they become more concerned with their own spiritual needs as well as committed to giving back to society. Those who have not successfully navigated the challenges of young adulthood may become resentful and bitter before resolving this crisis. Therefore, a woman who has not been married or reproduced and who feels unfulfilled in her career, may be especially resentful as she enters this stage.

Crystallized intelligence or the use of information gained by personal experience peaks later in life whereas fluid intelligence, or problem-solving abilities, declines. Creative abilities seem to increase with age and many authors, painters, sculptors, and poets peak in their middle or late adult years.

Late Adulthood

As individuals continue to live longer, many problems that historically have plagued the elderly can now be relieved by modern medical procedures. For example, while vision problems continue, many people may undergo laser surgery as treatment for cataracts, which in the past would have resulted in blindness. Shrinkage of the cerebellum does result in more accidents due to the loss of balance and coordination, but nutritional knowledge and testing have improved so that women at risk for osteoporosis may avoid bone loss and therefore decrease the risk of fractures that hindered elders in the past.

The loss of taste, smell, and—most notably—hearing, are also common. If the individual continues to be active and maintains some form of exercise, it is possible to delay or forego the loss of strength and reaction time that are common.

Many people shrink in old age and losses of 1 to 2 inches in height are common due to osteoporosis. However, in the 21st century, there are a plethora of treatments, injections, and supplements to enhance skin quality and maintain a youthful appearance (Winters-Smith, 2003).

Erikson's theory suggests that in late adulthood (60+) the individual may experience a crisis between ego identity and despair. At the end of life, one evaluates one's accomplishments and must face the challenges of changing lifestyles, including retirement, bereavement, and illness. If the individual failed to successfully navigate the earlier stages, this crisis is especially difficult.

Retired adults must find new ways to occupy their time once the work place is no longer part of the daily routine. Many people must establish new friendships after moving away to distant retirement communities or losing old friends to death.

The loss of a spouse is one of life's more stressful experiences and the elderly must deal with loss of their life partners while also facing their declining health and the new experience of loneliness. The geographic separation of families may also add to the distress experienced at this time. Social support is beneficial. Many modern religious practices, including the Jewish "shiva," provide the individual support as well as reintegration back into society (Santrock, 2002).

The most well known theory dealing with the experiences of death and grief is that proposed by Kubler-Ross. She described the 5 stages of dying: denial, anger, bargaining, depression, and acceptance, although modern researchers suggest that these may be experienced in any order (Santrock, 2002). Hospice services are now available to assist clients and their families in this process.

As the reader can see, human development is an integrative and holistic process that is clearly individualized. The OTA is greatly concerned with human development knowledge as it provides a foundation to treatment. The OTA working with children with disabilities is concerned with development and educational occupations. The teen receiving OTA services may need assistance in developing skills to bridge to adulthood. The OTA working with adults must first understand human development before collaborating with the client to find meaningful occupations as treatment approaches. In summary, an OTA who ignores human development theory is ill prepared to meet his or her client's needs.

LEARNING ACTIVITIES

1. Go to a day care center and observe the interactions between the caregivers and the children. List the verbal messages given by the caregivers to various toddlers. Note the behavioral responses of the toddlers to the verbal messages of the caregivers. List the nonverbal messages given by the caregivers to various toddlers. Note the behavioral responses of the toddlers to the nonverbal messages of the caregivers.

2. Observe children from 5 to 12 years of age in a playground at a local elementary school. What are the groupings of children? What kinds of games are they playing? What types of motor skills are evident among the children in the playground?

3. Interview some teens in a driver education class and find out what it might mean for them to have their own cars when they eventually get their licenses.

4. Interview 3 females and 3 males between the ages of 21 to 35. Identify how many belong to a health club. How often do they exercise, and what types of exercise do they do?

5. Interview 3 sets of parents between the ages of 35 and 60. How many still have children and/or grandchildren in their care? What are their plans for retirement?

6. Visit a nursing home and interview the social worker to get his or her perception of how the patients there give meaning to the end stage of their lives. With the permission of the social worker and nursing home staff, visit with some of the elderly patients to find out what kind of lives they may have lived in earlier years.

REFERENCES

Apgar, V. (1953). A proposal for a new method of evaluation in the newborn infant. *Current Research in Anesthesia and Analgesia, 32,* 260.

Bayley, N. (1949). Consistency and variability in the growth of intelligence from birth to eighteen years. *Journal of Genetic Psychology, 75,* 165-196.

Berk, L. A. (2002). *Infants and children: Prenatal through middle childhood.* Boston: Allyn & Bacon.

Brazelton, T. B. (1973). *The neonatal behavioral assessment scale.* Philadelphia: Lippincott.

Caldwell, B. M., & Bradley, R. H. (1994). Environmental issues in developmental follow-up research. In S. L. Friedman & H. C. Haywood (Eds.), *Developmental follow-up.* San Diego: Academic Press.

Feldman, R. S. (2003). *Child development.* New Jersey: Prentice Hall/Pearson Education.

Frankenburg, W. K., Dodds, J., Archer, P., Shapiro, H., & Bresnick, B. (1992). The Denver II: A major revision and restandardization of the Denver developmental screening test. *Pediatrics, 89,* 91-97.

Gardner, H. (1993). *Multiple intelligences.* New York: BasicBooks.

Goleman, D. (1995). *Emotional intelligence.* New York: Bantam Books.

Grubin, D. (2002) *Secret life of the brain.* PBS video series.

Hall, C. S. (1954). *A primer of Freudian psychology.* New York: The World Publishing Co.

Marcia, J. (1966). Development and validation of ego identity status. *Journal of Personality and Social Psychology, 3,* 551-558.

Myers, D. (2005). *Exploring psychology.* New York: Worth Publishers.

Papert, S. (1999). Child psychologist Jean Piaget. Understanding Psychology, Time reports. Retrieved December 7, 2004, from http:// www.time.com.

Santrock, J. W. (2002). *A topical approach to life-span development.* New York: McGraw Hill.

Thomas, A., Chess, S., & Birch, H. G. (1968). *Temperament and behavior disorders in children.* New York: New York University Press.

Winters-Smith., C. (2003). Normal human development. In K. Sladyk (Ed.), *OT study cards in a box* (2nd ed.). Thorofare, NJ: SLACK Incorporated.

Key Concepts

- International Classification of Function: World Health Organization's organized view of well being.
- Occupation: Activities of everyday life, named, organized, and given value and meaning by individuals and a culture.
- Occupational therapy domains: What occupational therapy uses to help clients engage in their occupations.
- Occupational therapy process: How occupational therapy helps clients fulfill their occupations.
- *Occupational Therapy Practice Framework*: AOTA's organized view of occupation.

Essential Vocabulary

activity: Goal directed but do not always assume a place of critical importance to a person.

activity demands: The specific features of an activity that affect skills and performance, including objects, space, social demands, sequencing or timing, required actions, and required underlying body functions and body structures needed to perform the activity.

areas of occupation: The broad range of occupations. These include activities of daily living (ADL), which are also referred to as basic activities of daily living (BADL), instrumental activities of daily living (IADL), education, work, play, leisure, and social participation.

client factors: Intrinsic factors that affect performance in occupations, including body structures and body functions.

context: Refers to the condition of a given occupation, which can be personal such as age, gender, and socioeconomic and education status.

engagement: Participation in occupations that connotes both subjective and objective performance, perceived by both the client and therapist as meaningful and necessary.

Framework: Refers to the *Occupational Therapy Practice Framework*, which includes language describing the domain and process of occupational therapy practice.

performance patterns: Patterns of human behavior related to daily occupations that include habits, routines, and roles.

performance skills: What a person "does" related to observable actions with specific purpose. These skills are described within 3 categories, including motor skills, process skills, and communication/interaction skills.

OCCUPATIONAL THERAPY PRACTICE FRAMEWORK: DOMAIN AND PROCESS— OUR LANGUAGE

Ben Atchison, PhD, OTR, FAOTA

INTRODUCTION

It was an interesting tour for the students in the OTA program as they observed several individuals involved in a variety of activities in a community-based program for persons with developmental disabilities. The OTA who was conducting the tour noted that one of the clients demonstrated difficulty with control of voluntary movement functions and was engaged in a fine motor coordination task. "So," asked a normally inquisitive student, "is he working on motor planning skills as well? "No," the tour guide responded, "actually, this is more related to eye-hand coordination. Praxis refers more specifically to the mental functions of sequencing complex movement." The student was confused and embarrassed for asking this question, but she distinctly recalled that her supervisor on her previous fieldwork assignment had explained that voluntary movement function referred to the development of praxis. "Why," she asked herself, "is this person using this term so differently than how I learned it?"

This student's experience is not uncommon. The language used to describe the many components of occupational therapy is not always consistent. Try this experiment: Ask a few OTAs to define ADL. Undoubtedly, several variations will be offered. The reason for this lack of consistency is that each of those persons you asked probably learned the definition from another person without reference to a standard set of terms. This presents a problem. When terms are used inconsistently among practitioners to describe occupational therapy practice, confusion results among clients, families, other members on the team, and third-party payers. The term *ADL* is often commonly used to refer to dressing, feeding, bathing, toileting, hygiene, and grooming. If the therapist is working with a person to engage in simple home repairs, care of pets, or helping a spouse understand safety needs in transfers, what is that called?

If the concept of ADL is limited to those typical activities mentioned, a very significant part of the kinds of activities that people engage in, or occupation, is not addressed. However, if all occupational therapists describe "ADL" in the same way, there is better assurance that the full spectrum of ADL will be addressed in intervention.

The lack of consistency in defining our practice is not unique to occupational therapy. In fact, legislation passed by Congress in 1977 (P. L.-95-142) mandated that health care facilities establish a uniform reporting system to ensure that health professions use common language when completing required documentation (Dohli & Leibold, 1998). In part, this law was passed in response to significant billing fraud and abuse in both the Medicare and Medicaid programs by all health-related disciplines. While the federal government never adopted these systems due to price-fixing concerns, the AOTA determined that consistency of language for communication among occupational therapists as well as with all other constituents was important and useful. In 1979, the AOTA created a task force to develop the *Uniform Terminology System for Reporting Occupational Therapy Services*. As a result, the *Uniform Terminology for Occupational Therapy* was developed and has been subsequently revised twice, in 1989 and 1994. With each revision, terms were updated and new domains or constructs were added to describe occupational therapy practice more accurately. The intent of *Uniform Terminology* was to "provide a generic outline of the domain of occupational therapy and... to create common terminology for the profession and to capture the essence of occupational therapy succinctly to others" (AOTA, 1994, p. 1047).

As was the practice in previous revisions, the Commission on Practice for AOTA initiated a review process that included feedback from all levels of the profession. The intent was to determine the changes and updates needed. Following the significant review of *Uniform Terminology 3rd edition* (UT III), major changes were felt necessary in response to changes in practice and the profession's evolving understanding of generic yet complex concepts. Moyers initially outlined and described these changing constructs of practice in *The Guide to Occupational Therapy Practice* (1999), which ultimately led to the development of the *Occupational Therapy Practice Framework: Domain and Process* (AOTA, 2002), more commonly referred to as the Practice Framework or Framework. In addition to incorporating language common to occupational therapists, the commission successfully included language that is recognized by others, such as the terminology used in the World Health Organization's (WHO's) *International Classification of*

Functioning, Disability, and Health (ICF) (2001). Interestingly, it was noted that *Uniform Terminology* had not included the concept of occupation in its terminology, and it was determined that this had to be emphasized in any revision that was going to occur. Therefore, the Framework was organized to focus on engagement in occupation to support participation in context. The use of occupation and related activities as a means of enabling participation in daily life is the unique domain that differentiates occupational therapy from other professions.

This chapter describes the 2 major parts of the Framework: domain and process with the concepts of occupation and client-centered practice embedded throughout. The term *client* is used as opposed to *patient* since this better describes the variety of individuals, groups, or populations that are served by occupational therapy.

THE DOMAIN OF OCCUPATIONAL THERAPY

When the public defines occupational therapy, it often does so with work or vocation as the central construct or with "occupying" folks with "things to do." As a pediatric neurologist once said to me, "You help people find jobs… this 3-month-old infant doesn't need a job!" or the psychiatrist who noted that "my role as an occupational therapist was to do activities to occupy patients." What is occupation? The definition included in the Framework is as follows:

> Activities… of everyday life, named, organized, and given value and meaning by individuals and a culture. Occupation is everything people do to occupy themselves, including looking after themselves, enjoying life… and contributing to the social and economic fabric of their communities. (Law, Polatajko, Baptiste, & Townsend, 1997, p. 32)

This definition makes an important distinction between occupation and activity. While closely related, each term has a distinct meaning and is experienced differently by each person. Occupations are activities having special meaning and purpose in one's life and in a sense, define who we are. Activities are goal directed but they do not always assume a place of critical importance to a person (Pierce, 2001). All of my occupational therapy students have to read books, write papers, prepare oral reports, memorize facts for exams, work with others on group assignments, perform clinical work, and complete other activities as a means of completing their degrees. While completion of related tasks is the goal, not all tasks necessarily take on special meaning for all students. While the activities of being a student must be accomplished, it is not correct to assume that a student views these as meaningful occupations. Perhaps the student is a dancer, musician, or artist and that is where his or her life is most enriched, then he or she would view this as his or her occupation. There are students who view some activities such as reading as "a necessary activity" and then others who view it as an "enriching activity and would perhaps describe themselves as an "avid reader." They see reading as germane to achieving competence and are fulfilled by what they would see as one of

their meaningful "occupations." This is an important distinction to make in considering the needs of clients. For one client, cooking is a mundane activity that must be relearned to fulfill the obvious need to eat. For another, cooking is an occupation that must be relearned because it brings great pride and satisfaction in preparing a wonderful gourmet dinner for others to enjoy. It is an occupation that defines in one way "who they are."

Engagement in Occupation to Support Participation in Context or Contexts

This section of the Framework describes the main focus of the domain. A central objective for occupational therapists and OTAs is to engage clients in meaningful occupations. A key concept that has emerged in the Framework is that of participation, which connotes both subjective and objective performance in occupations perceived by both the client and therapist as meaningful and necessary. Context is a critical component to consider as well, since the occupation takes on different meaning and requirements as the client goes from one "door frame" to another in his or her daily life. It is essential to understand how experience and performance requirements for clients shift with context.

Performance in Areas of Occupation

This section describes the broad range of occupations that individuals perform (Figure 5-1). These areas include ADL, which are also referred to as BADL, IADL, education, work, play, leisure, and social participation. ADL includes those activities that are oriented toward taking care of one's own body. These include bathing, showering, bowel and bladder management, dressing, eating, feeding, functional mobility, personal device care, personal hygiene and grooming, sexual activity, sleep and rest, and toilet hygiene. IADL are more complex activities that require interaction with one's external environment and include activities that allow participation in the care of others, care of pets, child rearing, communication device use, community mobility, financial management, health management and maintenance, home establishment and management, meal preparation and clean up, safety procedures and emergency responses, and shopping. Education includes activities needed to participate in formal education, which include academic categories such as reading and math and pursuit of a degree as well as nonacademic categories such as recess, extracurricular activities, and vocational preparation. This area also includes the identification of informal personal educational needs or interests and participation in informal educational activities. The area of work includes the process of identifying employment interests, pursuit and acquisition of job opportunities through exploration, and preparation for and participation in interviews. Job performance involves work habits and relationships as well as completion of assigned work and compliance with regulations of the work environment. Retirement preparation and adjustment and volunteer exploration and participation are included as essential components of the work area as well. The area of play includes play exploration and participation and is defined

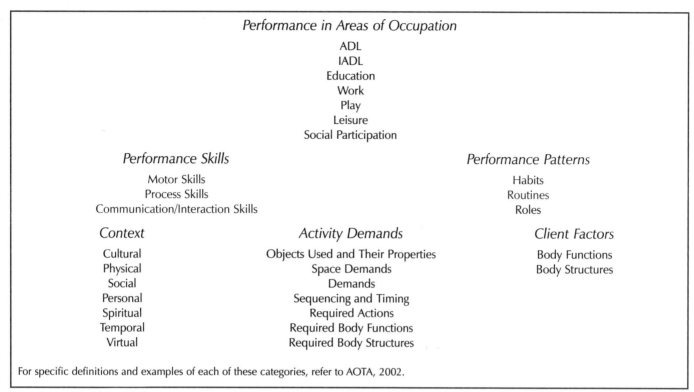

For specific definitions and examples of each of these categories, refer to AOTA, 2002.

Figure 5-1. Outline of the *Occupational Therapy Practice Framework*.

as "any spontaneous enjoyment, entertainment, amusement, or diversion" (Parham & Fazio, 1997, p. 252). Categories of play are described as practice play, pretend play, games with rules, constructive play, and symbolic play. Leisure is described as "nonobligatory occupations that one participates in during discretionary times" (Parham & Fazio, 1997, p. 250). Social participation describes activities that include successful interaction with community, family, and friends.

Performance Skills

Fisher and Kielhofner (1995) describe performance skills as what a person "does—not what a person has" and are related to observable actions with specific purpose. These are described by 3 categories, including motor skills, process skills, and communication/interaction skills. Motor skills refer to the skills in moving and engaging in a task and specifically involve posture, mobility, coordination, strength and effort, and energy requirements. Process skills include the ability to sustain a given task, including attending and accommodating to needed adjustments as the task demand continues.

Included in process skills is the energy needed to sustain task performance, the ability to gather and use task-related knowledge in order to succeed in the task, as well as temporal organization or that process needed to initiate, continue, sequence, and terminate the task.

The skills needed to organize necessary space and objects and adapt to and learn from errors that may arise during the task are part of process skill as well. Communication/interaction skills require the ability to express desire and needs while following expected social norms in the communication process. Skills involved include physicality, information exchange, and relations. Physicality involves the ability to effectively use the body

when communicating. This includes physical contact, visual communication, gestures, physical maneuvers, orientation to another when communicating, and physical position or posture. Information exchange refers to giving and receiving information and specifically considers speech articulation, asserting one's self, asking, engaging, expression of affect, voice modulation, sharing information, speaking skills, and sustained communication ability. Relations relate to collaboration, conformity, focus, development of rapport, and accommodating or respecting others' reactions and requests that emerge during the communication process.

Performance Patterns

This aspect of the domain includes habits, routines, and roles. Habits and routines are comprised of behaviors that make up daily life routines and are often addressed when providing intervention. Helping persons to re-establish habits and routines to support role functions is a consistent area addressed by occupational therapists and OTAs.

Context

Superimposed on performance skills and patterns is context. Context refers to the condition of a given occupation, which can be personal such as age, gender, or socioeconomic, and education status. Context includes temporal influences, which include time of day, time of year, or stage of life, as well as cultural, physical, and social aspects. Spiritual refers to the internal feelings that inspire and motivate. Virtual context refers to the social interaction and activities that occur in the absence of "real" physical contact such as tasks and communication that occur in "virtual" environments such as online computer use.

Activity Demands

Analysis of activity has long been a domain for occupational therapy practice and is explicitly included in the Framework. Activity involves various aspects, including the actual objects of the activity, space and social demands, sequencing or timing, and the requirements of body functions and structures to succeed in activity participation. Objects include the tools, materials, and equipment used to participate in the activity. Space demands relate to the physical requirements of the activity, including size, surface, noise, and temperature, while social demands include the rules and expectations demanded by the activity. Sequence and timing involve the process used to carry out the activity such as the steps needed to prepare a sandwich or make iced tea. To determine the required actions of an activity, consideration of the motor, process, and communication interaction skills is necessary, as are required body functions and body structures.

Client Factors

Client factors are internal to the person and include body functions and body structures necessary to engage in occupations. The authors of the Framework based the categorization of client factors on the ICF proposed by the WHO (2001). It is well understood by occupational therapists and OTAs that client factors influence the ability to perform occupations and that occupations can impact client factors. Specifically, client factors include body functions and body structures. While a description of these factors follows, it is suggested that occupational therapy students refer to the complete document published by the WHO.

Body functions are defined as "physiologic function of body systems including psychological functions" (WHO, 2001, p. 10). This includes mental functions, sensory functions and pain, and voice and speech functions. Systemic functions are included in body functions as well and are those related to cardiovascular, hematological, immunological, respiratory, digestive, metabolic, endocrine, genitourinary, reproductive, neuromusculoskeletal, skin and related structures, and movement-related functions.

Body structures refer to the anatomical parts of the body that support body functions. Included in the ICF are the structures of the nervous system; eye, ear, and related structures; voice and speech; cardiovascular, immunological, and respiratory systems; digestive, metabolic, and endocrine systems; movement systems; and skin and related structures (WHO, 2001, p. 10).

OCCUPATIONAL THERAPY PROCESS

The occupational therapy process includes evaluation, intervention, and establishing outcomes, which is not unlike other professions. The focus on participation in occupation, with an emphasis on context that is client centered throughout these categories, provides a distinct and unique process among health professions. Selection of evaluations, types of intervention, and goals or outcomes are focused on the occupations of the client. An example of this is illustrated in the case presentation on Dorothy on p. 49.

Evaluation

Evaluation begins with the formation of an occupational profile. This includes the client's needs, problems, and concerns related to engaging in occupations, which are identified in a collaborative manner, including the client's reasons for seeking services and desired outcomes. Questions needed to establish the profile include the client's past and current experiences and determining strengths and weaknesses as well as motivating factors that the client may express to enable him or her to reclaim or develop new occupations.

Determination of occupations that are considered to be both successful and problematic to the client is essential in this phase of the evaluation. In addition, an examination of the influence of contexts that facilitate or inhibit engagement in occupations is considered.

Starting the evaluation with the occupational profile sets the tone for a collaboration between the therapist and the client. Development of the profile allows the client to share that which is individually unique and important regardless of the referring diagnosis. The next phase of the evaluation is observation of engagement in occupations and a determination is made as to the need for a detailed analysis of performance. For example, an observation of a child in a classroom who is persistently inattentive may lead to the need for further assessment of sensory processing to determine the specific sensory mechanism that is interfering with the ability to attend to the teacher. On the other hand, the therapist may be able to determine the focus of intervention needed by observation alone.

Intervention

The second step of the occupational therapy process is intervention and includes the substeps of planning, implementation, and review. The planning step involves a collaborative process that includes the therapist, client, and family or significant others to determine goals. The goals, or expected outcomes, are matched with appropriate therapeutic or intervention approaches, and the method of service delivery is determined. Intervention approaches can include health promotion, remediation, maintenance, compensation, and prevention. The focus of intervention within these approaches can include necessary change in performance skills, performance patterns, context, activity demands, or specific client factors. In addition, the ways in which expected outcomes will be measured and development of the discharge plan is determined in this step. The implementation step puts the plan into action and includes internal and external factors that lead to effective change in occupational performance. Internal factors could include actual improvement in body functions such as perceptual functions (e.g., while external factors would include specific adaptations in the physical space in which occupations take place to enable participation).

The review step is not considered a single step in the intervention process. It is persistent throughout the implementation phase. In the course of intervention, the therapist and the client engage in a dialogue about the effectiveness of intervention and make adjustments to the plan as needed. In some settings, there may be a specific targeted point in the course of therapy when a review is conducted. In others, it is less formal and woven through the course of intervention. It is possible that the review can result in termination of occupational therapy and referral to a more appropriate service to better meet the need of the client or termination because goals have been attained.

Outcomes

From the initial point of contact with a client, the process of developing outcomes begins. The authors of the Framework suggest that the outcome targeted by occupational therapists and OTAs is "engagement in occupation to support participation" (AOTA, 2002). Engagement in occupation is defined as "the commitment made to performance in occupations or activities as the result of self-choice, motivation, and meaning, and includes the subjective and objective aspects of carrying out occupations and activities that are meaningful and purposeful to the person" (AOTA, 2002).

Participation is defined as "involvement in a life situation" (WHO, 2001, p. 10). These are not new concepts to occupational therapy as the profession has historically emphasized the need to "do with" and not "do to" the client in the course of intervention. The official inclusion of this term in the Framework underlines the core belief of the profession that health and well-being are achieved and maintained by actively participating in relevant and meaningful occupations that are client centered.

The specific ways in which outcomes of "engagement in occupation" are expressed in an outcome include:

- Occupational performance that is improved, such as increased function in dressing and bathing or the enhancement of performance that will prevent problems from occurring such as improved strength of the upper extremities for a person with lower extremity amputations to enable safe, independent transfers.

- Client satisfaction.

- Role competence, including the roles the client needs to engage.

- Adaptation, which allows the client to effectively respond to occupational challenges.

- Health and wellness: Health is a "complete state of physical, mental, and social well-being and not just the absence of disease and infirmity" (WHO, 1947, p 29).

- Wellness is defined as "a state of mental and physical balance and fitness" (*Tabers Cylopedic Medical Dictionary*,, 1997, p. 210).

- Prevention, which is defined as "promoting a healthy lifestyle at the individual, group, organizational, community, and governmental or policy level" (Brownson & Scaffia, 2001).

- Quality of life, which is defined as "a person's dynamic appraisal of his or her life satisfactions, self-concept, health and functioning, and socioeconomic factors" (AOTA, 2002).

Case Presentation

Dorothy, 55 years old, was diagnosed in 2001 with diabetic neuropathy, which is a complication of diabetes that results in loss of sensation and impaired motor function and further compromises circulatory function associated with diabetes. In Dorothy's case, her diabetic condition was very severe and led to multiple amputations over the next 2 years. When the home-care-based OT and OTA made their first visit to Dorothy's home in 2003, she was a quadrilateral amputee. She had bilateral knee amputations in addition to a left below elbow and right below metacarpophalangeal (MCP) amputation, leaving her metarcarpals and thumb intact. She had previously received extensive rehabilitation as an in-patient during the past year but was not able to continue outpatient services due to transportation difficulties.

In the course of the initial interview, the occupational profile completed by Dorothy and the occupational therapy team determined that she had received a Master's degree in Social Work and had worked with Children and Family Services until she could no longer tolerate the demands of the job. She lived in a well-kept, neat, accessible apartment that had been designed during the course of her progressive amputations. She had the assistance of a certified nursing assistant (CNA) who came to her home daily. Dorothy was able to meet all of her BADL needs with the assistance of the CNA and felt that any attempts to do these activities independently would be too time consuming and difficult. From her perspective, she was successful in this area of occupation. Her perceived needs were quite different from the team, who initially felt that the focus should be on personal self-care. They began suggesting adaptive devices that would enable Dorothy to perform some of the activities without assistance. Dorothy rejected this approach, indicating that this would expend too much physical energy and time that could be used to pursue other interests and needs. The team listened intently now as Dorothy outlined her occupational interests. She expressed strong interest in developing computer skills. She had recently acquired a personal computer with access to the internet. She enjoyed journaling and wanted to pursue the development of a book about her experiences. In addition to learning how to use word processing for writing, she was very interested in learning how to use email and to "surf the web." Dorothy was also concerned about the security of her apartment as she lived in a complex that was in a high crime area. She felt her disability heightened her vulnerability. She also expressed a desire to reclaim her involvement in her church's activities and had not been able to leave her apartment for the last few months as her van, which was equipped for a power wheelchair, was in need of repairs.

The team assessed performance in ADL by observing the collaboration between the CNA and Dorothy as she bathed, dressed, transferred to and from her wheelchair, and completed toileting and hygiene activities. Functional mobility issues centered on her ability to transfer from her wheelchair to bed and back, and a program was initiated to determine the feasibility of developing independent transfer skills, which Dorothy agreed would be helpful in terms of being able to change to positions of comfort. IADL observations included meal preparation and cleanup in which Dorothy actively participated by way of planning the menu and helping to clear the table when the meal was completed. After the meal, Dorothy phoned her sister on her voice activated speaker phone to confirm a card party that was planned at Dorothy's home for the next evening. Dorothy was particularly excited about the upcoming event because her sister was bringing along one of Dorothy's favorite male friends, Charles, who was a life-long friend that she knew from her church activities in the past.

Following an evaluation of performance and process skills related to Dorothy's interest in the use of a computer, the team developed a plan that included a program to provide appropriate adaptations and instruction in the use of her computer, including the use of word processing, email, and internet search tools. While teaching her the basics, the team suggested use of appropriate tutorial software for more in-depth use of applications that the computer software provided.

The discussion questions provide opportunity for a review of the Framework as it relates to this case, and readers are urged to answer each as a beginning to more in-depth understanding of the various parts of the framework.

SUMMARY

The *Occupational Therapy Practice Framework*, adopted by the Representative Assembly of the AOTA in 2002, replaced the UT III. The increasing recognition of the need to place "occupation" in the forefront of our professional language and to emphasize occupation-based practice was at the heart of this significant evolution in the official language of the AOTA. The domain of occupational therapy is outlined and described and incorporates language from the WHO, which was necessary in order to provide consistency with other health care services.

As stated by Youngstrom (2002), the Framework has 2 major components: domain and process. The domain describes the specific area of human activity that is the focus of the practitioner in occupational therapy and which forms the foundation of practice. The distinct component that the Framework adds, which was not part of the Uniform Terminology, is process. The process describes how the constructs in the domain are operationalized, which includes evaluation, intervention, and outcomes.

In each phase of the process, occupation is emphasized as the core element of practice with the threaded concept being "engagement in occupation to support participation in context or contexts" (AOTA, 2002). With the document, our official language finally emphasizes the concept of "occupation" and provides a framework for the profession that adds a clear and holistic presentation of what occupational therapy provides in attaining health and well-being.

LEARNING ACTIVITIES

1. If you were to participate with the occupational therapist in developing the Occupational Profile, what questions would you have specifically asked with regards to ADL? IADL? Education? Work? Play? Leisure? Social participation?

2. In what occupational areas was Dorothy most interested? What else would you want to know about that is not described in this case?

3. What specific performance skills and process skills would you have addressed with the occupational therapist during the ADL and IADL performance evaluation?

4. What activity demands would be considered in the use of a computer? Describe each one.

5. What body structures and body functions are involved in Dorothy's diagnosis?

REFERENCES

American Occupational Therapy Association. (1994). Uniform terminology for occupational therapy (3rd ed.). *American Journal of Occupational Therapy, 48,* 1047-1054.

American Occupational Therapy Association. (2002). Occupational therapy practice framework: Domain and process. *American Journal of Occupational Therapy, 56,* 609-633.

Brownson, C. A., & Scaffia, M. E. (2001). Occupational therapy in the promotion of health and the prevention of disease and disability. *American Journal of Occupational Therapy, 55,* 656-660.

Dohli, C., & Leibold, M. (1998). Uniform terminology and its application to OT evaluation. In J. Hinojosa & P. Kramer (Eds.), *Evaluation: Obtaining and interpreting data.* Bethesda, MD: American Occupational Therapy Association.

Fisher, A. G., & Kielhofner, G. (1995). Skill in occupational performance. In G. Kielhofner (Ed.), *A model of human occupation: Theory and application* (2nd ed., pp. 113-128). Philadelphia: Lippincott, Williams & Wilkins.

Law, M., Polatajko, H., Baptiste, S., & Townsend, E. (1997). Core concepts of occupational therapy. In E. Townsend (Ed.), *Enabling occupation: An occupational therapy perspective* (pp. 29-56). Ottawa, Ontario: Canadian Association of Occupational Therapists.

Moyers, P. (1999). The guide to occupational therapy practice. *American Journal of Occupational Therapy, 53,* 247-322.

Parham, L. D., & Fazio, L. S. (Eds.). (1997). *Play in occupational therapy for children.* St. Louis, MO: Mosby.

Pierce, D. (2001). Untangling occupation and activity. *American Journal of Occupational Therapy, 55,* 138-146.

Tabers cylopedic medical dictionary. (1997). Philadelphia: F. A. Davis.

World Health Organization (1947). Constitution of the World Health Organization. *Chronicle of the World Health Organization, 1*(1), 29-40.

World Heath Organization. (2001). *International classification of functioning, disability, and health* (ICF). Geneva, Switzerland: Author.

Youngstrom, M. J. (2002). The occupational therapy practice framework: The evolution of our professional language. *American Journal of Occupational Therapy, 56*(6), 607-608.

Key Concepts

- Activity analysis: Study of a task's subparts and process.

Essential Vocabulary

adaptation: Modifying a task to make it easier for a person to complete.
grading: Viewing an activity on a continuum from simple to complex, typically grading an activity more challenging as a person has gained skill.
therapeutic potential: The degree of likelihood that a therapeutic goal can be achieved.

ACTIVITY ANALYSIS: OUR TOOL

Sally E. Ryan, COTA, ROH, Retired and Karen Sladyk, PhD, OTR, FAOTA

INTRODUCTION

The meanings of activity, purposeful activity, and occupation are currently debated by OT educators and scholars. However, the role of activity analysis remains extremely important in OT. This process involves the "breaking down" of an activity into detailed subparts and steps, which is a necessary foundation for all ADL, play/leisure, and work tasks used in intervention. Activity analysis is an examination of the therapeutic characteristics and value of activities that fulfill the patient's many needs, interests, abilities, roles, and occupations. Without such analysis, it may be impossible to use the proper application of activity or to obtain the best treatment results to meet the patient's occupation needs. Skill in activity analysis is critical to determine the validity of the use of activities in OT assessment and treatment.

The type of activity analysis used will be determined, at least in part, by the individual therapist's or assistant's frame of reference (Crepeau, 1998). Such analysis will also be influenced by the use of particular techniques and variations in the use of equipment. While there is no universally accepted method of activity analysis, it is useful to consider the general categories of the *Occupational Therapy Practice Framework: Domain and Process* (AOTA, 2002). Other considerations should include factors such as the supplies and equipment needed, cost, the number of steps required for completion, time involved, supervision required, space needed, precautions, and contraindications. It is also helpful to think of functional requirements of the activity and then analyze them in terms of gradability. Functional requirements may be defined as components of an activity that require motor performance and behaviors for adequate completion. Gradability refers to a process whereby performance of an activity is viewed step by step on a continuum from simple to complex or slow to rapid (Holm, Rogers, & James, 1998).

The activity analysis yields the kind of data needed for determining therapeutic potential of a particular activity in relation to established patient goals, interests, and needs. Therapeutic potential is the degree of likelihood that therapeutic goals will be achieved. As specific techniques and equipment vary con-siderably for many activities, so will the results of an activity analysis. Once an activity is thoroughly analyzed, it can be adapted for therapeutic purposes.

HISTORICAL PERSPECTIVES

The profession of OT was founded on the notion that being engaged in activities promotes mental and physical well-being and, conversely, that the absence of activity leads to dysfunction (AOTA, 1980). Through their activities, human beings show their concern with how to survive, be comfortable, have pleasure, solve problems, express themselves, and relate to others. They come to know their strengths and they fulfill their roles in life. Thus the term *occupation*, as used in OT, is in the context of the individual's directed use of time, energy, interest, and attention (AOTA, 1980).

Activities being the foundation of the profession, historical definitions and other accounts place a strong emphasis on occupations or purposeful activities.

When William Tuke established the York Retreat in England in the late 1800s, employment in various occupations was a cornerstone of treatment in this facility for mental patients. Review of historical accounts of Tuke's work show that he had spent some time analyzing activities. For example, activities and occupations were selected to elicit emotions that were opposite of the condition; a melancholy patient would be given activities that had elements of excitement and were active, whereas a manic patient would be engaged in tasks of a sedentary nature. The habit of attention was a key element in using activities for treatment (Tuke, 1913).

Among the early pioneers of our profession, history records the work of Susan Tracy in relation to the process of analyzing activity. Tracy's work with mentally ill patients led her to believe that remedial activities "...are classified according to their physiological effects as stimulants, sedatives, anesthetics..." (Tracy, 1914). Over time, she analyzed the use of leather projects with patients and identified various components of a specific activity that would measure abilities in areas such as judgment, visual discrimination, spatial relationships, and making choices (Tracy, 1914). In 1918, she published a research paper, *Twenty-Five Suggested Mental Tests Derived From Invalid Occupations* (Tracy, 1918).

Eleanor Clarke Slagle's work in developing the principles of habit training certainly reflects her knowledge of activity analysis, as she placed particular emphasis on the gradation of activities and a balance among them (Slagle, 1922). The 1918 principles, established by the founders of our profession, also address aspects of activity that imply an ability to analyze the activity's properties. Emphasis was placed on the qualities of particular activities, with crafts and work-related activities being prominent; games, music, and physical exercise were also used (Dunton, 1918).

The terms *employment*, *labor*, *moral treatment*, *recreation*, *amusement*, *occupation*, *exercise*, and *diversion*, among others, have been used by different writers at various times to describe the forms of treatment used by OT personnel. The philosophy of the profession also places a strong emphasis on activities. Throughout our history, particular properties of activities were also addressed, giving strong roots to our basic belief in the activity analysis process. Activity properties are those characteristics of activities (e.g., being goal-directed, having significance to the individual, requiring involvement, gradability, adaptability) that contribute to their therapeutic potential.

Contemporary definitions of OT are summarized in the 1981 definition of the profession, developed for licensure purposes, which describes OT as the therapeutic use of self-care (ADL), work, and play/leisure activities to maximize independent function, enhance development, prevent disability, and maintain health. It may include adaptations of the task or the environment to achieve maximum independence and to enhance the quality of one's life (AOTA, 1981). Implicit in the latter statement is the ability to analyze activities. One must indeed know the particular properties and possibilities of a variety of activities to adapt the task to help the patient attain his or her goals. A related point, emphasized by Mosey (1986), is that activities used by OT personnel include both an intrinsic and a therapeutic purpose. This point is important to consider during activity analysis. Further, the reader should understand the OT process outlined by Moyers (1999).

ACTIVITY ENGAGEMENT PRINCIPLES

OT personnel must know various types of activities. Some of the categories of activities used in evaluation and treatment are the following:

- Crafts—Beading, ceramics, gifts
- Sensory awareness—Music, dance, hiking
- Movement awareness—Dance, drama
- Fine arts—Sculpting, painting, music
- Construction—Woodworking, electronics, computers
- Games—Bingo, checkers, parachute games
- Self-care—Dressing, feeding, hygiene
- IADL—Cooking, homemaking, community mobility
- Communication—Social activities, Internet
- Vocational—Collecting, reading

- Recreational—Sports, leisure interests
- Educational—Mathematics, writing, publishing

For activities to be considered purposeful and therapeutic, they must possess certain characteristics (Hopkins & Smith, 1983), which include the following:

- Be goal-directed.
- Have significance to the patient at some level.
- Require patient involvement at some level (mental, physical, or both).
- Be geared toward prevention of malfunction and/or maintenance or improvement of function and quality of life.
- Reflect patient involvement in life task situations (ADL, work, and play/leisure).
- Relate to the interests of the patient.
- Be adaptable and gradable.

The selection of appropriate activities for evaluation and treatment of patients must be based on sound professional judgment that is well grounded in knowledge and skill. As activity specialists, OTs and OTAs must have strong skills in this area (Punwar, 1994). A thorough knowledge of and experience in analyzing a wide variety of activities is an essential element of this process. The *Standards for an Accredited Educational Program for the OTA* states that analysis and adaptation of activities is a requirement for entry-level personnel (AOTA, 1998). Mosey (1986) stresses that purposeful activities cannot be designed for evaluation and intervention without analysis. Dunn (1989) states that if activities are to be the core of OT, they must be delineated, classified, and analyzed in terms of therapeutic value.

PURPOSE AND PROCESS OF ACTIVITY ANALYSIS

The purpose of activity analysis is to determine if the activity will be appropriate in meeting the treatment goals established for the patient. To analyze an activity with knowledge and skill, it is necessary to know how to perform the processes involved. It is also relevant to know the extent to which the activity fosters or impedes various types of human performance and interaction.

The patient must be receptive to the activity selected, in other words, it must be meaningful to the patient. Patients will be more motivated and participate if their interests, life tasks, and roles are considered. In addition, the patient's functional level should be considered. The individual may be interested in the activity and it may relate directly to his or her life tasks and roles, but due to performance deficits, it cannot be accomplished.

The process of analyzing an activity involves breaking it down to illustrate each step in detail that leads to the expected outcome. Consideration must be given to numerous factors that are used to achieve activity completion, as shown in examples later in this chapter.

An activity analysis can be helpful when determining the use of an activity for an evaluation or for treatment. When analyzing an activity intended for evaluative purposes, it must be broken down into separate components to determine what opportunities exist to objectively measure what is to be evaluated. For example, as Early (1993) points out, when the purpose of engagement in an activity is to measure decision-making skills, the activity selected must provide choices, as well as decision points, to allow it to be useful. She also stresses that OT personnel must know the exact responses and outcomes that might potentially occur and how they relate to the patient's ability to make decisions. An interpretation of observations of the individual's engagement in the activity (performance) would follow. When the activity is intended to be used for treatment, it again must be broken down into small units to determine which components (constituent parts) of the activity will help to achieve the treatment goals, such as to increase range of movement (ROM), to improve attention span, or to decrease isolative behavior.

The environment is also important to consider during analysis of an activity. Since many OTAs treat patients in their home, activity analysis in a home environment is likely to be more true and meaningful to the patient.

An accurate analysis of an activity allows OT personnel to select activities that will address the needs and goals of the patient therapeutically. This process also aids in determining the therapeutic potential of specific activities and their purposeful use. The absence of a thorough activity analysis is likely to prevent achievement of the best treatment results.

DEVELOPING SKILLS

Skill in activity analysis is critical to determine the validity of the use of activities in OT intervention programs. Prerequisite to achieving skill is the ability to understand the basic components of the activity (i.e., the fundamental processes, tools, and materials required for task completion). Self-analysis of a simple, frequently engaged in activity, such as bathing, is useful as an initial step. Asking questions, such as the following, is recommended:

- Why is the activity important to a person?
- What supplies and equipment are needed?
- What is the step-by-step procedure needed to complete this task?
- What other factors should be considered?

Once these questions have been answered, look at the information critically to determine if precise information was recorded. Recheck to be sure that no important factors were omitted. Ask a family member or peer to also answer these questions. In comparing results, differences in answers emphasize the uniqueness of the individual. Other questions can then be considered, such as how to adapt the activity for persons with various disabilities.

Experience in engaging in a wide variety of activities is also important in building skill, as it allows the OTA to make comparisons and formulate potential applications based on several possibilities. Practice in using several forms of activity analysis

and receiving objective feedback is also a way to develop skill. Once skill is achieved, the OTA can more easily select the most appropriate activity, that is of interest to the patient, relates to his or her life tasks and roles, is within the individual's functional capacity to perform, and provides opportunities for goal achievement (Trombly & Scott, 1995). Goal achievement is the accomplishment of tasks and objectives that one has set out to do.

RELATED CONSIDERATIONS

Frame of Reference

OT personnel use many approaches to analyze activities. The type of activity analysis is determined, at least in part, by the individual therapist's or assistant's frame of reference. For example, if a developmental frame of reference is used, activities are analyzed to determine the extent to which they might contribute to the age-specific development and related areas of occupational performance. If gratification of oral needs was a goal of treatment, it would be important to analyze the activity in terms of opportunities for eating, sucking, blowing, and encouraging independence, among other factors (Mosey, 1986).

Activity analysis is also influenced by the use of particular techniques and variations in the use of equipment recommended, such as in sensory integration and in the theoretical approaches of Rood, Bobath, or Brunnstrom. Additional information on theoretical frameworks and approaches may be found in Chapter 7.

Adaptation

To adapt an activity means to modify it (Early, 1993). It involves changing the components that are required to complete the task. Adaptations are made to allow the patient to experience success in task accomplishment at his or her level of functioning. For example, an individual who has had a stroke resulting in paralysis of one side of the body will need to use a holding device such as a lacing "pony" or a vice to stabilize a leather-lacing project. A change in positioning of the project, due to loss of peripheral vision and neglect of the involved side, is another important adaptation. Although few adaptations are required in this example, all of the components of the specific activity must be considered for potential changes to increase their therapeutic potential.

Grading

Grading of an activity refers to the process of performance being viewed step by step on a continuum that progresses from simple to complex. For example, a patient might begin by lacing 2 precut layers of leather together, using large prepunched holes and a simple whip stitch, to make a comb case. Once this is satisfactorily completed, additional challenges, such as the following, could be introduced over several treatment sessions:

- Use of saddle stitching, followed by single cordovan and double cordovan lacing, on other short-term leather projects.
- Use of simple stamping, followed by tooling and carving to decorate the project.
- Application of basic finishes, or more advanced techniques, such as antiquing and dyeing with several colors.

Activities may also be graded according to rate of time, varying from slow to rapid (e.g., a musician who wants to increase finger speed after hand surgery). An important concept is that the grading of activities builds on what has already been accomplished in progressive stages.

FORMS AND EXAMPLES

Although no universally accepted method of activity analysis exists, the following outline, checklist, and examples are provided to assist the reader in understanding the many diverse and complex factors inherent in the process of activity analysis. Study and use of these materials provides the OTA with opportunities to gain new skills or improve existing ones. Although every effort has been made to make these examples as complete as possible, other relevant aspects could undoubtedly be included. Some of the examples are formatted in such a way that they could be filled out and used as protocols for an OT clinic, thus ensuring that all personnel had information about a particular activity and its potential therapeutic uses. Those with limited experience in activity analysis should focus first on the general outline shown in Table 6-1. From time to time, unfamiliar terminology may be introduced. Definitions may be found by consulting a dictionary or reviewing the *Occupational Therapy Practice Framework* (AOTA, 2002).

An example of the narrative format of activity analysis shown in Table 6-1 is presented in Table 6-2. (Note: Each of the *Occupational Therapy Practice Framework* sections could easily be expanded with further justification of the practitioner's clinical thinking. The reader may want to further expand the format presented in the following figures.)

ACTIVITY ANALYSIS CHECKLIST

The Activity Analysis Checklist, shown in Table 6-3, is a faster method of determining the particular components of an activity, as it requires less writing than the narrative general activity analysis outline (see Table 6-1). The Activity Analysis

Checklist has a section to justify your thinking in a comment area. Students using the form for assignments may find it helpful to scan the form into a computer for future assignments. Table 6-4 shows the same form used to analyze the specific activity of brushing teeth.

SUMMARY

Activities are universal and historically have remained a primary foundation for the profession. Activity analysis is a deeply rooted concept, that has withstood the test of time and continues to be an important cornerstone for accurate assessment and effective intervention by OT personnel. The basic concepts and processes have been described to provide a fundamental understanding of the knowledge base and skills necessary for activity analysis. These skills include activity engagement principles, methods for developing skills, and concepts of grading and adapting activities. Forms and examples of the analysis of specific activities were also presented.

Emphasis was placed on the need for the activity analysis process and the information that may be gained through exploration of activity properties and possibilities. Skill in activity analysis is essential to determine the validity of the activities used for assessment and treatment. A thorough and accurate activity analysis allows the practitioner to select the most appropriate activity, which is of interest to the patient, relates to his or her life tasks and roles, and provides opportunities for goal achievement.

LEARNING ACTIVITIES

1. Discuss some of the reasons OT personnel use activity analysis.
2. Observe a person engaged in a work task. Identify the specific physical, cognitive, and social skills required.
3. List the general categories of information that should be a part of an activity analysis.
4. Working with a peer and using the format for brushing teeth (Table 6-4), complete an activity analysis for a dressing activity.
5. Using the format presented for brushing teeth (Table 6-4), complete an activity analysis for a cooking activity and a craft activity.

Table 6-1

General Outline to Structure an Activity Analysis in a Narrative Format

Name of activity:

Number of individuals involved:

Supplies and equipment: List all materials needed.

Procedure: List all steps required.

Cost: List costs and source for all materials. Separate consumable from nonconsumable.

Preparation: List any processes that need to be completed before the session.

Time: List time needed for each step in procedure, including set up and clean up.

Space needs or setting required: List space requirements including setting.

Activity qualities: To whom is this activity likely meaningful?

Occupation: What occupational roles would use this activity?

Supervision: List supervision requirements and degree.

Precautions: List safety issues.

Contraindications: List issues that indicate a person should not do this activity because it would be harmful.

Motor skills: Use the *Practice Framework* to consider sensory awareness, processing, neuromusculoskeletal, and motor issues.

Process skills: Use the *Practice Framework* to consider integrative and cognitive skills.

Communication/interaction skills: Use the *Practice Framework* to consider psychosocial and psychological skills.

ADL/IADL performance areas: How can this activity assist in ADL?

Work/education performance areas: How can this activity assist in work-type activities?

Leisure/play/social participation performance areas: How can this activity assist in leisure/play/social participation?

Adaptation: List the ways in which this activity can be made easier.

Grading: List the ways in which this activity can be made more challenging.

Disabilities: List the disabilities for which this activity could be recommended.

Goal: Write a primary goal that involves this activity.

Habits: How does this routine influence this?

Environmental aspects: Describe how physical, social, spiritual, temporal, virtual, personal, and cultural status influence this activity.

Other issues:

Adapted from American Occupational Therapy Association. (2002). The occupational therapy practice framework: Domain and process. *American Journal of Occupational Therapy, 56,* 609-633.

Table 6-2

An Example of a Narrative Format Activity Analysis

Name of activity: Volleyball.

Number of individuals involved: 8 to 15.

Supplies and equipment: Volleyball, net, poles, score pad, and pen. Optional: Refreshments and prizes.

Procedure: Stand in designated space. Reach (shoulder flexed, elbow extended, forearm supinated, wrist in neutral, fingers flexed) to hit the ball over the net when it approaches you. Move side to side and front to back within your designated space to hit the ball. Rotate to the space on your right after score is made. Optional: Start a new game after the established score is reached.

(continued)

Table 6-2

An Example of a Narrative Format Activity Analysis (continued)

Cost: None if equipment is available; otherwise about $60 (see Supplies and equipment).

Preparation: 5 to 10 minutes to obtain equipment and set up.

Time: 1 hour, 5 minutes—5 minutes to set up equipment, 5 minutes to instruct group (process, rules, scoring), 45 minutes for actual activity participation, and 10 minutes to clean up, pack, and store equipment.

Space needs or setting required: Outdoor area or large room free of obstacles and furnishings.

Activity qualities: Teens and young adults may find this meaningful. High potential for noise due to excitement and competitive behavior.

Occupation: Leisure interests such as exerciser. Social interests such as peer supporter.

Supervision: Direct to ensure proper follow-through and safety.

Precautions: Participants with low tolerance may need frequent breaks; participants with short attention span or memory deficits may need frequent cueing. Aggressive players may need limit setting. Thoroughly instruct in proper serving and other motions required to reduce potential for injury.

Contraindications: Avoid use with individuals with serious cardiopulmonary and respiratory problems. Not appropriate for the very young or those having pronounced perceptual and motor deficits.

Motor skills: Sensory awareness required. Sensory processing including tactile, proprioceptive, vestibular, visual, and auditory. Perceptual processing needed includes kinesthesia, pain response, body scheme, right-left discrimination, position in space, figure ground, depth perception, and spatial relations. Neuromuscular needs include reflex, range of motion, muscle tone, strength, and endurance. In addition, postural control and alignment are needed. Motor needs are gross, crossing the midline, laterality, bilateral integration, praxis, and visual-motor integration.

Process skills: Attention span, initiation, termination, memory for rules, sequencing, problem solving, and learning (if new to game).

Communication/interaction skills: Interests, self-concept, role performance, social contact, interpersonal skills, self-expression, coping skills, and self-control are needed.

ADL/IADL performance areas: Gross motor skills of volleyball can be helpful in dressing and functional mobility.

Work/education performance areas: If teen, volleyball may be helpful in physical education classes in school. If adult, volleyball has rules and structure helpful to adults working in gross motor jobs such as assembly line work of large items.

Leisure/play/social participation performance areas: Volleyball is an activity that can be continued as a leisure pursuit in most communities through local recreation programs.

Adaptation: Potential for adaptation or modification is very good. May use a foam ball, balloon, punching balloon, or a beach ball. May be played while seated. Instead of a net, 2 people can hold up a piece of crepe paper. Playing for points and rotations may be omitted (also see Grading). Use more people on one or both teams to reduce the area covered. Decrease emphasis on time; allow game to proceed as tolerated; add breaks.

Grading: Decrease time allocated and encourage increased participation. Decrease the number of people on the floor at any given time. Have players add wrist weights to hands or ankles.

Disabilities: People with gross motor issues that can tolerate resistive weight from hitting the ball. Teens with sensory integrative issues or conduct disorders. Adults with mental health issues such as schizophrenia or depression.

Goal: Within one OT treatment session, the patient will raise her hands over her head and hit a balloon 50% of the time the balloon is sent to her from the opposite team.

(continued)

Table 6-2

An Example of a Narrative Format Activity Analysis (continued)

Habits: Volleyball is typically a game played by teens and young adults; however, the game can be adapted for chronological, developmental, life cycle, and disability status issues.

Environmental aspects: Volleyball is typically played outdoors or in a large gym area. The game can be adapted to smaller rooms with chairs and balloons. The social aspects can be increased by having players call out names or socialize at each step of the game. Cultural aspects would have to be addressed on an individual basis as some cultures may not encourage people playing games.

Other issues: Prizes may be awarded for best serve, most points scored by a single person, good sportsmanship, etc.

Table 6-3

Activity Analysis Checklist

Name of activity:

Check the appropriate box

Skills and Subskills of Motor, Process, and Communication:	None	Min.	Mod.	Max.	Clinical thinking comment
Sensory awareness					
Tactile/touching					
Proprioceptive					
Vestibular					
Visual/seeing					
Auditory/hearing					
Gustatory/tasting					
Olfactory/smelling					
Voice and speech					
Stereognosis					
Kinesthesia					
Pain response					
R-L discrimination					
Form constancy					
Position in space					
Topographical orientation					
Reflex					
Range of motion					
Muscle tone					
Strength					
Endurance					
Postural control					
Postural alignment					
Soft tissue integrity					
Gross coordination					
Crossing the midline					
Laterality					
Bilateral integration					
Motor control					
Praxis					
Fine coordination/dexterity					
Visual-motor integration					
Oral-motor control					
Level of consciousness					
Orientation					
Recognition					

(continued)

Table 6-3

Activity Analysis Checklist (continued)

	None	Min.	Mod.	Max.	Clinical thinking comment
Attention span					
Initiation of activity					
Termination of activity					
Memory					
Sequencing					
Categorization					
Concept formation					
Spatial operations					
Problem solving					
Learning					
Generalization					
Values					
Interests					
Self-concept					
Role performance					
Social conduct					
Interpersonal skills					
Self-expression					
Coping skills					
Time management					
Self-control					
Habits and routines					
Cultural context					
Physical context					
Social context					
Spiritual context					
Personal context					
Temporal context					
Virtual context					
Bathing/showering					
Bowel/bladder management					
Dressing					
Eating					
Functional mobility					
Personal device care					
Personal hygiene					
Sexual expression					
Sleep/rest					
Toilet hygiene					
Care of others/pets					
Child rearing					
Communication device					
Community mobility					
Financial management					
Health management					
Home management					
Meal management					
Safety and emergencies					
Shopping					
Formal educational involvement					
Informal educational needs					
Informal educational involvement					

(continued)

Table 6-3

Activity Analysis Checklist (continued)

	None	Min.	Mod.	Max.	Clinical thinking comment
Work interests					
Employment seeking					
Job performance					
Retirement planning					
Volunteer experiences					
Play/leisure exploration					
Play/leisure performance					
Social in community					
Social in family					
Social in peers					
Narrative information of activity:					

This activity form is adapted from several sources including American Occupational Therapy Association. (2002). The occupational therapy practice framework: Domain and process. *American Journal of Occupational Therapy, 56,* 609-633; Jacobs, K., & Jacobs, L. (2004). *Quick Reference Dictionary for Occupational Therapy* (4th ed.). Thorofare, NJ: SLACK Incorporated; and Ryan, S. E., & Sladyk, K. (2001). *Ryan's Occupational Therapy Assistant: Principles, Practice Issues, and Techniques* (3rd ed.). Thorofare, NJ: SLACK Incorporated.

Table 6-4

Sample Activity Analysis Checklist

Activity: Brushing your teeth

Check the appropriate box:

Skills and Subskills of Motor, Process, and Communication:	None	Min.	Mod.	Max.	Clinical thinking comment
Sensory awareness			X		Receive sensory info
Tactile/touching			X		Feel brush in hand
Proprioceptive			X		Be aware of movement
Vestibular		X			Less impact unless dizzy
Visual/seeing			X		See sink, brush, water
Auditory/hearing	X				Less impact
Gustatory/tasting			X		Taste of toothpaste
Olfactory/smelling		X			Less impact unless smell
Voice and speech	X				Not required
Stereognosis			X		Find brush not comb/razor
Kinesthesia		X			Movement of brushing
Pain response	X				Not unless brush slips
R-L discrimination	X				Not required
Form constancy			X		Distractions might affect
Position in space				X	Relationship of body to sink
Topographical orientation	X				Possible surface issues
Reflex	X				Only if water hot/cold
Range of motion			X		For brushing movement
Muscle tone			X		For brushing movement
Strength			X		For brushing movement/cap
Endurance			X		For brushing movement
Postural control			X		To stand at sink
Postural alignment			X		Balance to stand/sit
Soft tissue integrity		X			If mouth/hands have sores
Gross coordination		X			More fine motor
Crossing the midline				X	Get both sides of teeth
Laterality			X		Can be done 1 handed
Bilateral integration			X		Opening toothpaste
					(continued)

Table 6-4

Sample Activity Analysis Checklist (continued)

	None	Min.	Mod.	Max.	Clinical thinking comment
Motor control			X		Control toothpaste
Praxis				X	Motor plan to mouth
Fine coordination/dexterity			X		Manage supplies, brushing
Visual-motor integration				X	Put paste on brush
Oral-motor control				X	Brush, rinse
Level of consciousness				X	Must be alert
Orientation	X				Not required
Recognition			X		Of supplies
Attention span			X		At least 3 to 5 minutes
Initiation of activity			X		To begin brushing
Termination of activity			X		To end brushing/rinse
Memory			X		Remember steps/all teeth
Sequencing			X		Order of steps
Categorization	X				Not required
Concept formation	X				Not required
Spatial operations	X				Not required
Problem solving			X		If drop cap/paste/brush
Learning		X			Likely learned early
Generalization		X			To other activities/eat
Values		X			All the psychosocial sub-skills
Interests		X			include some level of motiva
Self-concept		X			tion for the person to be
Role performance		X			interested in brushing their
Social conduct		X			teeth. In addition, clean teeth/
Interpersonal skills		X			breath is often related to social
Self-expression			X		and employment situations
Coping skills		X			
Time management			X		
Self-control		X			
Habits and routines				X	Healthy habit
Cultural context			X		May or may not be valued
Physical context				X	Healthy task
Social context				X	May affect social skills
Spiritual context	X				Not required
Personal context			X		May relate to self-image
Temporal context			X		May relate to self-image
Virtual context	X				Not required
Bathing/showering				X	Importance of grooming
Bowel/bladder management	X				Not required
Dressing				X	May be routine
Eating				X	Similar skills
Functional mobility			X		Get to bathroom
Personal device care			X		If dentures/retainer
Personal hygiene			X		Importance of grooming
Sexual expression			X		Important in relationship
Sleep/rest			X		Part of sleep prep
Toilet hygiene	X				Not required
Care of others/pets		X			Important in relationship
Child rearing				X	Model/care for kids teeth
Communication device	X				Not required
Community mobility		X			To buy supplies
Financial management		X			To buy supplies

(continued)

Table 6-4

Sample Activity Analysis Checklist (continued)

	None	Min.	Mod.	Max.	Clinical thinking comment
Health management				X	Prevent tooth/gum decay
Home management	X				Not required
Meal management	X				Not required
Safety and emergencies	X				Not required
Shopping			X		To buy supplies
Formal educational involvement			X		Fresh breath and clean teeth will affect all areas of education, work, and leisure as this typically involves other people who will not want to be with the client who does not address personal hygiene. Fresh breath and teeth is especially important in social situations in the community, family, and peers.
Informal educational needs			X		
Informal educational involvement			X		
Work interests	X				
Employment seeking			X		
Job performance			X		
Retirement planning	X				
Volunteer experiences			X		
Play/leisure exploration			X		
Play/leisure performance			X		
Social in community			X		
Social in family			X		
Social in peers			X		

Narrative information of activity: Supplies: Toothpaste, toothbrush, water, sink. Procedure: Open toothpaste, squeeze toothpaste, close toothpaste, open water, brush all teeth, rinse mouth, rinse brush/sink, close water. Generally the task can be completed in 5 minutes and for under $5, not including sink. This activity is likely meaningful to most people and often a prerequisite to many occupational roles such as spouse, worker, peer. Precautions: skin may be burned with hot water, child may gag on brush, paste may be too minty hot for sensitive mouth. Contraindications: severe oral problems. Adaptation for ease: Limited distractions, use of mirror, verbal cueing, adaptive equipment. Gradation for challenge can include finding supplies in medicine cabinet, making choices on supplies, using weights on wrists.

REFERENCES

American Occupational Therapy Association. (1980). *Reference manual of official documents of the AOTA.* Rockville, MD: Author.

American Occupational Therapy Association. (1981). Resolution Q: Definition of OT for licensure. Minutes of the 1981 AOTA Representative Assembly. *American Journal of Occupational Therapy, 35,* 798-799.

American Occupational Therapy Association. (1998). *Standards for an accredited educational program for the OTA.* Bethesda, MD: Author.

American Occupational Therapy Association. (2002). Occupational therapy practice framework: Domain and process. *American Journal of Occupational Therapy, 56,* 609-633.

Crepeau, E. B. (1998). Activity analysis: A way of thinking about occupational performance. In M. E. Neistadt & E. B. Crepeau (Eds.), *Willard & Spackman's OT.* Philadelphia, PA: Lippincott.

Dunn, W. (1989). Application of uniform terminology in practice. *American Journal of Occupational Therapy, 43,* 817-831.

Dunton, W. R. (1918). The principles of OT. In *Proceedings of the National Society for the Promotion of OT, second annual meeting.* Catonsville, MD: Spring Grove State Hospital Press.

Early, M. B. (1993). *Mental health concepts and techniques for the OTA.* New York, NY: Raven Press.

Holm, M. B., Rogers, J. C., & James, A. B. (1998). Treatment of occupational performance areas. In M. E. Neistadt & E. B. Crepeau (Eds.), *Willard & Spackman's OT.* Philadelphia, PA: Lippincott.

Hopkins, H. D., & Smith, H. L. (Eds.). (1983). *Willard & Spackman's OT* (6th ed.). Philadelphia, PA: Lippincott.

Mosey, A. C. (1986). *Psychosocial components of OT.* New York, NY: Raven Press.

Moyers, P. (1999). *Guide to occupational therapy practice.* Bethesda, MD: AOTA.

Punwar, A. J. (1994). *OT principles and practice*. Baltimore, MD: Williams & Wilkins.

Slagle, E. C. (1922). Training aides for mental patients. *Archives of OT, 1*, 13-14.

Tracy, S. E. (1914). The place of invalid occupations in the general hospital. *Modern Hospital, 2*(5), 386.

Tracy, S. E. (1918). Twenty-five suggested mental tests derived from invalid occupations. *Maryland Psychiatric Quarterly, 8*, 15-16.

Trombly, C., & Scott, A. D. (1995). *OT for physical dysfunction*. Baltimore, MD: Williams & Wilkins.

Tuke, S. (1913). *A description of the retreat: An institution near York for insane persons of the Society of Friends*. London, England: Dawson of Pall Mall.

Key Concepts

- Theory: A set of phenomena and relationships.
- Frame of reference: Guideline of practice based on theory.
- Model: Theoretical concepts used to guide practice in a specific arena.

Essential Vocabulary

what's functional?
what's not functional?

regarding change + intervention
states factors

function/dysfunction continua: The deficits addressed by the frame of reference.
indicators of function/dysfunction: Guidelines for identification of deficits through evaluation.
postulates regarding change: Guidelines for intervention.
theoretical base: The theoretical assumptions used as a foundation for the frame of reference.

THEORY THAT GUIDES PRACTICE: OUR MAP

Diane K. Dirette, PhD, OT

INTRODUCTION

Definitions

The terms explored in this chapter include *theory*, *frame of reference*, and *model*. A simplified definition of a theory is a description of a set of phenomena and the relationships among the concepts in those phenomena (Mosey, 1996). A frame of reference is a guideline for practice that provides direction for evaluation and treatment of particular deficits in the occupational therapy domain of concern. A frame of reference is not written to address a particular diagnosis such as spinal cord injury, but is designed to address deficits that may occur in a variety of diagnoses. Frames of reference link theoretical concepts to intervention.

The parts of a frame of reference include the theoretical base, the function/dysfunction continua, the indicators of function/dysfunction, and the postulates regarding change (Mosey, 1996). The theoretical base is the concept drawn from various theories that support the use of the guidelines. The function/dysfunction continua are the deficits addressed by the frame of reference. The indicators of function/dysfunction guide the therapist in the evaluation phase of the intervention. The postulates regarding change guide the intervention used to ameliorate the deficits.

Theories are used as the foundation for developing frames of reference. The theoretical foundation of occupational therapy comes from the biological sciences (such as anatomy and physiology), psychology, sociology, and medicine. For example, the biomechanical frame of reference discussed later in this chapter is based on anatomy, physiology, and kinesiology.

The Use of Frames of Reference in Occupational Therapy

The following discussion of frames of reference is separated into different practice areas. However, many individuals with whom the occupational therapists work will have deficits in many areas. For example, a person with a cerebrovascular accident (CVA) may have deficits in physical function, which leads the therapist to use the rehabilitation or NDT frame of reference. That same person may have deficits in social role functioning, which could lead the therapist to also use the role acquisition frame of reference. If the theoretical concepts of the frame of reference are not in conflict with one another, the frames of reference may be used in combination for a thorough treatment plan to address client factors, areas of occupational performance, performance patterns, performance skills, and/or the context in which the occupation is performed.

If the theoretical concepts are not compatible, the therapist would not be using these frames of reference simultaneously in intervention with the person. For example, the theoretical base of the psychodynamic frame of reference focuses on exploring underlying issues that lead to behaviors. The behavioral frame of reference is based on the concepts that address only outward behaviors without the need for exploration of underlying processes. Therefore, these frames of reference would not be used simultaneously when treating one individual.

The choice of frame of reference may also be determined by the setting in which the treatment occurs. According to Bruce and Borg (2002), the psychodynamic frame of reference is more likely to be used in a medical model setting. The approach may be determined by the psychologist, neuropsychologist, physician, or team that is treating the individual. The need for consistency of treatment may determine the frame of reference used. In addition, the time allowed to conduct the intervention may determine which frame of reference may be used. For example, when treating a client in the acute care setting, the occupational therapist may be limited to using a frame of reference that does not require long-term intervention, such as the rehabilitation frame of reference.

FRAMES OF REFERENCE FOR PHYSICAL FUNCTION

Biomechanical

Originated by Bolderin, Taylor, and Licht. Adapted from Dutton (1995).

Theoretical Basis

Anatomy, physiology, and kinesiology.

Theoretical Assumptions

1. Purposeful activity can be prescribed to remediate loss of ROM, strength, and endurance.
2. If ROM, strength, and endurance are regained, the person will automatically use these prerequisite skills to regain functional skills.
3. The body must be rested, then stressed.
4. The person must have an intact brain that can produce isolated, coordinated movements.

Function/Dysfunction Continua

Structural stability, endurance, edema, ROM, and strength.

Indicators of Function and Dysfunction

1. Structural stability (measured by observation of positioning and control).
2. Passive ROM (PROM) and active ROM (AROM) (measured by observation and goniometry).
3. Muscle strength (measured by manual muscle testing).
4. Peripheral edema (measured by observation, volumetry, and circumferential measures).
5. Endurance (measured by observation of the duration and/or intensity of activities performed).

Postulates Regarding Change

1. If the therapist uses orthoses and positioning, structural damage will be prevented.
2. If the therapist uses orthoses, positioning, and rest followed by stress, structural stability will be regained.
3. If the therapist prescribes increased duration and/or intensity of activities, then endurance will be gained.
4. If the therapist uses elevation, pressure, temperature control, and ROM, then peripheral edema will be reduced.
5. If the therapist uses PROM, active assisted ROM, AROM, scar prevention, orthoses, and positioning, then passive ROM will be maintained.

6. If the therapist uses heat, scar remodeling, passive stretch, active stretch, orthoses, positioning, and activities, then ROM will be increased.
7. If the therapist uses AROM and activities, then strength will be maintained.
8. If the therapist uses isometric, active assistive, active, and progressive or regressive resistive exercises, then strength will be increased.

Neurodevelopmental Treatment

Originated by Berta and Karl Bobath. Adapted from Dutton (1995).

Theoretical Basis

Neurology and developmental theories.

Theoretical Assumptions

1. It is important to remediate foundation skills that make normal skill acquisition possible.
2. Normal movement is learned by experiencing what normal movement feels like.
3. Postural control is essential for limb movement.
4. Normal movement cannot be imposed on abnormal muscle tone.
5. The brain has plasticity.

Function/Dysfunction Continua

1. Axial control (control of neck and trunk).
2. Automatic reactions (righting reactions, equilibrium reactions, protective limb extensions).
3. Limb control with specific focus on the scapula and pelvic mobility and stability.

Indicators of Function and Dysfunction

1. Reflex development (evaluated through observation).
2. Automatic reactions (evaluated using observation of the quality of movement).
3. Synergies (evaluated using clinical observation of positioning and movement patterns).
4. Muscle tone (evaluated using manual and visual observation of resistance to passive and active movements).

Postulates Regarding Change

1. If the therapist uses passive elongation, reflex inhibiting patterns, positioning, and weight shifts, then hypertonia can be inhibited.
2. If the therapist uses joint compression, joint traction, manual resistance, and weight shifts, then increased tone for hypotonia can be facilitated.
3. If the therapist uses passive elongation, active weight shifts, passive pelvic tilts, and active axial rotation, then axial control can be facilitated.
4. If the therapist uses reflex inhibiting patterns and desired combinations of movement patterns, then automatic reactions can be facilitated.

5. If the therapist uses dissociation of synergy patterns, reflex inhibiting patterns, limb weight shifts, place and hold, and postures and movements with rotational and reciprocal limb movements, then limb control can be facilitated.

Rehabilitation Frame of Reference

Originated by Dunton. Adapted from Dutton (1995).

Theoretical Basis

Systems theories and learning theories.

Theoretical Assumptions

1. A person can regain independence using compensation when underlying deficits cannot be remediated.
2. Motivation for independence cannot be separated from volitional and habitual subsystems.
3. Motivation for independence cannot be separated from environmental contexts.
4. A minimum level of emotional and cognitive prerequisite skill must be present to make independence possible.
5. Clinical reasoning should take a top down approach. Focus should first be on environmental demands and resources. Then, volitional and habitual subsystems should be considered followed by functional capabilities and then prerequisite skills/deficits.

Function/Dysfunction Continua

This frame of reference addresses ADL, work, and leisure activities.

Indicators of Function and Dysfunction

1. Ability to safely perform ADL in a timely manner.
2. Ability to safely perform home management tasks in a timely manner.
3. Work behaviors, work tolerance, general work traits, and/or specific work skills.
4. Ability to participate in meaningful leisure activities.

Clinical observations and interviews are used to evaluate these areas of occupational performance.

Postulates Regarding Change

1. If the therapist uses adaptive devices, orthotics, environmental modifications, wheelchair modifications, ambulatory aids, adapted procedures, and/or safety education, then independence in ADL, home management, work, and leisure will be maximized.

Proprioceptive Neuromuscular Facilitation

Originated by Kabat. Adapted from Voss, Ionta, and Myers (1985).

Theoretical Basis

Neurophysiology, anatomy, and kinesiology.

Theoretical Assumptions

1. Normal movement and posture are dependent upon a balanced interaction of antagonists.
2. The growth of motor behavior has cyclic trends as evidenced by shifts between flexor and extensor dominance.
3. Early motor behavior is dominated by reflex activity. Mature motor behavior is reinforced or supported by postural reflex mechanisms.
4. Normal motor development proceeds in a cephalocaudal and proximodistal direction.
5. Developing motor behavior is expressed in an orderly sequence of total patterns of movement and posture.
6. Normal motor behavior has an orderly quality with overlapping occurring.
7. Improvement of motor ability is dependent on motor learning.

Function/Dysfunction Continua

This frame of reference addresses movement patterns and postures.

Indicators of Function and Dysfunction

Smooth, controlled functional movement patterns of the head, neck, trunk, and extremities.

Postulates Regarding Change

1. If the therapist prevents or corrects imbalances between antagonists, then normal movement and posture are possible.
2. If the therapist assists the person through reversing movements, then there is interaction of the antagonists.
3. If the therapist uses reflex support, then voluntary movements are reinforced.
4. If the therapist has the person perform movement patterns in diagonal and spiral as well as forward, backward, sideward, and circular directions, then total patterns of movement and posture are achieved.
5. If the therapist uses appropriate sensory cues and demands, then learning of motor acts is enhanced.

FRAMES OF REFERENCE FOR PSYCHOSOCIAL FUNCTION

Role Acquisition

Originated by Anne C. Mosey. Adapted from Mosey (1986).

Theoretical Basis

Sociology, psychology, and behavioral learning theories.

Theoretical Assumptions

1. The individual has an inherent need to explore the environment.

2. What an individual must learn (roles) is specified by the society and cultural group in which he or she lives.

3. Learning basic skills, social roles, and temporal adaptation includes a socialization process and a learning process.

4. In the typical developmental process, the individual interacts in an environment where he or she is relatively free to explore and to acquire interests, goals, and competencies. Atypical development occurs when the environment is not conducive to learning, either in the past or at the present time.

5. Emphasis should be placed on purposeful activities, including both individual and group activities.

Function/Dysfunction Continua

The areas of concern can be viewed as hierarchical in nature, with task skills and interpersonal skills forming the base; family interactions, ADL, school/work, and play/leisure/recreation forming the middle; and temporal adaptation making up the top portion of the pyramid.

Indicators of Function and Dysfunction

1. Adequate participation in the physical, cognitive, and psychological aspects of tasks. Evaluation of task skills is usually accomplished through data gathered from a general interview and the Survey of Task Skills.

2. Initiation and participation in interpersonal interactions. Evaluation of interpersonal skills is typically accomplished through use of an interview, an evaluation group, and the Interpersonal Skill Survey.

3. Adequate family interactions, including the child role, the adolescent role, the parent role, and general family interactions. Evaluation tools include observation and general interview.

4. Participation in ADL. Evaluation includes observation and the Activities of Daily Living Survey.

5. Adequate participation in school or work roles. Evaluation is accomplished through interview, observation, and the School Survey or Work Survey.

6. Appropriate play/leisure/recreation participation. Evaluation includes interview, observation, and the Leisure/Recreation Survey.

7. Temporal adaptation for adequate participation in ADL and roles. Evaluation is accomplished through a general interview and the Activity Configuration.

Postulates Regarding Change

1. Long-term goals are set based on the client's expected environment.

2. The sequence of the change process is generally task skills, interpersonal skills, social roles beginning with ADL, and temporal adaptation.

3. The sequence, however, need not be rigidly adhered to and is often best determined by the client.

4. Task and interpersonal skills can be taught separately initially or they can be taught within the context of the learning of social roles.

5. An adequate repertoire of behavior is acquired through selected application of the principles of learning during activities that a) elicit the relevant behavior, b) are interesting to the client and allow for exploration and movement toward mastery, and c) include socialization.

6. Emphasis is on designing activities that will change the behavior and thus alleviate the problem rather than delving into intrapsychic reasons for the problem.

7. The therapist must know very specifically what kind of behavior he or she wishes to promote or enhance and can thus be accomplished through activity analysis and synthesis.

The Behavioral Frame of Reference

Adapted from Bruce and Borg (1993, 2002).

Theoretical Basis

The behavioral frame of reference is based on concepts drawn from experimental psychology, classical conditioning (Pavlov), operant conditioning (Skinner), and social learning theories (such as Bandura, Mischel, and Rotter).

Theoretical Assumptions

1. A person's behavior is predictable, measurable, and objective.

2. A person's verbalization and self-descriptions are behaviors.

3. The patient has a repertoire of behaviors (adaptive and maladaptive) that have been learned through selective reinforcement from the environment.

4. The patient's repertoire of behavior determines his or her ability to function in ADL, work, and leisure.

5. Through positive and differential reinforcement and the systematic application of learning techniques, the patient can learn to modify and control his or her behavior.

6. Only behavior that is demonstrated can be reinforced.

7. New behavior may be established through the use of continuous or frequent and predictable reinforcement; however, the most stable behavior is that maintained by intermittent reinforcement.

8. If maladaptive behavior is only occasionally reinforced, it is strengthened.

9. The strength of the patient's response is influenced by bodily conditions such as those related to emotions, drives, and the use of drugs.

10. The skills for adaptive functioning in the natural environment are independent and nonstage specific.

11. The environment gives positive or negative reinforcement of a person's behavior.

Function/Dysfunction Continua

The focus of this frame of reference is on the behaviors that elicit or inhibit functioning in the areas of ADL, work, and play/leisure. There is an emphasis on the stimuli that act as cues to the behavior and the reinforcers for specific behaviors.

Indicators of Function and Dysfunction

1. Age appropriate, culturally acceptable behaviors that contribute to or interfere with adaptive function.
2. Behaviors necessary for adequate function in the person's natural environment.
3. The frequency of specific adaptive and maladaptive behavior.
4. The ability of the person to discriminate among stimuli and to generalize learning effectively.

Evaluation is completed through a combination of observation and rating of task performance and interview using questionnaires or behavior checklists. Some examples of assessment tools include the Kohlman Evaluation of Living Skills, the Bay Area Functional Performance Evaluation, the Comprehensive Occupational Therapy Evaluation, Scorable Self-Care Evaluation, the Milwaukee Evaluation of Daily Living Skills, behavioral self-inventory, and behavioral database.

Postulates Regarding Change

1. If the therapist uses pleasurable activities, then adaptive behaviors are reinforced.
2. If the therapist uses negative reinforcement or ignoring of maladaptive behaviors, then those behaviors are decreased.
3. If the therapist grades activities to provide progressively more difficult learning challenges, then adaptive behaviors needed to function in the community environment are shaped.
4. If the therapist uses activity and occupation, then the client can learn new skills or refine present skills for occupational function.
5. If the therapist uses shaping, forward and backward chaining, scheduled reinforcement, modeling, and token economies, then adaptive behavior will be reinforced and learned.
6. If the therapist uses direct care, education and/or counseling, the client will increase his or her ability to transfer the behaviors learned during intervention to a broad range of environments and life situations.
7. If the therapist uses multiple settings and contexts, transfer of behavior will be enhanced.
8. If the therapist uses clear, concrete goals, then the client's understanding of the purpose of intervention and the achievement of occupational performance will be increased.
9. If the therapist uses clear, specific goals, then the intervention process will be expedited and the evaluation of the occupational performance outcome will be facilitated.
10. If the therapist uses intermittent and unpredictable reinforcement, then behaviors will be maintained and stable.
11. If the therapist uses modeling of desired behaviors, then the behavior is imitated and learned.
12. If the therapist provides a verbal label for behaviors, then that behavior is more successfully remembered and imitated.

The Psychodynamic Frame of Reference

Previously referred to as the Object Relations Frame of Reference. Adapted from Bruce and Borg (1993, 2002).

Theoretical Basis

The basis is an eclectic integration of principles from Freud, Jung, Hartmann, White, Rogers, Maslow, and Goldstein (Freudian, Jungian, neo-Freudian, existential-humanistic, and social and ego psychologies).

Theoretical Assumptions

1. A person is a valuable, unique individual.
2. The person is the expert on his or her life, including his or her feelings, emotions, and what he or she needs to change in order to function more successfully in the environment.
3. The person is capable of developing increased understanding of self and others, cause and effect and to learn from experience in a process referred to as insight.
4. Each person has an internal drive to love and be loved, to use unique skills, and to feel that life has meaning.
5. Human behavior is influenced by what is conscious and by what is not conscious in the individual.
6. Increased self-awareness contributes to one's ability to make satisfying choices.
7. The person who is more self-accepting and has less need to keep secrets from personal awareness has more energy to put toward establishing an abundance of satisfying object relationships.
8. The person has an innate tendency to restore internal equilibrium.
9. An individual needs to feel both physically and emotionally safe in order to be open to new perceptions and to make changes.
10. A person's most pressing needs will naturally emerge and need to be dealt with first.
11. Activities and objects have no meaning in and of themselves—people give them meaning.

Function/Dysfunction Continua

The focus of this frame of reference is on the inner workings of the human psyche. The concepts addressed include:

1. Self-awareness, self-identity, self-actualization, and adaptation to the real world.
2. Motivation for participation in meaningful occupations.
3. Use of defense mechanisms.
4. Engagement with human and nonhuman objects.
5. Self-control of impulses.
6. Social and occupational skills.
7. Responsibility for one's own actions.
8. Behavior that is consistent with personal values.
9. Ability to establish mature relationships.
10. Respect for the rights and boundaries of others.

Indicators of Function and Dysfunction

Function is indicated by:

1. The ability to make realistic assessments about what is going on in the environment.
2. Adaptation to environmental expectations, which include exerting self-control and deferring gratification.
3. Use of intellect, insight, and judgment to solve problems and satisfy personal needs in a socially acceptable way.
4. Has an accurate self-image and body image, including knowledge of one's strengths and limitations.
5. Has self-awareness and can alter self-image according to real information.
6. Uses skills/talents to meet needs in a manner that respects the rights of others.
7. Takes responsibility for his or her own behavior and occupational choices.
8. In pursuit of spiritual health, the person participates in activities that are meaningful to him or her and feels that he or she has a quality of life.

Dysfunction is indicated by:

1. The person views him- or herself or situations outside of the self in ways that are very different from how others see these.
2. The person is unaware of feelings that are shaping decisions.
3. He or she is not developing talents or skills or is making choices that are not in accordance with personal values.
4. The person is unable to function satisfactorily and meaningfully in either activities or daily life, in pursuit of personal interests, at work, and/or in social relationships.
5. Loss of self-motivation, feelings of helplessness, hopelessness, and/or anxiety.

Tools for evaluation include projective and expressive assessments such as the Azima Battery, the Shoemyen Battery, the Goodman Battery, the Lerner Magazine Picture Collage, the Barb Hemphill (BH) Battery, the Ehrenberg Comprehensive Assessment, human figure drawing, and Build A City.

Postulates Regarding Change

According to Bruce and Borg (1993), the intervention process occurs in individual and group situations with clients who are reality oriented and capable of logical thinking. To facilitate a dynamic understanding of behavior and problems, the occupational therapist uses creative media or semistructured experiences to help the patient project his or her thoughts, feelings, needs, fantasies, desires, and frustrations onto the end product (i.e., activity). The therapist uses activities and the discussions around him or her for one or more of the following:

1. To provide an avenue for self-exploration and for appropriate expression of feeling.
2. To provide an opportunity to improve ego function.
3. To provide a means to establish or re-establish a sense of self and control.
4. To provide a vehicle for learning new skills, improving skills, or gaining confidence in skills already held.
5. To provide an opportunity for trying out new roles or gaining confidence with already established roles.
6. To provide a vehicle for learning more about one's self, one's relationship to others, and what one needs to function optimally.
7. To provide a means toward increased self-acceptance with recognition, expression, and acceptance of one's thoughts and feelings.
8. To facilitate movement toward flexibility in approaching life tasks.
9. To enhance performance ability, including taking responsibility for one's own life, exhibiting improved functional problem solving, and being able to adapt to one's own circumstances.
10. To improve social skills, including communication skills and being able to cooperate with others in task performance.
11. To increase impulse control.
12. To connect to and find meaning in the world.

When increased learning, self-awareness, and self-satisfaction are goals, the process of doing an activity is as important as the outcome. The structure in activities can contribute to improved functional performance by people who have tenuous self-control and to enhanced feelings of safety in confused persons. Being able to actually do an activity rather than just talk about doing it is a powerful learning tool that allows the person to integrate what he or she thinks, knows, and believes. It can also change one's very identity in a way that introspection or talk alone cannot achieve.

According to this frame of reference, the client-therapist relationship significantly impacts the therapeutic process and the outcomes. Structure, predictability, and boundaries in this relationship and in the external environment help compensate for feelings of unpredictability, confusion, or tenuous internal boundaries within the person. The creation and maintenance of an atmosphere of mutual respect and regard contributes to the person's sense of safety and helps people function optimally in individual session and in a group milieu.

The Cognitive-Behavioral Frame of Reference

Cognitive-behavioral therapy is also referred to as cognitive therapy in the literature. Adapted from Bruce and Borg (1993, 2002).

Theoretical Basis

Based on principles from social learning, cognitive, and behavioral theories (such as Adler, Piaget, Beck, Bandura, Kazdin, and Wilson).

Theoretical Assumptions

1. A person makes decisions regarding behavior based in part on what he or she expects will be the outcome.
2. A person's emotions and feelings are interdependent with what he or she knows and believes.

3. The person develops as a result of the interaction of the cognitive system, behaviors learned, and the social and physical environments.

4. Being willing to explore one's environment and try out new behaviors depends in part on one's belief that it is safe to make mistakes.

5. A person has internalized "rules for living," life themes, and a style of problem solving that he or she may or may not be aware of but nevertheless characterize how he or she approaches life's tasks.

6. Cognitive change is a gradual process; changing one's knowledge base and one's attitudes toward the self takes time.

7. The person can learn skills and strategies that he or she can use independently to face problems and find solutions.

8. When the person masters the use of his or her body and objects, he or she has a resource for problem solving.

9. When a person learns new cognitive strategies to respond to the present, he or she is preparing to confront and solve future problems.

10. People are unlikely to participate in experiences in which they feel incapable. Increasing one's beliefs about being capable increases one's willingness to initiate tasks and risk change.

11. Beliefs about being capable and in control are more likely to increase when one experiences one's self successfully and is given responsibility for one's own learning.

12. One's thoughts are not always in conscious awareness; making thoughts aware makes them more amenable to change.

13. The self-monitoring process can be learned.

14. Self-regulation is a balance in which present knowledge, cognitive functioning, new learning, and challenges complement each other to facilitate growth, optimal function, and the quality of life.

Function/Dysfunction Continua

1. Self-knowledge.
2. Cognitive functioning, including an ability to understand the environment and effective or flexible problem-solving repertoire.
3. Sense of safety.
4. Emotional development, including dependence and independence, self-interest and interest in others, the ability to be empathetic, the ability to identify with others and establish an autonomous identity, and the ability to express and control feelings. 🐚
5. Feelings of competence.
6. Self-regulation.

Indicators of Function and Dysfunction

1. Optimum function reflects a balance of the 2 extremes for each of the continua in emotional development and is associated with feelings of competence. It depends on

flexible thinking, adequate knowledge, emotional health, the belief that one can meet life's challenges, and the ability to problem solve in multiple situations.

2. Self-regulation is evidenced by the person's ability to monitor relevant data that come from the self and the environment, to use these data to choose and implement new behaviors, and to practice these behaviors until they become automatic.

3. Dysfunction is usually seen when the predominant behaviors are at the extremes of the emotional continuum or when cognitive function does not enable the person to meet developmental, personal, and societal expectations and is associated with feelings of incompetence. This may include one or more of the following behaviors:
   - Insufficient, inflexible, or distorted self-knowledge.
   - Reasoning that may be illogical, not coinciding with reality, or involve inferences that do not have a basis.
   - Limited exploration of one's environment.
   - Failure to establish an autonomous identity.
   - Limited problem-solving skills.
   - Feelings of incompetence.

The person may think he or she is incapable of taking responsibility for his or her own life, lack a realistic understanding of his or her own abilities and limitations, have self-defeating beliefs or be unclear regarding his or her beliefs, or be unable to adapt and cope with changing circumstances.

Evaluation is viewed as an ongoing process and can include the use of observation, tests, and interviews to assess the effectiveness of the client's cognitive system for enabling occupational performance. The therapist evaluates life themes, person-environment match, and cognitive structures. Some assessment instruments that may be used with this frame of reference include the Task Check List, the Beck Depression Inventory, the Stress Management Questionnaire, and Rotter's Internal-External Scale.

Postulates Regarding Change

1. If thoughts and beliefs are changed or knowledge is enhanced, then behavior and occupational performance are improved.

2. If the therapist helps the client develop strategies that emphasize the interaction among thoughts, feelings, and behaviors, then the client can change behavior, build knowledge, develop problem solving, and improve occupational performance.

3. If the therapist arranges the learning environment to facilitate cognitive development and stimulate problem solving, then cognitive function is improved. ☜

4. If the therapist uses symbolic modeling, role reversal, and instructional models, assertive beliefs may be developed and personal rights may be identified. ☜

5. If the therapist uses role playing, including rehearsal, modeling, and coaching, then effective methods for responding to problematic situations will be learned.

6. If the therapist provides practice in multiple, varied, and real-life contexts, then learning is enhanced.

7. If the therapist provides a structured intervention setting that controls distractions and provides repeated opportunities for skill practice and problem solving, then learning and skills are improved.

8. If the therapist presents activities that provide a moderate challenge, then the client's interest will be improved and participation in the intervention will be facilitated.

9. If the therapist modifies the complexity of the tasks, then successful learning will be promoted.

10. If the therapist uses tasks with a high probability of success, then cognitive development will be stimulated.

11. If the therapist helps the client develop a broad knowledge base (of self, others, and the environment), skills to function competently in the environment, and the ability to use knowledge for problem solving, then the client will become a self-regulating system.

12. If the therapist helps the client develop adequate knowledge and skills to cope with a range of daily problems, then the client will experience him- or herself as competent.

Intervention can take place in both individual and group settings. The intervention does not eliminate the disorder but provides cognitive, affective, and behavioral learning experiences to teach skills, strategies, and methods of coping. Intervention is more effective when specific techniques and skills (activities) are learned than when only verbal methods are utilized. The therapeutic tasks used should consider the person's cognitive knowledge, level of function, and interests. Therapy should stress the highest degree of self-regulation, not the highest cognitive developmental level.

PEDIATRIC-FOCUSED FRAMES OF REFERENCE

Several of the physical dysfunction and psychosocial frames of reference listed above are used in pediatric practice. The following were developed for use with pediatrics but are also used in some settings for treatment of adults.

Motor Skills Acquisition

Originated by Gentile. Adapted from Kaplan and Bedell (1999).

Theoretical Base

Dynamic Systems Theory emerges from the interaction of many systems. The 3 general systems are the person, the task, and the environment. Motor Control and Learning and Development Theories (developmental level of child is also acknowledged, although do not aim to increase skills at one level before moving to next).

Theoretical Assumptions

1. Functional tasks help organize behavior (focus on tasks that are meaningful).
2. Successful performance of meaningful tasks emerges from the interaction of multiple personal and environmental systems.

3. Motor problems observed are the result of all the systems interacting and compensating for some damage or problem in one or more of those systems. (Don't always focus on underlying neurological problem in treatment.)

Function/Dysfunction Continua

This frame of reference focuses on the child's ability to perform a task. This is determined according to the needs of each individual.

Indicators of Function and Dysfunction

1. The indicators of function are those aspects of the task that the child is able to perform.
2. The indicators of dysfunction are those aspects of the task that the child is unable to perform (client factors and performance skills, characteristics of the task, or environment).
3. Stage of motor learning (early learning identified by problems in the performance skills and client factors such as speed, accuracy, and quality of movement).
4. Child-task-environment match.

The task can be analyzed and the task components that the child is able to do and unable to do can be identified. Function and dysfunction are determined by the environment within which the skill must be performed. The environment is also analyzed. Developmental expectations are also considered.

Postulates Regarding Change

1. If there is a match among the task requirements, environmental demands, and the child's abilities, then it is more likely that motor skill acquisition will be improved.
2. If the child understands what is to be achieved and is provided with clear information about the expected motor skill performance and outcome, then it is more likely that motor skill acquisition will be improved.
3. If the child is encouraged to independently problem solve to find his or her own optimal movement strategies to perform tasks, then it is more likely that motor skill acquisition will be improved.
4. If the child is provided with a task that is challenging (i.e., possible at the child's upper limit of capabilities or zone of proximal development) and motivating, it is more likely that motor skill acquisition will be improved.

Sensory Integration

Originated by Ayres. Adapted from Kimball (1999).

Theoretical Basis

Neuroscience and developmental theories.

Theoretical Assumptions

1. The central nervous system (CNS) is hierarchically organized. Cortical processing relies on adequate organization of inputs supplied by the lower brain centers.
2. Meaningful registration of stimuli must occur before the CNS can make a response to it and, therefore, allow for higher functioning to occur.

3. The brain is innately organized to program a person to seek out stimulation that is organizing or beneficial in itself.

4. Input from one sensory system can facilitate or inhibit the state of the entire organism. Input from each system influences every other system and the whole organism.

5. There is plasticity within the CNS.

6. Normal human development occurs sequentially.

Function/Dysfunction Continua

1. Sensory modulation
2. Functional support capabilities
3. End-product abilities

Indicators of Function and Dysfunction

1. Indicators of function in the sensory system modulation are noted by normal responses in the following areas: tactile system, auditory system, relationship to gravity, movement level, oral arousal, olfactory arousal, visual system, attention level, postrotary nystagmus, sensitivity to movement, proprioceptive sensitivity, and emotional arousal. Under-registration or over-registration, as noted by the level of response, would be indicators of dysfunction.

2. Indicators of function in the functional support capabilities would include normal responses in the following areas: suck-swallow-breathe, tactile discrimination, sensory discrimination, movement level, oral discrimination, olfactory discrimination, visual discrimination, proprioceptive discrimination, attention level, emotional discrimination, cocontraction, muscle tone, balance and equilibrium, developmental reflexes, lateralization, and bilateral integration.

   Dysfunction would be noted by poorly developed capabilities in the areas listed above.

3. Indicators of function in the end-product abilities would include adequate praxis, form and space perception, behavior, academics, language and articulation, emotional tone, activity level, and environmental mastery. Dysfunction would be noted by poorly developed skills in the areas listed above.

Evaluation is completed using clinical observations; parent, teacher, and child interviews; and several assessment tools, including one or more of the following: the Sensory Integration and Praxis Test, touch inventory for elementary school-aged children, tactile defensiveness checklist, Sensory Profile, and the Bruininks Oseretsky Test of Motor Proficiency.

Postulates Regarding Change

1. If intervention involves several sensory systems and requires intersensory integration, then it will be more powerful and more likely to bring about an adaptive response.

2. If the therapist provides a situation in which the child can act on his or her environment, then the child will be more likely to produce adaptive responses. The child's self-initiated actions also use the more efficient feed-forward neurological mechanisms that build motor patterns rather than only the neurologically less efficient feedback.

3. If the child moves his or her own body volitionally during therapy rather than being moved by someone else, then effective motor patterns are more likely to develop.

4. If the therapist provides a situation that requires an adaptive response that is developmentally appropriate, then the adaptive response is more likely to occur and more likely to promote growth.

5. If the activity presented to the child is challenging yet achievable, then it will facilitate an improved adaptive response.

6. If the therapist provides the child with a sense of emotional safety, then the child will be more likely to engage actively in the therapy process.

7. If the therapist provides the child with constant feedback during the therapy session, then the child will gain a greater understanding of what he or she is doing and what he or she has done.

8. If the therapist provides activities that involve controlled change and variety, then the child is more likely to make an adaptive response rather than develop a learned behavior.

There are also specific postulates regarding change that address each of the 3 levels of continua. They are not listed here. The postulates address function/dysfunction continua using the above guidelines. They are considered to be hierarchical, which means each of the levels should be addressed in order. For example, if there are deficits in sensory system modulation, they should be addressed before addressing functional support capabilities.

COGNITIVE/PERCEPTUAL FRAMES OF REFERENCE

Cognitive Rehabilitation

Developed by occupational therapists at Loewenstein Rehabilitation Hospital. Adapted from Averbuch and Katz (1998).

Theoretical Basis

Neuropsychological and cognitive theories (developmental and information processing).

Theoretical Assumptions

1. Each brain region is involved in various functions and interacts with other regions in completing a specific task.

2. Every normal act is a result of a dynamic balance between all brain structures.

3. Higher mental processes in the human cortex constantly change during child development and are influenced by the environment (learning and training process).

4. The functional system as a whole can be disturbed by a lesion in one area.

5. It can be disturbed differently by lesions in different localizations.

6. The normal intellect involves processing information from the environment, the memory, and the feedback received after an action.

7. The normal individual actively seeks and assimilates information in relation to his or her ability to understand and then remember it.

8. Perception, thinking, and memory are constantly interacting.

9. Impaired intellectual processes can be improved through cognitive retraining.

Function/Dysfunction Continua

This frame of reference addresses cognition (the acquisition, organization, and use of knowledge), perception, visual-motor organization, thinking operations (executive functions), memory, attention, and concentration.

Indicators of Function and Dysfunction

1. Basic cognitive task performance in the various cognitive subcomponents.

2. Comparison of current cognitive performance to premorbid information.

3. Sensorimotor function.

4. Functional performance of daily activities.

Assessment of cognition may be completed using various cognitive batteries, including the Loewenstein Occupational Therapy Cognitive Assessment, The Rivermead Behavioral Memory Test, the Behavioral Inattention Test, and/or the Neurobehavioral Cognitive Status Examination.

Postulates Regarding Change

1. In the first phase, component specific (perception, visual-motor organization, thinking operation, and memory) training is completed using specific tools in a "laboratory environment."

2. In this environment, the therapist instructs the person to complete tasks that are at the level of the person's capabilities for that specific component.

3. The level of difficulty for each task is increased when the person masters the task.

4. The person is trained to develop specific strategies for each specific component.

5. Once the person has internalized the given cognitive strategies and can manipulate them on different tasks, the person is trained to adjust and adapt them to activities of real life.

Dynamic Interactional

Originated by Toglia. Adapted from Toglia (1998).

Theoretical Basis

Concepts are drawn from neuropsychology and learning theories.

Theoretical Assumptions

1. Cognition is the individual's capacity to acquire and use information in order to adapt to environmental demands. Cognitive abilities are not conceptualized as specific components, but as the underlying strategies and potential for learning.

2. Cognitive function (i.e., the ability to receive, elaborate, and monitor incoming information) is influenced by the dynamic interaction between the individual (strategies, metacognition, the learner characteristics), the task, and the environment.

3. Cognitive abilities are modifiable and vary with the characteristics of the task, the environment, and the individual.

Function/Dysfunction Continua

1. Processing strategies.

2. Metacognition.

3. Learning capabilities.

4. Transfer of learning to varied tasks and environments.

Indicators of Function and Dysfunction

1. The ability to select and use efficient processing strategies to organize and structure incoming information.

2. The ability to anticipate, monitor, and verify the accuracy of performance.

3. The ability to link new information with previous experience.

4. Flexible application of knowledge and skills to a variety of situations.

Assessment methods include the use of the Dynamic Interactional Assessment, which includes awareness questioning, response to cueing and task grading, and strategy investigation; The Dynamic Visual Processing Assessment; and The Toglia Category Assessment.

Postulates Regarding Change

1. Task and environmental variables are systematically changed to enhance the person's ability to process, monitor, and use information across new tasks and situations.

2. The person is taught to use processing strategies for varied tasks.

3. The processing strategies are practiced in a variety of different situations to increase the person's understanding of the conditions in which the strategies are useful.

4. Strategies such as self-prediction, role reversal, self-questioning, self-evaluation, structured error monitoring systems, and videotape feedback are used to increase metacognitive function.

5. When the person has internalized the ability to estimate and self-monitor performance, he or she is moved from a cued to an uncued condition.

6. Motivation and individual personality characteristics are considered when selecting treatment activities.

7. Individual treatments need to be combined with group treatments to reinforce self-monitoring or task strategies.

The Neurofunctional Approach

Developed by Giles, Clark-Wilson, and Yuen. Adapted from Giles (1998).

Theoretical Basis

Neuroscience and learning theories.

Theoretical Assumptions

1. Deficits in memory, attention, processing, and frontal lobe functions interfere with a person's ability to perform daily functional skills.

2. The person's cognitive abilities and learning characteristics impact the manner in which daily functional skills can be retrained.

3. Damage to the cerebral cortex often results in deficits in adaptive behavior and the ability to reacquire adaptive patterns of behavior.

4. The extent and location of injury to the cerebral cortex places constraints on human learning, but the ability to acquire new behaviors is retained in all but the most profoundly impaired.

Function/Dysfunction Continua

This frame of reference focuses on performance in areas of occupation, including ADL, instrumental ADL, education, work and productive activities, and play or leisure activities.

Indicators of Function and Dysfunction

Function is defined as adequate completion of performance in areas of occupation in a naturalistic environment in which cues are not provided and demands are not specifically manipulated. Assessment methods include observation, standardized assessments, questionnaires, checklists, and rating scales. If the person is not able to perform tasks in a naturalistic environment, structure and cues are provided to obtain baseline information. If, despite careful observation, the origin of some functional skills deficits remains unclear, the occupational therapist may use standardized testing to attempt to elicit the true cause of the problem and develop an adequate treatment plan.

Postulates Regarding Change

1. Practice of functional skills leads to modification of the person's previous responses and replaces them with new and more adaptive ones.

2. New metacognitive control strategies can be formed through the development of a new and more accurate model of basic cognitive functioning.

3. Cognitive overlearning is used to focus the person's attention on the behavior or area of skills deficit and to develop a verbal label for the behavior.

4. Learning of functional skills is increased through reinforcements, task analysis (to determine the steps of the activity that need cueing), chaining, prompts, practice, shaping, antecedents, and overlearning (practicing a skill well beyond the point where the person is able to produce the behavior).

5. When the focus of therapy is on the person being able to set and pursue his or her own goals, the person can learn about his or her own cognitive abilities and develop effective metacognitive control strategies.

MODELS USED IN OCCUPATIONAL THERAPY

The term *model* is used in different ways in the occupational therapy literature. Some authors use the term interchangeably with the term *frame of reference* (Katz, 1998). Other authors use the term *model* to mean overarching concepts that guide the general approach to clinical practice (Christiansen & Baum, 1997; Kielhofner, 1995). Bruce and Borg (2002) use the term *model of practice* interchangeably with the term *frame of reference*. Kielhofner (2004) uses the term *conceptual practice model*, which he defines as a way of thinking about and doing practice. According to Kielhofner (2004), well-developed models include an interdisciplinary base, theory, technology for therapeutic application, and evidence of effectiveness. The term *conceptual practice model* is very similar to frame of reference. The examples provided, however, also include overarching concepts that guide practice without the specific guidelines for evaluation and intervention. Mosey (1996) concluded that the term *model* is a sometimes confusing term in an applied profession. For the purposes of this chapter, the term *model* is used as defined by the authors who present their work in the format of models or overarching concepts that are used in conjunction with frames of reference. These authors do not present specific guidelines for evaluation and treatment as done in frames of reference, but provide the profession with general ideas to guide clinical practice in a variety of settings.

Client-Centered Models

Originated by Law, Christiansen, and Baum. Adapted from Tufano (2003) and Kielhofner (2004).

Two models for practice in occupational therapy that focus on the client as the center of treatment include the Canadian Model of Occupational Performance (CMOP) and the Person-Environment-Occupation-Performance (PEOP) model. The CMOP is an open system-based model that focuses on the interaction of the environment, occupation, and the person. The environment includes social, cultural, institutional, and physical components. Occupation includes self-care, leisure, and productivity. The person includes cognitive, physical, and affective aspects with spirituality as the core. The CMOP is a generic model that was developed to guide practice with many types of clients in any type of therapy setting. The Canadian Occupational Performance Measure (COPM) is used to conduct evaluation and to guide the treatment process.

The PEOP model is also an open system-based model that focuses on ADL, motivation, and the personal characteristics that influence the person's ability to manage the environment. Performance is the result of complex relationships between the person and the environment and occupation facilitates adaptation. Stages of development influence motivation, skills, and roles.

According to both of these models, the client should be the center of treatment. The client identifies goals and meaningful occupations that are then used by the therapist to promote health. Occupation is addressed from intrinsic and environmental perspectives. Because of the general nature of these models, both the CMOP and the PEOP are used in conjunction with frames of reference that address the specific needs of the clients.

Model of Human Occupation

Originated by Reilly and Kielhofner. Adapted from Kielhofner (2002).

The Model of Human Occupation (MOHO) is based on general systems theory, existential/humanism, ego psychology, cognitive theory, sociology, and biology. Man is viewed as an open system with input, throughput (comprised of volitional, habituation, and performance capacity subsystems), output, and feedback. Information enters the human system as input, is processed as throughput, and results in output from the person. Occupation is viewed as behavior that is internally gratifying and used to fulfill a variety of culturally- and socially-accepted roles. Occupation is subject to feedback from the environment and is instrumental to one's self-development. Occupation is also viewed in terms of motivation, patterns, and performance. In MOHO, a person is not divided into physical and mental components but is viewed as an integrated total human being.

Using this model, assessment of occupation is completed through observation, interviews, and self-report. According to Kielhofner (2002), the focus of treatment from this model is effecting change in volition, habituation, and performance capacity through occupational engagement. Occupational engagement refers to the client doing, thinking, and feeling during performance of one or more occupational forms. The focus of treatment is not on the therapist providing restoration of client factors or modification of the environment for specific areas of occupation. Rather, the purpose of treatment is for the therapist to facilitate the client's accomplishment of his or her own change.

Occupational Adaptation

Originated by Schkade and Schultz. Adapted from Schultz and Schkade (2003).

Although Occupational Adaptation (OA) is sometimes referred to as a frame of reference, it is more congruent with the category of models as presented in this chapter. OA articulates overarching concepts that are based on systems theory and can be used in a variety of settings with a wide range of clients. It does not describe specific techniques for evaluation and intervention. The main concepts of OA are occupation and adapta-

tion. Occupation is used to promote adaptation and adaptation is accomplished to perform occupation. Adaptation is a process of change that occurs through interaction among the person, occupational environments, and occupational challenges. The therapist focuses on the internal adaptation process within the client through promotion of the person as the agent of change.

The therapist and the client work together to promote the client's ability to make adaptations in order to engage in occupational activities that are personally meaningful to the client. The therapist examines the client's ability to carry out activities related to self-selected occupational roles to determine the mechanisms that facilitate and those that deter mastery of the activities. Occupational readiness and occupational activities are then used as intervention. Occupational readiness addresses client factors to prepare the person to participate in occupational activities. Occupational activities are used to engage the person in tasks related to self-selected roles. The overarching principle in the intervention is that the therapist must always think holistically when planning and carrying out activities, keeping in mind the 3 systems of the person: sensorimotor, cognitive, and psychosocial.

Occupational Science

Originated by Yerxa. Adapted from Tufano (2003).

Occupational science is based on biological and social sciences, the humanities, and open systems theories. Human beings are viewed as complex multilevel systems who participate in their environment. Illness, disease, or other life experiences limit the person's ability to adapt to the environment and participate in occupation. Emphasis is placed on the human as a holistic being and not as the parts of the human.

The focus of treatment from this model is on the use of meaningful occupations to enable humans to achieve competency and a sense of efficacy. In keeping with the philosophy of occupational therapy, the therapist needs to be aware of each person's unique qualities in language, culture, experience, and spiritual meaning.

LEARNING ACTIVITIES

1. Make a chart of several frames of reference on the left column with assumptions and treatment focus on the top row. Compare and contrast the frames.
2. Review a simple case from the textbook. How would treatment change using different frames?
3. Write a treatment plan based on a specific frame of reference.
4. Pick your "favorite" frame of reference after an initial discussion of frames. Explain how your favorite frame of reference usually fits your frame of life. For example, students who like to analyze life are real "people watchers" and prefer psychoanalytic frames over biomechanical frames.
5. Write a poem, rewrite the words to a song, or do a skit that helps explain the theories to your classmates.

REFERENCES

Averbuch, S., & Katz, N. (1998). Cognitive rehabilitation: A retraining model for clients following brain injuries. In N. Katz (Ed.), *Cognition and occupation in rehabilitation: Cognitive models for intervention in occupational therapy* (pp. 99-124). Bethesda, MD: American Occupational Therapy Association.

Bruce, M. A. G., & Borg, B. (1993). *Psychosocial occupational therapy: Frames of reference for intervention* (2nd ed.). Thorofare, NJ: SLACK Incorporated.

Bruce, M. A. G., & Borg, B. (2002). *Psychosocial frames of reference: Core for occupation-based practice* (3rd ed.). Thorofare, NJ: SLACK Incorporated.

Christiansen, C., & Baum, C. (1997). *Occupational therapy: Enabling function and well-being* (2nd ed.). Thorofare, NJ: SLACK Incorporated.

Dutton, R. (1995). *Clinical reasoning in physical disabilities.* Baltimore, MD: Williams & Wilkins.

Giles, G. M. (1998). A neurofunctional approach to rehabilitation following severe brain injury. In N. Katz (Ed.), *Cognition and occupation in rehabilitation: Cognitive models for intervention in occupational therapy* (pp. 125-148). Bethesda, MD: American Occupational Therapy Association.

Kaplan, M. T., & Bedell, G. (1999). Motor skills acquisition frame of reference. In P. Kramer & J. Hinojosa (Eds.), *Frames of reference for pediatric occupational therapy* (2nd ed., pp. 401-430). Philadelphia: Lippincott, Williams & Wilkins.

Katz, N. (1998). *Cognition and occupation in rehabilitation: Cognitive models for intervention in occupational therapy.* Bethesda, MD: American Occupational Therapy Association.

Kielhofner, G. (1995). *A model of human occupation: Theory and application* (2nd ed.). Baltimore, MD: Williams & Wilkins.

Kielhofner, G. (2002). *Model of human occupation: Theory and application* (3rd ed.). Baltimore: Lippincott, Williams & Wilkins.

Kielhofner, G. (2004). *Conceptual foundations of occupational therapy* (3rd ed.). Philadelphia: F. A. Davis.

Kimball, J. G. (1999). Sensory integration frame of reference: Theoretical base, function/dysfunction continua and guide to evaluation. In P. Kramer & J. Hinojosa (Eds.), *Frames of reference for pediatric occupational therapy* (2nd ed., pp. 169-205). Baltimore: Lippincott, Williams & Wilkins.

Mosey, A. C. (1986). *Psychosocial components of occupational therapy.* New York: Raven Press.

Mosey, A. C. (1996). *Applied scientific inquiry in the health professions: An epistemological orientation* (2nd ed.). Bethesda, MD: American Occupational Therapy Association.

Schultz, S., & Schkade, J. K. (2003). Occupational adaptation. In E. B. Crepeau, E. S. Cohn, & B. A. Boyt Schell (Eds.), *Willard & Spackman's occupational therapy* (10th ed., pp. 220-223). Philadelphia: Lippincott, Williams & Wilkins.

Toglia, J. P. (1998). A dynamic interactional model to cognitive rehabilitation. In N. Katz (Ed.), *Cognition and occupation in rehabilitation: Cognitive models for intervention in occupational therapy* (pp. 5-50). Bethesda, MD: American Occupational Therapy Association.

Tufano, R. (2003). Frames of reference in occupational therapy. In K. Sladyk (Ed.), *OT study cards in a box* (2nd ed.). Thorofare, NJ: SLACK Incorporated.

Voss, D. E., Ionta, M. K., & Myers, B. J. (1985). *Proprioceptive neuromuscular facilitation: Patterns and techniques* (3rd ed.). Philadelphia: Harper & Row.

Key Concepts

- Referral: Request for occupational therapy services.
- Evaluation: Screening and assessment of an occupational therapy consumer.
- Intervention planning: Identifying problems, goals, and treatments.
- Treatment implementation: Putting the treatment plan in action and re-evaluating as needed.
- Program discontinuation: Ending services when goals are reached or consumer is unable to make further progress.
- Service management: Process of delivery of the therapeutic intervention.

Essential Vocabulary

activity analysis: Study of a task's subparts and process.
areas of occupation: ADL, IADL, education, work, play, leisure, and social participation.
context of performance: Environment of performance including cultural, physical, social, personal, spiritual, temporal, or virtual.
performance patterns: Habits and routines.
performance skills: Motor, process, and communication/interaction skills.

THERAPEUTIC INTERVENTION PROCESS

Sally E. Ryan, COTA, ROH, Retired

Chapter 8

INTRODUCTION

The profession of OT has developed a specific plan for therapeutic intervention known as the OT process (AOTA, 1998; Moyers, 1999). It is made up of 5 distinct procedural categories that should be carried out in a particular order. (Exceptions are noted in the discussion of each category.) Service management is considered a sixth category. These sections are as follows:

1. Referral.
2. Evaluation, including screening and assessment (AOTA, 1994).
3. Treatment planning.
4. Treatment implementation (including periodic re-evaluation).
5. Program discontinuation (including discharge planning and follow-up).
6. Service management.

The AOTA has established general standards of practice for OT service programs and OT practitioners providing direct service. These standards were developed as guidelines to assist members of the profession. They have been reprinted in Appendix B because they detail important aspects of the OT process in which the OTA serves an important role. In recent times, more specific standards of practice have been adopted in the areas of physical disabilities, developmental disabilities, mental health, home health, school settings, and other areas. These are published in the *Reference Manual of the Official Documents of the AOTA*, which is available from the products division of AOTA. Further detail of occupational practice can be found in AOTA's *Guide to Occupational Therapy Practice* (Moyers, 1999).

REFERRAL

Requests for OT services may come from many sources, including physicians, physical therapists, teachers, social workers, and other health professionals, as well as parents and patients themselves. Referrals may be initiated and/or received by the OT either before or after the patient's initial screening. All referrals must be documented in writing and become a part of each patient's permanent record. The OTA may initiate patient referrals in the area of ADL. When an OTA receives a referral, whether initiated or not, it must be given to the supervising OT who is ultimately responsible for any action taken regarding the referral (AOTA, 1998).

The AOTA does not require that a referral be received before services can be provided. When there is no referral, the OT must assume all responsibility for the delivery of services. In some instances, state laws or the requirements established by health care facilities mandate the receipt of a referral. For example, the Commission on Accreditation of Rehabilitation Facilities (CARP), the Joint Commission on Accreditation of Healthcare Organizations (JCAHO), and Medicare regulations require that a physician's referral must be obtained if OT services are to be provided (Punwar, 2000). Figure 8-1 shows an example of a referral form used in a major hospital.

EVALUATION

The process of evaluation includes both screening and assessment (AOTA, 1994) and must take place before individual program planning. Evaluation is used to describe the process of collecting and interpreting data. Assessment refers to specific tools (AOTA, 1994). A thorough assessment provides a comprehensive "picture" of the patient based on a complete analysis of all of the screening and evaluation data. It is a predictor of the need for OT or other services and the estimated duration of treatment.

Screening

Screening of individuals who may benefit from OT services can be carried out by various health care providers. For example, a physical therapist may believe that a young man has stress management problems that are contributing to his diminished physical condition. A recreational therapist may note that a child has difficulty maintaining balance when participating in

Patient _____   Date Referral Received _____
            Last   First   M. Initial

Address _____   Zip _____
Medicare # _____   Medicare # _____
Contact Person _____   Physician _____
Phone # _____   Phone # _____
Relationship: _____

Primary Diagnosis: _____
Date of Onset: _____
Secondary Diagnosis: _____
Restrictions and Precautions: ❏ None   ❏ Specify: _____
Medical Prognosis: ❏ Excellent   ❏ Good   ❏ Fair   ❏ Poor   ❏ Guarded
❏ Patient   ❏ Family   is aware of Diagnosis and Prognosis

Physician's Plan of Treatment
❏ Physical Therapy: ❏ Evaluation and Treatment   ❏ Other _____
Specify Rx/Modalities: _____
Rehabilitation Goals: _____
Frequency: _____   Duration: _____   Wk/Mos   Equipment: ❏ Yes   ❏ No

❏ Occupational Therapy: ❏ Evaluation and Treatment   ❏ Other _____
Specify Rx/Modalities: _____
Rehabilitation Goals: _____
Frequency: _____   Duration: _____   Wk/Mos   Equipment: ❏ Yes   ❏ No

❏ Speech Pathology: ❏ Evaluation and Treatment   ❏ Other _____
Specify Rx/Modalities: _____
Rehabilitation Goals: _____
Frequency: _____   Duration: _____   Wk/Mos   Equipment: ❏ Yes   ❏ No

❏ Social Work: ❏ Evaluation and Treatment   ❏ Other _____
Rehabilitation Goals: _____

Physician Certification: I ❏ certify   ❏ recertify that the above Skilled Rehabilitation Services are required and authorized by me.

Physician's Signature _____   Date _____

Figure 8-1. Outpatient, referral, and treatment care plan. Adapted from Irene Walter Johnson Rehabilitation Institute, St. Louis, MO. (Reprinted from Ryan, S. E. [1993]. *Practice issues in OT: Intraprofessional team building.* Thorofare, NJ: SLACK Incorporated.)

some play activities. Both of these individuals would be advised to seek an OT screening to determine the extent to which evaluation and treatment might alleviate or mediate the presenting problem.

The process of screening patients is necessary to determine whether a patient needs OT services. Screening involves the collection and analysis of specific data and facts. Information is obtained by observing the patient while he or she is performing tasks or engaging in social interactions; through interviews with the patient and family or significant others, such as a roommate or a close friend; or through a review of the patient's general history from sources that may include the medical chart, a psychologist's report, or a teacher's appraisal. The OTA collaborates with the supervising OT in the screening process by collecting and reporting selected information as requested. For example, he or she may use a structured interview form to gather information about the patient's educational background, employment history, hobbies, and ADL skills. If the OT's analysis of the screening information indicates that OT treatment would be beneficial, a comprehensive evaluation is performed.

Assessment

The purpose of an assessment is to determine the patient's current level of functional performance and to identify performance deficits. The OT is responsible for all aspects of the assessment; however, the OTA may carry out some evaluative tasks under supervision. These tasks may include administering an interest checklist or an activity configuration and summarizing the information in a written report. In addition, the OTA can observe the patient in a specific situation and report on interpersonal skills, coordination, strength, and endurance as they relate to ADL skills and tasks.

The profession of OT is concerned with function and uses specific procedures and activities to:

- Develop, maintain, improve, and/or restore the performance of necessary functions.
- Compensate for dysfunction.
- Minimize or prevent debilitation.
- Promote health and wellness (Punwar, 2000).

The *Occupational Therapy Practice Framework* (2002) by the AOTA provides a guide for assessment and treatment in OT. Areas of occupation are central to the document and include ADL, IADL, education, work, play, leisure, and social participation. To participate in these occupations, a person must have performance skills such as motor, process, and communication skills. In addition, personal patterns and external contexts impact the performance of an occupation. Occupational therapy assessment and treatment must consider all of these issues in the prevision of services. For example:

- Bathing (ADL): Requires motor and processing skills (performance skills). A person's habits and routines impact bathing (patterns). The place or environment (context) of bathing differs at camp, home, health club, or after PE class at school.
- Child Rearing (IADL): Requires motor, process, and communication skills (performance skills). Roles and routines (patterns) are key to managing parenting. Although some

aspects of parenting are universal, culture, social, and spiritual aspects (context) vary greatly.

- Leisure participation (Leisure): The skills necessary for a hobby are as various as the hobby itself (performance skills). Hiking requires high motor skills but less communication skills. Social club participation requires less motor skill and more communication skills. Adapting, organizing, and energy (process skills) also vary. Habits and routines (patterns) are extremely important in leisure. Games as hobbies are always performed in context from culture such as Bocce ball to virtual such as online card games.

Evaluation is necessary to determine the patient's strengths and weaknesses, needs, and the degree of change possible through OT intervention. OTs and OTAs use a variety of specific evaluations. Many are discussed in the individual case studies presented in Section II and the techniques of practice described in Section III.

The OT analyzes and interprets screening and evaluation data to determine the total assessment results. Recommendations for continuance or dismissal from OT are made. Services other than OT that may assist the patient are identified and referral may be made.

Information obtained through a comprehensive evaluation also assists OT practitioners in determining the activities that will be most beneficial in assisting the patient in performance deficit areas.

TREATMENT PLANNING

Treatment planning involves identifying the patient's problems and selecting goals that are reasonable to achieve and developing the methods to achieve them (Early, 1994). Hopkins and Tiffany (1981) stressed the need to use a problem-solving process in setting treatment objectives and carrying them out. This process is summarized as follows:

- Problem identification.
- Solution development.
- Development of a plan of action.
- Implementation of the plan.
- Assessment of results.

In the treatment planning process, both long- and short-term objectives and time lines are established. Specific activities related to the patient's occupations are analyzed, selected, and sequenced to assist the patient in meeting the goals. Specific frames of reference, methods, and approaches are also determined, and adaptations are planned. The patient's goals, values, cultural identification, stage of biological and mental development, and interests and abilities are all carefully considered as an integral part of the process. The active involvement of the patient, as well as family members and significant others, in all phases of treatment planning is important and influences the overall effectiveness of the plan. Motivation and cooperation often increase when the patient has a thorough understanding of the treatment process and feels that he or she has had an integral part in the planning.

Failure to include the patient in planning may result in ineffective or unnecessary intervention strategies. For example, if the patient is a woman who has had a stroke and needs to perform ADL tasks with one hand, it is often a common practice in OT to include goals related to meal preparation. This may be stereotypical planning in some cases, as evidenced by the report of one OTA. The woman was placed in a cooking group and later told the OTA that her husband did all of the cooking and related tasks and she "never set foot in the kitchen nor did she plan to!" Another area where stereotypical planning might occur is housework. Setting goals related to tasks such as cleaning and doing the laundry would be inappropriate for a person who always hires outside help to do them and has the necessary financial resources to continue to do so. These brief examples illustrate the importance of including the patient in the treatment planning process. Outcomes of intervention must relate to the needs and priorities of the individual.

A strong background in a variety of different activities, together with knowledge and skill in activity analysis, is a critical factor in effective treatment planning. The therapeutic potential of age-appropriate activities and their various properties, components, and potential for adaptation must be related to the specific treatment goals.

The OTA contributes to many aspects of the program plan; however, the OT is responsible for the final plan that will best meet the patient's needs and objectives and is acceptable to the patient (Early, 1994).

The long-term objectives of such a plan are to develop, improve, restore, or maintain the patient's abilities that allow for a more productive and meaningful life. They may be quite broad in focus and are written to reflect the expected outcome of treatment. The short-term objectives relate to the long-term objectives and contribute to their achievement. They must be stated in achievable, measurable outcomes and be met in a short enough time span to serve as a record of improvement. Short-term objectives address more immediate, specific goals. They may be viewed as "mini-steps" that will lead to the desired result (Punwar, 2000).

Treatment planning is a critical component of the OT process. It involves setting the problem and identifying the steps necessary in solving the problem (Parham, 1987). The former is the role of the OT, and the latter is a collaborative OT and OTA process, with the OT having the ultimate responsibility.

TREATMENT IMPLEMENTATION

All OT treatment is based on the treatment plan. Treatment implementation is putting the plan into action. Effective treatment requires the patient to participate in selected purposeful activities designed to achieve the established goals. The OTA, working under close supervision, may implement a program for acutely ill individuals, such as a patient who has had a recent stroke or someone who is depressed and suicidal. Close supervision is essential because of the complex problems and degree of change frequently seen that may require a modified treatment approach or re-evaluation by the OT (AOTA, 1999). If the patients are in a more stable, nonacute, or controlled condition,

the assistant may carry out treatment procedures with greater independence, as directed by the supervising OT. The OTA may also be responsible for monitoring the patient's performance and providing a summary report. It is the OTA's responsibility to keep the supervising therapist informed of all changes in patient performance and any other pertinent facts. As treatment progresses and changes are noted, the assistant may contribute suggestions for program modifications and additions that will help the patient reach the established goals.

In the event that the patient is not making satisfactory progress, the OT will conduct a re-evaluation to determine necessary changes in the program plan and the treatment procedures. Re-evaluation refers to repeating certain assessments and analyzing the findings. Results may indicate that objectives have been set at too high a level or are unrealistic (Punwar, 2000). Perhaps methods, activities, and/or time frames need to be modified. Specific aspects of the re-evaluation may be delegated to the assistant. Re-evaluation also takes place before discharge to determine discontinuation and discharge planning. Comparison of re-evaluation data with that obtained in the initial evaluation provides an objective means of measuring change.

PROGRAM DISCONTINUATION

Program discontinuation takes place when the patient has reached all of the established goals or it is determined that the patient can no longer benefit from OT services. Among other tasks, the OTA may assist in this process by providing specific information on progress or lack of progress to be included in a summary report. The OTA may also provide instructions for a home-based program, identify community resources and personnel, or recommend environmental adaptations that may assist the patient after discharge.

Although the Standards of Practice adopted by the AOTA (1998) do not specify that patient follow-up must occur, it is desirable to gather such information to determine the effectiveness of treatment; general adjustment outcomes; and the degree to which the patient is able to resume social, family, work, and leisure roles. This task could be performed collaboratively by an OT and OTA, with the OT determining the final conclusions. Follow-up also provides additional support to the patient in the transition from illness to wellness.

SERVICE MANAGEMENT

Service management is a process that involves planning, structuring, developing, coordinating, documenting, and evaluating the delivery of all OT services to ensure quality, efficiency, and effectiveness. It is the organizational framework and system that supports the OT process in therapeutic intervention. Service management is essential in the delivery of OT services. Because this area has so many specific components, it will be discussed in depth later in this book. Specific information relative to documentation may be found in Chapter 40.

SUMMARY

Therapeutic intervention follows a specific plan called the OT process. This process includes sets of tasks that should be carried out in a particular order. Referral, evaluation (including screening and assessment), treatment planning, treatment implementation (including re-evaluation), and program discontinuation (including discharge planning and follow-up) are presented. Service management is a system that allows the OT process to be carried out. The OTA may participate in all aspects of the process as directed by the supervising OT.

LEARNING ACTIVITIES

1. Review the history and evaluation data for several TV characters of varying ages with both physical and mental problems. Work with a peer to develop potential treatment plans in the area of ADL. Discuss your work with an OT.
2. Use the treatment plans developed in item 1 as a basis for recommending specific treatment activities. Identify areas where additional information, if any, is needed. Discuss your work with an OT.
3. Discuss specific roles the entry-level OTA can assume in the OT process.
4. What are some of the additional roles that may be assumed by experienced OTAs?

REFERENCES

American Occupational Therapy Association. (1994). Clarification of the use of the terms assessment and evaluation. *American Journal of Occupational Therapy, 48*, 1072-1073.

American Occupational Therapy Association. (1998). Standards of practice for OT. *American Journal of Occupational Therapy, 52*, 866-869.

American Occupational Therapy Association. (1999). Guide for supervision of OT personnel in the delivery of OT services. *American Journal of Occupational Therapy, 53*(6), 601-607.

American Occupational Therapy Association. (2002). The occupational therapy practice framework: Domain and process. *American Journal of Occupational Therapy, 56*, 609-633.

Early, M. B. (1994). *Mental health concepts and techniques for the OTA*. New York: Raven Press.

Hopkins, H. L., & Tiffany, K. G. (1981). OT—A problem solving process. In H. Hopkins & H. Smith (Eds.), *Willard & Spackman's occupational therapy* (7th ed.). Philadelphia, PA: Lippincott.

Moyers, P. (1999). *Guide to OT practice*. Bethesda, MD: American Occupational Therapy Association.

Parham, D. (1987). Toward professionalism: The reflective therapist. *American Journal of Occupational Therapy, 41*, 555-561.

Punwar, A. J. (2000). *OT principles and practice*. Baltimore, MD: Williams & Wilkins.

Key Concepts

- Occupation: The roles and tasks that give meaning and purpose to one's life.
- Disruptions in occupation: Environmental, community, culture, or tradition changes.

Essential Vocabulary

external environment: Contexts such as climate, community, and economics.
internal environment: Aspects such as motivation, wellness, and emotional state.
occupational performance areas: ADL, IADL, education, work, play, leisure, and social participation.

OCCUPATION:
AN INDIVIDUAL'S CHOICE

Bonnie Brooks, MEd, OTR, FAOTA

INTRODUCTION

One of the foundations of OT theory is that humans have a need to be active and participate in various occupations. Occupation is essential for basic survival and optimal mental and physical health. Occupation is also an integral part of survival and a basic drive of every person. Within this individual frame of reference, a person's activities and occupations enable him or her to function as a central part of a larger whole. It is the difference between existing and actively participating. Participation and optimal functioning within a person's environment provide an individual with feelings of purpose and self-esteem throughout his or her life span (Moyers, 1999).

What does the word *occupation* mean? To those in OT, it means engaging in purposeful activity. Occupations are effective in preventing or reducing disability and in promoting independence through the acquisition of skills, as the following examples illustrate:

- The occupation of a preschool child with a disability is learning the motor skills necessary to enter school.
- The primary occupation for a young adult may be planning for a career or vocation.
- Occupation for others may be providing for financial security through employment, which may require a variety of activities.
- Occupation for an individual with serious cardiac problems may include learning to conserve energy while doing daily activities.
- An occupation for the elderly may be prolonging participation in rewarding activities and maintaining personal independence.

An occupation may require a variety of activities and skills. For example, the occupation of self-care includes the activities of bathing, shaving, dressing, and feeding, each of which requires varying degrees of skill in gross and fine motor coordination and judgment.

OT is the art and science of directing an individual's participation in selected tasks to restore, reinforce, and enhance performance. OT facilitates teaming of skills and functions essen-

tial for adaptation and productivity, for diminishing or correcting pathology, and for promoting and maintaining health. The word *occupation* in the professional title refers to goal-directed use of time, energy, interest, and attention. OT's fundamental concern is developing and maintaining the capacity to perform, with satisfaction to self and others, the tasks and roles essential to productive living and mastering self and the environment throughout the life span (AOTA, 1979).

Three main types of occupation are necessary for the achievement of optimal performance and quality of life: ADL, work, and leisure. These areas are discussed in greater depth later in this book. Acquiring and maintaining skills in these areas enable a person to interact successfully with the environment. Activities and skills also enable a person to engage in a variety of occupations that result in the establishment of the individual's lifestyle.

OT provides service to those individuals whose abilities to cope with tasks of living are threatened or impaired by developmental deficits, the aging process, physical injury or illness, or psychological and social disability (Reed & Saunderson, 1999).

Intervention programs in OT are designed to enable the patient to become adequate or proficient in basic life skills, work, and leisure, and thereby competent to resume his or her place in life and interact with the environment effectively. As each patient is unique, each treatment approach must be individualized. With these goals in mind, this chapter focuses on case studies and examples of how OT intervention (AOTA, 2002) can be individualized in relation to the environment, society, change, and prevention.

CASE STUDIES IN OCCUPATION

The profession of OT recognizes that the level of optimal function to which a patient may aspire is highly individual and determined by all of the circumstances of the individual's life (AOTA, 2002). No 2 patients are alike, even if they are the same age and have identical problems or disabilities. Intervention programs should be individualized and focus on the uniqueness of the individual. To understand the multitude of factors that create an individual lifestyle, a description of John and Darlene follows. They will be referred to later in this chapter to illustrate various content areas.

Case Study 1

John is a 24-year-old obese man. He smoked 2 packs of cigarettes a day for 4 years and recently quit. He appears in good health.

Family Information

John is the oldest of 3 children. His sisters, aged 19 and 21, are away at college. His mother is 53 years old and in good health. His father is 57 years old and has high blood pressure. Three years ago the father experienced 2 severe heart attacks and was hospitalized both times. The following year the father had 3 minor attacks. He has generalized weakness and had been very depressed; however, he exhibited significant improvement recently.

Vocational Information

John graduated from college 2 years ago. He returned home to manage the farm because of his father's illness. The crop farm is located 25 miles outside a rural town in southern Minnesota. Employment opportunities were very limited for John in that particular region of the state, and he had just accepted a job to work as an accountant in Duluth. He plans to move there in 4 months.

Leisure and Socialization

During the winter, John watches television a great deal and plays cards. Recently, he decided to take half-hour walks twice a day to lose weight. In the summer, John plays softball on a local team, goes swimming, and meets socially with friends.

Case Study 2

Darlene is a 35-year-old woman in good health. She is slightly underweight because of constant dieting.

Family Information

Darlene is an only child. She lived in California and was married for 5 years, but divorced 2 years ago. She has no children. Her mother is 62 years old, her father is 65 years old, and both are retired. They are healthy and travel extensively, spending most of their time in Florida. Darlene currently lives in her parent's home located in a wealthy suburb of New York City.

Vocational Information

Darlene worked for a short time prior to her marriage at age 27. Before that time she took classes at a local college periodically and worked in her father's office part-time. Darlene completed a computer course 3 years ago and now works as a full-time programmer for a moderate salary. She pays no expenses while living in her parents' home; however, she does buy groceries and presents for her parents periodically. Her parents recently decided to sell their home and move to a condominium in Florida.

Leisure Information

Darlene is very active. She goes out every evening and frequently takes weekend trips. She is very fashion conscious, often attending fashion shows, and identifies shopping as a major interest. After shopping sprees, she and her friends frequently go to art galleries or the theater. Darlene belongs to a health spa, racquetball club, and country club. She enjoys golf and swimming.

John and Darlene have been introduced to provide a context to examine some of the factors that have impact on the development of their present lifestyles. These include the effect of the environment, sociocultural aspects, local customs, and economic implications. All of these factors must be considered to gain an understanding of individuals' current lifestyle, who they are, what roles they have, what they want and expect, and what they need.

ENVIRONMENTAL CONSIDERATIONS

A person's environment is comprised of all of the factors that provide input to the individual. The environment includes all contexts that influence and modify a person's lifestyle and activity level. Environmental considerations vary significantly in complexity. They can be as simple as climate, geographic location, or economic status or as complex as considering the sociocultural aspects of traditions, local customs, superstitions, values, beliefs, and habits.

Every individual has 2 environments that constantly provide input: external and internal. These environments are so closely integrated in an individual's life that it is often difficult to consider them separately. Both external and internal environments must be considered in designing a treatment intervention that will allow a person to function at maximum capacity. This coordinated approach is the essence of total patient treatment in OT.

External Environment

The external environment is comprised of a number of factors, including climate, community, and economic status. One of the most obvious external environmental factors is the climate. Some climates are warm or cold for most of the year and offer extremes in temperatures and weather hazards during several months. Many regions experience 4 seasons. In general, spring and fall are periods of transition, whereas winter and summer exhibit extremes in weather, such as floods, hurricanes, tornadoes, or blizzards. Individual responses to climates and weather conditions vary. Many people dislike the winter months and restrict their activities. It is very common for some people to gain weight during these months and then lose the added pounds when the weather permits them to resume their outdoor activities.

The Effects of Climate on John and Darlene

The impact of winter weather is greater for John than for Darlene. Darlene's work and leisure activities occur within a much smaller geographic area than those of John. Her suburban environment offers a variety of transportation options. The winter months impose more restrictions on John. This period of snow storms and icy conditions usually limits his transportation, which in turn restricts his opportunities for socialization. During severe weather, John restricts his leisure activities to watching television and playing cards, and he frequently gains weight during this period. Summer also affects John more than Darlene. Although Darlene experiences some changes, these have minimal impact on her activity level. John's farm work requires heavy labor as soon as the soil is workable, beginning with the first sign of spring and continuing well into the fall. He completely changes his leisure, recreation, and social activities, which include playing on a softball team, swimming, and meeting with friends.

External environment can affect a patient through secondary issues, such as the splinting problems seen in Case Study 3.

Case Study 3

A patient living in Georgia was required to wear a basic cock-up splint. During his monthly visits to the clinic, his splint always needed significant adjustments. It was discovered that he would frequently leave the splint on the back shelf of the car. The internal temperature of the closed car in a hot climate was excessive. The splint had been fabricated from a low temperature material, which tended to change shape in the high heat. A new splint was made from a heavier material that would withstand high temperatures, thus solving the problem.

Severe cold can also affect the selection of splinting materials. Some are made of plastic, which can become brittle and shatter on impact in extreme cold. Metal braces and splints can also be very uncomfortable in extreme temperatures. Special attention should be given to lining the splint to protect the skin that comes into contact with the device.

Community

Another important environmental consideration is the type of community in which the person lives. There are three basic types of communities: rural, urban, and suburban. Each type has different characteristics that can affect an individual's occupations, activities, and lifestyle.

The Effects of Community on John and Darlene

John is well-known in his small farming community. His neighbors know that he completed college and returned home to help his father. John knows the grocer, auto mechanic, drug store clerk, dentist, and physician personally.

Darlene shops and receives necessary services in a variety of places and therefore does not know many of these people personally. She knows the names of 2 women who work in her favorite boutiques. Personalized service and recognition can be status symbols if deliberately developed.

Internal Environment

One method of separating the internal and external environments is by considering the physiologic feedback provided by the various body systems. This feedback is the body's way of informing a person of his or her ability to respond to the daily requirements of the external environment. Moods and emotional states can be considered parts of an internal environment that influence the way a person responds to the external environment. Depressed persons frequently respond more slowly to their environment and may decrease social activities. Some may further restrict the environment by remaining at home. Self-image is another example of previous feedback from the external environment that creates an internal set or environment. These internal environments can exist long after the external environment has changed. Phobias are yet another example of adverse internal environments. They are defined as abnormal fears or dreads and are illustrated in the following case.

Case Study 4

Mrs. Anderson is 45 years old, married, and the mother of 2 children, aged 13 and 17. Her husband's job as an industrial consultant requires periodic travel for up to 4 consecutive weeks at a time. He is generally at home 1 week at a time between trips.

Approximately 8 years ago, Mrs. Anderson began to decline social invitations from friends when her husband was at home. She would excuse herself for some minor or nonexistent complaint or say that their time together was so limited that they needed to be alone as a family. Eventually, she reached the stage where she encouraged her husband to attend events without her because of headaches.

Mrs. Anderson no longer liked driving the car. She complained about heavy traffic, crowded grocery stores, and rude clerks in department stores. She located a small grocery store that would deliver orders, and she began buying mail-order clothing. Cosmetics and other items were ordered through door-to-door distributors. Her family became concerned and began encouraging her to go for rides or have an occasional dinner out. Mrs. Anderson was very uncomfortable and obviously in a state of anxiety. Finally, she simply refused to leave her home.

Mrs. Anderson was exhibiting symptoms of agoraphobia, a Greek term meaning fear of the marketplace, which, in current usage, refers to a fear of open or public places. In all probability, her agoraphobia had occurred as a result of previous environmental feedback; however, once the condition developed, it then became an internal environment affecting her occupation and effectiveness as a member of her family unit.

Economic Environment

The economic environment of the community and the economic status of individuals must also be considered. Values and standards vary greatly and affect OT treatment, as shown in the two case examples to follow.

Case Study 5

Susan was 16 years old when she was diagnosed as having juvenile arthritis, affecting her right hand. The rheumatologist referred her to OT to have a splint fabricated, which would block MCP flexion of all 4 fingers. A variety of splints were presented to the patient and her family. All were visually unacceptable. The patient agreed to wear the "ugly" splint when she was at home, but adamantly refused to wear it in public. Her family supported her in this decision, even though they understood the medical benefits that could be achieved by a regular wearing schedule. The parents requested that the OT work in collaboration with their local jeweler to design something more attractive.

Working with the jeweler, the OT designed rings for each finger, which were connected by chains to a large medallion on the back of the hand. The medallion was then connected by chains to a snug, wide bracelet. The design proved to be highly workable, although not ideal medically. The final product was made of 14-carat gold and studded with rubies and pearls. The patient wore it constantly and several of her friends requested similar jewelry. It seemed that the "splint" had become a status symbol in her social group.

Case Study 6

A diagnosis of rheumatoid arthritis had far reaching implications for Mrs. Kennedy, a 36-year-old woman employed as a bank clerk in a small community. Weight bearing had become very painful, and a total hip replacement and bilateral knee surgery had been recommended.

Several months before the diagnosis was made, persistent pain and stiffness had forced Mrs. Kennedy to give up her job in the bank, even though her salary was important to maintain the family's modest standard of living. She had allowed her health insurance coverage to lapse and was in the process of applying for coverage under her husband's policy when her condition was diagnosed. As a result, she was denied coverage.

Mrs. Kennedy was referred to OT for homemaking training and self-care activities before surgery. The evaluation revealed the need for a variety of adaptive equipment, including a wheelchair and a ramp to access her home. She also needed a commode, as the only bathroom was upstairs. A utility cart would be needed for basic kitchen activities.

When these recommendations were presented, Mrs. Kennedy began to cry. She explained that the family had already remortgaged their home to pay for her medical bills and the planned surgery. There was no money for the necessary equipment. She felt that in less than a year she had gone from being a contributing member of society to becoming a burden on her family. She was worried about the effects of financial stress on her husband and her inability to care for their 2 small children. The mere mention of possible sources of community assistance brought a fresh flood of tears.

The OTA working with Mrs. Kennedy had grown up in a small community and knew how important it was for people to maintain their pride and sense of self-worth. She also knew that friends and neighbors would welcome the opportunity to help Mrs. Kennedy and others like her who might need assistance. She suggested to the OT that they contact the local Kiwanis and Lions Clubs to propose the development of a community adaptive equipment bank. She also recommended that Mrs. Kennedy be asked to serve as coordinator of the equipment

bank, receiving requests from physicians and family members, arranging for purchase and delivery of equipment, and mainlining records and inventory. The OT approved the plan, which was put into action within 2 weeks. Mrs. Kennedy was pleased to have an opportunity to use her office and managerial skills and to have the use of the equipment until she recovered from her surgery.

SOCIOCULTURAL CONSIDERATIONS

Many communities contain diverse ethnic groups. People from the same cultural background have common traditions, interests, beliefs, and behavior patterns that give them a common identity. Frequently, these individuals tend to cluster in geographic areas to preserve their customs, values, traditions, and at times their native language. The ethnic neighborhood can be viewed as a society within a society. These clusters or environs provide individuals with opportunities for perpetuation of their culture and lifestyles.

Some cultures are matriarchal, or female controlled, whereas others are patriarchal, or male controlled. The roles and performance expectations of the oldest, middle, or youngest child can also vary among cultural groups. In some societies, the number of male children may determine the financial security of the parents in later life.

Customs

A custom is a pattern of behavior or a practice that is common to many members of a particular class or ethnic group. Although rules are unwritten, the practice is repeated and handed down from generation to generation. Cultural implications can have a significant impact on designing OT intervention techniques that enable a person to function at his or her maximum in the specific environment, as shown in Case Study 7.

Case Study 7

Mrs. Franko is a 61-year-old Italian woman who recently had a stroke. Her primary residual deficit was mild, right-sided hemiparesis. Mrs. Franko was also slightly dysarthric and difficult to understand, as her native language was Italian.

When she returned home from the hospital, Mrs. Franko was depressed, unmotivated, and not interested in beginning any ADL. When cooking activities were suggested, she became very upset and burst into tears. This behavior was discussed with one of her sons, and it was discovered that the entire family routinely gathered at the parents' home for Sunday dinner. Mrs. Franko greatly enjoyed this custom. She made her own pasta and canned homegrown tomatoes for sauce. She did not want her daughters-in-law to bring food or assist too much in meal preparation. Convenience foods and ready-made pasta had never been used, and the suggestion was totally unacceptable to the family.

In home care OT, Mrs. Franko was encouraged to regain her cooking skills, which required some minor adaptations. Her family bought her an electric pasta machine since she was no longer able to knead and roll her own pasta. Her heavy cooking pots were replaced with new, lightweight styles.

Once Mrs. Franko regained her cooking skills and resumed a role that was very important to her, she became receptive to relearning other aspects of ADL skills.

Traditions

Traditions are inherited patterns of thought or action that can be handed down through generations or can be developed in singular family units; they also may be perpetuated through subsequent generations. Many families develop their own special traditions during holidays, birthdays, vacations, and other occasions.

Customs and traditions may also occur on a daily basis and can be highly individualized. Their origin may be unknown and not related to any particular sociocultural custom or event, as illustrated by the following case.

Case Study 8

Mr. Wisneski is 50 years of age and was admitted to the Veterans Hospital with a diagnosis of multiple sclerosis. He was confined to a wheelchair and exhibited severe weakness of the upper extremities. His wife was 45 years old and they had 6 children all living at home who ranged in age from 4 to 16 years.

In OT, Mr. Wisneski participated in dressing activities, bathing, and transfer techniques and was actively experimenting with a variety of adaptive equipment that would assist him in resuming his previous employment. Although he was a very quiet, nonverbal person, he seemed highly motivated and always carried through on any requests made as a part of his treatment.

When the OTA suggested that he begin shaving techniques, Mr. Wisneski said that it simply was not necessary and told the assistant not to worry about it. The OTA reminded him of the accomplishments he was making in independent living skills and pointed out that this was one more activity in which he could achieve independence. He acquiesced and went along with the program to please the OTA. One day, when Mr. Wisneski had successfully shaved himself, the OTA asked him if he did not feel better shaving independently. Mr. Wisneski replied that "it felt okay;" however, in his family it was a tradition for the wives to shave their husbands. Mr. and Mrs. Wisneski felt that this daily activity reaffirmed their commitment to each other and was a daily declaration of their devotion.

Superstitions

Superstitions can be difficult to identify and define. They can be customs, traditions, and beliefs of a very small population that may be geographically localized. They can also be highly individualized and border on mental or emotional pathologic states. *Webster's New World Dictionary* defines them as "beliefs and practices resulting from ignorance and fear of the unknown" (Guralnik, 1994). They are also viewed as a statement of trust in magic. Superstitions are further defined as irrational attitudes of the mind toward supernatural forces.

It can be very difficult for OT personnel to deal with superstitions. It may be easy for a therapist or an assistant to point out how "ridiculous" superstitions are and to present facts that disprove such "ignorant" notions. The personal environment, standards, values, traditions, and beliefs of the OTA and OT can, at times, be in direct conflict with those of the patient. OT personnel must realize that the ultimate goal of OT is to return the individual to his or her lifestyle with all of its implications. The following case illustrates this point.

Case Study 9

Mrs. King is an 82-year-old woman who was admitted to the hospital with severe circulatory disturbances in her left leg. This condition resulted in surgical amputation of the lower left extremity.

The patient was referred to OT for generalized strengthening activities, cognitive stimulation, and reality reorientation. Although she frequently did not know where she was, past memory appeared to be intact. Mrs. King presented herself as a very pleasant person with a warm, personable manner.

During one of her initial treatment sessions, it was noted that she wore a small bag of coins tied tightly around her right thigh with several strips of gauze. When the OT questioned her about this, she explained that the bag of coins "kept evil spirits away" and made a person happy. She elaborated further, saying that she had always worn the bag on her left leg, but since the doctors had to remove that leg, she would now have to tie it to the right one. This situation had not been noted during prior medical examinations, as Mrs. King always removed the bag when she disrobed.

OT intervention consisted of introducing a 6-inch wide cohesive, light woven, elastic bandage, applied lightly on the thigh, with the small bag of coins attached with a safety pin. This solution was acceptable to Mrs. King. She also reported that all of the other family members also observed this practice. Therefore, all 12 family members were also instructed in this new method.

Values, Standards, and Attitudes

Values, standards, and attitudes are other aspects of an individual that develop through environmental transaction and influence lifestyle. These facets of a person's life usually result from feedback received from other people within one's work and leisure environments, as well as from the individual's sociocultural status, economic status, and self-image. They are very personal and become an important part of a person's internal environment. The presence of disease or injury can be very disruptive and require reassessment of all aspects of an individual's life and lifestyle, requiring some temporary or permanent adaptations. It is important for OT personnel to use intervention techniques that can be adapted to minimize the stresses that occur when the patient's values, standards, and attitudes are in jeopardy or must be compromised to some extent. Two case examples are presented to elaborate on these points.

Case Study 10

Mr. Hanson, a 50-year-old farmer living in a rural community in Indiana, had sustained a nerve injury to his left wrist. When his wrist was maintained in 50 degrees hyperextension, he could perform most precision patterns and his hand was functional.

All standard splints were unacceptable to Mr. Hanson, who stated that he would "feel like a sissy" and would not wear any of them in front of his friends. The solution was to fabricate a splint from a tablespoon, which was bent and angled to the correct medical alignment. The spoon was then riveted to a wide leather wrist band. Mr. Hanson wore the splint daily and enjoyed joking with his friends that he was "always looking for a meal." This adaptation was the change that convinced the patient to wear the appliance.

Case Study 11

Mrs. Nadeau was 60 years old when she had a stroke, which resulted in left hemiparesis. She had slight subluxation of the left shoulder. Shoulder subluxations are common, as the pull of gravity on the paralyzed or weakened limb frequently causes the ligaments surrounding a joint to stretch and the head of the humerus to pull out of the socket. Hemiplegic arm slings are sometimes recommended during ambulation to prevent this condition. These slings are very noticeable and not very attractive.

The patient was a very well-dressed, fashion-conscious woman of financial means. She frequently met with friends for luncheons and other social gatherings at her country club. Wearing the sling was an embarrassment for her. The solution involved adapting a leather shoulder bag to wear on these occasions. The bag was strong and large enough to support her forearm, and the strap was adjusted to a length that would support the humeral head in the shoulder joint. A wooden handle was attached to the bag, which maintained Mrs. Nadeau's wrist in hyperextension and held her thumb in opposition.

Consideration of these individual values and self-images enabled the OT to use everyday objects to fabricate necessary medical appliances in a form that was acceptable to both of the patients and compatible with their lifestyles.

Each OT and OTA has values, standards, and attitudes that may be in direct conflict with those of the patient, thus making it difficult to work with some individuals as noted in the example that follows.

Case Study 12

An OT was working one half day per week in a very small, rural general hospital. When she reported for work, she found 4 treatment requests for one patient, Mr. Smithe. Two were referrals from physicians requesting immediate initiation of feeding and toileting activities. There were also memoranda from the director of nursing and the hospital administrator requesting the same services. Mr. Smithe had been admitted for prostate surgery. He refused to use the toilet in his room, preferring instead a small, rectangular, plastic-lined wastepaper basket.

The patient was seen for an initial evaluation during the lunch hour. The meal consisted of cube steak with gravy, mashed potatoes, carrots, and a dish of sherbet. Mr. Smithe used no utensils; he ate with his fingers and licked up some foods. This behavior, together with his lip smacking and belching noises, was in total violation of the therapist's standards and values, as well as those of 2 female aides who cleaned up the food scatterings on the bed.

Limited information was available in Mr. Smithe's medical record. In addition to the problems discussed previously, nursing notes indicated that his behavior was that of a very hostile and angry person. It was difficult to determine whether Mr. Smithe was experiencing mental changes that required psychiatric intervention, whether his behavior was a reflected form of his personal lifestyle, or whether a combination of both was involved. Intake records revealed that Mr. Smithe refused to state his age or financial status.

Since there was no social worker available, the OT was requested to gather additional information from neighbors and the community. Mr. Smithe was described by his neighbors as an antisocial recluse. He had lived for at least 40 years in a large old toolshed on the back acres of a farm, which was a long distance from town. There had been windows in the building; however, he had covered them with roofing material many years ago. His home had no electricity or running water. He was always piling up wood and rubbish, so the neighbors felt certain that he had some sort of stove for cooking and heating.

The therapist visited a small grocery store nearby to see if Mr. Smithe bought food there. It was reported that he had indeed shopped there as long as the elderly owners remember. Mr. Smithe would slip a grocery list under the door and specify when he would pick up the items. He always paid in cash and requested that no females be present when he came to the store. He would talk with the male owner and periodically try new products that he recommended. If the owner's wife or other females were present, Mr. Smithe would slip in the back entrance, grab his groceries, pay, and leave hurriedly. With this information, the therapist made the following changes when she returned to the hospital:

- A male orderly was assigned to the patient.
- Mr. Smithe was informed that he could eat in any manner he chose; however, he would have to change his own linen. He began to cover himself with a large towel when eating and folded it neatly when finished.
- A portable commode was placed in his room. He liked it and stated that he had disliked the coldness of the toilet seat and the loud rushing of water. He also disliked 2 females taking him to the bathroom.

If Mr. Smithe had recently developed this lifestyle, intervention techniques may have been different. When an OT or OTA encounters a lifestyle that has existed for over 40 years, it requires different consideration. At times it can be difficult to understand how persons living in the same general environment respond in such highly individualized manners.

CHANGE AND ITS IMPACT

Changes in lifestyles, roles, and activity levels occur throughout the life cycle. Normal changes are expected at various ages. For example, a child is expected to walk and talk at a certain age, and a young adult is expected to begin a career when he or she has completed the necessary education.

Changes can be self-imposed or superimposed on an individual. Self-imposed and superimposed changes and their resulting influence on the individual can occur over a prolonged period or they can be very sudden. The length of time and timing of such change have an impact to varying degrees on lifestyles, roles, self-image, and activity levels.

Retirement, whether self-imposed or superimposed, is a change that affects most aspects of a person's life. Many professionals are becoming involved in pre-retirement planning. These programs are designed to help people consider the various aspects of their life and plan ahead. The emphasis is on all important areas, not just financial planning.

Stress

The potential for stress is inherent with any change. Individuals react very differently to what appears to be the same stress situation. People who have explored different environments and adapted to change may have some sense of mastery over their environment. They can recall and apply previous actions and thoughts that either worked successfully or were ineffective. This provides them with more resources and information to plan an action and respond appropriately.

John and Darlene: Follow-Up

Both John and Darlene will be experiencing significant changes in their environment. These changes will affect their activities, roles, and lifestyles. John's decision to relocate in Duluth is a self-imposed change. He has given a lot of thought to this decision to move and start a new career. This cognitive planning has prepared him for the changes in his environment, new roles, and a markedly different lifestyle from the one he has established on the farm.

Darlene's future change had been superimposed on her by her parent's decision to move. She must now identify and evaluate alternatives and make a decision. She could locate a place of her own or move to Florida with her parents. These 2 alternatives offer very different considerations in terms of finances, employment, social status, and activities, as well as the total physical environment.

As these changes occur, they will create stress for both John and Darlene. Individuals who have made significant changes in the past often find that they can draw on these past events in terms of future decision making and adjustment.

Severe Disruptions

Disruptions are sudden changes in a person's environment that require immediate attention and response. They are usually superimposed on an individual. Disruptions can be as simple and temporary as a common cold or loss of a job, or as complex and permanent as a stroke or death of a loved one. Most disruptions are high stress situations for the individual directly affected. Disruptions can also directly affect and cause stress for other persons in the client's environment.

Case Study 13

Michael, a mentally retarded young man functioning at about a 5-year-old level, had a severe disruption when his parents were in an automobile accident. Due to multiple injuries they both sustained and the length of time needed for rehabilitation, it was necessary to move Michael from his home to an institution. Michael's reaction to this abrupt change was evidenced by withdrawal and frequent tantrums. The OT at the facility visited the parents in the hospital to gain information that might assist in helping Michael to adjust to his new environment. She learned that Michael had particular food preferences, had favorite television programs, and enjoyed hearing bedtime stories. Other details of his daily routine were discussed. The therapist then made the appropriate changes in Michael's daily regimen, and Michael discontinued his tantrums and began relating to others.

SUMMARY

It is much easier for health care personnel to treat arthritis, a hand injury, a personality disorder, a suicide attempt, or an amputee than to treat the whole person. The latter requires knowledge and insight about the individual's development, values, lifestyles, environments, self-images, roles, and activities in planning and implementing purposeful and meaningful therapeutic programs.

The goal of OT is to return the person to his or her environment with the skills necessary to resume previous occupations and roles. OT is concerned with the quality of life, which is determined by the individual and his or her environment. The relationship between humans and their environs goes far beyond the simple stimulus-and-response theory. A total transaction occurs between the individual and the external and internal circumstances that make up the person's unique environment.

To effectively treat a person and not a disability, all members of the profession must know the sociocultural, economic, psychological, and physical aspects and view them in relation to the standards, values, and attitudes of the patient's total environment. OTs and assistants are performance specialists who design and implement highly individualized developmental, remediation, and prevention programs.

LEARNING ACTIVITIES

1. Identify some of the customs, traditions, or superstitions in your family and discuss how they might affect therapy.

2. Working with a peer, compare and contrast how your plan for therapy might be different in each of the following instances:

Patient Condition	*Patient Environment*
Arthritis	Well-to-do matron
	Bag lady
Stroke	Rancher in Texas
	Accountant in Chicago
Depression	Cambodian refugee
	American suburban housewife

3. Discuss common misuse and disuse syndromes with a classmate or peer. Determine what intervention techniques are likely to be most effective.

REFERENCES

American Occupational Therapy Association. (1979). *The philosophical base of occupational therapy, Resolution #531.* Bethesda, MD: Author.

American Occupational Therapy Association. (2002). The occupational therapy practice framework: Domain and process. *American Journal of Occupational Therapy, 56,* 609-633.

Guralnik, D. B. (1994). *Webster's new world dictionary.* New York, NY: Simon and Schuster.

Moyers, P. (1999). *Guide to occupational therapy practice.* Bethesda, MD: American Occupational Therapy Association.

Reed, K., & Saunderson, S. (1999). *Concepts of OT.* Baltimore, MD: Williams & Wilkins.

Key Concepts

- Learning: Acquiring knowledge or skill.
- Experiential learning: Learning through life experiences.
- Teaching and learning principles: Developed by Mosey to address learning in OT treatment.

Essential Vocabulary

Allen's cognitive levels: System to establish cognitive functioning from severely disabled to normal functioning.
andragogy: The study of adult education.
pedagogy: The study of teaching children.
transfer of training: The ability to take a learned skill or behavior and transfer it to other life needs.

TEACHING AND LEARNING

Karen Sladyk, PhD, OTR, FAOTA

INTRODUCTION

Everyone thinks they understand teaching and learning. After all, if you have a high school diploma, you have had at least 13 years of teaching and learning experience. If you have any additional schooling, you have had even more experience with the topic. But teaching and learning is much more than learning in school. Even for the healthy adult, who may never need rehabilitation services, most of what he or she "knows" did not come from school. In fact, when adults are asked to list everything they have learned and where they learned it, only about 25% of the list was learned in school (Sheckley, 1984). All the rest (75%) was learned experientially in life. This experiential learning fits nicely with OT because experiential learning is life bound and the occupation of OT is life bound as well.

Just because we learn through our life experiences does not mean that scholars have not tried to capture the educational experience. Just as there are many frames of reference in OT, there are many educational theories in learning. This chapter will briefly look at educational theories, Mosey's concepts on teaching and learning, Allen's view of cognitive disabilities, and applications in OT.

THEORIES IN ADULT LEARNING

Vast and numerous books have been written about educational theories. This section will look at theories specific to adults, commonly called *andragogy*. The educational foundations of your schooling through high school were based on pediatric theories, often called *pedagogy*. If you remember your medical terminology classes, you can see the word root focuses on the child or the adult.

Adults like to learn in different ways than do children. You may still use some of the skills learned in grade school in adulthood, such as making flashcards or lists for reminders, but you do not likely use every skill learned earlier now that you are an adult. Sometimes, teachers that use pedagogy techniques on adults actually insult the adult learner. An example of this is an experience I had recently.

Feeling that I was isolating myself in my work, I signed up for a holiday cookie class at the local adult education program. On the first night, I learned that we would be baking cookies in "teams of 3" and that there would be no cookies to take home because the class always ate them all. I was disappointed but I went along. My baking partners were significantly older than I was and they already had ideas of what we should make for the next week, so again I went along. After planning all the ingredients, I was sent to our assigned kitchen to find the 9x13-inch pan for next week. When I returned to the table with the pan, the teacher asked, "How do you know the size?" I started to explain how I estimated a 1-foot measurement then added an inch. I was handed a ruler to double check. I started to measure the bottom of the pan when one of my partners insisted I turn the pan over to measure the top. The pan was a half-inch short. I thought to myself, I'm here to relax, not worry over small details like this. I left the class and promptly withdrew. This educational experience had not met my needs.

I told this story to everyone at work the next day and besides all the ribbing I took from my peers, one physical therapist offered to show me how she makes her famous biscotti cookies. That was a perfect match for me. She showed me what I wanted and needed to know, not drilled me as I learned. Because of how I learned these skills, I was able to "transfer my training" to other tasks. The experience was positive.

The important lesson here is that adults learn differently. Some even like to learn the way they did in primary or secondary school, however, others want different approaches. The key to teaching adults is flexibility and continual assessment of meeting their learning needs.

Adult learners are a widely diverse group that encompasses many different styles, goals, and experiences (Cross, 1988). Understanding some of the major characteristics of this group can lead to more effective application of knowledge and transfer of learning to life situations. When interpreting major characteristics of adult learning, caution should be made to avoid labeling a diverse group with limited characteristics.

We live in a complex society in which continual learning is no longer a luxury, but a necessity (Cross, 1988; Wlodkowski, 1990). Adults are independent thinkers with a variety of thought and experiences that come with them when they embark on new learning. Addressing this diversity of experience and needs will help the educator or therapist succeed.

Adults come to each learning experience with an integration of all prior learning experience (Kolb, 1984). For example, if a teenager had negative experiences in high school, he is likely to come to a vocational training program with negative feelings. If a patient has had positive experiences all during her rehabilitation program, she is likely to be open to new experiences in an outpatient clinic. Formal and informal experiences (Bandura, 1978) are included in this integration of experiences, so academic success in the past is more than just good grades. It includes interactions with teachers, parents, and peers. As the adult gets older, work experiences are added to this integration. Have you ever been "forced" to go to a work inservice that was way over your head or so simple it was a waste of time?

Brookfield (1990) points out that adults learn best in situations of mutual respect. Fostering the growth of the learner along a path to an ideal goal is the job of the teacher. He advocates that teachers help students identify and challenge assumptions and context, imagine and explore alternatives, and view knowledge with reflective skepticism.

Simply providing the learner with information does not foster the transfer of knowledge. This learning situation does not foster mutual respect and clearly makes the teacher the powerful partner with "all the knowledge."

Chaffee (1998) says that the key to successful adult thinking consists of 8 steps:

1. Think critically.
2. Live creatively.
3. Choose freely.
4. Solve problems effectively.
5. Communicate effectively.
6. Analyze complex issues.
7. Develop enlightened values.
8. Think through relationships.

He encourages adults to transform themselves through thinking and to create a life philosophy to follow. This requires a strong commitment to self-analysis that many adults cannot call upon because of other factors.

Adult behavior is an interaction of person and environment (Bandura, 1978). Although most people believe that the learner's responsibility is to learn, the learner will act on his or her learning within the structure of his or her environment. In some cultures, women are not expected to be learners. Teaching a person from this environment may be extremely difficult.

When addressing the unique learning needs of adults, several themes emerge. Adults have an educational history that may be positive or not. Adults learn through their experiences (experiential learning). Motivation can support learning; however, adults typically learn within their own environments. Mutual respect plays an important role in adult learning. All of these factors can influence the transfer of training to life situations. All of these factors, if negative, can cause a negative loop that is recursive and self-fulfilling. The goal of the teacher is to manage these factors in a way that is positive to the adult learner.

Mosey's Teaching-Learning Process

Although teaching and learning have been a part of OT from the beginning, Mosey's (1986) book on psychosocial OT was one of the first to link educational theory and psychological theory with OT treatment. She details 16 principles to guide therapist/patient interaction in learning. She reminds practitioners that learning principles do not provide firm rules, but provide a base to begin to facilitate learning. A principle may carry more importance with one person than another. The therapist's judgment is the key to patient success. The following guidelines are adapted from Mosey's (1986) work:

When teaching in OT treatment, the practitioner will:

- Use good communication skills—Collaboration is a valued aspect of the therapeutic relationship that begins with the practitioner using good communication skills. The therapist should sit squarely toward the patient without crossing arms or legs. Good, comfortable eye contact and a relaxed approach will make the patient comfortable. Use open-ended questions in patient conversations. Open-ended questions are questions that require more than a one-word answer. This type of question should comprise the majority of the therapist's questions. Use open-ended questions to probe for details about a patient's life. For example, "What about that activity makes you tired, Seth?" Use closed-ended questions carefully and only when you need a specific answer. For example, "Where does the splint cause you pain, Annie?"

- Accept the client for who he or she is—All human beings have the right to good health. The practitioner should keep biases in check and be reflective of any behavior that appears judgmental. Remain the professional in the relationship and avoid behaviors that reflect friendship on a nonprofessional level.

- Begin treatment at the consumer's current level—This allows the person initial success before moving onto the next level. When the person is ready for the next level, provide what Allen, Earhart, and Blue (1992) call the "just-right challenge." Remember, everyone learns at different rates.

- Acknowledge the patient's current culture and environment—This can include heritage, country of origin, age, gender, and memberships. The person's assets and limitations are important to address in light of his or her culture and environment. All of these factors can have a positive and/or negative influence on returning to health. For example, membership in a street gang or social club can hinder a person remaining alcohol free, but membership in a church or fitness club can help.

- Communicate effectively in volume and pace—Consider how you are saying something as well as what you are saying. Patients with hearing problems usually hear better with their eyeglasses on because they pick up on the visual clues of speech. Confused patients perform better with simple, clear cues, such as "open the toothpaste."

- Encourage the learner to be an active learner—Empower the client to be the leader of his or her treatment. Encourage learning with all the sensorimotor components to reinforce the task.
- Control the consequences of learning—Pleasurable experiences reinforce the consumer to want to learn again. Always process the experience whether in a group or individually after the learning experience. Provide opportunities to make errors and then discuss how things could go better next time. If need be, stop an experience if safety is an issue because safety is always addressed first in treatment.
- Provide an opportunity for trial and error—This is empowering for the patient when consequences are controlled. Use first and last experiences to demonstrate how far the patient has improved. Stay open-minded to ways the patient wants to "try something out." The patient may know better than the practitioner.
- Provide opportunity for practice and repetition—No one likes to learn something by rote memory, but opportunities to practice skills provide mastery. Just like trial and error, use the first and last experiences to show the client his or her progress.
- Encourage the consumer to set his or her own goals—Too often practitioners write treatment goals in patient's records and the patients participated very little in the planning process. A practitioner should never solely develop goals for a patient even when goals may be influenced by insurance reviewers. The patient should always work with the therapist in developing goals for him- or herself because of motivation and responsibility. The practitioner's expertise is making sure the patient's goals are not too high or too low.
- Practice skills in different situations—Learning is often specific to an experience but practice in different situations allows the client to generalize the skill or transfer the training. For example, the electric dryer in the ADL kitchen is different from the electric dryer in the client's home or the gas dryer in the local laundromat.
- The learner should understand what is being learned—Too often the consumer does not understand what is being learned. This is especially true for head injured or confused patients. Too many times this leads to the patient making negative statements about OT, including to the media, who repeat the story without knowing the details of the situation. The practitioner must repeat the purpose of the task until he or she is sure the patient understands. Check for understanding during the processing stage of treatment to see the patient's understanding. Educate staff, family, and friends at every available opportunity.
- Learning moves from simple to complex—This integrates earlier discussions of helping clients succeed throughout their treatment process. The idea of learning moving from simple to complex is nicely illustrated by the rating system for ski slopes—bunny trail to black diamond.
- Encourage creative problem solving—Often times traditional approaches to a problem may not be the right answer for clients with nontraditional issues. The practitioner should role model and encourage his or her consumer to "think outside of the box."
- Acknowledge that everyone handles stress and anxiety differently—Learning is frustrating, stressful, and anxiety-producing. Remember anatomy exams? Learners deal with this stress in different ways. Some "shut down" and become very quiet. Some get loud and angry. Some get the giggles and laugh at everything. The practitioner needs to watch for signs that learning is causing stress or anxiety and process this information with the client.

LEARNING WITH A COGNITIVE DISABILITY

The cognitive disabilities frame of reference was developed on the belief that some patients have cognitive disabilities due to a biological or chemical defect in the brain. Because of this disability, cognitive functioning is impaired (Allen et al., 1992). These cognitive disabilities result in a decrease in the person's ability to learn. OT can assist with adaptation to maximize functioning but cannot improve cognitive functioning unless the patient has demonstrated a prior higher level. Medication can sometimes help improve functioning.

Allen's Cognitive Level Test (Allen et al., 1992) is a task-based assessment that provides information on a patient's cognitive functioning. Cognitive functioning is measured on a scale from 1 to 6, with 1 indicating severe impairment and 6 indicating normal cognitive functioning. In addition, each level is subdivided into smaller units to allow for scoring between levels. For example, a patient may score 4.6.

Each level indicates a higher level of cognitive functioning and is briefly summarized here:
- Level 1—Conscious but profoundly disabled. Stares, may sit, walk, or chew with simple commands. Needs 24-hour nursing care.
- Level 2—Actions related to comfort or discomfort. Short attention span of less than 10 minutes. May wander or be resistant to caregiver assistance. Needs 24-hour nursing care.
- Level 3—Manual actions. Pointless or destructive manipulation of objects. Behavior may be inappropriate or not goal-directed. Needs cues to groom.
- Level 4—Goal-directed with cues. Pace is slow and person pays little attention to environment. Needs support in community, as plans are often unrealistic.
- Level 5—Trial and error problem-solving. Often impulsive or careless. Fails to see consequences of behaviors, especially long-term.
- Level 6—Plans ahead. Thinks ahead before acting and can predict consequences of behavior. Independent and organized (Allen et al., 1992).

The cognitive level of a patient can help guide the practitioner in developing treatment goals (Allen et al., 1992). Patients with lower cognitive levels benefit most from changes to the environment to keep them safe. Patients with fluctuating cognitive functioning benefit from further evaluation and tasks that provide the just-right challenge. Patients with higher level scores benefit from learning activities within their cognitive functioning (Allen et al., 1992).

APPLICATION OF LEARNING THEORIES

Teaching and learning have been a foundation for OT from its early history. There are as many different theories on learning as there are different types of OT consumers. Choosing the right approach to each consumer requires clinical reasoning skills (Mattingly & Fleming, 1994). The practitioner must consider the procedures he or she is using, his or her interaction with the patient, and his or her understanding of the patient's world all at the same time. Learning theories can assist the therapist in his or her clinical reasoning.

Case 1

You are the OT personnel for a vocational program for young men leaving prison. This program accepts men 19 to 21 years old who have had one incarceration and a good behavior record while in prison. The vocational program trains these young men in cable TV installation and has an excellent record of job placement and work history. Your job is to evaluate basic skills in ADL and pre-work skills. You often find that your clients hold a high school diploma but lack skills in reading and social skills needed on the job. They are often resistive to "learning."

Discussion

Understand how the principles of adult learning can be applied here. Your clients are likely bringing with them negative learning experiences that have reinforced a negative attitude about new learning. What motivating factors might you use? What principles of Mosey's work might be useful?

Case 2

You are the primary practitioner for a home-based Alzheimer's program. This community-based program aims to keep cognitively impaired clients at home as long as possible. You work closely with an OT who comes in for periodic patient evaluation and provides collaborative supervision as you need it. Other members of the team include nursing, home health aides, and a physical therapist assistant. The team is concerned that a patient is no longer safe at home. He has wandered out of the home several times and locked his wife outside in the cold when she went to get the mail. His vision appears to be decreasing because he has had 2 recent falls. You ask the OT to come in for an evaluation and she uses the ACL test, modified with large holes. The patient scores a 2.4. Other professionals evaluate the client and agree that 24-hour nursing care is required. The problem is that his wife does not believe this and wants to keep him home because of their wedding vows. "I can teach him what he needs to stay safe, he trusts me," she says. She is clearly showing the strain of his care on her health.

Discussion

This is an interesting case because it involves learning on many levels. Allen et al. (1992) show us that a person functioning at 2.4 is not capable of learning even from someone he trusts. The 2.4 score is slightly higher than a 2.0 but can still require 24-hour nursing care. However, at this time, the patient's wife cannot see or understand his functioning.

Let's look specifically at the wife's learning. What reasons could be interfering with a clearer objective view of her husband's functioning? First reaction might say guilt, but this does not explain everything. She may have negative attitudes from earlier experiences about nursing homes that she brings to this experience. Similar to the young men in the case above, this appears in a "resistive" attitude. She may not understand the cognitive decline of her husband. The OT and OTA can work together to explain the process using Mosey's principles of learning. What other resources could the OTA call upon to assist the wife in objectively evaluating the home situation? How would the OTA use learning theories to prepare these other resources to address issues with the wife?

SUMMARY

Teaching and learning is a complex process of mutual respect, sharing information, guiding progress, and understanding adults. Educational theories help OT practitioners understand and practice teaching in treatment. OTs, including Mosey and Allen, help explain teaching and learning from the perspective of patient needs.

LEARNING ACTIVITIES

1. Students will teach a simple craft to classmates in 20-minute "groups." Evaluate the leader using Mosey's principles.

2. Go to preschool and senior centers to teach the same simple task. Write a reaction paper contrasting the experiences.

3. Show the class the ACL assessment and have them learn the single cordovan stitch. Discuss how difficult this stitch is to learn as the practitioner. Remind the class that not everyone is a level 6 24 hours a day.

4. Discuss a client from level I fieldwork in class. What teaching and learning theories or principles are an issue for that client?

5. Teach a simple task to the class using only demonstration or only verbal instruction. Discuss the differences.

References

Allen, C. K., Earhart, C. A., & Blue, T. (1992). *OT treatment goals for the physically and cognitively disabled*. Bethesda, MD: American Occupational Therapy Association.

Bandura, A. (1978). The self system in reciprocal determinism. *American Psychologist, 4,* 344-357.

Brookfield, S. D. (1990). *Understanding and facilitating adult learning*. San Francisco, CA: Jossey-Bass Publishers.

Chaffee, J. (1998). *The thinker's way: 8 steps to a richer life*. Boston, MA: Little, Brown and Co.

Cross, K. P. (1988). *Adults as learners*. San Francisco, CA: Jossey-Bass Publishers.

Kolb, D. A. (1984). *Experiential learning*. Englewood Cliffs, NJ: Prentice-Hall.

Mattingly, C., & Fleming, M. H. (1994). *Clinical reasoning: Forms of inquiry in therapeutic practice*. Philadelphia, PA: F. A. Davis Co.

Mosey, A. C. (1986). *Psychosocial components of OT*. New York, NY: Raven Press.

Sheckley, B. G. (1984). The adult as learner: A case for making higher education more responsive to the individual learner. Two part series. *CAEL News, 7*(8) and 8(1).

Wlodkowski, R. J. (1990). *Enhancing adult motivation to learn*. San Francisco, CA: Jossey-Bass Publishers.

OCCUPATIONS AND DISABILITIES

Key Concepts

- Early intervention laws: Laws providing services for newborns to 3 year olds.
- Family-centered approach: The family, and not just the child, is the consumer.
- Cultural implications: Performance context is specific to each family.
- Developmental evaluation: Children with visual impairments often have developmental delays.
- Program goals and objectives: Specific behavioral goals for treatment.
- Play and feeding activities: Encourage developmental skills.
- School adaptations: Providing learning in the most supportive environment.
- Transition planning: Promoting skills to transition to other areas of life.

Essential Vocabulary

Individualized Education Plan (IEP): Multidisciplinary, student-centered education plan documenting the student's present level of performance and how the student's educational needs will be met through special education, regular education, and related services.

Individualized Family Service Plan (IFSP): Multidisciplinary, family-centered treatment plan documenting how the infant's or toddler's developmental and family needs will be addressed through early intervention services.

Individualized Transition Plan (ITP): Plan of activities and instruction, based on student's individual needs, that will promote transition from school to postschool activities; ITP must be documented in student's IEP by age 14.

Clinical Summary

Etiology

"[Retinopathy of prematurity] ROP results from vascular damage to the retina.... In premature infants, this [retinal] blood vessel growth is incomplete. In the catching-up process, a ridge can develop, with some blood vessels growing into the vitreous (toward the center of the eye) instead of along the back wall of the eye on the retinal surface. These abnormal blood vessels eventually die, and the resultant scar tissue can constrict, pulling on the retina. This pulling can lead to a retinal detachment and loss of vision" (Miller, Menacker, & Batshaw, 2002, p. 174).

Prevalence

"Nearly one quarter of infants weighing less than 2,500 grams at birth will develop some degree of ROP... Despite treatment, many children with ROP will have visual impairments. These may include poor central vision, nearsightedness (myopia), strabismus, glaucoma, and even blindness" (Miller et al., 2002, pp. 174-175).

Classic Signs

- Infant doesn't visually fixate on people's faces or objects.
- Atypical eye movements or fixed gaze in one direction.
- Lack of response to bright lights (Miller et al., 2002, p. 185).

Precautions/Prevention

- Prevention of premature births.
- Use of lowest possible oxygen supplementation.
- Laser therapy or cryotherapy to prevent retinal detachment.
- Ophthalmological screening of premature infants (Miller et al., 2002, p. 174).

A Young Child With Visual Impairments

Chapter 11

Angela E. Scoggin, PhD, OTR, FAOTA; Dickson Rodriguez, MA-CVRT, OTR;
Mary Kathryn Cowan, MA, OTR, FAOTA; and Patricia K. Benham, MPH, OTR

Introduction

This chapter discusses a case study of a young child with a visual impairment within the context of early intervention services based on a family-centered model of care. Federal legislation that impacts services provided to children ages birth to 3 years and their families will be reviewed.

Concisely stated, "Visual impairments can result from problems with any part of the visual system, including the eyes, eye muscles, optic nerve, or the area of the cerebral cortex that processes visual information" (Gersh, 1991, p. 69). In order to be classified as legally blind in the United States, an individual must have 20/200 or poorer corrected visual acuity in the best eye or a visual field of 20 degrees or less. While a child with normal vision can clearly see a particular object that is 200 feet away, the legally blind child, with glasses or other correction, must be only 20 feet away to see the object with the same clarity. This means that the individual would most probably see shapes but not details. The definition of legal blindness is also met if the child's peripheral vision is limited to 20 degrees or less rather than the over 180 degrees in a normal visual field (Snow, 1996). A child classified as having low vision has acuity, or visual clarity, of 20/70 or poorer with correction. It is important to note that these criteria for measuring vision were developed with adults, and that measuring vision in infants and young children cannot be as precise and will also require observation of functional vision used during daily activities (Senitz, Bride, Adrian, & Semmler, 1990).

Although there are numerous factors that may be associated with visual impairments in infants and young children, hereditary disorders and the effects of prematurity are the most common causes (Senitz et al., 1990). Some of the most common conditions in children treated by OT practitioners include ROP (also referred to as retrolental fibroplasia), cataracts, and cortical blindness/visual impairment. ROP may occur in extremely premature infants, especially those with medical complications and those exposed to excessive oxygen. Children with healed ROP are also more likely to have myopia, strabismus, and amblyopia. In myopia, also referred to as nearsightedness, the child has much better vision at close range than farther away.

The child with strabismus demonstrates an inability of the eyes to converge on the same image. The term *amblyopia* refers to decreased vision most often resulting from the brain suppressing the visual image to one eye in order to prevent double vision (Berkow, 1992).

Chromosomal abnormalities and maternal diseases, such as rubella during pregnancy, are the most common causes of congenital cataracts. Congenital cataracts result in a cloudy or opaque, rather than clear, lens of the eye and require early surgical removal, followed by the use of visual correction such as glasses for the infant (Berkow, 1992). In cortical visual impairment (previously referred to as cortical blindness), the child's vision is functionally impaired because the visual cortex of the brain cannot process the visual information received from the eyes. This condition results from extensive neurological damage, as seen in children with severe cerebral palsy or victims of near drowning (Snow, 1996).

Regarding terminology, the term *blind* is only appropriate for someone who has no vision. The term *visual impairment* is most commonly used for children who have some residual vision, while the term *low vision* more commonly refers to adults/older adults who have lost visual abilities through conditions such as macular degeneration, glaucoma, or cataracts.

The Impact of Visual Impairment on Occupational Performance of Children

The effects of early visual impairment on a child's performance of occupational roles and activities vary greatly according to the extent of the visual impairment itself, as well as the number and extent of accompanying disabilities. However, considering visual impairment alone, it is known that developmental motor delays are common when infants with blindness are compared to sighted children (Adelson & Fraiberg, 1977). Touch and sound must provide the stimuli for reaching and movement behaviors in children with visual impairment, which will lead to normal play in infancy, and these do not stimulate the child to reach or move as early as visual stimuli will with sighted children (Senitz et al., 1990). Many social behaviors are learned through the visual experience, and then imitation of that experience occurs as the child evaluates his or her social world and develops his or her own repertoire of social behavior. Early visual impairment in and of itself is not a cause of any occupational performance problems, but rather an obstacle to overcome so that a child's true performance abilities may be developed and utilized and further disability prevented.

Occupational Performance Areas Affected by Visual Impairment

- Self-care—The development of independence in eating, drinking, and dressing may be delayed because children with visual impairment from birth may not have developed the necessary motor skills required for each task, or they have been unable to imitate the performance of other children or adults due to the lack of vision. Other areas of self-care that may be affected as the child gets older are the social aspects of grooming, eating in social situations, selecting food in cafeterias and stores, and mobility in the community.
- Play—Children with visual impairment may have underdeveloped play skills due to delays in motor/mobility skills, lack of exploratory behavior, or stimulation from the environment.
- School—As the child develops and attends primary and elementary school, mobility in the new environment can be limited by visual impairment, and all school skills that usually require vision will need to be monitored. These activities include reading and all materials presented in a visual manner (worksheets, instruction on a blackboard, teacher demonstration, etc.) and developing a method of communication through written format. Additionally, potential areas of limitation may also include the visual and social aspects of lunch and recess activities.

Occupational Performance Skills Affected by Visual Impairment

Although sensorimotor, cognitive, and personal/social performance skills are not part of the disability of visual impairment, a lack of development in these performance skills can occur if a child does not receive adequate environmental and interpersonal stimulation during infancy and early childhood. When other disabilities such as neurological impairment exist along with a diagnosis of early visual impairment or blindness, there can be significant impairment in sensorimotor, cognitive, and personal/social abilities from birth.

FRAMES OF REFERENCE

The *Occupational Therapy Practice Framework: Domain and Process* (AOTA, 2002, p. 615) states that "'engagement in occupation' is viewed as the overarching outcome of the occupa-

tional therapy process." Models that provide a theoretical framework for an occupation-centered approach include the Person-Environment-Occupation Model, the Model of Human Occupation, Person-Environment-Performance, Ecology of Human Performance, and Occupational Adaptation (Law, Missiuna, Pollock, & Stewart, 2001). Each of these models focuses on occupational performance and contextual factors and provides a framework for a top-down approach to assessment and treatment that can be the basis for the OT process for all individuals seen in OT.

Specific frames of reference/models that appear to be most appropriate for children born with severe visual impairment, and that can be congruent with the occupation-centered frameworks listed above, include the developmental and occupational behavior frames of reference and the coping model. The developmental frame of reference, as developed by Lela Llorens, views OT as the facilitator of development, which will help the child master each developmental life task and the ability to cope with life expectations. The occupational behavior frame, as developed by Mary Reilly, emphasizes play as the occupation of children, and within the world of play the child develops basic mastery and competence of all skills needed during the child's lifetime (Law et al., 2001). The coping model encourages self-initiation and the development of coping strategies to effectively deal with new challenges and learning. During intervention:

> The therapist continually evaluates whether the child's skills (internal resources) and environmental supports (external resources) are adequate to meet the demands of the activity. When the child exhibits ineffective coping strategies, the therapist adjusts the task demands and provides more human or environmental supports to enable the child to succeed in his or her coping efforts. (Law et al., 2001. p. 55)

If a child with visual impairment has other disabilities present, then neurodevelopmental, sensory integrative, and biomechanical frames of reference must be considered.

AMERICAN OCCUPATIONAL THERAPY ASSOCIATION POLICY, PUBLIC LAW, AND EARLY INTERVENTION SERVICE

AOTA supports the provision of early intervention services using a family-centered approach that incorporates professional collaboration, as outlined in *Position Paper: Occupational Therapy Services in Early Intervention and Preschool Services* (AOTA, 1998). Children make the most progress when their needs are constantly viewed within the context of the family. Purposeful, self-initiated activities continue to be the cornerstone of OT treatment, but parents are encouraged to actively participate in their child's treatment plan and to take satisfaction in their occupational roles as parents. OT practitioners strive for "best practice" by providing state-of-the-art treatment approaches while developing new and innovative strategies to better meet the needs of infants and their families. Prevention as well as intervention is stressed, and OT practitioners collaborate with community agencies to assist families in the many transitions that they face at this stage in their children's lives.

The position of AOTA is in agreement with the federal mandates regarding early intervention services. The U.S. Congress first enacted the Education of the Handicapped Act (EHA), also called P.L. 94-142, in 1975. This act mandated that public schools provide educational services for children with disabilities (Part B) and gave the states options for developing early intervention systems for infants, toddlers, and their families (Part H). Congress amended EHA in 1990, changing the name to the Individuals with Disabilities Education Act (IDEA) (Maruyama et al., 1999). The most recent amendments of IDEA, authorized in 1997, place increased emphasis on transition planning for school to work, team collaboration, and justification for instances when the child is placed in settings that do not include peers without disabilities. Mandates for early intervention are now included in Part C of IDEA. Other changes include the use of the terms *service coordinator* instead of *case manager* and *adaptive behavior* instead of *self-care* (Maruyama et al., 1999).

The purpose of IDEA is to ensure that children with disabilities ages 3 through 21 receive a free appropriate public education in the least restrictive environment. Part B addresses the needs of children with disabilities ages 3 through 21. Part H (now included in Part C) is the Early Intervention Program for Infants and Toddlers with Disabilities. It provides states with financial assistance to "...develop and implement a statewide, comprehensive, coordinated, multidisciplinary, interagency system of early intervention services for infants and toddlers with disabilities and their families; facilitate the coordination of payment for early intervention services from Federal, State, local and private sources" (34C.F.R. 303.1 [a][b], as cited in Maruyama et al., 1999, p. 13).

Since each state develops it own early intervention system, OT practitioners must be aware of the regulations and guidelines for the states in which they practice.

OT is a primary service in early intervention programs and a related service for children 3 through 21 years who are served through the public school system. As a primary service, OT can be provided either alone or in combination with other early intervention services to eligible children ages birth through 2 years. The goal of services is to enhance the child's functional ability and prevent or minimize future impairment by meeting the needs of the child and family as they relate to the child's development. Early intervention mandates require a multidisciplinary team model and a family-centered approach. Services should be provided in the child's natural environments and are based on a collaboratively developed IFSP. Eligible children include those who are developmentally delayed or who have a diagnosed condition that places them at risk of developmental delay (Maruyama et al., 1999).

In contrast, OT, as a related service under Part B of IDEA, is provided to children with identified disabilities who need OT in order to benefit from special education. A multidisciplinary, student-focused team model addresses the child's educational needs. Service delivery should be conducted in the least restrictive environment and in a regular educational setting with nondisabled peers to the maximum possible extent. Each child must have a written IEP that outlines how the student's educational needs will be met and how the school will ensure that needed services are provided (Maruyama et al., 1999).

Other federal legislation that may impact the OT practitioner working with infants and young children includes the Head Start Act of 1964. The Head Start program may assign at least 10% of its placements to preschoolers with disabilities. Additionally, the Early Head Start program provides family-centered services for low-income families with children age birth through 2 years. Title XIX of the Social Security Act of 1965 (Medicaid) and the Americans with Disabilities Act of 1990 (ADA) are additional federal laws that are relevant for OT service provision (Maruyama et al., 1999).

CASE STUDY

The following case study has been adapted from Benham (1993) and Cowan, Scoggin, and Benham (2001). Alejandro is a 15-month-old child with a diagnosis of retrolental fibroplasia (RLF); the current term for RLF is ROP. Retinal detachment may occur at that time or many years later.

Thomas (1997) defines ROP as:

A bilateral disease of the retinal vessels in preterm infants, some of whom have been exposed to prolonged periods of high postnatal oxygen concentrations. High oxygen concentration used in treating preterm infants, especially those weighing less than 1500 g, causes vasoconstriction of the immature retinal vessels and eventually occlusion of those vessels. This may be followed by fibrous proliferation and invasion of the vitreous. Retinal detachment may occur that time or many years later. Blindness develops within several weeks… Apnea, asphyxia, sepsis, nutritional deficiencies and many blood transfusions given over a short period have all been related to ROP. (p. 1673)

Referral

Alejandro was diagnosed as developmentally delayed and visually impaired as a result of RLF. He was born prematurely at 32 weeks gestation, weighing 3 pounds. He suffered severe respiratory distress and required oxygen, which resulted in a visual impairment diagnosed as RLF. When he was discharged from the hospital at 3 months of age, no motor impairments were noted and the extent of his visual impairment was unknown. At age 15 months, Alejandro was referred to his local Early Intervention Program by his pediatrician after an initial examination revealed delays in several areas on the Denver II Revised Developmental Screening Test (Frankenberg at al., 1992). A service coordinator was assigned and the early intervention team members began their assessments. Team members included a teacher of the visually impaired, developmental services interventionist, an OT, an OTA; and in some cases, especially for older children, an orientation and mobility specialist would also be involved.

Assessment and Evaluation Process

The Early Intervention Team Process

In early intervention settings, OT practitioners may be integral members of the team and participate in the team process. At the initial meeting with the family, a family needs survey is administered by the service coordinator. The results of the family needs survey determines which disciplines will be represented on the assessment team.

The Real Records section of this chapter provides an example of an IFSP based on the case study of Alejandro and his family. Any documentation must be in reader-friendly, layman terms, rather than in a medical model style. The IFSP process also requires that the IFSP be written at the actual meeting, with input from as many team members, including the parents, as possible. The parents are always seen as active and valuable members of the team. The professional team members build on the parents' goals by using their expertise to develop strategies to help the family meet their goals.

Although the following discussion of OT evaluation and treatment strategies uses professional terminology, when working with the family and team, OT practitioners would always present information in family-friendly terms. For instance, while talking with each other, the OT and OTA might discuss a suggested activity in terms of "present toys while he is in a prone position." When this activity is presented to the family or written on the IFSP, it would be stated as something like, "Give him toys while he is lying on his tummy."

The Occupational Therapist/ Occupational Therapist Assistant Team

When early visual impairment has been diagnosed by an ophthalmologist, an estimate of residual vision established, and the diagnosis of any accompanying disabilities completed, the OT/OTA team can discuss how each team member will be involved with the child. If blindness or severe visual impairment is the only disability present, the OT usually completes the evaluation with the assistance of the OTA, and program planning developed by the team may well be carried out by the OTA. If additional, increasingly complex disabilities exist (such as neurological problems), the OT may not only need to carry out the evaluation, but carry out the treatment program with the assistance of the OTA (AOTA, 1999).

Selected Evaluations

Considering the occupational performance areas that may be impacted by early visual deficits, tests of general development may be the first choice for assessment of young children since they can give a picture of a child's play, self-care, and personal social abilities, as well as motor abilities. If the child is school aged, more detailed evaluations of school, classroom, and environmental demands on the child will be required. This information can be obtained from interview of teachers, school checklists, self-care checklists, or formal evaluations such as the School Function Assessment (SFA) (Coster, Deeney, Haltiwanger, & Haley (1998) or the Pediatric Evaluation of Disability Inventory (PEDI) (Haley, Coster, Ludlow,

Haltiwanger, & Andrellos, 1992). If multiple impairments are present, more extensive evaluation of self-care (especially eating), sensory integrations, and motor functions may need to be completed by the OT for children of all ages.

It was decided by the OT and OTA that OT evaluation needs would include assessment of the following:

- Fine and gross motor development.
- Development of voluntary movement, including reflex maturation.
- Self-care or adaptive behavior activities.
- Sensorimotor development.
- Play development.

OT evaluations selected for Alejandro included the following:

- Developmental Programming for Infants and Young Children (Schafer & Moersch, 1981)
- The Milani-Comparetti Motor Development Screening Test (1992)
- Takata's Play History (Bryze, 1997)
- Sensory history

(The Early Coping Inventory [Zeitlin, Williamson, & Szczepanski, 1988] and the Infant/Toddler Sensory Profile [Dunn, 2002] are currently available tools that would also aid in evaluation of Alejandro).

Results of Family Interview

Alejandro's family includes his mother, father, and 2 older female siblings, ages 3 and 5 years. The family has recently moved to the United States from Honduras as a result of the father's employment opportunities. The father, who is Hispanic, and the mother, who is European-American, are professionals and employed outside of the home. The paternal grandmother takes care of Alejandro during the day and has a different view of Alejandro's condition than the mother. She believes that Alejandro's condition is a result of mal-puesto (bad luck) and that he should be accepted "as he is." The mother is aware of the possibilities for Alejandro in the future, due to volunteer experiences at a local high school for children with developmental disabilities. In general, the family would like to have more information about Alejandro's development and expressed a desire to have only one or two professionals involved in their son's care. Because the OTA speaks Spanish and English, she will work closely with the OT in assessment and programming for Alejandro. Both the OT and the OTA described in this study are practicing at the advanced level as defined by the AOTA document *Guide for Supervision of Occupational Therapy Personnel in the Delivery of Occupational Therapy Services* (AOTA, 1999).

Results of the Occupational Therapy Evaluation

Alejandro's gross motor, fine motor, self-help, and play development are delayed.

- Alejandro's gross motor development is typical of children with visual impairments (i.e., the milestones achieved are those that do not require self-initiated mobility). He sits alone briefly, but usually uses his arms for support. No trunk rotation was noted, and he is not able to achieve a sitting position independently. In a prone position, he moves by belly crawling, in an amphibian pattern. Occasionally, he will attempt to support himself on his hands and knees and rocks back and forth. He raises his head when in a prone position on extended arms, but has weak neck extensors and a lack of visual motivation to maintain the position. Rolling is achieved accidentally. If he hears his mother's voice, he will try to follow the sound, resulting in spontaneous rolling.

- Primitive reflexes appear integrated, with the exception of a slight Moro reflex reaction when startled by unexpected noises or a change in position. Righting reactions are emerging in prone, supine, and sitting. Muscle tone is slightly hypotonic.

- Fine motor development is in the 8-to 9-month range, due to resistance to tactile exploration and his visual impairment. He does not reach for objects by using sound location.

- Self-care or adaptive behavior activities are performed at the 9- to 11-month age range. He is able to chew and take food off of a spoon or finger feed himself. He refuses to try new foods and mealtime is often unpleasant.

- Play skills are limited primarily to solitary play. The OTA observed that his grandmother is very protective of him in regard to other children if they bump into him or try to engage him in play. He frequently engages in self-stimulating behaviors such as eye poking, waving his hands in front of his face, and rocking.

- The sensory history revealed that he does not enjoy "rough-housing" and cries when moved unexpectedly. He enjoys being rocked, but he does not like being held firmly or cuddled. Alejandro is orally defensive and does not readily mouth objects. He is resistive to tactile exploration of his parents' faces. He does not enjoy putting his hands in soft or "messy" textures.

- The teacher of the visually impaired assessed Alejandro's remaining vision using the *Functional Vision Inventory for the Multiple and Severely Handicapped* (Langley, 1980). Based on this assessment and the ophthalmologist's medical assessment of the child's eyes, Alejandro was thought to have remaining vision that he was not using optimally. The vision teacher made recommendations that were to be incorporated into the IFSP regarding optimal light conditions, distance of objects, object size, and visual field presentation.

General Goals

Child and family strengths that were identified by the team included the child's desire to participate in family interaction, the parents' desire to encourage independence, and the grandmother's interest in the child's well-being. The family identified the following areas of need:

- To visually localize, reach, and grasp toys.
- To have the child participate in play with siblings.
- To understand the child's condition and to have realistic expectations.

- To have the child become independent in feeding.
- To decrease the child's self-stimulation behaviors.
- To have the child walk independently.
- To have the parents and grandmother appreciate each other's point of view regarding treatment.

The family/team wrote the following treatment goals into the IFSP:

- Decrease stereotypical behaviors such as eye poking, waving his hands in front of his face, and rocking.
- Stimulate use of remaining vision.
- Decrease tactile defensiveness.
- Increase independence in feeding.
- Encourage typical play development and interaction with siblings.
- Increase tolerance for vestibular stimulation.
- Develop adequate righting and equilibrium reactions in sitting, kneeling, and standing.
- Enhance age-appropriate gross and fine motor development.

Writing Measurable Goals and Objectives

In early intervention and school programs, annual goals are written to the general area of need, and specific measurable objectives are written under each goal. Each objective must include 4 components:

1. The learner (the child).
2. The behavior or performance expected.
3. The conditions or circumstances under which the behavior will occur.
4. The criteria for measuring the degree of success of this objective.

Samples of Alejandro's Goals and Objectives

- Goal 1—Alejandro will feed himself using a spoon or fingers as appropriate with minimal assistance and compliant behavior, to increase independence with spoon feeding.
  - Objective 1—Alejandro will consistently tolerate his hand on the spoon using a hand-over-hand backward chaining technique as his grandmother directs food toward his mouth at mealtimes.
  - Objective 2—Alejandro will tolerate the introduction of one new food each week, as presented by his grandmother using a positive but firm approach.
- Goal 2—Alejandro will initiate a play activity by reaching for a toy given a sound or light cue, with minimal prompting, 2 out of 4 trials to increase independence with social play.
  - Objective 1—Alejandro will visually attend to toys for 45 seconds when a light is shone on them.
  - Objective 2—Alejandro will demonstrate a preference for social interaction by belly crawling toward a sibling playing nearby, with moderate verbal cues, to increase proximity to her, to increase independence in play.

Treatment Activities/Techniques

Play is the primary therapeutic medium with infants and young children, along with the introduction of technology to aid limited vision or blindness. Through play, body scheme, movement, and fine motor development are enhanced by using all forms of sensory stimulation and guided movements as needed. Children with visual impairment need maximal stimulation from sound, touch, movement, and remaining sight in order to develop the desire to move, to reach and manipulate objects, care for themselves, and lead productive occupational lives (Snow, 1996).

Treatment Activities for Alejandro

Literature describing treatment strategies consistent with Alejandro's needs are presented in Evidence-Based Treatment Strategies. The treatment activities, which focused on feeding and play, were carried out by the OTA, who worked well with Alejandro's grandmother. The OT would make a home visit once a week in the evening when both parents would be present. Treatment sessions would be videotaped to document progress and to ensure the accuracy of the home program instruction. Following are treatment activities developed from the sample goals and objectives previously written:

- During play time, place Alejandro's hand on a stacking cup and move him through the motions of banging the toy on various surfaces. Talk about the different sounds and whether the noises were loud or soft. To direct his visual attention to the object, wrap it with fluorescent tape. Initially, place him in a supported sitting position, as he is not able to maintain unsupported sitting. This will free his hands. As sitting balance improves, encourage him to sit with one arm support and gradually move to independent sitting with hands engaged in play at the midline. Gradually decrease the pressure of the "helping hand" on his hand until he is banging the stacking cup on various surfaces independently.

- During snack time, put yogurt or pudding on the spoon and encourage him to bring the spoon to his mouth. Initially, the spoon may need to be redirected 100% of the way, but the distance for which assistance is required should be gradually decreased. Children with visual impairments need to have experiences that will enhance body perception, so telling him about his hand and where it is in relation to his mouth is important. Because Alejandro is also orally defensive, thus decreasing the amount of oral play in which he engages, he needs assistance in developing proprioceptive awareness of the hand-to-mouth pattern.

- Encourage finger feeding by having Alejandro finger paint with whipped cream. He will benefit from variety in his sensory experiences, so add puffed rice cereal and fruit-flavored gelatin cubes to the whipped cream to add tactile and oral texture.
  - Make arrangements for the grandmother to visit a preschool classroom for children with visual impairments during lunchtime to observe independent self-feeding.

Also arrange to have a Spanish-speaking mother of one of the children talk to the grandmother about the progress her child has made with self-feeding.

- In a darkened room, shine a flashlight on a toy and direct Alejandro's face in the proper direction. Gradually increase the length of time he looks at the toy. Direct his hand toward the toy. Present toys while he is in a prone position, thereby also encouraging him to maintain neck extension for a prolonged period. This enhances visual attention and encourages use of remaining vision and to reach toward sound cues. Toys that light up in response to Alejandro's actions, such as Fisher-Price's Classical Chorus Star Stacker (Mattel, El Segundo, CA) or Playschool Lullabye Gloworm (Hasbro, Inc., Pawtucket, RI), would encourage him to use his developing fine motor as well as his visual abilities. As Alejandro gets older, a Lite-Brite (Hasbro, Inc., Pawtucket, RI) (for ages 4 and up) also could be used.

- Encourage sibling interaction by playing games such as "So Big" and "Patty Cake." Start out by engaging him in play with one sister initially to facilitate one-to-one interaction. Be sure that his sister is in close enough physical contact so that Alejandro can feel her presence. Gradually, increase the distance so that he will have to reach arm's length to pass a ball or tickle his sister. Be sure interactions are fun for both children.

- As Alejandro improves in his tolerance of vestibular stimulation, increase the use of activities that have physical and tactile components, such as rolling up in a blanket with his sister or riding "horsey back."

- The grandmother and the parents will need to be reminded to let the siblings comfort each other if there is an accident or hurt feelings during their play. This can be encouraged by having them hug or kiss the hurt or rub it to make it feel better as an additional tactile activity. Alejandro has been overprotected from the normal day-to-day bumps, bruises, and disagreements that occur among siblings. Efforts need to be made to allow the children to solve their own problems to empower the children and solidify Alejandro's family position.

Discharge Planning/Transition Planning

The service coordinator scheduled a meeting with the family and school district personnel in the family's home 120 days before Alejandro's 3rd birthday and anticipated date of discharge from the early childhood intervention program. Preschool services that Alejandro would be eligible for were also discussed. Segments of the videotape were reviewed, demonstrating the many goals that Alejandro had achieved. The parents and the grandmother indicated their appreciation and thought that the entire family had benefited from the intervention program. The service coordinator would continue to follow Alejandro and his family, assisting them in identifying appropriate community resources and groups as necessary. He would also receive services from the teacher of the visually impaired, primarily for premobility training.

CLINICAL PROBLEM SOLVING

- Alejandro demonstrated stereotypical behaviors. What activities would be appropriate to decrease these behaviors?

If stereotypical behaviors are present, purposeful activities should be used to distract the child, especially those activities using movement or proprioception. Stereotypical behaviors such as pressing or poking the eyes can cause dark circles under the eyes, the eyes sinking into the head, and even deform the bony structures around the eyes. If these patterns of behavior become established, they could have adverse effects on social interactions with others (Senitz et al., 1990).

- What precautions should be considered in carrying out feeding activities with Alejandro?

Refer to the evaluation of Alejandro's oral-motor functioning to make sure that he can chew and swallow the types of foods being introduced. Also be aware of any potential food allergies. For instance, peanuts are often a cause of allergy, and use of peanut butter should be discussed with the family before use in a feeding program. Honey is not recommended for children under 1 year of age, due to a possibility of causing infant botulism (Berkow, 1992). Finally, be aware of the possibility of latex sensitivity and the composition of toys that are presented to Alejandro, especially if he may be mouthing the toys (Scoggin & Parks, 1997). Some sources recommend using squeaky dog toys since they are easily obtained and inexpensive. However, be aware that pet toys do not meet the standards required of toys for children; they may be made of latex and the squeaky mechanism could come out and pose a choking hazard for the child.

ADDITIONAL CASE EXAMPLES

- Jason is 3 years old and, along with the diagnosis of cerebral palsy spastic quadriplegia, is considered to have cortical visual impairment. What additional considerations need to be made when considering the OT/OTA team relationship for this child?

If multiple handicaps are present, the OT will select and carry out appropriate neurodevelopmental, sensory integrative, or other specialized evaluations or treatment techniques that will treat underlying aspects of the child's occupational performance problems. Additional information on treatment of children with this condition is presented in Baker-Nobles and Rutherford (1995).

- John has a diagnosis of visual impairment due to ROP. He is in the third grade of a public school. What therapeutic interventions would you recommend for John? How would OT service be provided to John under IDEA 1997?

Self-care may need to be emphasized in terms of orientation to food and location of utensils. Social development may need to be enhanced and guided as John increasingly comes in contact with others in home, neighborhood, and school activities. Specialists in these areas provide mobility training, Braille reading and writing techniques, as well as low vision training; however, OT can prepare the child for learning these techniques by developing early perceptual/sensory sensitivity, manipulation, and mobility skills (Snow, 1996). For the child in a school-based program, the need for assistive devices or technology is usually decided by the child's IEP team and based on the recommendations of the specialists involved (usually the ophthalmologist, special education teacher, and OT). Magnification of images, increased light, reduction of glare, and increasing contrast are basic adaptation techniques used when there is visual impairment. Under the public law IDEA 1997, OT is provided as a "related service" for children with visual impairment as determined by the child's IEP team.

- Melanie is 15 years old, has a diagnosis of mild mental retardation, and has a visual impairment due to meningitis in early infancy. What occupational performance problems might you anticipate in her case? What services are required by IDEA 1997 at her age level? What type of an OT service plan would be appropriate for Melanie?

Some children with visual impairment, especially when combined with a cognitive disability, need guidance with reading social cues and behavior, developing independence and care in self-grooming, and appropriate social etiquette in eating and work situations. According to law, an ITP must be written at age 14, and vocational planning is essential. Working in the community will need to be discussed as an option, and the vocational counselor now becomes part of the planning team. The skills for selected jobs can be developed in OT. Assistive technology that will assist in development of job skills should be considered by the ITP team. Low technology devices, for example, may include magnifiers and bold-writing pens; high technology devices may include stand-alone print enlargement systems, character enlargement systems for computers, Braille output devices, voice output systems, audio tactile devices, scanning systems, note taking devices, and laptop computers (Mann & Lane, 1991). See Table 11-1 for a list of Web sites of organizations for persons with visual impairments.

LEARNING ACTIVITIES

1. Compare and contrast the 2 parts of IDEA (P. L. 94-142 and P. L. 99-457).

2. Choose a treatment goal from those listed and identify additional activities that would facilitate Alejandro's development in that area.

3. Work with a peer and develop a list of other activities that could be used for treatment with a visually handicapped child.

4. Visit a preschool program that provides services to visually impaired children. Observe the roles of at least 3 different professionals and describe some of the services they offer.

5. On the Internet, find resources for families of children with visual impairments. Make a list to use for future reference.

Table 11-1

Web Sites of Organizations Related to Visual Impairment

Early Intervention

Early Intervention Training Center for Infants and Toddlers With Visual Impairments
www.fpg.unc.edu/~edin

Vision Organizations

American Council of the Blind
www.acb.org

American Foundation for the Blind
www.afb.org

American Printing House for the Blind, Inc.
www.aph.org

Association for Education and Rehabilitation of the Blind and Visually Impaired
www.aerbvi.org

The Canadian National Institute for the Blind
www.cnib.ca

The Hadley School for the Blind
www.hadley-school.org

Lighthouse International
www.lighthouse.org

National Association for Visually Handicapped
www.navh.org

National Federation for the Blind
www.nfb.org

Royal Institute for the Blind
www.rnib.org.uk

---

6. Write to the American Foundation for the Blind and request information about the services offered.

ACKNOWLEDGMENTS

The authors would like to thank Elizabeth Reyna, ECI Manager, Easter Seals of the Rio Grande Valley (RGV), for her invaluable contributions in finalizing the IFSP "Real Records" section. The authors also acknowledge the following individuals for their contributions to the IFSP development process: Patricia Rosenlund, Executive Director, Easter Seals RGV; Roschel Servantes, Program Director, Easter Seals RGV; and, Kathy de la Pena, Director, Region I [Texas] ECI Program.

REFERENCES

Adelson, E., & Fraiberg, S. (1977). Gross motor development in infants from birth. In S. Chess & A. Thomas (Eds.), *Annual progress in child psychiatry and child development* (pp. 130-149). New York, NY: Brunner/Mazel Publishers.

American Occupational Therapy Association. (1998). Position paper: Occupational therapy services in early intervention and preschool services. In *The reference manual of the official documents of the American Occupational Therapy Association, Inc.* (7th ed.). Bethesda, MD: Author.

American Occupational Therapy Association. (1999). Guide for supervision of occupational therapy personnel in the delivery of occupational therapy services. Retrieved July 16, 2004, from http://www.aota.org.

American Occupational Therapy Association. (2002). Occupational therapy practice framework: Domain and process. *American Journal of Occupational Therapy, 56,* 609-639.

Baker-Nobles, L., & Rutherford, A. (1995). Understanding cortical visual impairment in children. *American Journal of Occupational Therapy, 49,* 899-903.

Benham, P. K. (1993). The child with visual deficits. In S. Ryan (Ed.), *Practice issues in OT: Intraprofessional team building* (pp. 27-34). Thorofare, NJ: SLACK Incorporated.

Berkow, R. (Ed.). (1992). *The Merck manual of diagnosis and therapy.* Rahway, NJ: Merck & Co., Inc.

Brown, S. L., & Donovan, C. M. (1981). Volume 3: Stimulation activities. In D. S. Schafer & M. S. Moersch (Eds.), *Developmental programming for infants and young children.* Ann Arbor, MI: The University of Michigan Press.

Bryze, K. (1997). Narrative contributions to the play history. In L. D. Parham & L. S. Fazio (Eds.), *Play in occupational therapy for children* (pp. 23-34). St. Louis: Mosby.

Burke, J. P., & Schaaf, R. C. (1997). Family narratives and play assessment. In L. D. Parham & L. S. Fazio (Eds.), *Play in occupational therapy for children* (pp. 67-84). St. Louis: Mosby.

Coster, W. (1998). Occupation-centered assessment of children. *American Journal of Occupational Therapy, 52,* 337-344.

Coster, W., Deeney, T., Haltiwanger, J., & Haley, S. (1998). *School Function Assessment.* San Antonio, TX: The Psychological Corporation.

Cowan, M. K., Scoggin, A. E., & Benham, P. K. (2001). A baby with visual deficits. In K. Sladyk & S. E. Ryan (Eds.), *Ryan's occupational therapy assistant: Principles, practice issues, and techniques* (3rd ed., pp. 109-117). Thorofare, NJ: SLACK Incorporated.

Dunn, W. (2002). *Infant/Toddler Sensory Profile.* San Antonio, TX: Harcourt Assessment, Inc.

Edwards, M. A., Millard, P., Praskac, L. A., & Wisniewski, P. A. (2003). Occupational therapy and early intervention: A family-centered approach. *Occupational Therapy International, 10*(4), 239-252.

EVIDENCE-BASED TREATMENT STRATEGIES

Treatment Strategies	Authors
Promote self-feeding	Brown & Donovan, 1981; Coster, 1998; Humphry, 2002; Klein & Delaney, 1994
Encourage exploratory play in family context	Burke & Schaaf, 1997; Hinojosa & Kramer, 1997
Promote optimal use of vision and fine motor development	Brown & Donovan, 1981; Griffin, Williams, Davis, & Engleman, 2002; Hyvärinen, 1995
Family collaboration/education	Edwards, Millard, Praskac, & Wisniewski, 2003; Moxley-Haegert & Serbin, 1983
Improve sensory processing	Roley & Schneck, 2001

Frankenberg, W. K., Dodds, J., Archer, P., Bresnick, B., Maschka, P., Edelman, N., et al. (1992). *Denver II Training Manual*. Denver, CO: Denver Developmental Materials, Inc.

Gersh, E. S. (1991). Medical concerns and treatments. In E. Geralis (Ed.), *Children with cerebral palsy: A parent's guide* (pp. 57-89). Bethesda, MD: Woodbine House.

Griffin, H. C., Williams, S. C., Davis, M. L., & Engleman, M. (2002). Using technology to enhance cues for children with low vision. *TEACHING Exceptional Children, Nov/Dec*, 36-42.

Haley, S., Coster, W., Ludlow, L., Haltiwanger, J., & Andrellos, P. (1992). *Pediatric Evaluation of Disability Inventory*. San Antonio, TX: Psychological Corp.

Hinojosa, J., & Kramer, P. (1997). Integrating children with disabilities into family play. In L. D. Parham & L. S. Fazio (Eds.), *Play in occupational therapy for children* (pp. 159-170). St. Louis: Mosby.

Humphry, R. (2002). Young children's occupations: Explicating the dynamics of developmental processes. *American Journal of Occupational Therapy, 56*, 171-179.

Hyvärinen, L. (1995). Considerations in evaluation and treatment of the child with low vision. *American Journal of Occupational Therapy, 49*, 891-897.

Klein, M. D., & Delaney, T. A. (1994). *Feeding and nutrition for the child with special needs: Handouts for parents*. Tuscon, AZ: Therapy Skill Builders.

Langley, B. M. (1980). *Functional vision inventory for the multiple and severely handicapped*. Chicago, IL: Stoelting Co.

Law, M., Missiuna, C., Pollock, N., & Stewart, D. (2001). Chapter 3: Foundations for occupational therapy practice with children. In J. Case-Smith (Ed.), *Occupational therapy for children* (4th ed., pp. 39-70). St. Louis: Mosby.

Mann, W. C., & Lane, J. P. (1991). *Assistive technology for persons with disabilities*. Rockville, MD: American Occupational Therapy Association.

Maruyama, E., Chandler, B., Clark, G. F., Dick, R. W., Lawlor, M. C., & Jackson, L. L. (1999). *OT services for children and youth under the Individuals with Disabilities Education Act* (2nd ed.). Bethesda, MD: American Occupational Therapy Association.

Miller, M. M., Menacker, S. J., & Batshaw, M. L. (2002). Vision: Our window to the world. In M. L. Batshaw (Ed.), *Children with disabilities* (5th ed., pp. 165-192). Baltimore, MD: Paul H. Brookes Publishing Co.

Milani-Comparetti Motor Development Screening Test (3rd ed.). (1992). Omaha, NE: Meyer Rehabilitation Institute.

Moxley-Haegert, L., & Serbin, L. A. (1983). Developmental education for parents of delayed infants: Effects on parental motivation and children's development. *Child Development, 54*, 1324-1331.

Roley, S. S., & Schneck, C. (2001). Sensory integration and visual deficits, including blindness. In S. S. Roley, E. I. Blanche, & R. C. Schaaf (Eds.), *Understanding the nature of sensory integration with diverse populations* (pp. 313-344). San Antonio, TX: Therapy Skill Builders.

Scoggin, A. E., & Parks, K. (1997). Latex sensitivity in children with spina bifida: Implications for occupational therapy practitioners. *American Journal of Occupational Therapy, 51*, 608-611.

Schafer, D. S., & Moersch, M. S. (Eds.). (1981). *Developmental programming for infants and young children*. Ann Arbor, MI: University of Michigan Press.

Senitz, C., Bride, B. M., Adrian, J., & Semmler, C. J. (1990). Visually impaired children. In C. J. Semmler & J. G. Hunter (Eds.), *Early OT intervention—Neonates to 3 years* (pp. 262-274). Gaithersburg, MD: Aspen.

Snow, E. (1996). Services for children with visual or auditory impairments. In J. Case-Smith, A. S. Allen, & P. N. Pratt (Eds.), *OT for children* (3rd ed., pp. 717-742). St. Louis, MO: Mosby.

Thomas, C. L. (Ed.). (1997). *Taber's cyclopedic medical dictionary*. Philadelphia: F. A. Davis.

Zeitlin, S., Williamson, G., & Szczepanski, M. (1988). *Early Coping Inventory*. Bensenville, IL: Scholastic Testing Services, Inc.

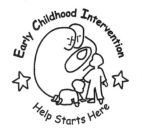

p. _1_ of _7_

Individualized Family Service Plan
IFSP
(Plan of Care)

Child's Name: _Alejandro_   IFSP Date: _6-30-02_

Parents, Guardians, Surrogate Parents: _

☑ Initial   ☐ Annual   ☐ Other: _____

Service Coordinator: _Elizabeth Reyna_   Translated for Parents: ___Yes _✓_No

INTEGRATED SUMMARY

(Includes a summary of pertinent medical history and current health status including vision, hearing and nutrition. Describes the child's development in each area: communication; cognitive; gross and fine motor; social/emotional; and self help/adaptive in functional terms. Describes the settings in which the child lives and plays, who else is in these natural environments, and how the child functions in these natural environments. Includes a review of the need for assistive technology assessments, services, and devices which support the child's ability to function in his/her natural environments.)

Alejandro is a happy 15 month old toddler who lives at home with mom, dad and two older sisters ages 3 and 5. He spends most of his day with grandma while mom and dad go to work. He is seen for his well baby care by his pediatrician Dr. Martinez and has been diagnosed by his opthalmologist Dr. Smith with retrolental fibroplasia. Alejandro's immunizations are current and has not had any recent hospitalizations. He is currently not on any medication. Alejandro has started sitting alone for brief periods and is also able

Real record 11-1A. Real record for a client with visual impairments. (Reprinted with permission from the Texas Early Childhood Intervention Program of the Department of Assistive and Rehabilitative Services.)

Case #: _____

INTEGRATED SUMMARY
(Continued)

to move by crawling on his belly. He turns at the sound of mom's voice and often smiles. He attempts to support himself on his hands and knees when in a crawling position. Alejandro enjoys being carried and will reach to touch mom's face. He is able to finger feed himself and has no problems chewing his food. He smiles and kicks his legs and waves his hands when he hears his older sisters. He is able to say single words like "more", "ball" and frequently uses body motions to express himself. Alejandro is a picky eater and sensitive to soft foods. In the evenings before going to bed, Alejandro enjoys being rocked to sleep

Real record 11-1B. Real record for a client with visual impairments. (Reprinted with permission from the Texas Early Childhood Intervention Program of the Department of Assistive and Rehabilitative Services.)

Case #: _____   p. __3__ of __2__

STRENGTHS AND NEEDS OF YOUR CHILD

STRENGTHS	NEEDS
(what we are going to build on)	*(where we are going to go next)*

STRENGTHS:
- He is able to chew
- attempts to crawl
- began to sit
- turns to sounds
- finger feeds himself
- belly crawls
- participates with family
- smiles

NEEDS:
- to explore more
- to play with his sisters
- to sit independently and walk
- to eat a variety of foods
-

Real record 11-1C. Real record for a client with visual impairments. (Reprinted with permission from the Texas Early Childhood Intervention Program of the Department of Assistive and Rehabilitative Services.)

Case #: _____   p. 4 of 7

FAMILY CONCERNS, PRIORITIES AND RESOURCES

(including those things that will enhance your child's ability to function in a natural environment)

Concerns/Priorities	Resources
- Would like information on Alejandro's condition - would like for grandmother and parents understand eachother's point of view regarding treatment - For Alejandro to play with sisters	Health insurance Dr. Martinez - pediatrician Dr. Smith - opthalmologist family support, home, transportation

Family Outcome: To learn more about Alejandro's condition

Strategies: - Provide family with information on retrolental fibroplasia
- obtain medical reports from opthamologist
- review information with family and other team members

Family Outcome: For mom, Dad, and grandmother to be able to understand eachother's opinion on alejandro's condition

Strategies:
1. Invite grandmother to medical appointments.
2. Provide grandmother with information in Spanish on Alejandro's condition
3. Have all family members participate in sessions so everyone will be able to see Alejandro's progress and to see what works and does not work

~~Family Outcome:~~ Outcome; For alejandro to play and interact more with his sisters

Strategies:
1. include Alejandro's sister's in implementing the strategies
2. Have siblings talk to him and explain/describe the activity they are doing - no sudden movements.
3. Describe Alejandro's vision impairments ex. ask siblings to close their eyes, tell a story about vision impairment.

Real record 11-1D. Real record for a client with visual impairments. (Reprinted with permission from the Texas Early Childhood Intervention Program of the Department of Assistive and Rehabilitative Services.)

Case #: _____ p. 5 of 7

OUTCOMES, CRITERIA, STRATEGIES

OUTCOME (*I want my child to*): For Alejandro to be able feed himself independently

CRITERIA (*the above outcome has been achieved when*): When Alejandro is able to eat a meal with minimal assistance

ROUTINE: feeding time / snack time

STRATEGIES (*activities that will help my child to achieve the outcome*):

1. Allow Alejandro to play (explore) a spoon
2. Apply "sticky" food items to spoon such as peanut butter, and use hand over hand technique to work on hand to mouth motion
3. Allow Alejandro to touch different types of textured foods

ROUTINE:

STRATEGIES:

ROUTINE:

STRATEGIES:

Real record 11-1E. Real record for a client with visual impairments. (Reprinted with permission from the Texas Early Childhood Intervention Program of the Department of Assistive and Rehabilitative Services.)

Case #: _____   p, 6 of 7

OUTCOMES, CRITERIA, STRATEGIES

OUTCOME (*I want my child to*): For Alejandro to be to sit on his own

CRITERIA (*the above outcome has been achieved when*): When Alejandro is able to sit without support when playing or eating

ROUTINE: Feeding

STRATEGIES (*activities that will help my child to achieve the outcome*):

1. Place Alejandro in a high chair with minimal support gradually decreasing supports ex) begin with the use of pillows or a towel for support along with feeding tray on high chair)

ROUTINE: Play-time

STRATEGIES: 1. Place Alejandro on the floor in front of mom while in a sitting position

2. Place toys within reach to distract him from supporting himself with his hands

3. Use pillows for support while sitting with his sisters

ROUTINE: Dressing

STRATEGIES:

1. Allow Alejandro to assist with pulling off and on his shirt while sitting on the bed

2. Encourage him to pull off his socks using hand over hand technique.

Real record 11-1F. Real record for a client with visual impairments. (Reprinted with permission from the Texas Early Childhood Intervention Program of the Department of Assistive and Rehabilitative Services.)

Name:
There is medical documentation in this record that these services **are not** covered by the DRS program.   yes ☐   no ☑

p. ___ of ___

SERVICES

Service	Discipline	Frequency	Intensity	Location*	Method	Duration Start Date	Duration End Date	Payment*
Service Coordinator	Elizabeth Reyna, EIS	when necessary		home	individual	6-30-02	6-29-03	FCS
Occupational therapy	Martha Smith OTR	8x month	45 minutes	home	individual	6-30-02	6-29-03	FCS
Vision impairment services	John Hunt	4 x month	1 hour	home	individual	6-30-02	6-29-03	FCS
developmental services	Elizabeth Reyna EIS	2 x month	45 minutes	home	individual	6-30-02	6-29-03	FCS

The services in this IFSP include developmentally appropriate individualized skills, training and support to foster, promote, and enhance the child's 1) participation in daily activities; 2) functional independence; and 3) social interaction. In addition, assistance to caregivers is included to identify and utilize opportunities to incorporate therapeutic intervention strategies into daily life activities that are natural and normal for the child and family. Continuous monitoring of child progress in the acquisition and mastery of functional skills will be done in order to reduce or overcome limitations resulting from disabilities or developmental delay.

* See Family Cost Share Agreement for details

Assistive Technology is ☐   is not ☑ (check one) planned as a strategy as part of this IFSP

* Describe how and why any location of services was determined if services are not provided in the child's natural environment, and how these services will be generalized to support the child's ability to function in his/her natural environment _____

OTHER RESOURCES AND SUPPORTS ACCESSED BY FAMILY:

None at this time

The *ECI Family Rights Handbook* has been reviewed with me, I understand that my consent is voluntary and may be withdrawn at any time, I understand that my consent may be given for some services and not for others, I understand that the consequence of refusing services is that my child/family will not receive the services, I understand that my signature grants permission for my child to receive services, I understand that services subject to the Family Cost Share will begin once I have signed my Family Cost Share Agreement.

Signature of Team Members	Discipline	Date	Present	Reviewed
Victoria	Mom	6-3-02	✓	
Elizabeth	EIS/BSW	6-30-02	✓	
Martha	OT	6-30-02	✓	
Claude	OT	6-30-02	✓	
John	VI	6-30-02	✓	

G:\Program Services\Administration\ECI Policy & Procedures\FY 2003 P&P\Proposed IFSP Grid (DRS) added fees

Real record 11-1G. Real record for a client with visual impairments. (Reprinted with permission from the Texas Early Childhood Intervention Program of the Department of Assistive and Rehabilitative Services.)

Key Concepts

- Diagnosis: Previously termed pervasive developmental disorder (PDD), but now termed *autism spectrum disorder*.
- Medically based services: Paid for by insurance carrier upon medical necessity.
- School system practice: Guided by federal law for a free and appropriate education.
- Medical vs. educational services: Differences in service delivery models and team approaches.
- OT/OTA collaboration: Intricate interactions between 2 practitioners who each have necessary information and understanding of performance.

Essential Vocabulary

autistic spectrum disorders: Common name for a variety of autistic disorders.

***Diagnostic and Statistical Manual of Mental Disorders* (4th ed.) (DSM-IV):** Nationally used manual outlining diagnostic criteria.

Asperger's syndrome: Characterized as high-functioning autism with impairments noted in social interactions.

occupational behavior: Acquiring skills to meet the demands of the environment.

pervasive developmental disorders (PDD): The name of the category of disorders identified in the DSM-IV used to describe autistic features. The term *autism spectrum disorder* is now more commonly used to refer to this group of disorders.

sensory defensiveness: Misperception of sensory experiences; results in fight, flight, or fright response.

sensory integration: A clinical theory and frame of reference developed by Dr. A. Jean Ayres that is based on extensive research of normal development, experimental neuroscience, studies with children diagnosed with learning disabilities, concepts on mind-brain-body, and open systems theory.

sensory modulation: The ability to maintain an alert and focused state.

A Toddler With Autism Spectrum Disorder

Tara J. Glennon, EdD, OTR, FAOTA

INTRODUCTION

The field of autism research has expanded exponentially in the past 10 years. Unfortunately, however, the most recent manual to outline the conditions necessary for the official diagnosis was published in 1994. A matter that clearly illustrates this issue is the name of the disorder itself. While the fourth edition of the *Diagnostic and Statistical Manual of Mental Disorders* (DSM-IV) (American Psychiatric Association [APA], 1994) delineated the criteria for the diagnoses termed autism or PDD, current literature refers to this classification as autism spectrum disorders. Additionally, the criterion specified in the DSM-IV does not seem to assist with recent attempts to develop a system of early diagnosis (Glennon & Miller-Kuhaneck, 2004). For example, failure to develop peer relationships, failure to initiate or sustain conversational interchange, and lack of varied spontaneous make-believe or social imitative play would be quite difficult to identify in very young children.

In terms of presenting concerns, here is what we know. The categories identified in the DSM-IV (APA, 1994) include qualitative impairment in reciprocal social interactions, qualitative impairment in verbal and nonverbal communications and imaginative play, restricted repertoire of activities and interests, and onset prior to age 3. In addition, experts include disturbances in developmental rates and sequences that affect motor, cognitive, and socioemotional areas; and disturbances in response to sensory stimuli as evidenced by hyperreactivity, hyporeactivity, or extreme alternating between these 2 states. It is also important to note that these characteristics can be observed with other developmental disorders and should be considered as additional diagnoses in order to be addressed accordingly.

The DSM-IV (APA, 1994) outlines 3 categories of functioning. In order for the diagnosis of autism to be made, at least 2 items from Category 1 and one item from both Categories 2 and 3 need to be identified. However, there are many children who demonstrate several of the criteria without meeting the number or combination required to meet the diagnosis of autism. If the child does not meet the autism criteria, the diagnosis of PDD would be made. With so many possible combinations, it has been long speculated, and currently considered likely, that different etiologies also exist. Therefore, there should be no "norm" for intervention. Rather, the symptomatology should be identified, specific research information should be analyzed, and various interventions should be considered.

The last point to be addressed with regard to autism spectrum disorders is severity. Again, based on the combination of symptoms and the severity of each symptom, there is a wide range of disability. For example, one child may be intellectually average, or even superior, and possess several communicative and interactional limitations. Another child may function in the mentally deficient range with no ability to participate in self-care activities. For this reason, each child who carries an autism spectrum diagnosis needs to be treated on an individual basis with no preconceived notions with regard to maximum level of independence.

HISTORICAL PERSPECTIVE

Henry Maudsley, the first psychiatrist to pay specific attention to very young children with severe issues in the developmental processes, considered these issues to be psychoses. This thought was commonplace until 1943, a mere 60+ years ago, when a paper titled *Autistic Disturbances of Affective Contact* was written by Dr. Leo Kanner (Kanner, 1943). Kanner, who first coined the term *infantile autism*, was a psychiatrist at Johns Hopkins Medical Center when he established the hallmarks of the disorder. At the time, he was working with a group of 11 patients who demonstrated similarities in their symptoms. The original concept of the disorder was described as a lack of responsiveness on the part of the child to environmental input and an inability to relate to people and situations from the beginning of life. As this original concept continued to be refined and clarified, DSM revisions reflected the changes in perspective (Sponheim, 1996), and intervention plans were modified and clarified.

At the time of original identification, intervention was minimal and inadequate, as the preliminary theories identified the mother as part of the problem. It was thought that the child ceased to interact because the mother was "cold" to the child.

Unprepared and uneducated physicians cited this theory as late as 1990. In fact, before 1980, children with any PDD were classified as having a type of childhood schizophrenia (Petty, Ornitz, Michelman, & Zimmerman, 1984). Physicians, pediatricians, and psychologists who are now current with the literature understand that autism spectrum disorders are considered to be neurobiological disorders. Additionally, with more refined diagnostic information, the incidence of autistic spectrum disorders has been reported as high as 1 in every 500 births (Ritvo et al., 1990). These numbers imply that autism spectrum disorders are more common than cystic fibrosis, which occurs 1 in every 2,500 births, and Down syndrome, which is 1 in every 1,000 births (Cohen & Volkmar, 1997).

RESEARCH CONSIDERATIONS RELATED TO OCCUPATIONAL THERAPY

Studies emerging with the technological advances in the 1970s have continued with full force today, secondary to the increased incidence of the disorder. Discovering the etiology or etiologies of autism spectrum disorders, which could lead to prevention and more effective interventions, has been a challenge. While much progress has been documented, there continues to be much work ahead. However, most researchers agree that many factors interplay in order to have the disorder express itself (Table 12-1). Although technological advances in neuroimaging and neurochemical analysis have advanced this cause, the results have also been mixed with regard to the site of neurological dysfunction. Researchers have provided us with conflicting information and a variety of possibilities. Therefore, this section will focus on anatomical findings that would be considered to directly impact the role of OT personnel.

Researchers have identified neurological abnormalities in the limbic system, cerebellum, thalamus, and reticular formation (Bauman & Kemper, 1994, 2003; Brambilla et al., 2003; Courchesne, Yeung-Courchesne, Press, Hesselink, & Jennigan, 1988; Fatemi et al., 2002; Hardan, Minshew, Harenski, & Keshavan, 2001). Rimland (1985), a pioneer in the field and a leading researcher even today, cited that the symptomatology might be secondary to a deficit in perceptual capacities, possibly due to brainstem dysfunction, especially in the reticular formation. Rimland theorized that this results in "perceptual inaccessibility" as evidenced by a lack of preparedness to respond. Ornitz and Ritvo (1968) reflect on the possibility of faulty sensory modulation. Modulation, a term that will be discussed later in the chapter, refers to a lack of response or exaggerated response to certain environmental stimuli. Ornitz and Ritvo identify a lack of orientation and attention to stimuli; inconsistent responses to sensory input; increased sensitivity to sensory input, which is termed *defensiveness*; and possible increased awareness of sensation coupled with a tendency to seek the input.

The limbic system, which is actually several structures that function together, includes the hippocampus circuits and the amygdaloid complex. These structures function with the adjacent neocortices, hypothalamus, brainstem, and reticular sys-

tem. As a review, the limbic system is involved in survival mechanisms, including frustration, anger-rage-violence continuum, hormonal and immune systems, and long-term memory. Bauman and Kemper (1985) identified smaller neurons and issues with cell density within the limbic system structures of individuals diagnosed as autistic, while Brambilla et al. (2003) also noted abnormal sizes within these structures.

Several researchers have also identified cerebellar irregularities (Bauman and Kemper, 1985; Fatemi et al., 2002; Hardan et al., 2001). The cerebellum, which has distinct regions responding to different sets of input, has been found to be 20% to 30% smaller in person's diagnosed on the autism spectrum. The Purkinje cells, which typically have extensive dendrite trees whose axons go down into the white matter of the cerebellum, are the sole output of the cerebellar cortex. With the diagnosis of autism spectrum disorder, however, Purkinje cells have been noted to be fewer in number and have immature axons. The result of these cerebellar findings is pertinent for OT, as information being processed within the cerebellum is compromised secondary to the defects in the Purkinje cells. Additionally, the 2 hemispheres of the cerebellum are divided by the vermis, which functions as a relay station. The sections of the vermis found to be affected in the autistic population carry information related to visual and vestibular information. Therefore, communication between the 2 halves of the cerebellum through the vermis regarding visual and vestibular information is compromised.

Frames of Reference

Despite the frame of reference utilized on behalf of the child with an autism spectrum disorder, any interventionist must always consider the child's role within the environment. Identifying the facilitators and barriers to successful participation in one's life roles is the basis of our profession. It is imperative that environmental adaptations be completed and opportunities presented so that the child can acquire the skills necessary to meet the demands of the environment. This concept is universal to many frames of reference, based on developmental principles, acquisitional considerations, and coping concepts, so that the child is able to take care of his or her own needs.

The most common intervention strategy for OT staff working with this diagnosis is Ayres' sensory integration. This approach, developed by Dr. A. Jean Ayres, was outlined for parents in *Sensory Integration and the Child* (Ayres, 1972). Sensory integration is a clinical theory and frame of reference based on extensive research of normal development, experimental neuroscience, studies with children diagnosed with learning disabilities, concepts on mind-brain-body, and open systems theory. It should be noted that Ayres' groundbreaking clinical insights initially met with resistance in the late 1960s. The information, however, eventually altered the way OTs and OTAs work with children. Ayres' sensory integration theory emphasizes the importance of sensory processing as a foundation for learning within all developmental sequences. Ayres developed the Southern California Sensory Integration Test (SCSIT) and was instrumental in the creation and interpretation of the Sensory Integration and Praxis Tests (SIPT), an updated senso-

Table 12-1

Etiology, Prevalence, and Classic Signs and Precautions

Etiology: Currently Unknown

The current scientific view suggests that a variety of factors, both genetic and environmental, interplay to create the conditions necessary for the expression of autistic symptomatology (Miller-Kuhaneck & Glennon, 2004).

Genetic: Gene susceptibility, which makes an individual more susceptible to, rather than directly causing, the disorder. In fact, there appear to be several chromosomal regions that may contain genes related to the autism spectrum disorder diagnosis.

Environmental: As genetics do not fully explain the existence of this disorder, researchers continue to look at additional environmental causes. These include the possibility of:
- Pre- and perinatal factors.
- Early toxin exposure.
- Viral or bacterial infections.
- Vaccinations (although this is currently not considered to be valid).
- Autoimmune concerns.

Prevalence: Rapidly Rising

Recent reports suggest significant increases in this country and abroad.

- Merrick, Kandel, and Morad's (2004) synopsis cites that the prevalence before 1985 was 4 to 5 per 10,000 children for the broader autism spectrum, and about 2 per 10,000 for the classic autism definition. Recently, the numbers have been as high as 40 per 10,000 in 3- to 10-year-old children for autistic disorder and 67 per 10,000 children for the entire autism spectrum.

- United Kingdom: From 1991 to 1996 increases of 18% per year of classic autism and of 55% per year of other autism spectrum disorders in preschoolers (Powell et al., 2000).

- Australia: 200% increase between 1989 and 1997, despite a decrease in population of 0.5% (Baker, 2002).

Arguments given for recent increases include:
- Greater public awareness.
- Increased training of pediatricians to identify the signs and symptoms.
- Better diagnostic procedures.
- Expanded diagnostic criteria found in DSM-IV.

Despite these arguments, indicators from governmental agencies, private research foundations, the National Institute of Health, and the Centers for Disease Control all indicate a significant rise in the incidence of the diagnosis in the past 15 years. A recent study by the M.I.N.D. institute in California found that these increases are not due to factors other than a true increase in the number of cases (Byrd, 2002).

Classic Signs and Precautions

As the term *autism spectrum disorder* implies, there are a wide range of signs and symptoms.

Hallmarks of the disorder include the following:
- Qualitative impairment in reciprocal social interactions.
- Qualitative impairment in verbal and nonverbal communications and imaginative play.
- Restricted repertoire of activities and interests.
- Onset prior to age 3.

In addition, experts include the following:
- Disturbances in developmental rates and sequences that affect motor, cognitive, and socioemotional areas.
- Disturbances in response to sensory stimuli as evidenced by hyperreactivity, hyporeactivity, or extreme alternating between these 2 states.

It is also important to note that these characteristics can be observed with other developmental disorders and should be considered as additional diagnoses in order to be addressed accordingly.

Precautions
- This diagnosis requires intensive intervention by a variety of professionals, so be sure to make appropriate referrals.
- Coordinate with the speech pathologist so that you can utilize the appropriate verbal cues.
- Investigate the teaching approach utilized so that it can be supported when appropriate.

ry integrative assessment tool published in 1989. While these assessment tools are only to be administered by OTs, the results are also valuable for the OTA. Additionally, while OTAs are not able to become certified in the administration and interpretation of the SIPT, the theory course of the certification track is open to OTAs. This course is offered through a collaborative effort of the University of Southern California and Western Psychological Services (USC/WPS). For additional information on the sensory integrative frame of reference, please see Chapter 13.

The role of the OTA can be quite extensive within home-, school-, and clinic-based therapy and institutional environments. The intricacy of this frame of reference requires intense cooperation between the OT and OTA. The primary emphasis of OT staff working with children on the spectrum would be to educate other team members on the utilization of sensory integrative techniques so that these strategies can be incorporated into everyday experiences (Hanschu, 1997; Wilbarger & Wilbarger, 1991).

Dr. Mary Reilly, an OT, developed a concept of play that has expanded how we value the play experience (Parham & Fazio, 1997). She believed that play gave meaning to the daily life of a child and provided opportunities to learn rules, develop interactions, and form the basis for adult competencies. The play experiences chosen by clinicians working with a child diagnosed on the autism spectrum must provide opportunities for the child to grow and develop socially and emotionally. Within this framework, capitalizing and expanding upon what the child finds intriguing is a useful technique in expanding the child's play sequences as well as motor planning opportunities. As attempts are made to provide an environment in which the play experience is meaningful and accessible for these children, the therapist would need to incorporate sensory integrative components.

Assessment

Within the arena of pediatric practice, the evaluation process for a child on the autism spectrum is always complex. Due to the fact that the effects are pervasive, as noted in the diagnosis, full team evaluation and intervention planning often occurs, particularly within the educational system. This interdisciplinary approach is often considered to be most appropriate for these children. This section will focus on the assessment tools utilized by OT personnel. Once this information is identified, it can be incorporated into the full team evaluation. As the OTA may in fact be the therapist assigned to this team, full understanding of what assessment tools have been utilized is essential. In addition, if the child is referred for a medically-based evaluation, a full team evaluation may not be available. In that case, the OT would assess the child and the results would be shared with the OTA for collaboration and intervention planning. Therefore, this section is offered to the OTA not only to understand his or her role within this process, but to appreciate the evaluation tools completed by the OT. Please also refer to the chapter regarding the pediatric diagnosis of cerebral palsy (see Chapter 14) for additional information

regarding the pediatric evaluation process and the tools utilized under medical and educational scenarios.

Despite the assessment tool identified for use, the OTA can play an integral role in the initial phase of the process. Observations of functional performance within the classroom or home environment would be important to complete. Additionally, conversations with the parent or teacher to determine their concerns regarding the child's performance cannot be emphasized enough. It is the parent and teacher who are part of the child's natural environment and are able to share pertinent information that might not be readily observed by a third party. During these observations, the assistant's knowledge of task analysis is helpful when attempting to identify areas of concern through observation of functional performance. This initial phase of the evaluation process should also include a chart review. It is quite important to review the observations of other team members in order to document how areas of deficit noted within those reports impact varying domains of function. For example, if the speech pathologist identifies a language processing disorder, this would impact how the child follows through on commands related to occupational performance. Additionally, this review would also allow the OTA to gain preliminary information as to where OT concerns might be impacting performance in other domains of functioning. For example, if the OT or OTA determines sensitivities to auditory stimulation, this might relate to the teacher reporting that the child retreats to the corner during music class. Therefore, any information obtained by the OTA should be shared with the OT as the more formalized stage of the evaluation begins.

With the autism spectrum disorder diagnosis, the level of severity would impact the assessment procedure chosen. When choosing an assessment tool, it should be remembered that children who are significantly impaired would not be able to complete standardized assessments. In fact, many standardized assessments should not be implemented if a known diagnosis interferes with the child's ability to complete the required tasks. If the child is able to attend successfully, understand the directions, follow the commands, and plan his or her responses, then a standardized tool might be implemented.

The first area to be assessed should be sensory processing. If standardized assessment tools are possible, the SIPT (Ayres, 1989) might be chosen. This assessment, only appropriate for children aged 4 to 8 years 11 months, requires a specialty certification to administer and interpret. The therapist certified to administer this assessment tool would be able to make an educated decision as to whether the tool is appropriate or not. Additionally, the Sensory Profile (Dunn, 1999) would be appropriate in order to gather additional information from the caregiver.

If the child is not able to participate in a standardized procedure, there are several formalized, but nonstandardized, tools focusing on sensory processing. Each of the following tools is designed for a particular age group:

- The Test of Sensory Functioning in Infants (TSFI) (DeGangi & Greenspan, 1989) is for children birth through 18 months. This tool of quantified observations is helpful if there are concerns noted in the young child.

- The DeGangi-Berk Test of Sensory Integration (TSI) (DeGangi & Berk, 1983) was created by the same primary author as the TSFI but is used for children 3 to 5 years. There is a more formalized scoring of the identified quantified observations, which results in a score classification of normal range, at risk, or deficient. The areas addressed include postural control, bilateral integration, and the influences of residual reflexes.
- Reisman and Hanschu (1992) created the Sensory Integration Inventory of Individuals with Developmental Disabilities (SII-DD), a formalized questionnaire to identify issues in specific areas of sensory processing. This tool, which is not age specific, is designed as a formalized questionnaire that can be completed by the family or educational staff. The SII-DD is used to identify sensory processing issues that present as behaviors that might interfere with functional participation within the environment. The results of the questionnaire need to be interpreted by the OT secondary to the complicated and evolving theory of sensory integration.

In addition to the tests of sensory processing, traditional standardized motor assessments could be helpful. These include the following:

- Test of Visual Perceptual Skills-Revised (TVPS-R), by Gardner (1996), is a nonmotor test assessing 7 areas of visual perceptual functioning. There are upper and lower divisions of the test depending on the child's age, 4 to 12 years for lower division and 12 to 17 years 11 months for upper division.
- Test of Visual Motor Skills-Revised (TVMS-R), also by Gardner (1995), has upper and lower divisions. The revised test has categories of visual motor functioning, such as intersecting lines, the ability to close or connect designs, angulation, and change of direction of the strokes.
- The Beery Developmental Test of Visual-Motor Integration (VMI) (Beery, 1997) is another test of visual motor functioning.
- The Bruininks-Oseretsky Test of Motor Proficiency (BOTMP) (Bruininks, 1978) is used for children 4.5 years to 14.5 years. This tool is useful in assessing underlying skills such as speed and dexterity, upper extremity control, and response speed.
- Miller and Roid (1994) created the Toddler and Infant Motor Evaluation (TIME) for children 4 months to 3.5 years. The intent of the tool is to identify motor delays and deviations in 8 domains related to motor abilities. This assessment tool may be useful if the referred child is younger than 4 years and therefore ineligible for most other standardized tools.
- Peabody Developmental Motor Scales-2 (PDMS-2) (Folio & Fewell, 2000) is also appropriate for younger children who might not be able to complete other assessment tools. The PDMS is utilized for children birth to 6 years 11 months.

With the diagnosis of autism, there are numerous occasions when a child appears to possess the motor ability to complete a task but does not demonstrate the skill within the appropriate context. For example, a child may be noted to climb up on high furniture and balance with extreme precision. However, the child is unable to complete a prerequisite skill of standing on one foot for a specified amount of time. Again, the role of OT would be to assess occupational performance. Therefore, the certified assistant should develop competencies in and be able to implement criterion-referenced assessments. These tools are designed to gain descriptive information of functional domains of performance, outline components of skills that are present or absent, and describe the child's current functioning while providing guidelines for future skill emergence. During these observations, the OTA should remember to clinically observe sensory processing, including defensiveness, modulation, registration, and motor planning. If a criterion-referenced tool is used, the OTA may in fact complete most of the data gathering and collaborate with the OT to write up a formal report. The following criterion-referenced tools might be appropriate:

- The Brigance Diagnostic Inventory of Early Childhood Development (Brigance, 1991), a tool for children birth to 6 years, is particularly appropriate for school settings because it allows for other disciplines to complete additional sections related to other domains of functioning. Domains appropriate for OT include fine motor, dressing, and feeding. The certified assistant is able to complete these portions of the evaluation and share the findings with the OT for analysis and coordination with other assessment findings.
- The Hawaii Early Learning Profile (HELP) (Vort Corporation, 1995) outlines skills for 2 age groups: birth to 3 years and 3 to 6 years. As this evaluation tool provides an in-depth task analysis of all daily living skills (e.g., dressing, feeding, fine motor, and visual motor skills), it is an appropriate tool for the OTA to complete. Again, this tool would be helpful because the child with autism may have the necessary motor skills to complete a task but may not demonstrate active participation in functional activities.

Case Study

Review of Medical Records Pertinent to Educational Intervention

Ethan is a 3-year 2-month-old boy that was referred to the Board of Education. He has received medically-based OT services since being diagnosed with autism spectrum disorder at 2.5 years of age. Based on the initial occupational profile and the client factors determined to be interfering the most with functional participation, the services identified as the most pressing at the time of initial evaluation were sensory integrative in nature. Ethan's family arranged for him to receive services at a clinic that specializes in Ayres' sensory integration. At the time of the original referral, Ethan was not able to be assessed via standardized measures. The following clinical issues, which will require coordination with the educationally-based services, were presented in the medically-based OT report:

- Defensive responses to tactile, vestibular, and auditory inputs. The following definition, noted within the medical report, should be shared with the educational team in order to understand how Ethan may be responding to sensory experiences within the educational environment.

  All of us have a protective system in our bodies that responds to certain sensations that are interpreted as potential danger. For example, touching a hot stove or having a spider crawl on our arm makes us react by quickly removing our arm, getting an internal response of fear or anxiety, or brushing our skin until the "annoying touch" goes away. Certain people, however, have what is termed *tactile defensiveness* (i.e., an overactivation of this protective sense). These people, due to a misperception of the tactile experience, respond "protectively" to certain touches that most people would not find annoying, noxious, or potentially dangerous. For example, individuals with tactile defensiveness can be described as avoiding, sometimes overactive, emotional, or responding with behavioral outbursts. It is also important to recognize that the literature supports that people who are defensive to tactile stimuli are often sensitive to sights, sounds, movements, tastes, and/or smells. If more than one sensory system is involved, it is termed *sensory defensiveness*.

- Decreased body awareness in space secondary to inefficient proprioceptive processing.

  The proprioceptive system refers to the perception of joint and body movement, as well as position of the body, or body segments, in space. It enables us to check on the spatial orientation of our bodies or body parts in space, the rate and timing of our movements, how much force our muscles are exerting, and how much and how fast a muscle is being stretched. When considering the educational implications, OT personnel decided that fine motor functioning should be investigated due to the influence that efficient proprioceptive feedback has on the development of fine motor skills.

- Decreased motor planning skills were identified via clinical observations and parent report. As the educationally-based OT and OTA discussed this issue, it was determined that a functionally-based, criterion-referenced assessment tool should be utilized rather than standardized assessment tools.

Educational Assessment and Staff Training

Upon referral to the local school district, Ethan was assessed with the Childhood Autism Rating Scale (CARS) by the special education teacher and the speech language pathologist. This assessment tool (Western Psychological Services, 1988) contains several categories including relating to people, imitation, body use, object use, adaptation to change, and responses to sensory experiences. Based on the results, a referral to OT as

a related service was initiated. A related service is defined as that which is necessary to support the special education instruction. OT, as an educationally-based related service, is not intended to be a medical service but rather must be necessary for educational performance. The law that outlined OT services as a related service was written in the early 1970s. Although the laws have been revised, expanded, and redefined since that time, OT has always remained as a related service for the child to benefit from special education.

During the assessment period, the team decided that the OT/OTA should begin training the educational staff based on the information provided by the medically-based OT, which also coordinated with the CARS results and preliminary clinical observations within the classroom setting. The following 2 concerns were focused upon by the therapists for initial staff training:

1. Sensory defensive responses to tactile, vestibular, and auditory inputs were identified in the medically-based report and supported within the CARS results. With reference to intervention, literature supports that this issue needs to be addressed first. Therefore, training was implemented at the earliest opportunity. It was important to emphasize that negative responses to sensory experiences might not be readily apparent to the staff at the moment of occurrence. Defensiveness, which has cumulative effect, can impact the individual without being noticed by staff until a dramatic behavioral response is demonstrated. The primary procedure to address defensiveness, called the Wilbarger Protocol (Wilbarger & Wilbarger, 1991), requires strong doses of deep touch pressure followed immediately by quick joint compressions. The Wilbarger Protocol is ideally implemented every 2 hours for maximum effect. The OT or OTA is responsible for training and monitoring staff implementation of the protocol on a regular basis. Although every 2 hours is ideal, the constraints of a classroom routine may influence this schedule. In an attempt to follow this schedule as closely as possible, the other team members were trained in carrying out the program.

2. Sensory modulation concerns were mentioned within the medically-based OT report but not emphasized. This may have been due to the fact that within a one-on-one environment, modulation concerns were not readily apparent. However, within the hustle and bustle of a classroom environment, Ethan's modulation concerns were quite evident. His sensory seeking behaviors appeared to be associated with modulation difficulties. Modulation is the ability to regulate/maintain arousal so that a person can orient, focus attention on meaningful sensory events, and maintain an alert but relaxed state. It is this optimum level of arousal that allows us to function meaningfully within our environment. It was determined by team observations that Ethan was seeking out sensory experiences that appeared to have an organizing effect. These experiences included movement (e.g., running, rocking, and swinging), as well as proprioceptive input such as pulling, pushing, biting toys, poking his fingers into peo-

ple, and hiding under the pile of pillows in the reading corner.

It was important to emphasize to the staff that the protocol for defensiveness works best within the context of a sensory program to address modulation. This program, often called a sensory "diet" to reflect the concept of many inputs provided in a well-balanced format, can occur within the natural context of the classroom (Wilbarger & Wilbarger, 1991). Components are not meant to be different from the typical classroom routine. Rather, these components are meant to augment naturally occurring situations. This diet emphasizes the exact types of inputs that Ethan was seeking on his own, but provides the experiences in a more socially appropriate manner. Frequent movement breaks, gross motor tasks, input to muscles and joints, and heavy work experiences are the main components of the sensory diet. This input should occur frequently, some say as often as every hour, to maintain the system in a calm, yet attentive state.

Although a sensory diet is individualized and must be flexible to respond to a child's fluctuating sensory needs, it was important to provide the staff with structured suggestions. The sensory diet outlined for Ethan is exhibited in Figure 12-1. Additionally, based on Ethan's auditory sensitivities, a program of therapeutic listening (Frick, 1998) was outlined. This program can be flexible within the educational environment. In addition, it would possibly assist with transitions, another area of concern noted within the CARS results, as it provides grounding and organization.

Documentation of Educationally-Based Services

As with any federally-funded program, a legal document must be designed in order to outline the necessary services. Within the school system, the IEP is the legal document that addresses the child as part of his or her educational environment (Blossom, Ford, & Cruse, 1996). The IEP is designed by a group identified as the Pupil Planning and Placement Team (PPT). Members of this team include parents, special and regular educators, an administrator, special service providers such as the OT or OTA, the student if appropriate, and other invited members, which could include an attorney, parent or child advocate, or other parent support. The IEP serves as a tool for measuring progress, ensuring communication, and providing ongoing evaluation of the child.

The IEP, which is updated at least every year, must include the child's current level of educational performance, annual goals, short-term/behavioral objectives, the services required to meet the objectives, and criteria to assess whether objectives have been met (AOTA, 1997). It is imperative that the goals and objectives be specifically related to education. Each year, at the annual IEP meeting, the previous goals are measured to determine progress, continued or additional services are decided, and new goals are developed as appropriate. At that time, the OT and OTA are to collect data and provide information to the team to assist with discussions and the decision-making process. Throughout each of these phases, the OT staff must remember to translate technical information into educational terms so that interdisciplinary team members can utilize this information effectively.

For Ethan, the delivery of educationally-based OT services by a certified assistant is appropriate. In addition to educating the team on sensory strategies, the OTA is able to address the fine motor and daily living concerns found as a result of the criterion-referenced assessment process. The goals and behavioral objectives outlined in Ethan's IEP included the following:

- Following the Wilbarger Protocol, Ethan will be able to maintain a seated position for 5 minutes of circle time for 4 out of 5 consecutive school days.
- Through the use of a sensory diet and vestibular stimulation, Ethan will sustain eye contact with the speech pathologist during a 2-turn reciprocal imitation game in 3 out of 4 consecutive attempts.
- Through sensory strategies and backward chaining techniques, Ethan will execute all steps of putting on his coat with assistance for zipper engagement in 4 out of 5 consecutive school days.
- While sitting at the table with 2 classmates, Ethan will cut on a line within a ½-inch deviation in 3 out of 4 attempts.

Service Delivery

Through a team discussion, it was decided that the educationally-based OT intervention would be delivered within the classroom environment. The parents agreed to this model of service delivery for several reasons. First, they planned to continue the specialized OT service at the private clinic. Second, they valued the idea that the OTA would function as a role model for the implementation of sensory strategies, as well as assist the staff with understanding the nonverbal sensory messages demonstrated by Ethan throughout the school day. Additionally, classroom delivery would allow the therapist to address the fine motor, visual motor, and daily living skills as they naturally occur for all of the children.

SUMMARY

The incidence of autistic spectrum disorders, also referred in previous literature and in the DSM-IV as PDD, is on the incline. As practitioners with unique knowledge of sensory processing, we are in a position to positively contribute to the intervention plans for these children. The therapist's ability to facilitate play and motor development, as well as the ability to task analyze and focus on specific skill development, is specifically useful when program planning for the child with an autism spectrum disorder. The multiple issues involved, including sensory processing, motor planning, relating to others, and adaptation to change, emphasize the need for intense cooperation between the OT and OTA. Each professional collects specific information with respect to the child's level of functioning, after which collaboration and synthesis is necessary in order to develop a comprehensive plan of action. Several frames of ref-

---

Child's Name: Ethan W.   Date: September 2004
Therapist: Tara G.

Please implement checked items.

Morning Routine:
- ❑ Push the car door closed
- ❑ High five to bus driver upon greeting
- ❑ Carry heavy object from bus to classroom (object: _____)
- ❑ Walk around school building (up/down the hills/stairs) while deep breathing
- ❑ Hold open the school door for the other children
- ❑ Pull open the classroom door
- ❑ Vigorous handshake with teacher or assistant when entering classroom
- ❑ Brisk rub over back by staff while coat is on (remember to ask permission)
- ❑ Joint compressions (as instructed by therapist) after coat is removed
- ❑ Shoulder squeezes after coat is removed
- ❑ Wall push-ups after coat is removed
- ❑ Remove chairs from on top of the table and put in correct location at table
- ❑ Errand of pushing cart or pulling the wagon while delivering a message to office
- ❑ Push something while delivering attendance
- ❑ Pull a friend in a wagon
- ❑ Apply wrist or ankle weights
- ❑ Put on weighted vest

Circle Time:
- ❑ Drag chairs to and from the circle area
- ❑ Carry containers with circle time materials to and from circle area
- ❑ Carry stack of carpet squares to the circle area
- ❑ Greet each child with a handshake or high five
- ❑ Play with squeezy ball (or other fidget) while at circle time
- ❑ Therapy band or lycra around legs of the chair
- ❑ Lycra around the trunk of the child to encapsulate
- ❑ Provide long strokes down back while seated in chair
- ❑ Provide shoulder/trunk compressions (as instructed by therapist)
- ❑ If sitting on floor, provide own personal space
- ❑ If sitting on floor, provide back support
- ❑ Allow for movement up and down for changing the calendar, etc.
- ❑ Carry containers to put materials away

Figure 12-1. Sensory diet outlined for Ethan.

erence are appropriate, some requiring more intensive training than others. For example, the use of Ayres' sensory integration requires intense and consistent attention on the part of the therapist through professional development opportunities. For this approach, although extensive clinical experience is considered optimal for medically-based intervention, educationally-based services are more manageable for the assistant. For within the educational environment, occupational behavior predominates as the basis or our profession and is inherent in the role of the assistant.

CLINICAL PROBLEM SOLVING

- Jenny, a 39-year-old woman, has resided in the state's institution for individuals with mental retardation since

she was 25. Her diagnoses include autism, mental retardation, and receptive/expressive receptive language disorder. The institution recently received a state grant to provide augmentative communication devices for 20 clients. The OTA, who had been working with Jenny for the past 6 months utilizing sensory integrative techniques, identified Jenny to the speech language pathologist as a candidate. Based on the observations that Jenny's interactions and relatedness improved following sensory integrative interventions, the OTA felt that this would be an ideal time to require more formalized communication from Jenny. Based on collaboration between the speech pathologist and certified assistant, a simple device requiring Jenny to press a switch with a picture attached was developed. The plan was to train Jenny to press the switch when she wanted more of a desired sensory activity. This was mastered fairly quickly based on its simple cause-and-effect nature. At that point, the device was adapted for 2 pictures. The intent of this step was for Jenny to identify which activity she wanted based on a choice of 2 activities. If this was accomplished, the device could be expanded to include more choices. Based on the fact that the sensory input was desired by Jenny, and also had a positive organizing effect, the potential for using a communicative device during these activities was optimum. The OTA would continue to provide sensory possibilities for Jenny, while the speech pathologist would continue to provide access to communication.

Considering the living and community environment, what types of sensory diet activities could Jenny naturally participate in during her day? Remember that sensory diets include frequent movement breaks and heavy work experiences, which are incorporated into the naturally-occurring experiences. If you were able to order $500 worth of equipment from a catalog, what would you order for Jenny?

- William Z., an 8-year-old boy with Asperger's syndrome, was referred for an educationally-based OT evaluation. Mrs. Z. indicated difficulties at home, which included meltdowns some afternoons, decreased ability to manage family events, and difficulty following verbal instructions. The OT completed 3 standardized assessments that were mastered at or above age level. Based on the fact that children within the autism spectrum often possess skills that they are unable to functionally utilize within a more distracting environment, the certified assistant was asked to observe William within his natural environments. The OTA observed William and interviewed his teachers. When discussing the outcomes with the OT, it became apparent that William functioned appropriately within his classroom, art class, physical education, and in the cafeteria, but he did have some difficulty organizing himself on the playground. While not minimizing Mrs. Z.'s concerns, William did not qualify for educationally-based OT services. Strategies to address the playground concerns included outlining the activities in which William should participate, organizing a group game prior to the children going outside, and monitoring and redirecting by the playground aide should William appear to be nonproductive. At the meeting to discuss the outcome of the evaluation, Mrs. Z. continued to express concerns regarding William's home performance. The school administrator outlined the laws governing educationally-based OT and stated that she may wish to consult her pediatrician for a medically-based referral. Additionally, although the educational system was not responsible for providing medically-based services, they were responsible for assuring that sensory issues did not interfere with participation in school, home, and community. As a result, the school did provide a sensory diet for use at home that the mother could implement as necessary. The OTA met with Mrs. Z. to demonstrate the Wilbarger Protocol and emphasized implementation before leaving for school, upon his return from school, and just after dinner time. Additionally,

since the fall season provides many opportunities for outdoor activities, Mrs. Z. received a list of suggested activities. These activities included raking, digging up the summer plants, pushing the wheelbarrow around to pick up the fallen twigs, and bagging the leaves. All of these tasks would provide heavy muscle work as well as a variety of head positions to activate the vestibular system.

What other activities could be suggested as part of an 8-year-old boy's typical afternoon or weekend? It was suggested to William's parents that he be enrolled in body-oriented, extracurricular activities. The possibilities included swimming, karate, horseback riding, yoga, and gymnastics. What are the sensory experiences in each of these activities that support the sensory diet concepts?

- Carlos was 25 years old when he was referred for a medically-based OT consultation by the state. The intent of the referral was to determine if OT could diminish Carlos' self-abusive behaviors. The assistant working within the state system had gone to a conference regarding the topic and thought that this might be a worthwhile investigation. Carlos' history included seeking large amounts of vestibular input, whirling himself, obsessing on spinning objects, banging on his ear or head to induce vibratory stimulation, crashing against the furniture, falling or throwing himself on the floor or against the wall, scratching and rubbing his arms and face until they were raw, and excessive mouthing of objects. Additionally, Carlos demonstrated a decreased tolerance of everyday noises such as the hairdryer or vacuum.

The state's OTA had already implemented structural changes within Carlos' day in an effort to help him manage his environment. These strategies included organizing his vocational work environment in zones for different activities, implementing structure and routine to his day, organizing picture card symbols to help him transition from one activity to the next, providing timers to help with preparation with transitions, and minimizing the extraneous stimuli within his environment by setting up his work station in a less distracting part of the work area. The consulting OT confirmed the OTA's thought that sensory integrative strategies were appropriate. The Wilbarger Protocol, the most effective for sensory defensiveness, was shared with the assistant. As part of this program, it was emphasized that the possible fear reactions that Carlos might demonstrate be respected. If someone has functioned in a defensive manner for what could have been the past 25 years, therapy needs to be supportive and not invasive. Therapeutic listening (Frick, 1998) was also outlined for implementation based on Carlos' auditory issues. It was suggested that this program begin prior to the Wilbarger Protocol in order to begin modulating Carlos' level of arousal. In addition to the Wilbarger Protocol and therapeutic listening, the concepts of the sensory diet were discussed based on the assistant's understanding from the seminar. The plan was for the assistant to implement these strategies and call the OT to discuss observations and possible revisions.

EVIDENCE-BASED TREATMENT STRATEGIES

Treatment Strategies	Authors
Social and peer interaction (including social stories)	Barry et al., 2003; Jackson et al., 2003; Laushey & Heflin, 2000; Nikopoulos & Keenan, 2004; Orsmond, Krauss, & Seltzer, 2004; Thiemann & Goldstein, 2001
Play	Jarrold, 2003; Kok, Kong, & Bernard-Opitz, 2002; Stahmer, Ingersoll, & Carter, 2003; Van Berckelaer-Onnes, 2003
Functional impact of sensory experiences	Baraneck, 2002; Case-Smith & Bryan, 1999; Case-Smith & Miller, 1999; Dawson & Watling, 2000; Hogg, Cavet, Lambe, & Smeddle, 2001; Ingersoll, Schreibman, & Tran, 2003; Linderman & Steward, 1999; Olson & Moulton, 2004; Watling, Deitz, & White, 2001
Communication	Hetzroni & Tannous, 2004; Kravits, Kamps, Kemmerer, & Potucek, 2002

If Carlos spends each day in a workshop setting, identify sensory diet activities that might be appropriate. Remember to include opportunities within self-care, vocational, and maintenance activities. Are there any suggestions that could be shared with the transportation staff with regard to noise on the van, seat placement, or the amount of touch provided when assisting Carlos on and off the van?

LEARNING ACTIVITIES

1. Visit a preschool and observe children playing. Observe the sensory components of the child's environment and the types of social interactions these children have spontaneously and with teacher prompting.

2. Interview the parents of a child with autism spectrum disorder. Ask them to tell "their story" from pregnancy to current time. Pay particular attention to the signs that caused them concern before the child actually received the diagnosis. Also, obtain information on the process of getting therapeutic support for their child.

3. Check the Internet for organizations that provide diagnostic and therapeutic information, offer support to families, and/or offer current research information. Evaluate each site for trustworthiness.

REFERENCES

American Psychiatric Association. (1994). *Diagnostic and statistical manual for mental disorders* (4th ed.). Washington, DC: Author.

American Occupational Therapy Association. (1997). *OT services for children and youth under the Individuals with Disabilities Education Act*. Bethesda, MD: Author.

Ayres, A. J. (1972). *Sensory integration and the child*. Los Angeles, CA: Western Psychological Services.

Ayres, A. J. (1989). *Sensory Integration and Praxis Tests*. Los Angeles, CA: Western Psychological Services.

Baker, H. C. (2002). A comparison study of autism spectrum disorder referrals: 1997 and 1989. *Journal of Autism and Developmental Disorders, 32*(2), 121-125.

Baraneck, G. T. (2002). Efficacy of sensory and motor interventions for children with autism. *Journal of Autism and Developmental Disorders, 32*(5), 397-422.

Barry, T. D., Klinger, L. G., Lee, J. M., Palardy, N., Gilmore, T., & Bodin, S. D. (2003). Examining the effectiveness of an outpatient clinic-based social skills group for high-functioning children with autism. *Journal of Autism and Developmental Disorders, 33*(6), 685-701.

Bauman, M. L., & Kemper, T. L. (1985). Histoanatomic observations of the brain in early infantile autism. *Neurology, 35*, 866-874.

Bauman, M. L., & Kemper, T. L. (1994). *The neurobiology of autism*. Baltimore, MD: Johns Hopkins University Press.

Bauman, M. L., & Kemper, T. L. (2003). The neuropathology of the autism spectrum disorders: What have we learned? *Novartis Foundation Symposium, 251*, 112-122.

Beery, K. E. (1997). *The Beery developmental test of visual-motor integration-revised*. Parsippany, NJ: Modern Curriculum Press.

Blossom, B., Ford, F., & Cruse, C. (1996). *Physical therapy and OT in the public schools*. Rome, GA: Rehabilitation Publications and Therapies Inc.

Brambilla, P., Hardan, A., di Nemi, S. U., Perez, J., Soares, J. C., & Barale, R. (2003). Brain anatomy and development in autism: Review of structural MRI studies. *Brain Research Bulletin, 61*(6), 557-569.

Brigance, A. H. (1991). *Brigance diagnostic inventory of early development-revised*. North Billerica, MA: Curriculum Associates Inc.

Bruininks, R. H. (1978). *Bruininks-Oseretsky test of motor proficiency*. Circle Pines, MN: American Guidance Service.

Byrd, R. S. (2002). The epidemiology of autism in California: A comprehensive pilot study. Report to the Legislature on the Principal Findings.

Case-Smith, J., & Bryan, T. (1999). The effects of occupational therapy with sensory integration emphasis on preschool-age children with autism. *American Journal of Occupational Therapy, 53*, 489-497.

Case-Smith, J., & Miller, H. (1999). Occupational therapy with children with pervasive developmental disorders. *American Journal of Occupational Therapy, 53*, 506-513.

Cohen, F., & Volkmar, F. R. (1997). *Autism and pervasive developmental disorders: A handbook.* New York, NY: Doubleday.

Courchesne, E., Yeung-Courchesne, R., Press, G. A., Hesselink, J. R., & Jennigan, T. L. (1988). Hypoplasia of vermal lobules VI and VII in autism. *New England Journal of Medicine, 318,* 1349-1354.

Dawson, G., & Watling, R. (2000). Interventions to facilitate auditory, visual and motor integration in autism: A review of the evidence. *Journal of Autism and Developmental Disorders, 30,* 415-421.

DeGangi, G. A., & Berk, R. A. (1983). *DeGangi-Berk test of sensory integration.* Los Angeles, CA: Western Psychological Services.

DeGangi, G. A., & Greenspan, S. (1989). *Test of sensory functioning in infants.* Los Angeles, CA: Western Psychological Services.

Dunn, W. (1999). *The sensory profile.* San Antonio, TX: Psychological Corp.

Fatemi, S. H., Halt, A. R., Realmuto, G., Earle, J., Kist, D. A., Thuras, P., et al. (2002). Purkinje cell size is reduced in cerebellum of patients with autism. *Cellular and Molecular Neurobiology, 22(2),* 171-175.

Folio, M. R., & Fewell, R. R. (2000). *Peabody developmental motor scales-2.* Austin, TX: Pro-ed.

Frick, S. (1998). *Listening with the whole body workshop.* Hamden, CT: Author.

Gardner, M. F. (1995). *Test of visual-motor skills-revised.* Hydesville, CA: Psychological and Educational Publications Inc.

Gardner, M. F. (1996). *Test of visual-perceptual skills-revised.* Hydesville, CA: Psychological and Educational Publications Inc.

Glennon, T. J., & Miller-Kuhaneck, H. (2004). Introduction to autism and pervasive developmental disorders. In H. Miller-Kuhaneck (Ed.), Autism: A comprehensive occupational therapy approach (2nd ed.). Bethesda, MD: AOTA Press.

Hanschu, B. (1997). *Evaluation and treatment of sensory processing disorders.* Bridgewater, NJ: Author.

Hardan, A. Y., Minshew, N. J., Harenski, K., & Keshavan, M. S. (2001). Posterior fossa magnetic resonance imaging in autism. *Journal of the American Academy of Child and Adolescent Psychiatry, 40(6),* 666-672.

Hetzroni, O. E., & Tannous, J. (2004). Effect of a computer-based intervention program on the communicative functions of children with autism. *Journal of Autism and Developmental Disorders, 34(2),* 95-113.

Hogg, J., Cavet, J., Lambe, L., & Smeddle, M. (2001). The use of "Snoezelen" as multisensory stimulation with people with intellectual disabilities: A review of the research. *Research in Developmental Disabilities, 22(5),* 353-372.

Ingersoll, B., Schreibman, L., & Tran, Q. H. (2003). Effect of sensory feedback on immediate object imitation in children with autism. *Journal of Autism and Developmental Disorders, 33(6),* 673-683.

Jackson, C. T., Fein, D., Wolf, J., Jones, G., Hauck, M., Waterhouse, L., et al. (2003). Responses and sustained interactions in children with mental retardation and autism. *Journal of Autism and Developmental Disorders, 33(2),* 115-121.

Jarrold, C. (2003). A review of research into pretend play in autism. *Autism, 7(4),* 379-390.

Kanner, L. (1943). Autistic disturbances of affective contact. *Nervous Child, 2,* 217-250.

Kok, A. J., Kong, T. Y., & Bernard-Opitz, V. (2002). A comparison of the effects of structured play and facilitated play approaches on preschoolers with autism: A case study. *Autism, 6(2),* 181-196.

Kravits, T. R., Kamps, D. M., Kemmerer, K., & Potucek, J. (2002). Brief report: Increasing communication skills for an elementary-aged student with autism using the Picture Exchange Communication System. *Journal of Autism and Developmental Disorders, 32(3),* 225-230.

Laushey, K. M., & Heflin, L. J. (2000). Enhancing social skills of kindergarten children with autism through the training of multiple peers as tutors. *Journal of Autism and Developmental Disorders, 30(3),* 183-193.

Linderman, T., & Stewart, K. (1999). Sensory integrative-based occupational therapy and functional outcomes in your children with pervasive developmental disorders: A single subject study. *American Journal of Occupational Therapy, 53,* 207-213.

Merrick, J., Kandel, I., & Morad, M. (2004). Trends in autism. *International Journal of Adolescent Medicine and Health, 16(1),* 75-78.

Miller, L. J., & Roid, G. H. (1994). *The toddler and infant motor evaluation.* Tucson, AZ: Therapy Skill Builders.

Miller-Kuhaneck, H., & Glennon, T. J. (2004). Examining the etiology and neurologic basis of the autism spectrum disorders. In H. Miller-Kuhaneck (Ed.), Autism: A comprehensive occupational therapy approach (2nd ed.). Bethesda, MD: AOTA Press.

Nikopoulos, C. K., & Keenan, M. (2004). Effects of video modeling on social initiations by children with autism. *Journal of Applied Behavioral Analysis, 37(1),* 93-96.

Olson, L. J., & Moulton, H. J. (2004). Use of weighted vests in pediatric occupational therapy practice. *Physical and Occupational Therapy in Pediatrics, 24(3),* 45-60.

Ornitz, E. M., & Ritvo, E. R. (1968). Neurophysiologic mechanisms underlying perceptual inconsistency in autistic and schizophrenic children. *Archives of General Psychiatry, 19,* 22-27.

Orsmond, G. I., Krauss, M. W., & Seltzer, M. M. (2004). Peer relationships and social and recreational activities among adolescents and adults with autism. *Journal of Autism and Developmental Disorders, 34(3),* 245-256.

Parham, L. D., & Fazio, L. S. (1997). *Play in occupational therapy for children.* St. Louis, MO: Mosby-Year Book Inc.

Petty, L., Ornitz, E. M., Michelman, J. D., & Zimmerman, E. G. (1984). Autistic children who become schizophrenic. *Archives of General Psychiatry, 41,* 129.

Powell, J. E., Edwards, A., Edwards, M., Pandit, B. S., Sungum-Paliwal, S. R., & Whitehouse, W. (2000). Autistic spectrum disorders in preschool children from two areas of the West Midlands, U.K. *Developmental Medicine and Child Neurology, 42(9),* 624-628.

Reisman, J., & Hanschu, B. (1992). *Sensory integration inventory-revised for individuals with developmental disabilities.* Hugo, MN: PDP Press.

Rimland, B. (1985). The etiology of infantile autism: The problem of biological versus psychological causation. In A. Donnellan (Ed.), *Classic readings in autism.* New York, NY: Teachers College Press.

Ritvo, E. R., Freeman, B. J., Pingree, C., Mason-Brothers, A., Jorde, L., Jenson, W., et al. (1990). The UCLA-University of Utah epidemiologic survey of autism prevalence. *American Journal of Psychiatry, 146,* 194-199.

Sponheim, E. (1996). Changing criteria of autistic disorders: A comparison of the ICD-10 research criteria and DSM-IV with DSM-III-R, CARS, and ABC. *Journal of Autism and Developmental Disorders, 26(5),* 513.

Stahmer, A. C., Ingersoll, B., & Carter, C. (2003). Behavioral approaches to promoting play. *Autism, 7(4),* 401-413.

Thiemann, K. S., & Goldstein, H. (2001). Social stories, written text cues, and video feedback: Effects on social communication of children with autism. *Journal of Applied Behavioral Analysis, 34*(4), 425-446.

Van Berckelaer-Onnes, I. A. (2003). Promoting early play. *Autism, 7*(4), 415-423.

Vort Corporation. (1995). *HELP checklist*. Palo Alto, CA: Author.

Watling, R. L., Deitz, J., & White, O. (2001). Comparison of Sensory Profile scores of young children with and without autism spectrum disorders. *American Journal of Occupational Therapy, 55*(4), 416-423.

Western Psychological Services. (1988). *The childhood autism rating scale*. Los Angeles, CA: Author.

Wilbarger, P., & Wilbarger, J. (1991). *Sensory defensiveness in children ages 2-12: An intervention guide for parents and other caregivers*. Santa Barbara, CA: Avanti Educational Programs.

SUGGESTED READING

American Occupational Therapy Association. (1989). *Guidelines for OT services in school systems*. Bethesda, MD: Author.

Blanche, E. I., Botticelli, T. M., & Hallway, M. K. (1995). *Combining neurodevelopmental and sensory integration principles: An approach to pediatric therapy*. Tucson, AZ: Therapy Skill Builders.

Bundy, A., Lane, S., & Murray, E. A. (2002). *Sensory integration theory and practice* (2nd ed.). Philadelphia: F. A. Davis.

Case-Smith, J., Allen, A. S., & Pratt, P. N. (2001). *Occupational therapy for children* (4th ed.). St. Louis, MO: Mosby-Year Book Inc.

Dunn, W. (1991). *Pediatric occupational therapy*. Thorofare, NJ: SLACK Incorporated.

CENTER FOR PEDIATRIC THERAPY

CONSENT FORM

CHILD: _Ethan_

PARENT: _Janet_

no   CPT may videotape my child for the sole purpose of education and instruction.

X   CPT may release or share information concerning my child with the below listed individual(s):

X   CPT may obtain information concerning my child with the below listed individual(s):

	NAME	ADDRESS	PHONE
Pediatrician:	Dr. Bartholomew	Fairfield	
Neurologist:	Dr. Frank Martin	New Haven (going next wk)	
Other:	—		
Insurance Co.:	Cigna Healthcare		
Board of Ed:			
Therapist:	—		

Janet
Parent's Signature

Dec 2, 2003
Date

Tara J. Glennon, EdD, OTR/L, BCP
Executive Director

Real record 12-1. Real record for a client with autism spectrum disorder.

Center for Pediatric Therapy

◆ Executive Director: Tara J. Glennon, EdD, OTR/L, BCP, FAOTA

INTAKE   ☐ Out Of Network   ☒ OT ☐ PT ☐ SPEECH

Child's Name: Ethan	Date of Intake: 11/13/03
DOB:	Date of Eval: 12/2/03
Diagnosis Code: no dx; investigating c̄ MD *if applicable*	Therapist: CR
Medications: Ø ; hx of antacids for reflux	
Parents' Names: Janet *mother* Richard *father*	Home: 255-
	Work: 212-
Home Address: 27 Old Ftd.	Cell: 414-
School Program: Ø	Grade: Ø
Insurance Co.: Cigna	Phone:
	Group #: ⎫ will find out
Subscriber Name: Richard	ID #: ⎭ husband has info
MD Script: ☐ bringing day of evaluation ☒ faxing	
Pediatrician: Dr. Bartholomew *first last*	Phone: 215-
Dr.'s Address: ftd. *street unit* *city zip*	
Other therapists: Ø	
Other Physicians: Ø	

Referred By: Mary *psychologist neurologist* (neighbor whose child comes *other*
Reason for Referral: hard time tolerating things here)

ADDITIONAL COMMENTS:
- hx of reflux, vomit after chunky food; car sick - can't go anywhere in the car.
- was always a fussy baby; even tantrums
- can't play c̄ other kids
- always on the go or just sits & stares
- never really "plays" c̄ toys; has a room full but doesn't use them
- going to neurologist next wk. bec' Dr. B said might be neurological issue
- husband says that he is fine, but something is going on.

Available evaluation times: any am is ok	TOTAL TIME: 19 days.
Available treatment times: same	

Real record 12-2. Real record for a client with autism spectrum disorder.

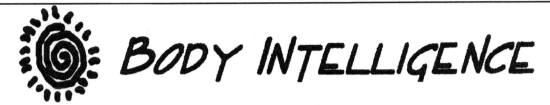

BODY INTELLIGENCE

facsimile transmittal

To: Mary Jones - Speech   Fax: _____

From: Debra   Date: 3-7-04

Re: Jenny   Pages: 1

CC: —

Notes:

Mary,

I heard from DMR that you will be evaluating Jenny next month. Jenny has been receiving therapeutic massages for approximately 3 months. I have been communicating with Kim Suleivan, Jenny's OTA, and we have both seen positive results of the massage. I would be happy to speak with you as well. Please feel free to call with any questions.

Thanks,

Debra McMurphy, LMT

a place of comfort and health —

enabling you to connect with the healer within...

Real record 12-3. Real record for a client with autism spectrum disorder.

Key Concepts

- Sensory integration (SI): The term is used in 2 primary ways. It is a term used to denote the convergence and perception of multiple stimuli in the CNS, and a theory and frame of reference developed by A. Jean Ayres and used in OT.
- Adaptive response: Sensory integration provides a foundation for the development of skills essential for engagement in meaningful, needed, and desired occupation and co-occupations. The outcomes expected from OT using Ayres' SI approach are functional outcomes, improved occupational performance, and increased engagement in appropriate co-occupations.
- Advance training: An OT or OTA using Ayres' SI approach should have advanced training, as the process is complex and requires ongoing assessment and continual clinical reasoning based on theory.

Essential Vocabulary

adaptive response: An effective adjustment to an environmental demand (Spitzer & Smith Roley, 2001)

arousal: Alertness or wakefulness.

dyspraxia: A developmental condition in which the ability to plan novel motor tasks is impaired (Bundy, Lane, & Murray, 2002).

praxis: The ability to plan and execute a novel motor task. Includes ideation, planning and execution (Ayres, 1985).

sensory defensiveness: A fight or flight reaction to sensation others would not find noxious (Bundy & Murray, 2002); one type of sensory modulation dysfunction.

sensory integration: The neurobiological process of organizing sensations and using them effectively (Ayres, 1972); a theory and frame of reference originated by A. Jean Ayres developed within the profession of OT.

sensory integration intervention: A therapeutic approach originally designed by A. Jean Ayres used within OT practice primarily in pediatrics. This intervention highlights playful, child-directed activities guided by a specially-trained therapist that are rich in vestibular, tactile, and proprioceptive sensations. These activities encourage planning and organizing of behavior and elicit increasingly complex and generalizable adaptive responses.

sensory integrative dysfunction: Difficulty with the processing of sensation, which is manifested as poor praxis, poor modulation, or both (Bundy et al., 2002)

sensory modulation: The capacity to regulate and organize the degree, intensity, and nature of responses to sensory input in a graded and adaptive manner (Miller & Lane, 2000).

sensory modulation dysfunction: A pattern of dysfunction whereby an individual over or under responds to sensory input (Bundy et al., 2002).

sensory processing: Functions relating to the CNS, including the receipt, modulation, integration, and organization of sensory stimuli (Bundy et al., 2002).

sensory strategies: Techniques or methods designed by trained therapists and used to assist a child maintain self-regulation, attention, and focus and increase skilled performance within his or her home, school, and community.

Clinical Summary

Etiology

Currently unknown. Experts in the area of SI believe it to be a brain-based disorder, as did A. Jean Ayres. Further research is needed to clarify the etiology of these disorders and document them as individual disorders, differentiated from other disorders.

Theory Base

Sensory integration theory is built upon research in multiple professional fields such as anatomy, neuroscience, psychology, motor control, education, and occupational science.

Prevalence

There has been little research in this area. However, Miller (2004) suggested from her research that perhaps 5% of the general population might have sensory modulation disorder, one type of SI dysfunction.

Observable Signs and Symptoms

The largest body of research in SI supports the identification of specific types of sensory integrative deficits, specifically vestibular-based postural and bilateral disorders; tactile-based praxis disorders; visual-motor and visual construction disorders; and sensory modulation deficits. Some possible signs include clumsiness, poor coordination, poor balance, limited play skills, repetitive use of materials or toys, fear of sensations, extreme over or underreactions to sensation, and difficulty regulating arousal level and behavior in response to sensations.

A KINDERGARTNER WITH SENSORY INTEGRATION DYSFUNCTION

Heather Miller Kuhaneck, MS, OTR, BCP and Susanne Smith Roley, MS, OTR, FAOTA

Robby, a 5.5-year-old boy, is a loving and sensitive child who becomes extremely upset when he realizes he has done something that makes others unhappy. He loves playing with other children and cannot understand why they don't want to play with him. He tries very hard to make friends but often becomes frustrated when his attempts to enter into play with his peers are unsuccessful.

He was referred for an OT evaluation by his kindergarten teacher, who is concerned with Robby's ability to participate with his peers at school. His peers are wary of him because he is unpredictable and plays too roughly. His teacher also reports concerns with his writing and cutting skills. She says the other children in the class are drawing and writing some letters, but Robby expresses no interest in these activities at all. In fact, he refuses to draw and will give the crayons to others, saying, "You make it for me."

His mother, Liz, also notes that he prefers to be helped rather than doing things on his own. She reports that Robby occasionally knocks down his little sister while playing and sometimes hugs her too hard. He has trouble keeping up with the neighborhood children on his bike, which bothers him tremendously. He refuses to consider removing his training wheels. She reports that although she has other children, he consumes most of her attention. It is often easier to leave him out than include him in typical family events such as dinner out because of his behavior. She is concerned that Robby gets into a lot of trouble at school and may be falling behind.

INTRODUCTION

Children like Robby often have deficits in SI and praxis that affect their ability to engage in occupations and negatively impact their ability to learn, attend, and behave appropriately. In turn, the occupational engagement patterns of the whole family are affected by the difficulties of the child. Therefore, parents commonly seek out OTs knowledgeable in the SI approach, to identify potential causes of their child's behaviors and for strategies that will help their child and the family. An OT, Dr. A. Jean Ayres, originated the theory and methods called SI, and their further development has continued primarily within the profession of OT. OTs are best equipped to use the SI frame of reference because of the significant impact of these deficits on all aspects of the child's occupational performance. This chapter will introduce the core concepts of SI theory and provide information to the OTA regarding its use in practice.

A THEORY AND FRAME OF REFERENCE IN OCCUPATIONAL THERAPY

SI is a term known in OT as both a theory and an intervention approach. Dr. Ayres refined her theory over many years, through her study of neurobiological and related literature, her research, and her innovative test development (see Bundy & Murray, 2002). She was a scholar and a clinician whose ideas have heavily influenced pediatric practice in multiple fields. Dr. Ayres' unique playful, child-directed intervention approach embodied her personal philosophy of empathy and respect for her clients (Spitzer & Smith Roley, 2001).

Ayres defined SI as the neurobiological process of organizing sensations and using them effectively (Ayres, 1972). She proposed that SI is a crucial part of our development and is essential even before birth. Sensation and action are intimately linked, with one leading to the other (Spitzer & Smith Roley, 2001). Ayres believed that the individual has a drive to be purposeful and to interact in an adaptive fashion within the environment. SI, therefore, is not merely about the receipt of sensation by the body; it is about the individual's ability to use the information received to act effectively on the environment (Ayres, 1972, 1979; Spitzer & Smith Roley, 2001). As a mediator between the child's sense of self and the world, SI provides a critical foundation for learning, motor development, skill acquisition, and engaging in meaningful occupations and co-occupations (Parham, 2002).

THE CONTRIBUTIONS OF SENSATION TO FUNCTION

Humans acquire knowledge and process information through multiple senses starting very early in life and continuing throughout the life span. In fact, the sensory receptors are fully formed and begin functioning at or before birth (Bear, Connors, & Paradiso, 2001). Sensory receptors provide information about what is outside the body (i.e., exteroceptors), where and how the body is positioned and moving (i.e., proprioceptors), and what is going on inside the body (i.e., interoceptors). The exteroceptors include the tactile sense, or touch; the auditory sense, or hearing; the visual sense, or vision; the olfactory sense, or smell; and the gustatory sense, or taste. The proprioceptors include proprioception, or awareness of muscle and joint position and muscle force; and the vestibular sense, or awareness of movement and head position in relation to gravity (Blanche & Schaaf, 2001; Cohn, 1999). The interoceptors, or internal sensations, provide information about bodily states such as hunger, pain, and the need for elimination (Bear et al., 1996; Kandel, Schwartz, & Jessell, 2000).

Human beings need to be able to discriminate the temporal and spatial qualities of sensation in order to determine where a sound came from, how fast we are moving, or how much force we are using to throw a ball. We also use our senses to know if the object in our mouth feels sharp and dangerous or if we just stepped onto something that is unstable. We use sensation to anticipate and plan our activities and to provide feedback when we move, eat, work, and play. While each sensory receptor system has an important primary function for the body, the senses do not function independently. Rather, the senses work in concert to provide a 3-dimensional view of the world needed to navigate and perform (Calvert, Spence, & Stein, 2004; Lewkowicz & Lickliter, 1994).

Sensory experiences are essential for learning. Learning takes place through the interactions of experiences and the perception and memory of these experiences. Each person is unique in his or her sensory and perceived experience depending on his or her genetics, interests, abilities, and experiences (Jacobs & Schneider, 2001; Kraemer, 2001). When the individual has accurate and efficient sensory processing, these perceptions are accurate. Over time, the developing child has increasing perceptual memories that form the basis for future action plans. As adults, it is easy for us to see something and know the texture, weight, distance, and smell just from looking at it as a result of these multisensory memories. We can also navigate through space without much conscious thought because we have done it before and know what to do before we even start (Mailloux & Smith Roley, 2004).

SI is an ongoing process. An individual's inner drive to be involved in meaningful activity leads to activity. Activity produces sensations and feedback as action occurs. The sensations are integrated; responses are planned and executed; and if the demands of the environment are met, feedback from within and without allows learning to occur. Therefore, more and more complex behaviors can be generated. As SI occurs and adaptive interactions take place, the individual learns to believe in his or her skill level and gains a sense of mastery and control. This in turn provides meaning and satisfaction, motivation, and self-direction, eventually leading to self-actualization (Bundy & Murray, 2002).

THE RELATIONSHIP OF SENSORY INTEGRATION TO OCCUPATION

SI is one of many factors that potentially affect occupational performance. Performance is influenced by an individual's capacities, desires, opportunities, environmental supports, and a myriad of other factors. A child may choose or avoid specific activities because of the way that he or she perceives the sensory aspects of those tasks. While poor SI is only one of many factors that creates ineffective occupational performance, it has a pervasive influence over time, and therefore may be a significant factor in shaping a person's occupational choices, the possibilities of occupational engagement for the individual and their friends and family, and sense of one's self as an occupational being (Parham, 2002).

Spitzer and Smith Roley (2001) proposed a model of SI as a critical foundation for occupation. The model depicts the dynamic and nonlinear nature of SI at the center of development like the hub of a spinning wheel. The core functions of sensory modulation and sensory discrimination are separate, but interact and affect each other. The ability to modulate sensation affects primarily social-emotional development and behaviors, while the ability to discriminate sensory data affects primarily postural control, motor skills, and praxis. Dynamically interacting, these functions influence and are influenced by the individual's ability to adapt to the sensory environment, their motivations and desires, and their internal and external organization of behavior. Interacting well, these functions allow engagement in occupation through the physical, cultural, temporal, and social environments. Through engagement in occupations and co-occupations, the individual becomes more integrated, ready to engage further in satisfying necessary and increasing complex activities.

USING SENSORY INTEGRATION THEORY IN OCCUPATIONAL THERAPY PRACTICE

Currently, many parents seek OT services specifically for evaluation and intervention highlighting SI function and dysfunction. Typically, the parents will report confusing sensory-seeking behaviors, sensory-avoiding behaviors, or inadequate sensorimotor skill development in addition to areas of concerns related to social-emotional development and motor planning. OT using the SI frame of reference requires specialized knowledge of the sensory systems, typical and atypical development, and the contribution of sensation to occupation. Knowledge of SI theory supports clinical reasoning, allowing the OT to take into consideration typical fluctuations in day-to-day sensory processing abilities and its impact on occupational performance.

When a child is referred for OT specifically for issues related to SI, it is important for the OT to ensure that:

- The referral is related to concerns regarding engaging in needed and desired occupations.
- The evaluation by the OT guides the use of SI or any other of the many methods used.
- The goals and objectives of OT are to improve occupational performance.
- The practitioner knows when to refer a child to a specialist who is certified in SI and the Sensory Integration and Praxis Tests (SIPT) to provide a thorough evaluation and intervention.
- The OT using Ayres' SI approach is specially trained and uses these methods in an appropriate, safe environment. The environment must have access to specialized equipment, providing the possibility for vestibular, tactile, and proprioceptive sensations, as well as the ability to rearrange items within the environment to engage the child in active play and build praxis skills.
- OTs knowledgeable in the SI frame of reference create the home programs, environmental modifications, and/or sensory strategies used in settings such as the home or the school that may be carried out by the OTA.

Occupational Therapy Evaluation Including Sensory Integration

The evaluation process often begins with the occupational profile and then the analysis of occupational performance (AOTA, 2002). The information from the occupational profile guides the OT in the selection of the types of assessments appropriate to the child and the areas of concern. While the OTA may complete specific aspects of the assessment, it is essential that the OT selects the appropriate tools and interprets the data to determine the presence and nature of SI deficits.

The primary SI deficits have been classified into 3 primary areas: vestibular-proprioceptive processing and motor skill deficits; tactile discrimination and praxis deficits; and sensory modulation, arousal, and self-regulation deficits (Ayres, 1989; Windsor, Smith Roley, & Szklut, 2001). The symptoms presented can vary based on the specific type of sensory disorder. Some possible signs of vestibular-proprioceptive processing issues may include clumsiness, poor coordination, poor balance, and fatigue during sustained sitting or standing. Possible signs of tactile discrimination and praxis deficits may include limited play skills, repetitive use of materials or toys, and disorganization. Possible signs of sensory modulation, arousal, and self-regulation deficits include fear of sensations, extreme over- or under-reactions to sensation, and difficulty regulating alertness. In children, the SI disorders found via assessment are rarely a single type (Parham & Mailloux, 2001).

Assessment Methods

A detailed evaluation of SI requires an OT with specialized training to administer and interpret the assessments. Because we cannot directly observe the functioning of the brain, it is essential to use assessment tools and observations of behavior that specifically focus on the child's ability to effectively use sensory information to create an appropriate response. The OT will choose one or more sensory history questionnaires, standardized tests, and structured and unstructured observations of underlying sensory and motor processes in order to determine the nature and extent of the SI dysfunction (Windsor et al., 2001). Through the use of these measures, the OT constructs a hypothesis about the problem.

The "gold standard" for assessing praxis is the SIPT (Ayres, 1989). However, there are other tools such as the Sensory Profile (Dunn, 1999) and the Evaluation of Sensory Processing (Parham & Ecker, 2000) to examine other aspects of sensory processing. The Test of Sensory Function in Infants (DeGangi & Greenspan, 1998) and the DeGangi-Berk Test of Sensory Integration (Berk & DeGangi, 1987) are designed for use with younger children. The Miller Assessment for Preschoolers also provides very useful information for the younger age group. The clinical observations of motor performance (COMPS) (Wilson, Pollack, Kaplan, & Law, 2000) is a standardized tool based on several of Ayres' original clinical observations. Blanche (200a) provides a more comprehensive review of clinical observations based on SI theory.

Unstructured Observations

The OTA can support the OT by alerting him or her to any observed behaviors that are commonly associated with SI dysfunction. The OTA may observe behaviors that indicate either poor sensory awareness or unusual sensitivities to sensation. The OTA will document these observations and provide this information to the OT who will then add these data to other unstructured observation data. For example, during a fine motor task, the OTA may observe difficulty with crossing the middle of the body, poor alignment of the body to the table, extreme pressure when drawing with the pencil, and an incredibly tight writing grasp. She might also notice extreme fidgetiness in the chair, a tendency to slump or lean, or difficulty maintaining a seated position. She might take note of the child using unusual head positions in order to look at the pictures or directional confusion when drawing, often associated with visuomotor deficits. None of these observations in isolation would indicate a sensory integrative disorder; however, when the variety of evaluation information is compiled, these observations might support additional findings of difficulties with sensory processing. In this example, the OT may hypothesize that the child has poor head, neck, eye, and postural control often associated with vestibular-proprioceptive processing deficits. The child may also have poor discrimination and is therefore seeking proprioceptive feedback to assist with his or her writing skills. A standardized evaluation will assist the therapist in confirming or negating these hypotheses.

Table 13-1

Observations Possibly Related to Vestibular Proprioceptive Processing and Visual Motor Control

- Slumping in seat
- Falling out of the seat
- Low muscle tone
- Difficulty holding a body position
- Poor balance and falling
- Poor endurance or fatigue
- Difficulty watching a moving target
- Leaning head or hands on the desk
- Extreme fidgetiness while seated at the desk
- Wrapping legs around the legs of the chair
- Rocking or bouncing in the chair
- Avoiding playground equipment
- Difficulty with ball skills (catching, throwing, or kicking/hitting)

Table 13-2

Observations Related to Poor Discrimination and Motor Planning

- Poor grasp and tool use
- Writing too lightly or with too much pressure
- Frequently breaking objects like chalk, crayons, or pencil leads from pushing too hard
- Holding the pencil very tightly or very loosely
- Difficulty with precise manipulation of small objects
- Dropping objects frequently
- Difficulty cutting smoothly
- Difficulty using 2 hands together (cutting shapes, stringing beads, using a ruler)
- Sitting on legs while in chair
- Difficulty imitating a body position
- Poor coordination
- Poor timing and sequencing of motor tasks
- Clumsiness
- Inefficiency when doing things
- Difficulty playing cooperative games and organized sports
- Negative comments regarding abilities "I can't" or "I'm no good at that."

Please see Tables 13-1 to 13-3 for further examples of observations that may indicate difficulties with aspects of SI.

Interpretation and Sensory Integrative Dysfunction

Ayres' research determined that there were vestibular-based bilateral integration and sequencing deficits, somatosensory-based praxis deficits, visual perceptual and visuomotor deficits, and sensory modulation deficits. She also identified that many children demonstrated a pattern of dysfunction that indicated primarily a language disorder, dyspraxia on verbal command (Ayres, 1989; Parham & Mailloux, 2001). Mulligan's research with 10,000 children (Mulligan, 1998) supported these patterns and also found that these individual patterns were all highly related to a single factor that she called SI and praxis. It is beyond the scope of this chapter to thoroughly cover all of the types of sensory integrative dysfunction and their indications. However, careful interpretation of the data gathered through the OT evaluation may lead the OT to suspect one or more of these sensory-based disorders (Windsor et al., 2001). When this is the case, OT using Ayres' SI approach may be one of the

---

Table 13-3

Observations Related to Sensory Modulation, Arousal, and Self-Regulation

- Poor attention
- Frequent attempts to get up from the chair
- Kicking or pushing with legs onto chair, desk, or other objects (wall, table)
- Refusing hand-over-hand assistance
- Chewing on shirt, excessive mouthing, or picking at skin
- Extreme fidgeting with objects off of the table
- Withdrawal from the nearness of the therapist or from touch
- Extreme reactions to unexpected touch
- Extreme reactions to smells, tastes, bright lights, or loud noises
- Highly active, extremely fidgety
- Very lethargic and hard to get moving
- Functions well in a quiet supported setting but poorly in noisy or crowded places

---

many methods selected for intervention. The supervising OT is responsible for the interpretation of all of the assessment data and creating the intervention plan that leads to occupationally relevant outcomes. The OTA knowledgeable in the SI frame of reference is better prepared to understand the implications of the assessment for ongoing intervention.

Robby's evaluation began with his occupational profile. The OT, Julie, interviewed Robby, his mother, his father, his teacher, and his school-based OT. Julie found that Robby wanted desperately to play with the other boys in his classroom and repeatedly attempted to join in. However, he had difficulty reading their cues regarding his behavior and often played too roughly. She also found that he frequently hugged the other children too hard and wouldn't let go. However, when others approached him unexpectedly, he occasionally would react with pushing or yelling. Robby's teacher reported that he was disruptive in class because he was out of his seat constantly. She felt he was easily distracted and inattentive. She reported that he avoided many classroom tasks and activities such as arts and crafts or building with constructive toys. He was behind the others in his ability to write his name and draw pictures from his imagination.

Robby's mother, Liz, reported that Robby was adopted from another country. She had noted that he was a poor sleeper and a very fussy eater from the start. He achieved all of his motor milestones appropriately, but he never seemed to play like other children. They had often left play dates early because of his escalating behavioral difficulties. Liz mentioned the difficulties he was having with riding his bike and how important that was for Robby and the family. She also mentioned how difficult it was for the family to go out to dinner with Robby because of his behaviors in the restaurant. He would not remain in his seat and attempts to keep him occupied and eating at the table often would escalate his disruptive behaviors until he was yelling, crying, or having a tantrum. She was also still concerned that he was not sleeping sufficiently. She suggested that his behaviors varied based upon the amount of sleep that he had gotten the night before.

When Robby came to the clinic, Julie completed a variety of evaluations in addition to a play observation. Julie examined Robby's fine and visual perceptual motor skills and also his sensory-processing abilities and praxis. For this evaluation she chose the following assessment tools. Donna, the OTA, was assigned to administer portions of these evaluations.

- The Sensory Profile (Dunn, 1999) (Completed by the OT)
- Portions of the Bruininks-Oseretsky Test of Motor Proficiency (BOTMP) (Bruininks, 1978) (Completed by the OT)
- The COMPS and other structured and unstructured observations based on SI theory (Completed by the OT)
- The Test of Visual Motor Integration (VMI) (Beery, 1997) (Completed by the OTA)
- A Human Figure Drawing Assessment (Completed by the OTA)

Julie discussed the test results with Donna, who informed Julie about her observations of Robby's performance during the portions of the assessment that she completed. The results suggest that Robby has both a fine motor and a visuomotor delay in relation to other children his age. Julie hypothesizes that perhaps his difficulties with writing and drawing could be due to these delays. However, she also has noted things from the interview and her observations that suggest Robby may have dyspraxia, which could also explain the difficulties with writing, drawing, and cutting, as well as his difficulties with other play activities. His difficulties creating drawings from his imagination and building with constructive toys may reflect difficulties with ideation in particular. She is considering discussing the use of the SIPT with Liz to further examine Robby's abilities with praxis.

Robby's excessive hugging and frequent rough play suggest to Julie that perhaps he has poor sensory discrimination. Also, his human figure drawing is immature, suggesting poor body awareness perhaps also due to poor sensory discrimination. Liz's answers on the Sensory Profile and Julie's observations of his movement patterns and overall coordination support this. Lastly, Julie had noted extreme sound sensitivity during her evaluation that was supported by his Sensory Profile and further questioning of Liz. Julie believes that perhaps this sound sensitivity may be related to his distractibility in the classroom and even perhaps his disruptive behavior in restaurants.

Throughout the assessment process, Julie is generating hypotheses based on her knowledge of SI theory, neurological processes, activity analysis, and occupational performance. She systematically attempts to fit the evaluation data with her hypotheses and then rejects those that do not explain the results adequately. Julie's hypotheses consist of explanations of his difficulties in occupational performance, including the types of SI dysfunction that Robby may be experiencing, as well as the potential impact of certain environments or environmental characteristics. Over the course of the assessment and throughout intervention as well, Julie revises her clinical opinion as she gets to know Robby better, and he makes changes related to the intervention.

Children with SI deficits are not all the same and they almost never fall into a single category of dysfunction. Sometimes children will have symptoms of multiple types of sensory integrative problems. Types of sensory integrative dysfunction have been categorized and labeled by a variety of authors since Ayres, based upon their own research and ideas or through collaboration with many experts in the field (Bundy et al., 2002; Dunn, 1997; Hanft, Miller, & Lane, 2000; Miller, Cermak, Lane, Anzalone, & Koomar, 2004; Miller & Lane, 2000; Royeen & Lane, 1991). Although new research continues to provide information to guide our thinking regarding the nature of SI dysfunction, the original research completed by Ayres forms the backbone for identifying certain patterns or clusters of difficulties we call SI dysfunction.

Occupational Therapy Intervention Using Ayres' Sensory Integration Approach

The goal of all OT intervention is improved engagement in occupations to support participation in life. Whatever intervention strategies are used, they must always relate back to the needed and desired occupations identified by the family and also the funding agency. Often, it is helpful to think about the behaviors and concerns that initially brought the parent to OT when contemplating goal areas. For example, if the parent is concerned with Johnny's picky eating and behavioral outbursts, whether the problem is neuromotor deficits, tactile discrimination deficits, or auditory sensitivity, the goals and objectives will focus on improving Johnny's eating habits and behaviors. In Robby's case, the initial concerns related to appropriate play, behaviors, and participation with his family as well as peers.

Liz and Julie met to discuss the findings from Robby's OT evaluation. Together they decided upon appropriate goals for his outpatient OT. Additionally, Julie spoke with Robby's school-based practitioner to provide collaborative services for Robby. Robby's intervention with Julie and Donna will work toward the following goal areas:

- Robby will play with his peers without hugging, hitting, or pushing them.
- Robby will be able to eat at the table in a restaurant for an entire meal.
- Robby will improve his sleep patterns.
- Robby will be able to ride his bike with his peers.
- Robby will draw simple pictures from his imagination.

His goals on his IEP reflect his difficulty with the educational aspects of his performance such as cutting, writing, and playing with peers on the playground or in the classroom.

Julie suspects, and her evaluation data support, that Robby has difficulties with SI that are affecting his occupational performance. However, note that the goals are occupationally-related goals and not goals specific to the underlying sensory processing or motor deficits even though these skills and abilities are believed to reflect sensory integrative deficits. For example, Robby's inability to ride a bike could reflect inadequate vestibular proprioceptive processing, leading to poor balance and bilateral motor control. His poor cutting with scissors and writing could also reflect inadequate tactile discrimination. Robby's sleep patterns and behavior in the restaurant reflect inadequate self-regulation, sensory modulation, and arousal, especially in high stimulus environments. Julie recommends OT twice weekly in a specialized setting using Ayres' SI approach.

Julie begins Robby's therapy and develops activities appropriate for his needs. Over time, as Robby becomes more consistent in his responses, requiring less frequent and imperative changes to the interventions "on the spot," Julie is able to have Donna assume portions of Robby's direct intervention. While Julie is responsible for the OT sessions using Ayres' SI approach, Donna is able to complete other OT activities with Robby that also address his areas of need. For example, Donna works with Robby on sensory-based approaches to establishing and practicing specific motor skills. Julie feels comfortable with Donna's ability and has assessed her competence in the interventions she will be providing.

General Principles of Intervention Using Ayres' Sensory Integration Approach

OT using Ayres' SI approach is different from many of the other intervention methods used in OT (Mailloux & Smith Roley, 2004). It is highly individualized and not protocol based. The actual activities chosen and the order in which they are completed will vary tremendously from child to child and even session to session for the same child. Ayres' SI approach requires an environment in which the child is free to move safely through space and one in which the child can change the location of objects and people to create the just-right challenge. The approach requires a skilled OT who continually is evaluating, adjusting the activities, and altering the challenges based on the responses being observed at that moment.

Additional hallmarks of Ayres' SI methods are as follows:

- The child is actively engaged in child-directed activities.
- The sessions occur in an environment rich in tactile, vestibular, and proprioceptive opportunities.

- The activity taps into the child's inner drive so that the activity is its own reward.
- The therapy is provided within the context of play.
- The activities elicit an adaptive response.
- The activities provide a "just-right challenge."

Ayres' SI approach is not passive. Ayres believed that the individual has a drive to be purposeful and to interact in an adaptive fashion within the environment. SI, therefore, is not merely about the receipt of sensation by the body, but is about the individual's ability to use the information received to act effectively on the environment. A key concept in the SI frame of reference is the adaptive response (Ayres, 1972, 1979; Spitzer & Smith Roley, 2001). Being adaptive requires that individuals generalize knowledge to different environments and different challenges requiring different actions. The nature of the adaptive response changes based upon the situation and the individual. What is an adaptive response for one child may not be for another. The adaptive response for one individual changes over time as well. What is an adaptive response at one moment may become habitual if repeated over and over without any change to the environment, creating additional challenges.

Another key concept is that the approach is child directed. A child-directed approach does not mean that the child does whatever he or she wants. Rather, the child's desires and motivations are continually taken into account as the therapist very carefully and artfully crafts the activities within the sensory-rich environment. The child typically enjoys the activity as its own reward and the therapist alters the activities so that the child experiences challenges but also success. Opportunities for cooperative and imaginative play are typically present. The intervention approach uses play to create a safe space with the therapist, encouraging the child to willingly attempt more challenging tasks and experience greater successes. OT using Ayres' SI approach is fun, creative, active, and motivating. It fosters self-esteem and a "can-do" attitude. Using Ayres' SI methods is often fun for the therapist as well.

The link from theory to intervention is an art requiring the creativity and careful planning and implementation of a vigilant OT. Activities provide specific types of sensorimotor experiences that will engage the child and promote development in the appropriate areas of performance. While the intervention may look simple, it is in actuality incredibly complex and changes moment to moment. For this reason, the OT must engage in ongoing dynamic assessment to find the right level and types of activities that will benefit the child. The practitioner's skill in reflection and activity analysis is crucial in OT intervention using Ayres' SI approach.

Robby has dyspraxia, particularly difficulties with ideation and sequencing along with inadequate tactile discrimination and poor vestibular-proprioceptive processing. He also demonstrates mild tactile defensiveness, and extreme sound sensitivity. Julie feels that it is important for Robby to engage in appropriately complex activities that provide heavy work (intense input to his muscles and joints through movement) and deep touch pressure, in addition to vestibular-rich activities. She also wants to provide appropriate motor challenges to his balance and postural control and visuomotor challenges. She designs a variety of sequenced motor activities and opportunities for him to create and explore new games and motor challenges. She also realizes how much Robby needs a "playmate" to help him learn to play with his peers more appropriately. She will model ways to enter play and create peer play experiences at the clinic to allow him to practice with children his own age.

Robby's outpatient OT sessions are playful, and he doesn't seem to notice all the hard work he is doing. Julie structures the environment in the room to provide appropriate play activities that allow for vestibular, proprioceptive, and tactile inputs, along with visual and motor challenges. At times, specific skills such as writing or cutting are used during their pretend adventures, but the specific skills are not the focus of the sessions. His ability to discriminate and perceive sensations accurately, allowing for motion, action, the development of body awareness, and improved praxis, is the focus of the sessions. In addition, Julie focuses on reducing his sensitivity to sounds (sensory defensiveness) with activities that provide heavy work and deep touch pressure through active play.

Robby enjoys the activities Julie has created for him. One of Robby's favorite activities is "space defenders." Robby sits on a square platform swing, which is suspended from one point so that it may move freely in multiple directions and arcs. A variety of cardboard "bricks" are used to build space cities around the area in a circle around his "spaceship." Other objects are "aliens" that are placed around the room as well. Robby chooses a variety of sufficiently heavy objects as the spacebombs to place onto his spaceship, and then he too gets on board. Robby "blasts off" by pulling his spaceship into motion with a nearby bungee cord, which he calls the slingshot. Once he has been "slung" into space, Robby must protect the cities by knocking down the aliens. During this game he must balance his body while moving, adjust for the speed and direction of his movement to accurately target the aliens with the spacebombs, and visually track and scan the environment as he moves. Julie continually determines how to alter the difficulty and motor challenge of this game by changing his speed, body position, position and size of the aliens, weight and size of the spacebombs, and many other factors as well. Robby seems to truly enjoy being the hero and saving the cities. However, Julie is constantly alert for any behavioral or physiological signs of overstimulation and any indication that she needs to rapidly alter or end the activity.

Each activity in a session using Ayres' SI approach may not address EACH area of need. The OT structures the entire session, however, so that the child's needs are met through the range of the activities they complete for that session. The OT may also use other methods of intervention besides Ayres' SI approach. Specific skills may need to be taught and another frame of reference may be more appropriate at those times. The desired outcome of the OT intervention is to meet the goals identified and improve occupational performance; therefore, the most appropriate methods should be used to meet those goals. Often the OTA may provide those portions of the intervention in collaboration with the OT.

The Occupational Therapist and Occupational Therapy Assistant Interactions

OT using Ayres' SI approach requires continual assessment and therefore is outside the realm of competence for OTAs. However, depending upon the child's needs and deficits, the OTA can often provide portions of the intervention supporting sensorimotor skill development using other methods. The interaction between the OT and the OTA will vary greatly depending upon the setting, the OTA's competencies, and most importantly, the child's needs.

Robby has been attending OT sessions with Julie for quite some time and he now willingly works on specific motor skills that are still difficult for him. Donna, the OTA, frequently completes the OT sessions with Robby by practicing skills or specific tasks when Robby and Julie are done with their portions of the session. Donna's intervention with Robby is equally playful and silly, as this approach seems to work well with Robby. However, Donna focuses specifically on his fine motor skills and his ability to ride his bike, both areas of concern to Robby's family. She also occasionally cotreats with Julie and another child so that Robby and the other child can practice their newly learned social and play skills with a peer.

Additionally, the OTA may have a role in implementing specific OT intervention based upon the SI frame of reference. These can be called sensory-based strategies.

The Continuum of Intervention: Sensory-Based Strategies

As stated, there are certain hallmarks of Ayres' SI approach that require a specific type of environment not readily available everywhere. Therefore, many OTs have generated strategies based upon their knowledge of the SI frame of reference that address the interactions between the child, activity, and environment that are useful in the community, schools, and home. Some of these strategies may be more passive in their approach than is typical of Ayres' SI method, but many are believed to be effective, particularly in assisting children with self-regulation and arousal. The practitioner recommending these strategies should be knowledgeable in the SI frame of reference.

An important aspect of Julie's intervention will be collaboration with all the other people on Robby's team. Julie will assist Robby in finding interests and activities in the community that will help him participate with others, help his self-esteem, and support his ongoing development. His mother, Liz, must be able to understand Robby's difficulties so that she can anticipate sensory challenges and notice possibilities available during daily routines and occasions when Robby is not in therapy. The school-based OT and OTA, with Julie's consultation, will design and implement classroom strategies and environmental modifications to assist Robby in dealing with the functional impact of his SI deficits in school. For example, his sound sensitivity may be affecting his classroom performance and ability to attend. The use of headphones or earplugs might be helpful. A variety of calming sensory inputs could be used to assist him in regulating his level of arousal and attention, allowing him to participate more effectively in his education. Altering his seating to a seat that allows some motion (a ball chair or a Move 'n

Sit cushion for example) may assist him to stay in his seat and attend to instruction. The school OT via collaboration with Julie will also educate the staff at school about Robby's difficulties with sensory processing and the ways in which they all can help him perform more effectively.

Every child is different; however, various methods are known for the effect that they have on most people. Certain types of inputs are generally calming such as dim lights; soft, quiet music; slow rocking; warm baths; chewy foods or sucking candies; and deep touch inputs to our skin. Other inputs are generally alerting or arousing such as strong smells, strong tastes, bright lights, rapid or unpredictable motion, light tickly touch, and very cold temperatures. Other types of inputs are very variable. Knowledge of a child's reactions and responses to inputs and their typical arousal levels in certain environments can assist the therapist in educating others to provide the "right" types of inputs when they are needed. Please see Table 13-4 for a description of some of the strategies that may be suggested and their rationale.

Precautions

Sensory-based interventions have a powerful effect on a child's CNS. This is especially true of children with irregular CNS functioning. Therefore, it is important to study the signs of autonomic nervous system activity and adjust the activities accordingly. The therapist must be a careful observer at all times. Signs of overstimulation in a child can include autonomic nervous system reactions such as changes in skin color, yawning, hiccuping, pupil dilation, fight or flight responses, and pretending to sleep. Over stimulation may also cause behavioral changes such as significant increases or decreases in activity level, yelling, crying, striking out, withdrawing, hiding, or staring blankly. The therapist must respond immediately to any indication of overstimulation. Behavioral strategies are often unnecessary if the therapist anticipates the child's discomfort and can change the task demand or the environmental stressors. It may be difficult to determine how to assist the child in regaining a calm alert state. Discuss strategies appropriate to the individual child with the supervising therapist. Be prepared to immediately stop the activity and engage the child by employing calming, noninvasive activities. If treating a child using sensory-based strategies or Ayres' SI approach, be sure you have discussed with the OT the child's specific precautions and the methods to be used if the child shows signs of distress.

Ongoing Assessment and Documentation of Effectiveness

Since SI is a dynamic and nonlinear process, it can be difficult to accurately predict the specific improvements that occur in any one child (Spitzer & Smith Roley, 2001). However, generally the therapist can look for improvements in the following areas:

- Adaptive responses (increased frequency or duration).
- Increased complexity of interactions with people and objects.
- Greater self-confidence and self-esteem.

Table 13-4

Sensory-Based Strategies That May be Used in the Home or School

Strategy	Rationale
Deep touch pressure For example, pressure garments such as exercise gear or lycra clothing under regular clothes, sitting under a large bean bag chair, weighted vest or blanket, massage, using different types and qualities of brushes on the skin	Deep touch pressure is believed to reduce sensory sensitivities and is thought to be calming and organizing to the nervous system. It may also help to improve discrimination of body boundaries, improving body awareness and motor execution.
Heavy work For example, carrying heavy items or heavy backpacks; wearing weighted vests; using weighted pens; helping to move classroom chairs; holding open heavy doors for peers; eating chewy foods or chewing on chew tubes, chewing gum, or necklaces; placing theraband around the legs of the chair; hanging from monkey bars; using clay in art; squeezing balls	Believed to be calming and organizing for the nervous system and to assist in improving body awareness via improved sensory discrimination of force, body position, and motion.
Movement For example, sitting on a ball chair or seat cushion, allowing extra time on the playground, using a rocking chair in classroom, participating in gymnastics, engaging in other therapist-guided movement activities such as those on suspended equipment	Movement may regulate arousal level being both alerting and calming depending on the type of movement and the specific child. Motion such as that provided by a ball chair or cushion uses the vestibular system's connections throughout the CNS to potentially increase postural muscle tone, allowing the child to remain seated upright for longer periods.
Vibration For example, a vibrating pen or pillow	Vibration is carried by many different sensory receptors and can assist in heightening sensory discrimination, thereby improving body awareness.
Auditory attention For example, listening to music, using headphones	Soft, slow music can be calming and organizing for the nervous system. Rhythmic music with a definite beat can help organize movements and increase alertness. Headphones can reduce outside and background noises.
Visual attention For example, use of study carrel, dimmed lighting, wearing a cap or sunglasses	Reducing visual input may reduce visual distractions and the orienting responses caused by peripheral visual inputs, perhaps reducing arousal level and distractibility.
The Alert program (Williams & Shellenberger, 1994)	This cognitively-based program educates the child about his or her level of alertness and teaches self-regulatory strategies.
Classroom jobs For example, pushing a cart of books to the library, watering plants, or holding doors for the line	Classroom jobs primarily use "heavy work" in a way that typically provides calming and reduced motor activity, allowing for better attention in the classroom.
Community activities For example, rock-climbing, bowling, swimming, or horseback riding	Community activities that provide sensorimotor experiences can be very beneficial for the family to engage in outside of therapy time. When chosen appropriately, they can assist in regulating arousal level and reducing other sensory-seeking behaviors.
Household chores For example, helping to carry groceries, run the vacuum, or carry laundry	Household chores can also provide additional appropriate sensory inputs for a child in the home, when outside of therapy time. When chosen appropriately, they can assist in regulating arousal level and reducing other sensory-seeking behaviors.

- Improved fine and gross motor skills.
- Improved self-care skills and independence in daily habits and routines.
- Improved social skills.
- Improved cognitive, language, or academic performance (Parham & Mailloux, 1996).

The therapy practitioner using any approach should be consistently monitoring the effectiveness of his or her methods in regards to progress in goal attainment.

After 6 months of therapy, Robby has made significant changes and Liz is extremely pleased with his progress. Together, Julie and Donna created a system of data collection that would be easy to complete quickly and would provide information specific to Robby's goal attainment. Julie and Donna have both been keeping very specific records on the frequency of certain behaviors, as has his OT at school.

Through general observation and discussion with Liz, it appears that Robby is now able to play with peers without pushing them. He is riding his bike with his friends in his immediate neighborhood, and he is writing the letters of his name. He is not yet able to independently create a novel picture and still struggles with complex cutting tasks, but he is much more willing to try and does so more frequently. The data demonstrate progress more specifically and concretely. For example, his frequency of being too rough with other children at school (reported and recorded by his teacher) went from an average of 3 times per day when he began therapy to a current average of once per week. He also went from very limited play with peers, an average of 2 successful attempts per week, to a current average of twice per day. In the clinic, he has changed from requiring Julie's assistance to create or alter a game or activity an average of 2 times per session to a current average of only twice per month. He has gone from being unable to ride his bike without training wheels for any distance to being able to ride around his block several times in a day. He went from being able to copy 5 letters of the alphabet, to being able to copy the entire alphabet and write his name independently. He also recently sat through an entire meal at a restaurant and Liz was thrilled. These are all measures of his progress toward both his school and outpatient goals. Therefore, Julie feels confident that the approach she has taken with Robby has been appropriate and also that both she and Donna have been successful in the implementation of the intervention.

Summary

The SI frame of reference offers a rich foundation upon which to interact with clients. OT using Ayres' SI approach is a playful intervention method ideally suited and originally developed for children, but also used with adolescents and adults. To be maximally effective, the use of Ayres' SI approach requires additional training,* supervision, and mentoring. This training is imperative in order to support theoretical knowledge; under-

standing of the research; and the clinic reasoning used to design, implement, and effectively modify the intervention. OT using Ayres' SI approach is one of many intervention methods that may be used during OT. The use of this frame of reference allows the practitioner to enhance the foundational abilities on which the child builds perception, improves motor performance, gains praxis and organization of behavior and allows engagement in increasingly complex occupations and co-occupations.

Clinical Problem Solving

1. You are an OTA working in an outpatient clinic where you often collaborate with the OT to do the final portion of sessions with children who have just finished activities using Ayres' SI approach. You typically focus on fine and visual-perceptual motor skills or ADL. On this day, you are seeing Carl who typically is a pleasant and cooperative child. However, today he is not himself and he is becoming increasingly agitated as you attempt to intervene. When his OT brought him to you after his session, she said that everything had gone well. She mentioned, though, that one of the games they had played had involved lots of movement. What do you need to know about Carl? What do you need to observe right now? What do you need to do?

2. Mark is a little boy with autism who has been using sensory strategies in his preschool classroom successfully for over 2 months. When you enter his room to check in one morning, the teacher seems relieved to see you and tells you that he is having an awful day. She just tried to use some of the sensory strategies that she has seen you use, but they made his behavior worse. Initially, he was upset, but as she tried things with him he became agitated. She says that he started crying and yelling and would not let her come near him. He is now hiding under a table in the classroom that has a curtain around it and he will not come out. She wants you to see what you can do. What do you need to find out from her first? What might you do in this situation? What are some precautions to be aware of?

3. Imagine you are the OTA working with a family of a child named Johnny. Johnny has been receiving OT at an outpatient clinic where the therapist is providing OT using Ayres' SI approach. You see Johnny in the school and you are responsible for implementing his sensory strategies in that environment. You recently received a phone call from Johnny's mother asking you to speak to her husband. Apparently, he does not believe there is anything "wrong" with Johnny that a little firm discipline wouldn't fix. Johnny's mom has been very pleased with his progress in both school and outpatient OT, but she is frantic now because her husband wants him to stop receiving services. He feels that they are wasteful and doesn't see any differ-

---

* This education may be pursued through an advanced degree program or through certification in SI including the SIPT. The certification process endorsed by the Franklin B Baker/A. Jean Ayres Trust is the University of Southern California/Western Psychological Services certification program. See www.wpspublish.com/Inetpub4/w0903.htm for more information on these courses.

EVIDENCE-BASED TREATMENT STRATEGIES*

Treatment Strategies	Authors
Ayres' SI approach to treat sensory modulation disorders	Miller, 2003, 2004
Ayres' SI approach with various types of children	Daems, 1994; Ottenbacher, 1982; Vargas & Camilli, 1999
Ayres' SI approach with children with autism	Ayres & Tickle, 1980; Case-Smith & Bryan, 1999; Linderman & Stewart, 1999
Ayres' SI approach with children with Down syndrome	Uyanik, Bumin, & Kayihan, 2003
Ayres' SI in combination with therapeutic riding to positively alter behaviors	Candler, 2003
Deep touch pressure to reduce arousal level and anxiety and improve attention and behavior in children with autism (hug machine, massage)	Edelson, Goldberg, Edelson, Kerr, & Grandin, 1999; Escalona, Field, Singer-Strunck, Cullen, & Hartshorn, 2001; Field et al., 1997
Weighted vests for calming and to improve attention, decrease distractibility, and increase task behavior in children with attention deficit hyperactivity disorder and autism	Fertel-Daly, Bedell, & Hinojosa, 2001; Olson & Moulton, 2004a; 2004b; VandenBerg, 2001
Therapeutic listening to decrease behavioral difficulties in children with autism	Edelson et al., 1999
Therapeutic listening for calming and to improve attention	Smith & Watkiss, 2004
Vestibular stimulation	Arnold, Clark, Sachs, Jakim, & Smithies, 1985; Ayres & Mailloux, 1981; Ayres & Tickle, 1980
Reframe the child's behavior in a new light for parents using knowledge of SI frame of reference	Cohn, 2001

* Please see www.nasponline.org/publications/cq315sensory.html for an excellent review of the state of sensory integration research as of 2003.

ence in Johnny at all. You have been keeping data to establish the effectiveness of the strategies and you are confident that they have been helpful. What do you do?

4. You are an OTA working in the schools with a newly hired OT who is trained in SI. She is very experienced and you have a wonderful working relationship. She often makes recommendations for sensory strategies in the classroom and you collaborate to design and implement the plans. However, you feel that the teachers in your school are averse to using these strategies in the classroom because they are uncertain if they will be worthwhile. You are also certain that the school administrator does not believe in SI intervention and does not want it used in his schools. What do you do?

LEARNING ACTIVITIES

1. Complete a sensory history. Compare results and discuss if these sensory "differences" interfere with occupational performance.

2. Conduct observations of "typical" children and of children with identified sensory issues.

3. Participate in a sensory lab:
   - Spin on a swing—How long does it take to become dizzy?
   - Feel cooled spaghetti and gelatin with vision occluded.
   - Wearing gloves, try to pick up cereal or other small objects.
   - Walk an obstacle course wearing prism glasses.
   - Trace a star or complete a maze by looking at the reflection in a mirror

4. Interview families working with an OT or OTA trained in SI. Questions may include:
   - What is the parents' definition of SI?
   - How long has the child been receiving intervention?
   - What is the progress to date?
   - What are the components of the home program?

REFERENCES

American Occupational Therapy Association. (2002). Occupational therapy practice framework: Domain and process. *American Journal of Occupational Therapy, 56,* 609-639.

Arnold, L. E., Clark, D. L., Sachs, L. A., Jakim, S., & Smithies, C. (1985). Vestibular and visual rotational stimulation as treatment for attention deficit and hyperactivity. *American Journal of Occupational Therapy, 39*(2), 84-91.

Ayres, A. J. (1972). *Sensory integration and learning disorders.* Los Angeles, CA: Western Psychological Services.

Ayres, A. J. (1979). *Sensory integration and the child.* Los Angeles, CA: Western Psychological Services.

Ayres, A. J. (1985). *Developmental dyspraxia and adult onset apraxia.* Torrance, CA: SII.

Ayres, A. J. (1989). *Sensory integration and praxis tests.* Los Angeles, CA: Western Psychological Services.

Ayres, A. J., & Mailloux, Z. (1981). Influence of sensory integration procedures on language development. *American Journal of Occupational Therapy, 35*(6), 383-390.

Ayres, A. J., & Tickle, L. S. (1980). Hyper-responsivity to touch and vestibular stimuli as a predictor of positive response to sensory integration procedures by autistic children. *American Journal of Occupational Therapy, 34*(6), 375-381.

Bear, M. F., Connors, B. W., & Paradiso, M. A. (2001). *Neuroscience: Exploring the brain* (2nd ed.). Philadelphia: Lippincott, Williams & Wilkins.

Beery, K. E. (1997). *Developmental test of visual motor integration.* Parsippany, NJ: Modern Curriculum Press.

Berk, R., & DeGangi, G. (1987). *DeGangi-Berk test of sensory integration.* Los Angeles, CA: Western Psychological Services.

Blanche, E. I. (2001). The evolution of the concept of praxis in sensory integration. In S. Smith Roley, E. I. Blanche, & R. C. Schaaf (Eds.), *Understanding the nature of sensory integration with diverse populations* (pp. 125-132). Tuscon, AZ: Therapy Skill Builders.

Blanche, E. I. & Schaaf, R. C. (2001). Proprioception: A cornerstone of sensory integrative intervention. In S. Smith Roley, E. I. Blanche, & R. C. Schaaf (Eds.), *Understanding the nature of sensory integration with diverse populations* (pp. 109- 123). Tuscon, AZ: Therapy Skill Builders.

Bruininks, R. H. (1978). *Bruinincks-Oseretsky test of motor proficiency.* Circle Pines, MN: American Guidance Service.

Bundy, A., & Murray, E. A (2002). Sensory integration: A. Jean Ayres' theory revisited. In A. Bundy, S. Lane, & E. A. Murray (Eds.), *Sensory integration theory and practice* (2nd ed., pp. 3-34). Philadelphia: F. A. Davis.

Bundy, A., Lane, S., & Murray, E. A. (2002). *Sensory integration theory and practice* (2nd ed.). Philadelphia: F. A. Davis.

Calvert, G., Spence, C., & Stein, B. (2004). *The handbook of multisensory processes.* Cambridge, MA: MIT Press.

Candler, C. (2003). Sensory integration and therapeutic riding at summer camp: Occupational performance outcomes. *Physical and Occupational Therapy in Pediatrics, 23*(3), 51-64.

Case-Smith, J., & Bryan, T. (1999). The effects of occupational therapy with sensory integration emphasis on preschool-age children with autism. *American Journal of Occupational Therapy, 53,* 489-497.

Cohn, H. (1999). *Neuroscience for rehabilitation* (2nd ed). Baltimore: Lippincott, Williams and Wilkins.

Cohn, E. S. (2001). Parent perspectives of occupational therapy using a sensory integration approach. *American Journal of Occupational therapy, 55,* 285-294.

Daems, J. (Ed.). (1994). *Reviews of research in sensory integration.* Torrance, CA: SII.

DeGangi, G., & Greenspan, S. (1998). *Test of sensory function in infants.* Los Angeles, CA: WPS.

Dunn, W. (1997). The impact of sensory processing abilities on the daily lives of young children and their families: A conceptual model. *Infants & Young Children, 9,* 23-35.

Dunn, W. (1999). *The sensory profile.* San Antonio, TX: Psychological Corp.

Edelson, S. M., Arin, D., Bauman, M., Lukas, S. E., Rudy, J. H., Sholar, M., et al. (1999). Auditory integration training: A double blind study of behavioral and electrophysiological effects in people with autism. *Focus on Autism and Other Developmental Disabilities, 14,* 73-81.

Edelson, S. M., Goldberg, M., Edelson, M. G., Kerr, D. C., & Grandin, T. (1999). Behavioral and physiological effects of deep pressure on children with autism: A pilot study evaluating the efficacy of Grandin's hug machine. *American Journal of Occupational Therapy, 53,* 145-152.

Escalona, A., Field, T., Singer-Strunck, R., Cullen, C., & Hartshorn, K. (2001). Improvements in the behavior of children with autism following massage therapy. *Journal of Autism and Developmental Disorders, 31,* 513-516.

Fertel-Daly, D., Bedell, G., & Hinojosa, J. (2001). Effects of a weighted vest on attention to task and self-stimulatory behaviors in preschoolers with pervasive developmental disorders. *American Journal of Occupational Therapy, 55*(6), 629-640.

Field, T., Lasko, P. M., Hentleff, T., Kabat, S., Talpins, S., & Dowling, M. (1997). Autistic children's attentiveness and responsivity improve after tough therapy. *Journal of Autism and Developmental Disorders, 27,* 333-339.

Hanft, B. E., Miller, L. J., & Lane, S. J. (2000). Toward a consensus in terminology in sensory integration theory and practice: Part 3: Observable behaviors: Sensory integration dysfunction. *SI SIS Quarterly, 23*(3), 1-4.

Jacobs, S. E., & Schneider, M. L. (2001). Neuroplasticity and the environment: Implications for sensory integration. In S. Smith Roley, E. I. Blanche, & R. C. Schaaf (Eds.), *Understanding the nature of sensory integration with diverse populations* (pp. 29-42). Tuscon, AZ: Therapy Skill Builders.

Kandel, E. R., Schwartz, J. H., & Jessell, T. M. (2000). *Principles of neural science* (4th ed.). New York: McGraw-Hill/Appleton & Lange.

Kraemer, G. W. (2001). Developmental neuroplasticity: A foundation for sensory integration. In S. Smith Roley, E. . Blanche, & R. C. Schaaf (Eds.) *Understanding the nature of sensory integration with diverse populations* (pp. 43-56). Tuscon, AZ: Therapy Skill Builders.

Lewkowicz, D. J., & Lickliter, R. (Eds.). (1994). *The development of intersensory perception: Comparative perspectives.* Hillsdale, NJ: Lawrence Erlbaum and Associates.

Linderman, T. M., & Stewart, K. B. (1999). Sensory-integrative-based occupational therapy and functional outcomes in young children with pervasive developmental disorders: A single subject study. *American Journal of Occupational Therapy, 53,* 207-213.

Mailloux, Z., & Smith Roley, S. (2004). Sensory integration. In H. Miller-Kuhaneck (Ed.), *Autism: A comprehensive occupational therapy approach* (pp. 215-244). Bethesda, MD: American Occupational Therapy Association.

Miller, L. J. (2004). Planning and implementing effective treatment using Ayres' sensory integration approach. American Occupational Therapy Association Presentation, May, 2004, Minneapolis MN.

Miller, L. J. (2003). Empirical evidence related to therapies for sensory processing impairments. *NASP Communiqué, 31,* 5.

Miller, L. J., Cermak, S., Lane, S., Anzalone, M., & Koomar, J. (2004). Position statement on terminology related to sensory integrative dysfunction. Retrieved July 15, 2004, from http://www.sinetwork.org.

Miller, L. J., & Lane, S. J. (2000). Toward a consensus in terminology in sensory integration theory and practice: Part 1: Taxonomy of neurophysiological processes. *SI SIS Quarterly, 23,* 1-4.

Mulligan, S. (1998). Patterns of sensory integrative dysfunction: A confirmatory factor analysis. *American Journal of Occupational Therapy, 52,* 819-828.

Olson, L. J., & Moulton, H. J. (2004a). Use of weighted vests in pediatric occupational therapy practice. *Physical and Occupational Therapy in Pediatrics, 24*(3), 45-60.

Olson, L. J., & Moulton, H. J. (2004b). Occupational therapists' reported experiences using weighted vests with children with specific developmental disorders. *Occupational Therapy International, 11*(1), 52-66.

Ottenbacher, K. (1982). Sensory integration therapy: Affect or effect. *American Journal of Occupational Therapy, 36*(9), 571-578.

Parham, L. D. (2002). Sensory integration and occupation. In A. Bundy, S. Lane, & E. A. Murray (Eds.), *Sensory integration theory and practice* (2nd ed., pp. 413-434). Philadelphia: F. A. Davis.

Parham, L. D., & Ecker, C. J. (2002). Evaluation of sensory processing research—Version 4. In A. Bundy, S. Lane, & E. Murray (Eds.), *Sensory integration: Theory and practice* (2nd ed., pp. 194-196). Philadelphia: F.A. Davis.

Parham, L. D., & Mailloux, Z. (1996). Sensory integration. In J. Case-Smith, P. N. Pratt, & A. S. Allen (Eds.), *Occupational therapy for children* (3rd ed., pp. 307-356). St. Louis: Mosby.

Parham, L. D. & Mailloux, Z. (2001). Sensory integration. In J. Case Smith (Ed.), *Occupational therapy for children* (4th ed., pp. 329-381). St. Louis: Mosby.

Royeen, C. B., & Lane, S. J (1991). Tactile processing and sensory defensiveness. In A. G. Fisher, E. A. Murray, & A. C. Bundy (Eds.), *Sensory integration: Theory and practice* (pp. 108-136). Philadelphia: F. A. Davis.

Smith, M. J., & Watkiss, J. (2004). The effectiveness of therapeutic listening: A pilot study. Materials presented May 20, 2004 at AOTA's national conference, Minneapolis, MN.

Spitzer, S., & Smith Roley, S. (2001). Sensory integration revisited: A philosophy of practice. In S. Smith Roley, E. I. Blanche, & R. C. Schaaf (Eds.), *Understanding the nature of sensory integration with diverse populations* (pp. 3-28). Tuscon, AZ: Therapy Skill Builders.

Uyanik, M., Bumin, G., & Kayihan, H. (2003). Comparison of different therapy approaches in children with Down syndrome. *Pediatrics International, 45*(1), 68-73.

VandenBerg, N. L. (2001). The use of a weighted vest to increase on-task behavior in children with attention difficulties. *American Journal of Occupational Therapy, 55*(6), 621-628.

Vargas, S., & Camilli, G. (1999). A meta-analysis of research on sensory integration treatment. *American Journal of Occupational Therapy, 53*(2):189-198.

Williams, M. S., & Shellenberger, S. (1994). *"How does your engine run?": A leader's guide for the alert program for self-regulation.* Albuquerque, NM: Therapy Works, Inc.

Wilson, B. N., Pollack, N., Kaplan, B. J., & Law, M. (2000). *Clinical observations of motor and postural skills* (2nd ed.). Framingham, MA: Therapro.

Windsor, M. M., Smith Roley, S. S., & Szklut, S. (2001). Assessment of Sensory Integration and Praxis. In S. Smith Roley, E. I. Blanche, & R.C. Schaaf (Eds.), *Understanding the nature of sensory integration with diverse populations.* San Antonio, TX: Therapy Skill Builders.

Robby   9/2003
Observation notes

    — consistently uses too much force
     while playing

    — fell off of equipmt into crash mats mult. times
     no fear though got right back on
     seemed to enjoy the falls

    — needs mult. cues to create activities

    — flinched when I touched him   x /

    — covered his ears when the door buzzed

    — seemed a little low tone — slumped seq position often

    — ↓ endurance, fatigued quickly
     especially in prone

    — appears happy and did not seem
     to be easily frustrated today

Real record 13-1. Real record for a client with sensory integration dysfunction.

Robby : Data chart for week of March 8th

Completed by
Audrey - classroom aide

	Mon	Tue	Wed	Thurs	Fri
initiates play w/ peers during recess	√√√	√√√	√√√√	√√	√√√
successfully plays w/ peers for 5 min or >	√√	√√√	√√√	√	√
hits or pushes peers during play	√ (pushed)	∅	∅	∅	√ (pushed) while in line
letters copied from board	7 words	5 words	∅ refused today	6 words	6 words

Real record 13-2. Real record for a client with sensory integration dysfunction.

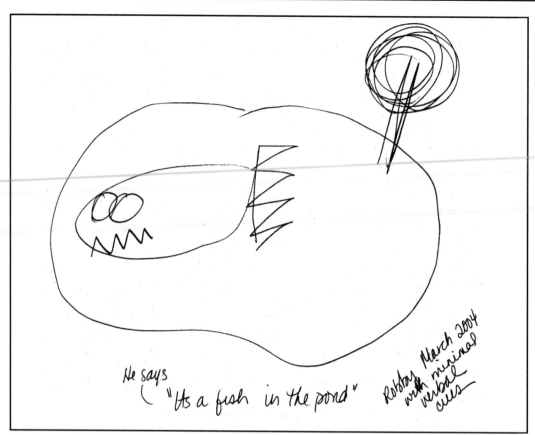

Real record 13-3. Real record for client with sensory integration dysfunction.

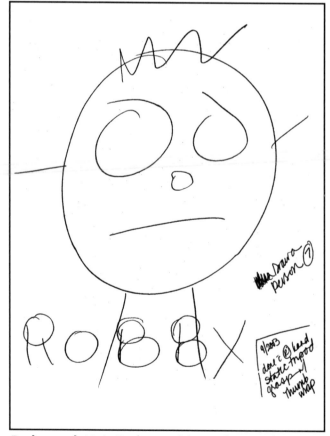

Real record 13-4. Real record for a client with sensory integration dysfunction.

Key Concepts

- Medically-based services: Paid for by insurance carrier upon medical necessity.
- School system practice: Guided by federal law for a free and appropriate education.
- Medical vs. educational services: Differences in service delivery models and team approaches.
- OT/OTA collaboration: Intricate interactions between 2 practitioners who each have necessary information and understanding of performance.

Essential Vocabulary

ataxic: Characterized as a disturbance of balance secondary to abnormal muscle tone.

athetoid: Characterized as fluctuating tone with decreased proximal stability.

cerebral palsy (CP): Collective term for brain injury prior to, during, or just after birth.

family centered: The child functions within the family as a unit.

hypotonic: Low tone that often masks underlying spasticity or athetosis.

neurodevelopmental: Developmental theory that emphasizes symmetry and righting reactions.

occupational behavior: Acquiring skills to meet the demands of the environment.

spasticity: High tone often resulting in synergistic patterns of the upper and lower extremities.

Two Children With Cerebral Palsy

Tara J. Glennon, EdD, OTR, FAOTA

Introduction

Cerebral palsy (CP) is a category name for brain injury that occurs prior to, during, or just after birth. The causes of the damage are often associated with intracranial hemorrhage, loss of oxygen, infections, trauma, delivery complications, or metabolic disorders. In some situations, however, the cause of the CP is unidentifiable, and thus termed etiology unknown. The reader should appreciate that medical and technological advances have both increased and decreased specific instances of CP (Table 14-1). It is logical for one to understand that medical testing and pre-emergency interventions have decreased the incidences of brain injuries. However, medical interventions have also resulted in a higher frequency of babies surviving a fragile pregnancy. These babies, surviving despite low birth weight and prematurity, often show a higher incidence of abnormal tone and motor issues. Despite the cause(s), the neurological effect results in motor deficits that can be observed by early childhood. The specific location of the brain damage results in distinct types of motor and tonal problems. Thus, there are differing types of CP reported (Table 14-2).

Frames of Reference

Despite the frame of reference utilized on behalf of the child with CP, any interventionist must always consider the facilitators and barriers to a child's participation within the environment. Occupational behavior is the basis of our profession and a child has roles to fulfill while at school. It is imperative that environmental adaptations be completed and opportunities presented so that the child can acquire the skills necessary to meet the demands of the environment. This concept is universal to many frames of reference, based on developmental principles, acquisitional considerations, and coping concepts so that the child is able to take care of his or her own needs.

The most common intervention strategy for this diagnosis, despite the specific type of CP observed, is the neurodevelopmental treatment (NDT) approach. This approach, developed by Dr. and Mrs. Bobath in the 1940s, was originally designed for children with CP and is primary within the medical model. Although NDT is considered a developmental theory, it does not encourage the development of typical motor milestones. Rather, the theory emphasizes foundational skills such as symmetry, righting and equilibrium reactions, and weight shifting as precursors to acquiring motor skills. The NDT frame of reference outlines specific, intricate treatment strategies that focus on precise handling techniques to promote normal movement patterns. Extensive clinical experience and a strong foundational knowledge of normal and abnormal movement patterns provide the framework of treatment implementation. In preparation for work with children diagnosed with CP, these complex intervention strategies are outlined in an 8-week, advanced certification course offered to OTs, PTs, and speech language pathologists. Despite the complexities of direct therapeutic intervention, the NDT frame of reference consistently emphasizes carryover within the natural context of the child's day and participation in functional tasks. The role of the OTA can be quite extensive within home- or school-based therapy, as well as within institutional environments. The intricacy of this frame of reference requires intense cooperation between the OT and OTA.

The use of sensory integrative (SI) techniques is also critical when understanding the child's responses to movement inputs and other sensory experiences. Sensory integration theory emphasizes the importance of sensory processing as a foundation for learning within all developmental sequences. Motor skill acquisition is among the most identifiable of these sequences. NDT and SI techniques are often utilized together.

Dr. Mary Reilly developed a theory of play that has expanded how we value the play experience. She believed that play gave meaning to the daily life of a child and provided opportunities to learn rules, develop interactions, and form the basis for adult competencies. As clinicians working with a child diagnosed with CP, the play experiences chosen must provide opportunities for the child to grow and develop socially and emotionally. The child with CP, therefore, presents a unique challenge that may require the use of environmental modifications, technology, adaptive equipment, and toy modification so that the child's curiosity is stimulated. The focus is providing

Table 14-1

Etiology and Prevalence

General Principles

Etiology

1. Significantly greater incidence as the number of births increases: twins more than singles; triplets more that twins; and quadruplets more than triplets.
2. Possible issues:
   - Developmental and metabolic abnormalities
   - Infection
   - Autoimmune and coagulation disorders
   - Trauma and hypoxia in the fetus
   - Prematurity
   - Multiple births
   - Uterine rupture
   - Tightened umbilical cord
   - Premature placental separation

Obstetrics and Gynecology Literature

Etiology

1. Blickstein (2004) cites the following:
   - Epidemiological studies suggest that only 10% are thought to be part of an intrapartum event.
   - Only CP involving spastic quadriplegia is associated with an acute interruption of the blood supply, while purely dyskinetic or ataxic CP generally is genetic in origin.
   - Epidemiologic studies have clearly demonstrated a causal relationship between premature birth and CP.

Prevalence

1. The Florida Obstetric and Gynecological Society (2004) cites the following:
   - Despite a reduction in the maternal death rate by more than 95% and in the neonatal death rate by more than 66% over the last 50 years, the incidence of CP has changed little.
   - Even with the tremendous improvements in obstetric, neonatal, and surgical care of the last 25 years, the incidence of CP remains unchanged.
   - The incidence of CP appears consistent between developed and underdeveloped nations. Based on the fact that current obstetric technologies, including electronic fetal monitoring and the capability of emergent cesarean section, are not available in underdeveloped nations, CP must be primarily a developmental issue.
2. Williams, Hennessy, and Alberman, (1996) cite the frequency as follows:
   - 3.2% among live births at less than 29 weeks' gestation
   - 2.8% at 29 to 32 weeks
   - 0.3% at 33 to 36 weeks gestation
   - 0.07% at 37 or more weeks

UCP Research and Educational Foundation

Etiology

1. The Research Status Report (UCP Research and Educational Foundation, 2002) cites the following:
   - 70% of the cases occur prior to birth (prenatal).
   - 20% occur during the birthing period (perinatal).
   - 10% occur during the first 2 years of life (postnatal).

Prevalence

1. The Research Status Report (UCP, 2002) cites the following:
   - The number of new cases has increased 25% during the past decade.
   - There are 9,750 new cases each year.
   - There are 550,000 to 764,000 persons in the United States with this diagnosis.

Table 14-2

Classic Signs and Related Issues

Type of Tone: Spastic; hypertonic	Type of Tone: Hypotonic; low tone; flaccid	Type of Tone: Ataxic	Type of Tone: Athetoid
Tonal Patterns	**Tonal Patterns**	**Tonal Patterns**	**Tonal Patterns**
• Presents as low tone in the trunk and high tone more distally.	• Markedly low at birth or in infancy.	• Described as a disturbance of balance.	• Characterized by writhing, worm-like movements.
• Increased flexor patterning of the upper extremities.	• Low tone typically masks underlying spasticity, athetosis, or ataxia.	• Underlying muscle tone usually hypotonic or slightly increased in the lower extremities and more distally.	• Fluctuating tone.
• Extensor patterning of the lower extremities.	• Flat or "pancake" chest, which makes the child prone to upper respiratory tract infections.	• Tone changes with emotion and excitement.	• Demonstrates decreased proximal stability.
• Tone increases with effort or quick movements, emotion, excitement, and attempts at speech.			• Abnormal tone noted in all extremities.
• Severe tone constant cocontraction.	**Movement Patterns**	**Movement Patterns**	**Movement Patterns**
	• Affects trunk and all limbs with resulting hypermobile joints.	• Dysmetria: Clumsy, unstable, and uncoordinated; presents as low tone in the trunk and high tone in extremities.	• Movement in extreme ranges.
Movement Patterns	• Decreased gradation of movement.	• ROM is not an issue.	• Movements appear bizarre and purposeless.
• Mild/moderate cases: Child is able to walk but may demonstrate stereotypical movements as total movement synergies; associated reactions noted with movement attempts; range limitations occur more distally.	• May be noted to utilize anatomic structures rather than active muscular control.	• Decreased coordination, control of muscles, and balance.	• Movements may be uncontrollable.
	• Decreased righting, equilibrium, and protective extension responses.	• Lack of a point of stability negatively influences the execution of equilibrium and righting reactions.	• Lacks midrange control.
• Decreased midrange control.	• Primitive reflexes persist.	• May need to utilize a wide base of support.	• Demonstrates increased movements with emotion and excitement.
• Primitive reflexes persist, such as ATNR, STNR, TLR, positive support, Moro, and startle.		• Uses more gross patterns.	• Secondary joint fixing when attempting to increase stability.
• Moderate/severe: Decreased postural reactions, protective responses, and righting and equilibrium reactions; joint tightness and contractures can lead to orthopedic deformities.	**Related Issues**	• Decreased performance of fine and gross motor skills.	• Hypermobile distal joints that can sublux.
	• Decreased tactile, proprioceptive, and vestibular processing.		
	• Decreased postural control affects respiration and the suck-swallow-breathe mechanism.	**Related Issues**	**Related Issues**
Related Issues	• Decreased oral motor status secondary to decreased stability.	• Oral control is compromised, may use his or her teeth to stabilize cup.	• Possible hearing loss.
• Postural issues may affect respiration, suck-swallow-breathe, and oral motor control.	• Can also be diagnosed learning disabled or MR.	• Decreased manipulation of food in mouth.	• Possible learning disabled.
• Seizure disorders occur in approximately one-half the individuals with CP, most likely with spasticity.	• May demonstrate decreased motivation, frustration, have difficulty with change, and poor self-image.	• Decreased articulation.	• Less likelihood of MR than with other types of CP.
• Mental retardation (MR), visual perceptual difficulties, hypersensitivity to environmental stimuli.	• May be fearful of movement.	• Nystagmus.	• Emotionally labile.
• Play skills slow to develop.		• Sensory problems.	• Easily frustrated.
• Psychosocial issues: Self-esteem, behavioral, and social skills.		• May have diagnosis of MR.	• Possibly has poor self-image and low self-esteem.
		• Difficulty developing social relations.	
		• Difficulty with pre-vocational tasks and life skills.	

the child with the possibility of pressure-free mastery of the environment. As we attempt to provide this accessibility to play experiences, the therapist may also wish to remember the biomechanical approach. ROM, strength, and endurance must be factors in the designing of play experiences. The more accessible the activity, the more the child will be invested, and the more meaningful and organizing the activity is for the child.

ASSESSMENT

Within the arena of pediatric practice, the evaluation process is complex. When presented with a child with CP, the collaboration between the OT and OTA is quite involved. For this reason, this section is offered to the OTA not only to understand his or her role within this process, but to appreciate the evaluation tools completed by the OT.

The first step in the assessment process is determined by who is asking for and paying for the evaluation and for what reason. There is a distinct difference between medically- and educationally-based services; therefore, the evaluation tools must reflect those differences. Within the medical realm, standardized evaluation tools, analysis of adaptive living skills within the home environment, and the identification of underlying quality of skills would be emphasized. The educational system focuses on functional outcomes within the academic environment to determine eligibility for services (AOTA, 1989a, 1989b). Through either evaluation process, the collaboration between both therapists allows for the identification of strengths and weaknesses, possible causes of problems, intervention needs, and appropriate plans for intervention. The role of the OTA can be essential if managed effectively with the OT.

Quite often, when concerns are raised about a child's performance, a screening might occur. The screening is often considered to be the initial step in the evaluative process, in order to rule in or out the need for specific evaluations. However, within the medical realm, a screening is not generally utilized when a child has a diagnosed condition because it is assumed that the child will demonstrate rehabilitative or occupational concerns. A child with CP, therefore, moves directly to the assessment process. Within the educational environment, a screening may occur in order to determine if the child's deficits are interfering with classroom performance. If the child's classroom functioning is compromised, the child would move to the assessment phase. As this screening is not formalized, it can typically be completed by the OT or OTA. Observations of functional performance within the classroom environment, conversations with the teacher to determine his or her concerns regarding the child's performance, and chart review of other team member evaluations to document areas of deficits can be completed by the OTA as the initial phase in the evaluation process (Blossom, Ford, & Cruse, 1996).

For the child with CP, the degree of involvement would determine the appropriate assessment tools (Case-Smith, 1993; Case-Smith, Allen, & Pratt, 1996). For example, if the child is severely involved, there are 2 distinctly different types of evaluation tools that would need to be reviewed for possible use. First,

standardized assessment tools specifically designed to evaluate the quality of movement are uniquely appropriate for the child with motor impairments. These include the Toddler and Infant Motor Evaluation (TIME) (Miller & Roid, 1994) and the Alberta Infant Motor Scale (AIMS) (Piper & Darrah, 1994). Given the complexity and intricacy of these tools, an OT or PT's implementation, judgment, and rating are necessary. However, while these tools provide valuable information regarding the movement patterns of these children, they do not necessarily address occupational performance or movement within the context of functional life tasks (Dunn, 1991).

The second cluster of evaluation tools, standardized instruments commonly utilized with other children, is available to the OT in order to assess fine motor, visual motor, or perceptual skills. However, these tools do not typically provide for the needed modifications with regard to a child with significant motor impairments. Therefore, in addition to the standardized qualitative observations of motor performance mentioned above, criterion-referenced tools, nonstandardized assessments, and adaptive skill checklists are often appropriately utilized for this population of children. Several of these tools can be completed by the OTA and shared with the supervising therapist for review and analysis. Again, the role of the OTA within the evaluation process is substantiated due to the need for extensive information regarding functional skills within a variety of environments. For it is the information related to occupational performance that will substantiate the need for intervention and focus the plan of action.

As part of the overall assessment process, the OTA might utilize nonstandardized tools for a child with CP. These include gathering historical information from the chart regarding other medical assessments and/or teacher reports and completing interviews with parents and/or teachers. In addition, questionnaires should be implemented that might identify areas of difficulty not readily observed within a clinic or school environment, investigate child/family history, document developmental milestones, obtain pre- and postnatal birth history, and outline pertinent hospitalizations. A specific inventory/observation tool that may be used is the Sensory Integration Inventory of Individuals with Developmental Disabilities (SII-DD) (Reisman & Hanschu, 1992). This tool is not age specific and is designed as a formalized questionnaire that can be completed by the family or educational staff. The SII-DD is used to identify sensory-processing issues that present as behaviors that might interfere with functional participation within the environment. The results of the questionnaire need to be interpreted by the OT secondary to the complicated and evolving theory of SI.

Based on the fact that children with CP are frequently unable to functionally complete a task and demonstrate poor quality of skills, the certified assistant should develop competencies in and implement a criterion-referenced assessment. These tools are designed to gain descriptive information of functional domains of performance, outline components of skills that are present or absent, and describe the child's current functioning, while providing guidelines for future skill emergence. The following is a list of criterion referenced assessments that would be appropriate for a child with CP:

- The Brigance Diagnostic Inventory of Early Childhood Development (Brigance, 1991), a tool for children birth through 7 years, can be used for the child with CP. This assessment is particularly appropriate for school settings as it allows for other disciplines to complete additional sections related to other domains of functioning. Domains appropriate for OT include fine motor, dressing, and feeding. The OTA is able to complete these portions of the evaluation and share the findings with the OT for analysis and coordination with other assessment findings.

- The Hawaii Early Learning Profile (HELP) (Vort Corporation, 1995) outlines skills for 2 age groups: birth to 3 years and 3 to 6 years. This tool is specifically designed for children with multiple handicaps or developmental delays and can be used for severely delayed children up to 12 years of age. As this evaluation tool provides an in-depth task analysis of all daily living skills (e.g., dressing, feeding, fine motor, and visual motor skills), it is an appropriate tool for the OTA to complete.

- Therapy Skill Builders publishes comprehensive books authored by Rhoda Erhardt (Erhardt, 1994). The Erhardt Developmental Prehension Assessment (EDPA) and the Erhardt Developmental Vision Assessment (EDVA), highly descriptive approaches to observing children birth to 6 years, are particularly appropriate for children with CP. The intricacy of these tools is appropriate for the OT to complete due to the quantified observations. Both age levels and outlines of the sequences of development are provided.

CASE STUDY 1—LAUREN, A 1.5-YEAR-OLD CHILD WITH SPASTIC TYPE CEREBRAL PALSY

Background Information Concerning Early Intervention

Federal legislation from the 1980s significantly impacted services to young children. Based on a collection of principles that recognizes that the family is the constant in the child's life, a family-centered system was created placing the emphasis of services on the child within the context of his or her environment. The focus of early intervention services is to promote interaction, collaboration, and sharing of information between the family and the professionals (AOTA, 1989a). Through these interactions, the professionals can recognize and appreciate family strengths and individuality, with respect for diversity and various cultural backgrounds, while attempting to meet the family's concerns. For these reasons, the evaluation is typically completed by 2 professionals. This team utilizes permitted standardized evaluation tools to look at many variables, such as the degree and type of disability, personality, temperament, and behavior of the child, as well as family interactions, needs, and strengths. This allows the parents to express their concerns and

the priorities of their child's intervention program. The OTA, regardless of the level of experience, would not be appropriate to evaluate the child's needs as extensively as the early intervention process mandates. As attempts are generally made to minimize the number of professionals entering the family's home, it would not be appropriate to perform a joint evaluation with the OT. Additionally, the system intends to foster relationships with critical individuals, thus decreasing the number of people with which the family needs to interact.

This process of outlining the child's needs, as seen by the parents, results in the formal document of services called the IFSP. This plan ensures that partnerships with the family are established and family goals are outlined and prioritized. The IFSP is reviewed at 6-month intervals until such time as the child no longer requires intervention or until the child turns 3 years and exits the program. Throughout this process, the team must determine the most natural environment for the services to be delivered. Typically, the child's home or day care environment is the most appropriate. However, there are situations where community-based services, which emphasize specialized play group experiences with therapeutic support, can also be outlined. Regardless of the location, it is of primary importance that the interventionist functions as an educator for all people who are naturally a part of the child's life.

For the reasons stated above, the early intervention specialist must be flexible and responsive to family-identified needs in an ongoing situation. Additionally, because communication is key, the primary interventionists are typically identified so that the family is not bombarded with the input of many people. The transdisciplinary model of one primary interventionist or the interdisciplinary approach of a small team of people who collaborate and prioritize goals together is most often utilized. The role of the OTA within this model is dependent on several factors. First, the level of experience is critical. If one is delivering services within the home environment, with no others immediately available for discussion and collaboration, the practitioner must be sufficiently adept at answering all of the parent's potential questions (Finnie, 1974). Therefore, the therapist must have suitable experience in order to manage the situation effectively. If the child receives services within a community setting, with many professionals or the supervising OT readily available, the OTA has the necessary supports and is therefore an appropriate service provider.

The next series of considerations include the priorities identified by the parents, the extent of the child's limitations, and the other service delivery personnel identified to participate in the child's plan. In order for the OTA to be identified as the OT service provider, all of these factors would need to be discussed and resolved to the satisfaction of the entire team of professionals working on behalf of the child.

Case Presentation

Lauren, the only child of William and Sarah, has been determined eligible by the state's Birth-to-Three system for therapy services following a referral from her pediatrician. The parents, who own their own business and work from home, have identified several priorities for their child. Positioning and handling at home to make caring for her easier during functional tasks such as mealtime, bathing, dressing, and play was a major concern. Additionally, they felt that physical, occupational, and speech language therapies should be provided away from the home environment. Their concern, secondary to the fact that they work within the home, was that they would be unable to work effectively if Lauren was having difficulty with the therapies. They appeared fragile in terms of the difficulties that lie ahead of Lauren and did not believe that they would be able to endure her possible crying or resistance to the therapeutic processes. Instead, they would prefer that one parent accompany Lauren to her community program while the other parent worked at home.

The OTA employed by the early intervention facility had 3 years experience working with children and had worked intricately with the OT throughout. Because of this, and considering the fact that the primary intervention would take place within a community setting with other professionals readily available, she was assigned this case following the eligibility process. The team of therapists working directly with the child completed the HELP so that a baseline of each domain of functioning was established and progress could be measured by this tool in the future.

The priorities identified by the parents shaped the goals recorded on the IFSP. These goals, outlined for a 6-month period, focused on functional tasks. Each professional, in combination with the parents and team, outlined the behavioral objectives that would be utilized to measure Lauren's progress toward the goal areas. For Lauren, as with all children, a behavioral outcome is required to identify an observable, behavioral statement and to identify under what conditions or circumstances the child would be expected to master the behavioral statement. For all outcomes, criteria were documented to determine how the team would measure Lauren's success. Lauren's behavioral outcomes were as follows:

- When provided with upright support within her mother's ring sitting position on the floor, Lauren will:
  - ○ Push her arm three quarters of the way through a sleeve (shirt, coat) as it is held open for her, in 3 out of 4 attempts.
  - ○ Pull the shirt down over her head as it rests on top of her head, using 2 hands, in 3 out of 4 attempts.
  - ○ Push her leg into the pant opening as her leg is held at the beginning of the opening by the caregiver in an effort to achieve correct placement, in 3 out of 4 attempts.
- When in a 90-90-90 sitting position in her Rifton chair (Rifton Equipment, Chester, NY) with foot rests, hip strap, shoulder harness, and tray, Lauren will reach for and obtain a preferred toy using palmar grasp in 4 out of 5 consecutive attempts.
- While in a supported side-lying position, Lauren will activate a single switch positioned 6 to 12 inches in front of her, with the hand or the upper arm, to activate a preferred toy for at least 30 seconds.

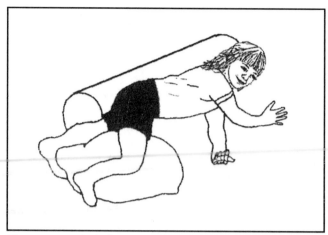

Figure 14-1. Side-lying position.

Within the direct sessions, the NDT focus was on postural control and weight shifting in order to allow for more functional reach patterns. Weight bearing and trunk rotation activities were consistently incorporated so as to decrease the tonal influence on upper extremity movements (Blanche, Botticelli, & Hallway, 1995). Throughout these sessions, the practitioner focused on expanding play opportunities for Lauren, as well as increasing participation in daily living tasks following therapeutic handling techniques. Although Lauren's mother was present during all sessions to allow for training and carryover, several visits were made to the home. During these sessions, positioning for function and handling techniques were outlined based on the specific contextual factors of the home environment. The practitioner utilized home programming sheets from the OT files in order to outline what the parents could do at home. These sheets included information concerning relaxation of muscles, encouraging movements in as normal a pattern as possible, positioning in proper alignment to prevent deformities, lifting and carrying alternatives that minimized abnormal tonal responses, and positioning options for play (Figure 14-1) and daily task involvement. When in the home, the practitioner needs to be as supportive as possible. This includes respecting and encouraging beneficial ways in which the family was already facilitating the child's development; making suggestions that are practical and relevant to their family life; and making sure not to give the family more than they could physically, emotionally, or logistically handle.

CASE STUDY 2—MARY, A 5.5-YEAR-OLD DIAGNOSED WITH MILD, HYPOTONIC CEREBRAL PALSY

Background Information Concerning School System Practice

In the early 1970s, OT services were mandated within the educational system. Although these laws have been revised, expanded, and redefined since that time, OT has always remained part of the law as a related service for the child to benefit from special education (AOTA, 1989b). A related service is defined as that which is necessary to support the special education instruction. OT, as an educationally-based related service, is not intended to be a medical service. Despite the rehabilitative concerns, the therapist must determine if the therapeutic intervention is necessary for educational performance.

The intent of special education is to educate the child in the typical classroom with peers who do not have special needs. This part of the law is referred to as the least restrictive environment (LRE). For the child with CP, this creates a unique challenge. The role of practitioner is critical in outlining modifications and adaptations within the classroom environment, so that the child is able to be educated with his or her peers.

As with any federally-funded program, a legal document must be designed in order to outline the necessary services. For Birth-to-Three, this was called the IFSP with the child within the family unit as the focus; whereas in the school system, the IEP is the legal document that addresses the child as part of his or her educational environment. The IEP is designed through the process of a group identified as the PPT. Members of this team include parents, special and regular educators, an administrator, related service providers such as an OT or OTA, the student if appropriate, and other invited members who could include an attorney, parent or child advocate, or other parent support. The IEP serves as a tool for measuring progress, ensuring communication, and providing ongoing evaluation of the child.

The IEP, which is updated at least every year, must include the child's current level of educational performance, annual goals, short-term/behavioral objectives, the services required to meet objectives, and criteria to assess whether objectives have been met. It is imperative that the goals and objectives be specifically related to education. Each year, at the annual IEP meeting, the previous goals are measured to determine progress, continued services are decided, and new goals are developed as appropriate. At that time, the roles of the OT and OTA are to collect data to answer these questions. Throughout each of these phases, the therapy staff must remember to translate technical information into educational terms so that interdisciplinary team members can utilize this information effectively.

For the child with CP, educationally-based OT services are uniquely appropriate for the certified assistant. A focus on environmental modifications and adaptive skill development is important as the therapist strives to facilitate the development of functional skills for use within the educational environment. When considering the child's level of physical involvement, environmental issues include seating and positioning, utensil adaptation, modification of learning and play/leisure materials, use of technology to access learning materials, and/or accessibility in and around the school building. Self-care activities within this environment are also critical in allowing the child every opportunity to meet his or her own needs and master occupational performance.

Although the services discussed within this section are prescribed through educational laws, OT must also address what might be considered more medically based or rehabilitative in nature, if these issues impact activities within the educational environment. These concerns might include safety secondary to possible seizures, oral motor skill development in order to ensure safety during lunch and snack time routines, strength and ROM as related to participation endurance, wheelchair training for building accessibility, and/or postural control in order to maintain an upright "ready for learning" position.

Case Presentation

Mary, the second of Barbara and Joseph's 3 children, began special education services at age 3, as outlined by the educational laws. Upon entrance, Mary, diagnosed with mild, hypotonic CP, was identified as having fine motor, visual motor, and oral motor concerns that were determined to have potential negative effects on her educational program. Since that time, Mary has received OT services in order to address the above mentioned issues.

At present, Mary is entering kindergarten and is to be included within the regular classroom. Based on the issues identified within Mary's current IEP, several types of service delivery methods were discussed by the team. For OT, direct intervention and monitoring within the classroom environment were determined to be appropriate, while consultation to the team was inherent in the monthly team meeting process.

Prior to arrival in kindergarten, the OT department, with assistance from physical therapy, was responsible for ordering appropriate positioning devices that would allow Mary access to educational materials and situations. Collectively, it was determined that Mary would require a Rifton chair, stander with a tray (Figure 14-2), and tumbleform supportive seating device (Figure 14-3) for use during floor time, daily circle time, and music class. Additionally, equipment for the playground was ordered in order for Mary to fully participate in these naturally occurring play-based experiences. These included a swing system that allowed for the wheelchair to lock in place, as well as the adapted see-saw and merry-go-round seat, which offered full support and a harness system. The therapists ordering and providing these devices for Mary's use were accountable for the functional and safe implementation of this equipment. Therefore, both therapists designed a program for use, in-serviced the classroom staff, and outlined a system to monitor how the equipment was being used within the classroom. For OT, the focus was on how this equipment supported Mary's ability to participate in educationally-related activities.

Mary's direct service, the most basic form of service provision that implies hands-on contact, was discussed by the team. While Mary's parents were not opposed to pull-out services, if necessary, they would prefer for her interventions to occur within the classroom environment. This thought was consistent with the inclusion model outlined on her IEP. For the OTA assigned to Mary's case, the scheduling of intervention was critical. Since fine and visual motor goals were outlined on Mary's IEP, it was determined that the therapist would provide services within the classroom during morning "drawing" time and during free play. This would allow the therapist to address the fine and visual motor skills as they naturally occur for all of the children. During the first weeks of the school year, the OTA set up the

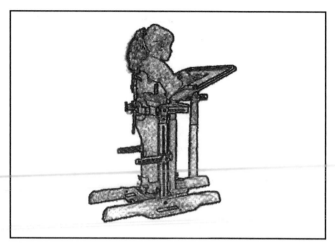

Figure 14-2. Stander with tray.

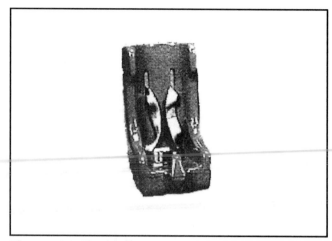

Figure 14-3. Tumbleform seat.

tabletop situation where Mary does her work. This included lowering the table to the proper height, ensuring that her feet were able to be firmly placed and supported on the floor when sitting all the way back in her chair, and providing a tabletop surface that was angled approximately 30 degrees. The 90-90-90 position was encouraged for all functional tasks presented to Mary.

The part of Mary's IEP that outlined oral motor goals was also discussed by the team. Although Mary was physically able to get food to her mouth, either with her fingers or with the spoon, safety was a concern during feeding. Therefore, 2 methods needed to be outlined for meal and snack time at school. For snack in the classroom, Mary was provided with foods that were safe for her to eat independently. This allowed Mary to sit at the table with her friends and develop socialization skills that might typically occur during mealtime. During lunch time, when the other children went to the cafeteria, Mary would receive therapeutic feeding. The discussions that led to this decision involved several factors:

- Oral motor skills were identified as a primary concern.
- The cafeteria was particularly loud and distracting for Mary.
- Therapy would be intrusive.

When therapeutic feeding strategies were discussed, Mary's parents felt that direct therapy for feeding was inappropriate for lunchroom implementation. The decision was based on the fact that the intense intervention might be disturbing for Mary to receive in view of the other children. For Mary, delayed oral movements, low tone, and postural issues affecting the suck-swallow-breath mechanism made choking a possibility. Additional difficulties included drooling, food loss, decreased tongue movements, decreased involvement of cheeks to manage food, and limited ability to chew. These issues required both NDT and sensory integrative approaches (Blanche et al., 1995).

The oral motor interventions were designed and implemented through the collaboration of OT, OTA, speech language pathologist, teacher, and parents. In addition to direct intervention by the therapy staff, a plan for training all staff included a written plan and videotape of a session. Daily implementa-

tion of strategies could be ensured when all staff involved with program implementation were adequately trained.

The first issue, proper positioning, was one of the most critical issues for Mary due to decreased tone and limited postural control. Providing stabilization allowed Mary to concentrate on eating rather than maintaining her posture. It also allowed for alignment of internal organs necessary for digestion and for ease of swallowing to prevent aspiration. The program also identified that the person feeding Mary should ideally be directly in front of Mary, at or below eye level, to allow for observation of jaw, mouth, and tongue movements. This also enhanced midline orientation and facilitated interaction between Mary and the caregiver.

The actual feeding part of Mary's program was quite specific to prevent variation and reduce safety concerns. A shallow-bowled spoon was provided as it was the appropriate size to fit between her teeth, was rubberized, and had a shallow bowl (Figure 14-4). This shallow bowl, along with the feeder placing small to moderate amounts of food on the spoon, allowed for greater ease when Mary attempted to remove the food from the spoon. The program emphasized presenting the spoon at midline and pressing the bowl of the spoon on the front third of tongue. This technique facilitated the proper tongue movements to manage and propel the food backward for Mary to swallow safely. The feeder was not to remove the spoon until Mary's mouth was ready to close, waiting for the lips to close around the spoon. Then the spoon was to be removed straight out.

For cup drinking, Mary's juice was thickened with gel thickener, yogurt, or applesauce, as she demonstrated difficulty managing and swallowing thin consistencies. The recommended technique was to bring the cup to the lips, rest the cup on Mary's lower lip, and wait for Mary to come to the cup to obtain the juice. Instructions were provided to watch fluid flow, easily observed with the use of a cut-out cup (see Figure 14-4), and provide jaw control during this process. Jaw control variations, outlined on the home program sheets, were outlined to teach normal jaw movements, provide proprioceptive feedback during drinking and swallowing, and promote lip/jaw closure and gradation.

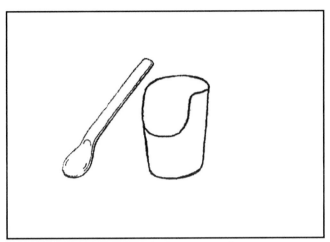

Figure 14-4. Shallow-bowled spoon and cut-out cup.

SUMMARY

The diagnosis of CP, the category name for brain injury resulting in abnormal muscle tone, is a unique challenge for the OTA. The multiple issues involved, including postural control, upper extremity functioning, oral motor skills, daily living skills, and ability to access the environment, emphasize the need for intense cooperation between the OT and OTA. Each professional collects specific information with respect to the individual's level of functioning, with synthesis necessary in order to develop a comprehensive plan of action. Several frames of reference are appropriate, some requiring more intensive training than others. For example, NDT outlines specific handling techniques to promote normal movement patterns. For this approach, extensive clinical experience is considered optimal. Occupational behavior, on the other hand, is inherent in the role of the certified assistant and is the basis of our profession.

Also important for the delivery of OT services, the interventionist must remember to view the child within the context of his or her environment. Varying laws regulate how services are delivered, based on the environment in which the child must function. These laws need to be clearly understood and adhered to. Working with this population of children is not only intricate, but fascinating in all its complexities.

CLINICAL PROBLEM SOLVING

1. Barry, a 35-year-old man who is severely medically involved, has spastic type CP and significant oral motor difficulties. He resides in a group home for the mentally retarded and has a history of frequent pneumonia. Based on his medical status, oral motor programming is critical to prevent aspiration. The procedures mentioned above continue to be appropriate, but the carryover portion of feeding intervention would need to be more structured. Based on the fact that there are 3 shifts of caregivers and the therapists are not always available, training and monitoring are critical. Frequent in-service sessions need to be implemented, and documentation of training must be part of the record for liability reasons and to keep track of the schedule of training sessions. Photos and diagrams, easily accessible to the caregiver, would assist with correct implementation of the plan. The formal program, outlined in the chart with specific detail, must be consistently followed by every caregiver working with Barry. Therefore, a formal chart of documentation would need to be outlined so that the therapist can track implementation. What suggestions could be used to develop this?

2. Carlos, a 6-year-old Hispanic boy, presented with athetoid type CP, average intelligence, and primitive oral motor patterns. He was the youngest of 5 children, ages 6 through 12. Although the therapist made many attempts to facilitate independence during self-care activities, Carlos' mother, Alicia, continued to complete these tasks for him. At school, he was fed using the strategies designed by OT. These techniques were shared with the staff and Carlos' family. However, Alicia continued to feed Carlos with a bottle at home. As the therapist assigned to this case began to understand the cultural background and values of Carlos' family and his role as the youngest child, she began to modify her original plans. The revised plan, intended to elicit a match with Alicia that respected her cultural beliefs, first focused on Carlos' health and safety. By designing activities that would not significantly disrupt the family's routine at home, play and leisure were expanded. Alicia enjoyed watching Carlos learn to play with toys and interact with his siblings. As Carlos demonstrated increased curiosity, motivation, and independence, other activities were added. What activities could be suggested to enhance the mother-son relationship? How else could you elicit cooperation from Alicia to promote oral motor development?

3. Brian, a 13-year-old boy with athetoid type CP, presented with perceptual and motor deficits, as well as a seizure disorder that resulted in unanticipated drop seizures. He received medically-based occupational and physical therapy services within a clinic environment. During physical therapy, Brian worked toward independent ambulation with the use of a walker weighted at the base for stability. At school, Brian received only OT services. Since he was able to independently negotiate the school environment with his wheelchair, he was not eligible for educationally-based physical therapy. Toward the end of the school year, as Brian had mastered the use of the walker, his mother requested that he be able to use the walker in school. The school administrator asked the OTA to develop safety mechanisms for using the walker. First, data were collected regarding the seizures to determine if any precipitating events could be identified. It was determined that seizures were most associated with the onset of illness, lack of sleep, and when over-aroused. The protocol for walker use that was outlined, in collaboration with the OT, identified that communication between home and school would be imperative so that illness or decreased sleep could be identified and the walker would not be used. Additionally, Brian was restricted from using the walker in the hallway

EVIDENCE-BASED TREATMENT STRATEGIES

Treatment Strategies	Authors
Environmental barriers and facilitators	Hammal, Jarvis, & Colver, 2004; Hemmingson & Borell, 2002; Mihaylov, Jarvis, Colver, & Beresford, 2004
Participation in recreation and leisure	King et al., 2003
Family-centered service	King, Teplicky, King, & Rosenbaum, 2004; Palisano, Snider, & Orlin, 2004
School participation	Hemmingson & Borell, 2002; Mancini & Coster, 2004; Richardson, 2002
Quality of life	Houlihan, O'Donnell, Conaway, & Stevenson, 2004
Psychosocial adjustment	Day & Harry, 1999; McDermott et al., 2002; Richardson, 2002; Witt, Riley, & Coiro, 2003
Employment	Murphy, Molnar, & Lankasky, 2000
Botox and the management of spasticity	Gooch & Patton, 2004; Wallen, O'Flaherty, & Waugh, 2004; Wong, 2003
Upper extremity management (including casting)	Boyd, Morris, & Graham, 2001; Law et al., 1991; O'Flaherty & Waugh, 2003; Yasukawa, 1990
Constraint-induced therapy	Crocker, MacKay-Lyons, & McDonnell, 1997; DeLuca, Echols, Ramey, & Taub, 2003; Eliasson, Bonnier, & Krumlinde-Sundholm, 2003; Pierce, Daly, Gallagher, Gershkoff, & Schaumburg, 2002; Taub, Ramey, DeLuca, & Echols, 2004
Functional results of a rhizotomy	Bloom & Nazar, 1994; Kim, Choi, Yang, & Park, 2001; Kinghorn, 1992; Mittal et al., 2002

when changing classes and in the cafeteria. These situations were identified as too over-arousing, with many people moving erratically and too much noise. When using the walker in specified situations, Brian would have to wear a hard helmet for protection, as well as be closely supervised by educational staff. What other options might be available? How could it be arranged for Brian to navigate the hallways but not be put at environmental risk?

4. John, a 13-year-old with ataxic type CP, has received OT since the age of 2. Early on, his direct OT program focused on NDT techniques to gain more control of his extremities for functional use. As John advanced in the grades and continued difficulty with controlled upper extremity was observed, the use of technology gained importance. At the most recent IEP meeting, the parents and team decided to focus on vocational skills needed for the upcoming years. John's regular and special education teachers presented the district's curriculum for review by the team. Secondary to motor, perceptual, and cognitive limitations, the role of the OT outlined by the team included environmental modifications, task analysis, assistive technology, and assistance with program development. This consultative role was considered to be more beneficial to the team rather than direct services. What might the consultant suggest for modifications? What other frames of reference would be important to utilize

now that John is older and moving into another phase in his life?

LEARNING ACTIVITIES

1. Compare the 2 cases in the chapter for similarities and differences.

2. Interview a child or adult with CP. What occupational roles are important to that person?

3. Design clothing that would be easy for a parent to use with a 3-year-old with CP. What developmental issues do 3-year-old children have with dressing?

4. What recommendations could a student make so that the children in this chapter could participate in community activities such as scouts or swimming at the community pool?

5. Locate vendors of adapted toys for children with limited mobility. Make a simple switch to turn a toy on or off.

REFERENCES

American Occupational Therapy Association. (1989a). *Guidelines for OT services in early intervention and preschool services.* Bethesda, MD: Author.

American Occupational Therapy Association. (1989b). *Guidelines for OT services in school systems*. Bethesda, MD: Author.

Blanche, E. I., Botticelli, T. M., & Hallway, M. K. (1995). *Combining neurodevelopmental and sensory integration principles: An approach to pediatric therapy*. Tucson, AZ: Therapy Skill Builders.

Blickstein, I. (2004). Cerebral palsy: A look at etiology and new task force conclusions. OBG Management Online/Dowden Health Media, Retrieved July 6, 2004, from http://www.obgmanagement.com/content/obg_featurexml.asp?file=2003/05/obg_0503_00040.xml

Bloom, K. K., & Nazar, G. B. (1994). Functional assessment following selective posterior rhizotomy in spastic cerebral palsy. *Child's Nervous System, 10*(2), 84-86.

Blossom, B., Ford, F., & Cruse, C. (1996). *Physical therapy and OT in the public schools*. Rome, GA: Rehabilitation Publications and Therapies, Inc.

Boyd, R. N., Morris, M. E., & Graham, H. K. (2001). Management of upper limb dysfunction in children with cerebral palsy: A systematic review. *European Journal of Neurology, 8*(Suppl. 5), 150-166.

Brigance, A. H. (1991). *Brigance diagnostic inventory of early development-revised*. North Billerica, MA: Curriculum Associates Inc.

Case-Smith, J. (1993). *Pediatric OT and early intervention*. Newton, MA: Andover Medical Publishers.

Case-Smith, J., Allen, A. S., & Pratt, P. N. (1996). *OT for children*. St. Louis, MO: Mosby-Year Book, Inc.

Crocker, M. D., MacKay-Lyons, M., & McDonnell, E. (1997). Forced use of the upper extremity in cerebral palsy: A single-case design. *American Journal of Occupational Therapy, 51*(10), 824-833.

Day, M., & Harry, B. (1999). "Best friends": The construction of a teenage friendship. *Mental Retardation, 37*(3), 221-231.

DeLuca, S. C., Echols, K., Ramey, S. L., & Taub, E. (2003). Pediatric constraint-induced movement therapy for a young child with cerebral palsy: Two episodes of care. *Physical Therapy, 83*(11), 1003-1013.

Dunn, W. (1991). *Pediatric OT*. Thorofare, NJ: SLACK Incorporated.

Eliasson, A. C., Bonnier, B., & Krumlinde-Sundholm, L. (2003). Clinical experience of constraint induced movement therapy in adolescents with hemiplegic cerebral palsy—A day camp model. *Developmental Medicine and Child Neurology, 45*(5), 357-359.

Erhardt, R. P. (1994). *Developmental hand dysfunction: Theory, assessment, and treatment* (2nd ed.). Tucson, AZ: Therapy Skill Builders.

Finnie, N. R. (1974). *Handling the young cerebral palsied child at home*. New York, NY: Penguin Books USA, Inc.

Florida Obstetric and Gynecologic Society (2004). Talking points: Cerebral palsy and newborn encephalopathy. Retrieved August 5, 2004, from http://www.flobgyn.org/services/cpalsy.php

Gooch, J. L., & Patton, C. P. (2004). Combining botulinum toxin and phenol to manage spasticity in children. *Archives of Physical Medicine and Rehabilitation, 85*(7), 1121-1124.

Hammal, D., Jarvis, S. N., & Colver, A. F. (2004). Participation of children with cerebral palsy is influenced by where they live. *Developmental Medicine and Child Neurology, 46*(5), 292-298.

Hemmingson, H., & Borell, L. (2002). Environmental barriers in mainstream schools. *Child Care, Health, and Development, 28*(1), 57-63.

Houlihan, C. M., O'Donnell, M., Conaway, M., & Stevenson, R. D. (2004). Bodily pain and health-related quality of life in children with cerebral palsy. *Developmental Medicine and Child Neurology, 46*(5), 305-310.

Kim, D. S., Choi, J. U., Yang, K. H., & Park, C. I. (2001). Selective posterior rhizotomy in children with cerebral palsy: A 10-year experience. *Child's Nervous System, 17*(9), 556-562.

King, G., Law, M., King, S., Rosenbaum, P., Kertoy, M. K., & Young, N. L. (2003). A conceptual model of the factors affecting the recreation and leisure participation of children with disabilities. *Physical and Occupational Therapy in Pediatrics, 23*(1), 63-90.

King, S., Teplicky, R., King, G., & Rosenbaum, P. (2004). Family-centered service for children with cerebral palsy and their families: A review of the literature. *Seminars in Pediatric Neurology, 11*(1), 78-86.

Kinghorn, J. (1992). Upper extremity functional changes following selective posterior rhizotomy in children with cerebral palsy. *American Journal of Occupational Therapy, 46*(6), 502-507.

Law, M., Cadman, D., Rosenbaum, P., Walter, S., Russell, D., & DeMatteo, C. (1991). Neurodevelopmental therapy and upper-extremity inhibitive casting for children with cerebral palsy. *Developmental Medicine and Child Neurology, 33*(5), 379-387.

Mancini, M. C., & Coster, W. J. (2004). Functional predictors of school participation by children with disabilities. *Occupational Therapy International, 11*(1), 12-25.

McDermott, S., Nagle, R., Wright, H. H., Swann, S., Leonhardt, T., & Wuori, D. (2002). Consultation in pediatric rehabilitation for behavior problems in young children with cerebral palsy and/or developmental delay. *Pediatric Rehabilitation, 5*(2), 99-106.

Mihaylov, S. I., Jarvis, S. N., Colver, A. F., & Beresford, B. (2004). Identification and description of environmental factors that influence participation of children with cerebral palsy. *Developmental Medicine and Child Neurology, 46*(5), 299-304.

Miller, L. J., & Roid, G. H. (1994). *The toddler and infant motor evaluation*. Tucson, AZ: Therapy Skill Builders.

Mittal, S., Farmer, J. P., Al-Atassi, B., Montpetit, K., Gervais, N., Poulin, C., et al. (2002). Functional performance following selective posterior rhizotomy: Long-term results determined using a validated evaluative measure. *Journal of Neurosurgery, 97*(3), 510-518.

Murphy, K. P., Molnar, G. E., & Lankasky, K. (2000). Employment and social issues in adults with cerebral palsy. *Archives of Physical Medicine and Rehabilitation, 81*(6), 807-811.

O'Flaherty, S., & Waugh, M. C. (2003). Pharmacologic management of the spastic and dystonic upper limb in children with cerebral palsy. *Hand Clinician, 19*(4), 585-589.

Palisano, R. J., Snider, L. M., & Orlin, M. N. (2004). Recent advances in physical and occupational therapy for children with cerebral palsy. *Seminars in Pediatric Neurology, 11*(1), 66-77.

Pierce, S. R., Daly, K., Gallagher, K. G., Gershkoff, A. M., & Schaumburg, S. W. (2002). Constraint-induced therapy for a child with hemiplegic cerebral palsy: A case report. *Archives of Physical Medicine and Rehabilitation, 83*(10), 1462-1463.

Piper, M., & Darrah, J. (1994). *Alberta infant motor scale*. Oakland, NJ: W. B. Saunders.

Reisman, J., & Hanschu, B. (1992). *Sensory integration inventory-Revised for individuals with developmental disabilities*. Hugo, MN: PDP Press.

Richardson, P. K. (2002). The school as social context: Social interaction patterns of children with physical disabilities. *American Journal of Occupational Therapy, 56*(3), 296-304.

Taub, E., Ramey, S. L., DeLuca, S., & Echols, K. (2004). Efficacy of constraint-induced movement therapy for children with cerebral palsy with asymmetric motor impairment. *Pediatrics, 113*(2), 305-312.

UCP Research and Educational Foundation. (2002). *Diagnosis of cerebral palsy: A research status report*. Washington, DC: Author.

Vort Corporation. (1995). *HELP checklist*. Palo Alto, CA: Author.

Wallen, M. A., O'Flaherty, S. J., & Waugh, M. C. (2004). Functional outcomes of intramuscular botulinum toxin type A in the upper limbs of children with cerebral palsy: A phase II trial. *Archives of Physical Medicine and Rehabilitation, 85*(2), 192-200.

Williams, K., Hennessy, E., & Alberman, B. (1996). Cerebral palsy: Effects of twinning, birth weight, and gestational age. *Archive of Disease in Childhood, 75*, 178-182.

Witt, W. P., Riley, A. W., & Coiro, M. J. (2003). Childhood functional status, family stressors, and psychosocial adjustment among school-aged children with disabilities in the United States. *Archives of Pediatric and Adolescent Medicine, 157*(7), 687-695.

Wong, V. (2003). Evidence-based approach of the use of Botulinum toxin type A (BTX) in cerebral palsy. *Pediatric Rehabilitation, 6*(2), 85-96.

Yasukawa, A. (1990). Upper extremity casting: Adjunct treatment for a child with cerebral palsy hemiplegia. *American Journal of Occupational Therapy, 44*(9), 840-846.

SUGGESTED READING

American Occupational Therapy Association. (1997). *OT services for children and youth under the Individuals with Disabilities Education Act*. Bethesda, MD: Author.

Dunn-Klein, M., & Delaney, T. A. (1994). *Feeding and nutrition for the child with special needs*. Tucson, AZ: Therapy Skill Builders.

Henderson, A., & Pehoski, C. (1995). *Hand function in the child: Foundations for remediation*. St. Louis, MO: Mosby-Year Book, Inc.

Parham, L. D., & Fazio, L. S. (1997). *Play in OT for children*. St. Louis, MO: Mosby-Year Book, Inc.

Sheda, C., & Small, C. (1990). *Developmental motor activities for therapy: Instruction sheets for children*. Tucson, AZ: Therapy Skill Builders.

World Health Organization. (1993). *Promoting the development of young children with CP*. Geneva, Switzerland: Author.

OT for Kids, LLC
www.otforkids.com

Monthly Running Notes

CHILD's NAME: Mary Castro

Month/Year: March 03	1	2	3	4	5	6	7	8	9	10	11	12	13	14	15	16	17	18	19	20	21	22	23	24	25	26	27	28	29	30	31
ADLs:	30							30	15							30							0	15	10					30	
Fine Motor:		✓						✓	✓						✓	✓														✓	
Graphomotor:																															
Visual Motor:		✓						✓	✓							✓														✓	
Perceptual:									✓	✓																					
Oral Motor:								✓	✓	✓																					
Postural Control:		✓						✓								✓							✓	✓	✓					✓	
Balance/ Equilibrium:																															
Gross Motor:		✓						✓								✓								✓						✓	
Strength:																															
Sensory Processing:																															
Vestibular/Proprioceptive:																															
Bilateral Coordination:																															
Motor Planning:																															
Parent/ Family Education:																															
Home Program:									✓																						
THERAPIST's INITIALS:	MM							MM	MM						MM	MM							MM	MM	MM					MM	

ADDITIONAL COMMENTS:

March 3: MrsC requested home prog for Mary. I'm that we would get that to her w/in wk. (MM)

March 10: Worked in cafe ṽ SLP for oM. (MM)

March 11: Fl-up ṽ Mrs C. @ home prog. She understands consent.

March 24: Worked ṽ it to get more postural supports as Mary was weak after her illness. Used foam inserts for the day. Will check in Monday.

March 26: no need for extra supports today. Teacher will keep in case Mary is fatigued at end of day.

THERAPIST: Meaghan

Real record 14-1. Real record for a client with cerebral palsy.

Child's Name **Mary**

School: **John**

Date: **March 2003**

Grade: **K**

Fine Motor Tasks - Facilitate a Mature Grasp:

☑ Play-Doh (be creative… use tools, kneed, pinch, roll into big balls or pinch into pea sized balls, flatten).

☑ Trigger type spray bottles (food coloring to make designs; draw a picture in marker, spray and watch the colors melt; hit targets; water plants; wash windows) -- smaller handles promote the "skill side" of the hand.

☐ Use eyedroppers to make pictures with colored water on paper towels or coffee filters.

☐ Shaking dice with cupped hands

☐ Flipping cards

☑ Pik-Up Sticks

☐ Paper mache

☐ Tops

☐ Jacks

☑ Monkeys in a barrel

☑ Pop beads, snap blocks, Velcro blocks, bristle blocks

☐ Open and close lids and containers or Ziploc bags

☐ Hole punchers (make confetti, or put circles in clear cup and cover for shaker)

☑ Lacing and sewing activities

☐ Stringing beads, macaroni and cheerios

☐ Tissue paper ball pictures

☑ Playing games with small manipulatives (buttons, coins, checkers, marbles, small pieces).

☐ Pick up small objects using fingers, tweezers, tongs, or clothespins.

☑ Peg boards

☐ Finger games, finger walking

☑ Popping bubble wrap with fingers tip to tip

☐ Finding hidden beads or treasures in Play-Doh or theraputty

☐ Tearing paper or newspaper

☐ Using toy tool set tools of different sizes - hammer, screwdriver etc.

☑ Wringing out sponges, wash clothes.

☐ Cooking activities require fine motor manipulation.

☑ Finger puppets

☐ Wind-up toys

☐ Fishing with magnets

☐ Transferring objects from palm to fingers and vice versa without other hand assistance.

☐ Using fingers in isolation to activate cause and effect toys.

☐ Building blocks and other construction toys.

☑ Self help skills - let the child dress, undress, snap, button, fasten as much as possible.

☐ Painting, Drawing, Finger painting.

☐ Magnet Letters

☑ Lite Brite

☑ Magna Doodle (put eraser lever at the top)

☑ Peg boards

☐ Chalkboards (writing or painting with water)

☐ Ink stamping

☐ Felt Boards

☐ Sticker Pictures

☐ Cut junk mail to start

☐ Eye Spy

☐ Matching games

☐ Sorting games

☐ Puzzles

☐ Shape Sorters

☐ Facilitate appropriate grasps on all utensils, even with glue sticks!

NOTES

Mrs. Castro -
   You can start with these activities. Remember to keep it fun - always a game vs. "homework". Don't forget to have her in a secure seated position before working on fine motor tasks.
   Call with any questions
                              Meaghan

Center for Pediatric Therapy

Real record 14-2. Real record for a client with cerebral palsy.

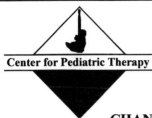

Center for Pediatric Therapy   ◆ Executive Director: Tara J. Glennon, EdD, OTR/L, BCP, FAOTA

CHANGE OF STATUS

Date: August 20, 1999   Date of last session: August 19, 1999

Child's Name: John Smith

John is now almost 10 years old and has received OT at this facility since the age of 7.

Date Therapy Initiated: October 22, 1996 eval'd

Who is requesting discontinuation? Mutual decision

parent

therapist

If parent, please provide reason for request.

Mrs. Smith knows that she can reinstitute therapy at any time. At this time, it is felt by both parents and therapist that John's needs can be met in school.

Please list remaining areas of concern.

1. The need for technology to support continued participation.
2. Continue home programs.
3. Continue community based activities including swimming and horseback riding.
4. Remain in touch for any wheelchair concerns.
5. Therapy team be available to the school team.

Erin Johnson, OTR/L

Real record 14-3. Real record for a client with cerebral palsy.

Key Concepts

- Oppositional defiant disorder (ODD): A psychiatric disorder characterized by recurrent patterns of negativistic, defiant, disobedient, and hostile behavior toward authority figures.
- Conduct disorder: A psychiatric disorder characterized by repetitive and persistent patterns of behavior in which the basic rights of others, societal norms, or rules are violated.
- Occupational behavior: A frame of reference that targets the broad parameters of play, student role, and socialization as the primary concern of OT practitioners working with children of this age.
- Task performance: An assessment of attention span, ability to make decisions, follow directions, sequence steps, use tools and materials, solve problems using a craft or activity.
- Individual Educational Plan: An individualized education plan aimed at improving the child's educational performance. It contains specific instructional objectives, including specific services and modifications needed to achieve the objectives.
- Discharge planning: The process of suggesting and arranging for services beneficial after discharge.
- Behavioral frame of reference: A frame of reference in which learning is based on environmental consequences and leads to either positive or adaptive behavior or negative or maladaptive behavior.
- Grading activities: The process of analyzing activities along specific dimensions (e.g., cognitive, motor, social complexity) to achieve therapeutic goals.

Essential Vocabulary

cognitive, motor, social complexity: Used in grading activities according to problem-solving processes, visuomotor skill, and social exchange required.

interdisciplinary treatment plan: A plan of care, includes goals and interventions of all disciplines working with a patient.

learning disability: A chronic condition of unknown cause that interferes with learning/working.

legal hold: A court-ordered restraint often associated with a belief that an individual is a danger to self or others.

middle childhood: The years from 6 to 12.

open seclusion: Temporary placement in an isolated room with no windows or furniture, door open.

post traumatic stress disorder (PTSD): Symptom pattern following exposure to an extreme situation often involving threatened death or serious injury that produces intense fear, helplessness, or agitation.

residential treatment facility: A setting in which individuals live temporarily for therapeutic benefit.

social skills: The ability to produce mutually reciprocal interactions with others.

Clinical Summary

Etiology

There is no specific etiology of this disorder. High reactivity in preschool, high motor activity, marital discord, and disrupted child care may contribute to this condition.

Prevalence

ODD is more common in boys than girls before puberty, but after puberty the rates in both genders are equal (U.S. Department of Health and Human Services [DHHS], 1999).

Classic Signs

A recurrent pattern of negativistic, defiant, disobedient, and hostile behavior toward authority figures, including parents, teachers, and other adults.

Precautions

ODD is often a precursor of conduct disorder, which is characterized by a repetitive and persistent pattern of behavior in which the basic rights of others, societal norms, or rules are violated (DHHS, 1999). The course of conduct disorder is variable, but children with early onset are at increased risk for antisocial personality and substance-related disorders (APA, 2000).

15

A Second-Grader With Oppositional Defiant Disorder

Linda Florey, PhD, OTR, FAOTA

Introduction

ODD is the diagnostic name given to a recurrent pattern of negativistic, defiant, disobedient, and hostile behavior toward authority figures, including parents, teachers, and other adults. Children with ODD typically display persistent fighting and arguing, are deliberately annoying or spiteful to others, refuse to comply with requests or rules, and blame others for their own mistakes. Children with this disorder are repeatedly angry and resentful, stubborn, and frequently test limits. These behaviors cause significant difficulties with family and friends and at school (DHHS, 1999). This disorder is of great concern because of the high degree of impairment and antisocial behavior. ODD, conduct disorder, and attention deficit hyperactivity disorder (ADHD) are collectively referred to as disruptive disorders.

Tony is an 8-year and 7-month-old boy admitted to the child inpatient service of a teaching hospital for combative behavior at school and increasingly aggressive behavior at home. He had thrown furniture in the classroom, punched a teacher in the stomach, hit other children at school, and had made increasing verbal threats to harm his younger brother and mother. Tony lived with his mother, stepfather, and his 4-year-old biological brother. His mother was 6 months pregnant with another child.

Tony was born in Florida and was of mixed ethnicity. His mother was Latino-American and his biological father was Caucasian. Tony had been abused both physically and mentally by his biological father, who was an alcoholic. He had also witnessed beatings of his mother by his father. His parents divorced when he was 5, and his mother moved him and his brother to California to seek asylum from the father. His mother met and married his stepfather, a Latino-American, who had no children of his own.

Tony had problems in the first and second grades and had been dismissed from school on 3 occasions for physically fighting with others. The teachers said that he would not follow the rules of the classroom and routinely argued with teachers and his peers. He picked on the younger children on the playground, and they regarded him as a bully. He had been sent to the principal's office at least once weekly for these behaviors since the first grade. Aside from his poor behavior on the playground and

during class, he was not a good student. He achieved poor marks but the teachers did not know if he was really trying or too busy misbehaving to concentrate on schoolwork. At home, Tony swore, broke toys, and often threatened his younger brother. His stepfather tried to be buddies with him and felt that he was just acting "normal" as anyone would if they had been abused so young. His mother became increasingly afraid that Tony might harm her, her unborn baby, and her younger son. He had threatened her with a kitchen knife on 2 occasions.

On the day of admission, Tony had thrown a chair across the room in class and started to physically attack 2 other boys. The police were called, and Tony was brought into the emergency room of a medical hospital and placed on a 72-hour legal hold, which meant that he had to remain at the hospital for 72 hours because he was a danger to self and others. His parents were notified. He was transferred to the psychiatric section of the hospital and admitted as an inpatient. His parents agreed to a voluntary admission, which meant that the legal hold could be cancelled.

Theory That Frames Practice

The frame of reference used in this chapter is occupational behavior. This frame of reference targets the broad parameters of play, student role, and socialization as the primary concern of OTs in working with children and adolescents. Play, work, and role are major theoretical principles that contribute to an understanding of an individual's occupational behavior (Reilly, 1966). There is a developmental progression in the manner in which work and play are incorporated into an occupational role—from player to student to worker, homemaker, or volunteer to retiree. Occupational role focuses on a combination of societal expectations and individual achievements in productive daily activities or occupations of individuals (Florey, 2003). In middle childhood, the ages of 6 to 12 years, work, play, and major daily activities focus on the role of student. The role of student is much broader than solely mastering the expectations of the curriculum. This role includes the learning and mastery of both academic and social expectations, which include those formally taught in school and those informally learned on the playground, gym, and other social settings. A major clinical focus for OTs is to determine the extent to which a psychiatric disorder has disrupted or impoverished occupational behavior and to identify steps to ameliorate dysfunction and to foster new learning (Florey, 2003).

Assessments and treatment techniques drawn from additional frames of reference may be used to ameliorate dysfunction in occupational role and socialization. The behavioral frame of reference is very useful in working with children with disruptive behavior disorders.

ASSESSMENT

The overall focus of inpatient hospitalization for children is to stabilize behavior, identify major problems, clarify diagnosis, and initiate medication trials if indicated. The treatment of long-term psychiatric problems or family issues is not done at the inpatient level, but at a less expensive level of care such as in a partial hospital program or as an outpatient. The length of stay on the child service at the hospital to which Tony was admitted is 10 to 14 days. In that setting, the OT practitioners work as part of an interdisciplinary team. The focus of the assessments of all team members is to quickly determine direction for intervention as an inpatient and at discharge. The initial OT assessment is documented in the chart within 48 hours of admission. Additional evaluations may be performed to probe deficit areas first identified.

The typical OT assessment includes several separate evaluations. These include an interview regarding patterns of daily activity, play activity check list, observation of task performance, observation of social interaction, and an assessment of visual-motor integration. This latter evaluation is routinely done as many of the children have deficits in this area and their attempts to "cover" for deficits may spark behavior problems in the school situation. The OT and OTA engaged in separate and joint evaluations of Tony. The purpose of the evaluations and the results follow. These are separated to highlight the OT personnel responsible.

Evaluation by the Occupational Therapist

The OT administered a typical day interview and the McDonald Play Activity Inventory-Revised (MPAI-R) (McDonald, 1987). The purpose of this evaluation is to determine typical patterns of daily living, school, play interests, and friendship patterns and to probe play activities and determine if they are dominantly gross motor, fine motor, social, or solitary in nature.

Initially, Tony refused to answer questions about chores, school, and play, stating, "It's none of your business." Although this is not typical of all children with ODD, this pattern of refusal to engage in what adults request occurs frequently. The OT then used the MPAI-R. This is a play activity inventory in which children are asked to circle the activities they enjoy from a list of 48 activities. The activities are divided into 4 categories of gross motor, fine motor, social group, or solitary passive. The

inventory can also be used as a probe to elicit information from children who do not or are unable to spontaneously identify activities in which they like to engage. In this case, it was used as a probe and this seemed less threatening to Tony. The activities he circled were distributed nearly equally in all areas and included a mix of sports, crafts, card, and team games. He also used the items to indicate activities he wished to do in the future. For example, he circled "play baseball" saying that he wanted to be on a team. He circled several items concerning friends. When asked what he and his friends did, he named 2 of the children on the unit and referred to a game they had played earlier in the hospital day. When asked about friends away from the hospital and at home, he said, "I just told you."

Tony responded to questions concerning additional likes and school activities but responses were negative and minimal. For example, he said he hated school and that school "sucked" but could not detail what he did not like about school. Additional information was gained through a brief interview with the mother during visiting hours. His mother reported that he was able to handle his self-care and that he had responsibilities at home of setting the table, making his bed, and cleaning the garage with his stepfather. He received an allowance of $2.00/week. He had not received his allowance in several months as he refused to do his chores. She said that he had behavior problems in school and had trouble controlling his temper with other children. He did not do well sharing TV time at home with her younger son and always wanted things his way. There were not any boys his age in the neighborhood so she knew that he didn't have any friends there and assumed he did not have any at school because of his behavior.

Evaluation by the Occupational Therapy Assistant

The Beery-Buktenica Developmental Test of Visual-Motor Integration (VMI) (Beery & Beery, 2004) is a structured test using form copying. The purpose is to determine developmental or age equivalent status of visual-motor skills.

Tony printed his name on the VMI booklet, and then threw it on the floor, saying, "I'm not doing this crap." The OTA gave him a count of 5 to pick it up or he would have a time out of the area. This is part of the general behavioral program for noncompliance and will be covered under the treatment activities/techniques section. After the 2 minute time-out, the OTA picked up the book and again explained the purpose as seeing how his eyes and hands worked together and that it was not a test of his drawing ability. He achieved an age equivalent score of 5 years 9 months, indicating impairment in visual-motor integration.

Evaluation by Both the Occupational Therapist and Occupational Therapy Assistant

Task performance and social behavior were evaluated by both practitioners using checklists to record observed behaviors. Key areas of task performance include ability to make a decision, to follow directions, to solve any problems that arise, and to attend to a task. Key areas in social behavior include the frequency and content of interactions with peers and adults.

Tony was observed working on craft projects on 2 separate occasions. He was seen individually and with a peer. When seen individually, the OT initially gave him a choice of 2 "failproof" activities: stain-a-frame or copper tooling with a template. Easy 1-step activities are initially given to assess task performance and to give children a feeling of success and promote positive feelings about OT. Tony selected copper tooling and chose a pirate template from the template choices. He eagerly started out and then said that he had "messed up" and wanted to start over. When assured that he had not made any mistake, he seemed unsure and needed to be coached and encouraged to finish.

The OTA worked with Tony and another boy on a simple craft project. They each were making a treasure box by painting a cigar box and then decorating the box with objects of their choice. Tony wanted to decorate his box with shells immediately after painting and did not want to wait until the paint had dried. He had difficulty accepting this limit and said he didn't want it anyway as it was "dumb." In task assessment, the therapist noted that he was able to select from alternatives, was able to attend to the activity, and was able to share the attention of the therapist with another child. He frequently thought he had made a mistake on projects that contained little margin for failure, and he needed encouragement and coaxing to complete projects and to wait for results. He did not display any pleasure with his end product.

To assess peer interaction, Tony was observed during activities of dodge ball, a community meeting, and informal activities on the unit. Tony displayed 2 styles of interaction with peers. He was either isolative and distanced himself from others unless specifically included in activities, or he was intrusive, bossy, and dominating with others. With adults, he was mainly negative and oppositional, testing and challenging the limits. At other times, he was pleasant and laughed but he seemed to convey a general demeanor of distrust and responded best on a one-on-one level with an adult working with him in a playful manner. He also seemed to gravitate toward the male staff on the unit.

FUNCTIONAL IMPACT AND GOAL SETTING

The functional impact of a disorder is the extent to which the disorder interrupts or impoverishes current and future occupational behavior. For a child, this includes the extent to which a disorder is interrupting normal learning in play, school, and daily living skills within many environments. Goals are then formulated to address deficit or at-risk areas and to build upon any areas of strength. The OT summarized the evaluation findings and presented them to the treatment team. The primary concerns identified by the OT and OTA were his social distancing and/or bossiness with peers, lack of peer friendships in the home and school setting, fear of failure in task situations,

difficulty waiting for results in tasks, and poor visual-motor integration. He had strengths in that although negative, he would engage in activities and had identified many activities with friends, perhaps indicating that he wanted friends but did not know how to make or retain them. He was currently at risk for learning in both the academic and social aspects of school and for learning the give and take of social relationships in play.

Nursing and recreation therapy had observed similar social interaction problems with peers, and additionally, Tony had 2 open seclusions for physical aggression against peers and attempting to kick staff. School testing revealed that he was functioning below grade level in all areas. Psychology had completed cognitive testing and although Tony was in the dull normal range, there was a 15 point differential between verbal and performance IQ, with verbal higher, suggesting a potential learning disorder.

Based on his low performance on the VMI, and the point differential between verbal and performance IQ, The OT decided to pursue additional visual-motor testing in this short hospitalization to tease out more information that might be useful for securing services as part of his IEP. The psychiatrist on the team had administered a depression inventory in which Tony had scored as clinically depressed. This was not surprising as he was not doing well in school and had interactional difficulties. Depression is also not unusual with children with ODD and is often manifested as irritability. The physician was also concerned with the potential for PTSD given his early history of physical abuse. Tony was placed on a small dose of antidepressant medication to help with the depression. Social work was concerned with the stepfather's minimizing Tony's aggression and threats as "normal" and "macho."

The entire team was concerned with the functional impact of his behaviors and skill deficits on his ability to adapt in the school and home setting both currently and in the future. He was having academic and social difficulties in school and was defiant and aggressive in the home. The goal was to further identify any deficits contributing to his poor performance, to teach more productive coping mechanisms, and to make recommendations postdischarge that would enable Tony to make friends, do schoolwork, achieve positive feelings about himself, and generally fit in both at home and school. The team was concerned that placement in a regular class might not be the best option for Tony, given his behavioral difficulties, and the potential of a learning disorder. They felt that the mother and stepfather should request an IEP at school.

General OT goals included that Tony follow the rules of activities, initiate positive contacts with peers, resolve problem situations by using words instead of fighting, and that he successfully complete simple projects to gain a feeling of accomplishment and mastery in tasks. Additional visual-motor testing to determine if his difficulties were more in the visual or motor realm was also a goal. Nursing was teaching principles of behavior management to the parents to deal with Tony's noncompliance and aggression, and social work was also working with the parents to help them initiate an IEP and to help the stepfather gain a more realistic picture of Tony's problems.

TREATMENT ACTIVITIES/TECHNIQUES

Treatment activities focus on constructing a pattern of typical childhood occupations within the hospital environment to the extent that this is possible. The OT practitioners work closely with other disciplines in developing a variety of occupations throughout the day and week. OT goals for each patient are developed within the context of the existing program, which is broadly designed to promote goals for most child patients while addressing individual needs.

The program assumes a "top down" approach in that the focus is on providing typical play and work occupations in middle childhood and assisting patients to achieve goals within those occupations. The specific needs/OT goals of each child are tailored and addressed within these occupations. Specific features of the occupations within a program for children follow.

- Play and task environments in which occupations are dominant should be populated with peers. It is critical for children to be able to work within a peer group, and it is the peer group in which many children with psychosocial dysfunction have difficulty. In the peer group, children learn and practice the sharing of materials, equipment, space, and the attention of others. One-on-one intervention with an adult may be necessary as children may benefit from learning the specifics of a craft or game, but as soon as feasible, peers should be included.

- Social skills learning should be part of play and work occupations. There is a social nature to occupations and this is a natural arena for the learning and relearning of social skills. Social skills are part of social competence in which social skill is one component. Social competence refers to mutually reinforcing social relationships and these are developmental in nature (Cartledge & Milburn, 1995; Cox & Schopler, 1996.) In middle childhood, fostering positive social relationships may include sharing and compromising, giving affection and praise to others, helping others, learning to enter ongoing peer activities, and changing behavior in response to the needs of others. OT practitioners model and frame interactions by giving praise—"I like the way everyone is working together"—or by correcting negative interactions when they occur— "How else could you have said that?"

- Programs should be conducted within natural childhood activities dominated by toys, crafts, and games and embedded within natural childhood models. The overall process of the activity should be emphasized and not the final product, although an end product is necessary to assist children to visualize the goal they are working toward. The end goal in using toys, crafts, and games is focusing on ways in which children can benefit, such as sharing materials, engaging in social banter, and achieving a sense of pride in workmanship rather than simply making a coin purse. Florey and Greene (1997) suggest that activities be graded according to cognitive complexity (problem-solving process required), motor complexity (motor and visual-motor skill required), and social complexity (social exchange such as opportunities for peer

interaction and cooperatively using space and materials). Often, social goals with children cannot be attained as the activity may be too complex along other dimensions and this triggers poor social strategies.

Natural models for this age range include club, scout, and small group formats that have a distinctive identity. Children of this age seek to belong and be part of a larger social environment. At the UCLA Neuropsychiatric Hospital, a Cub Scout Den chartered under the Boy Scouts of America has been in operation since 1971, and there has been an informal liaison with the Girl Scouts as well. With dramatically shorter lengths of stay, both boys and girls are combined into a general scout program. The children wear t-shirts and shirts representative of scouts and work on scouting principles, such as citizenship, rather than specific badges and pins.

Groups are conducted on the inpatient unit, in other parts of the hospital, and in the immediate community to gain an idea of how the children are able to maintain safety and social cues in less restrictive spaces.

- Occupations used should be varied. They should be graded to the developmental skills of each child and they should allow individual choice. The functional level of an activity is one of the most difficult to determine. Children with ODD or other psychiatric disorders may have learning, cognitive, or speech disorders in addition to previous failures that result in a general resistance to trying new activities. The starting point for any occupation is to have clear steps and to sequence steps from simple to complex. There should also be individual choices within occupations so that children may learn skills and activities of their interest.

- Expectations for behavior should be explicit and known. Expectations for behaviors are best phrased as rules. Children of this age are beginning to understand rules and enjoy constructing rules. Rules for general safety and conduct as well as consequences for rule violations should be known. Principles of the behavior management system may be incorporated in the rules.

There is a behavioral program on the child inpatient service to insure consistent expectations for behavior and consequences for loss of control for all children by all staff. Children are given a prompt or reminder for unacceptable behavior and if they fail to comply, then they are given a 2-minute time out of the area or activity to cool off. If they are unable to voluntarily take the time out and if their behavior continues to escalate, they may be placed in the seclusion room, which is barren, containing no windows or furniture. The door of the room is open or closed depending on the severity of the tantrum or behavioral dyscontrol. Children are released into the milieu after they have calmed to the point that they can talk about the events that led to their escalation.

Tony was involved in a number of OT programs during his 13-day hospitalization. These included community meetings, "problem solvers not problem starters club," the scout troop, and a lunch cooking group, which the OTs co-lead with recreation therapy. He was also involved in task/craft, newspaper, free play, and baking groups and in a special group that focused on spiritual needs of children in which the OT and OTA work with the chaplain. The OT and OTA work together in most of the groups but also divide functions as well. Tony's mother attended 2 OT sessions and the OT worked with her to learn how to present activities at his level and to set limits on his noncompliant and aggressive behavior while the OTA served as a model. Parental participation was arranged in conjunction with nursing, and it gave parents an opportunity to practice the behavioral strategies in an activity context.

Tony's participation and the specific goals in the baking, task, and free play groups are reviewed, as these give a snapshot of his patterns of behaving in different situations.

Baking Group

The purpose of this group is to teach skills, to simulate being part of a family work group, and to interact positively with others. Tony worked with 3 other children in preparing after dinner snacks for all of the children on the inpatient unit. Specific goals for Tony included working with others in taking turns, sharing, and using words to express his anger instead of physically fighting. The group was baking and frosting cupcakes. The OT and OTA had organized the tasks so that as one pair mixed the cake batter, the other pair placed cupcake papers in tins and both pairs then filled the cups. At first, Tony did not want to participate and then rapidly changed to wanting to do everything. He needed specific direction as to what his job was and required prompts to stay within those limits. The group played a simple table game while the cupcakes were baking and cooling. Tony wanted to dominate the game, choosing the color of his marker and announcing that he would go first but was responsive to therapists' suggestions to settle color and turns in a fair manner. Throughout the game, he tried to cheat by moving ahead spaces, became angry, and denied that he was cheating when his errors were pointed out to him. He needed continual prompting to keep from dominating his peers. He worked better on frosting the cupcakes, a solo task, in which each member was responsible for frosting and decorating a set number of cupcakes.

Task Group

The goal for Tony in this group was to follow directions, complete a simple craft, and say one good thing about how he had done. The OT led the task groups. Tony's response was typical throughout his stay. During task groups, he typically refused to engage, saying that the craft was "stupid" or babyish. With encouragement and cajoling, he would engage. He made real or imagined mistakes and had little tolerance for any error or frustration. When he made an error, he wanted to begin again instead of attempting to fix his mistake and when told that the mistake could be corrected, he threw the project across the table. He would allow the OT to fix the mistake, and then he could continue after a great deal of encouragement. He could not find anything good to say about his performance, and when the OT suggested that he was learning to try hard things, he replied, "Whatever, I guess." Tony was very sensitive to failure

of any kind and anticipated failure in most activities that he attempted.

Free Play

The purpose of the free play session was to observe how children were able to select play activities without an adult directing them and how they approached settling any disputes that occurred. The OTA set up the free play situation that was a mix of board games, creative media, dress up clothes, and selected crafts. Three to 4 children were in the group. There were few stated rules for this group except for the obvious ones of no hitting or fighting. The OTA began the session by saying that the number one rule of the playroom was to have fun but in order to have fun, they would have to share materials and take turns. She also told them that they had responsibilities in that they had to return play items to their storage spaces and they had to clean up for themselves. She also stated that although she was in the playroom, she would not be able to teach a craft or play a game with anyone as she was making a list of needed supplies. The goal for Tony was to observe his overall pattern and to see to what extent he could negotiate positively with peers on his own.

Tony either isolated himself and wandered around the playroom touching materials, or he gravitated toward the play of others. He seemed to have little capacity to generate ideas on his own. He abruptly entered situations in which others were playing and announced that he would play too. He was bossy, domineering, and had very little tolerance for doing anything other than his way. The OTA needed to prompt him several times to stop annoying others before the situation escalated to Tony losing control. It was as if he had 2 modes: loner or boss, and he needed the modeling of others to select play activities.

DISCHARGE PLANNING

There was a meeting of all the disciplines with the mother and stepfather at discharge in which different team members presented their findings and recommendations. The team told the family that Tony's persistent pattern of aggressive behavior was called ODD and that there were many factors that contributed to this clinical picture. He may have sustained some "soft" neurological damage during periods of physical abuse and this may have contributed to a learning disorder. A learning disorder is suspected when there is a difference in verbal and performance IQ, which often suggests a processing problem. The poor performance picture also fit with the OT extended testing on the motor and visual subtests of the Berry-Buktenica in which he was below age equivalent in both components but lower in fine motor areas. Although he did not display any pronounced fine motor deficits in simple tasks, his fear of making a mistake and exposing a deficit may have made him hesitant to attempt new activities.

The team explained that a learning disorder may help explain some of his behaviors in the school setting, as he had a very low tolerance for frustration and his behavior focused attention on his interactional rather than academic difficulties.

He also showed some evidence of depression, a disorder of mood, which may have been due to a poor self-image. This was manifest largely by his irritability, which is typical of children with depression. The physician recommended that he be continued on the antidepressant initiated early in the hospital stay.

Tony also had an ingrained distrust of adults, which made it difficult for adults to like engaging with him. His peer interactional difficulties and his noncompliance leading to aggression were paramount and evident in the reports of all clinical disciplines. His stepfather was still of the conviction that he was only sticking up for and asserting himself, but he did agree that without strict limits on his aggressive outbursts, there could be danger to the younger son in the family, his pregnant wife, and the newborn baby.

The team focused on discharge recommendations centering on the school and home. They recommended that Tony have an IEP. The team felt he may qualify for a learning disabled class and would probably need additional testing in the school system to pinpoint the learning problem. He would also qualify for an emotionally disturbed (ED) class based on his behavioral difficulties, but it was the hope of the team that dealing with his underlying learning disorder may help with his behavioral difficulties. The OT recommended that Tony have OT in the school to address his fine motor difficulties and that structured social skills be included in the IEP so that he could learn positive ways of working with other children.

At home, the team advised the parents to continue the behavioral training program they had learned in the hospital, which was a system of earning privileges for good behavior and the withdrawal of privileges for poor behavior. He also needed to be included in family chores and needed some special time with both his mother and his stepfather so that he could begin to trust adults. The occupational and recreation therapists suggested games and activities that Tony could easily do such as cards, baking cookies, planting flowers, and playing catch, which his parents could do in their special time with him. This was important for him, as Tony made working with him difficult and pushing people away was part of his strategy of not getting hurt first. It was also important to find activities in which he could succeed so that he could begin to generate some positive feelings about himself. The OT also recommended that Tony attend a camp for children with behavior problems in the summer. This camp worked exclusively with children with social problems and had daily structured activities in which competition with others was eliminated. The focus instead was on process and this would be a good direction for Tony.

CLINICAL PROBLEM SOLVING

Tony

Having followed Tony through this treatment program, review the notes in the case section. What are some of the issues of importance documented? Choose a day of notes, if the OTA were to see Tony for a second session following the session documented, what activities might be appropriate? See the * on the second page of notes. What does this likely mean? Do you understand all the language in the notes?

Ben

Ben is a 9-year-old boy admitted to the child inpatient service for increasingly violent and aggressive behavior and a suicidal threat. Ben was admitted from a residential treatment center where he had been for the past 3 months. He was born out of wedlock to an 18-year-old woman who had abused alcohol and cocaine during her pregnancy. He had been removed from the mother and placed in a foster home at that time as the mother was unable to care for him. He had had no contact with his biological mother. He had been adopted by his first foster mother.

Ben's behavior problems began in preschool. He was aggressive, hyperactive, and diagnosed as having ADHD at age 5. He was placed on a stimulant to control his hyperactivity. Ben had been suspended from schools on several occasions because of fighting and destroying school property. His adopted mother had other children in the home, and she was increasingly unable to handle his behavior problems. He had been moved from one foster home to another as foster parents were unable to handle his impulsive and aggressive behavior. He had also been placed on an antipsychotic medication in addition to the stimulant because of his increasing rage attacks. He was placed in a group home for children for behavior problems but had run away. He was placed in a locked residential treatment facility as this was felt to be the most therapeutic option for him. He was admitted to the inpatient service because he had thrown furniture, hit staff, and was threatening to kill himself by jumping out of a 2-story window.

How would the OT and OTA evaluate Ben? What effect does in utero exposure to drugs and alcohol have on an individual? What types of recommendations does one make to a residential treatment facility? Is there a way to influence this negative and self-defeating cycle that Ben is exhibiting?

LEARNING ACTIVITIES

1. Discuss some of the factors contributing to the behavior problems of both Tony and Ben.
2. Analyze the cognitive, motor, and social complexity of preparing lunch, making a lanyard, and making a birdhouse in a group and describe how to upgrade or downgrade these components.
3. Interview normal 8-, 9-, and 10-year-old children about their typical day including the types of activities in which they engage and with whom. Compare and contrast these descriptions with those of Tony.
4. Describe different ways a COTA could educate and work with parents or caretakers as a continuation of a treatment plan.
5. How does the OT elicit information from a child or adolescent who is resistant to an interview situation?

EVIDENCE-BASED TREATMENT STRATEGIES

Treatment Strategies	Authors
Top down treatment approach	Burke, 1996; Coster, 1998; Humphry, 2002
Childhood play as major occupation	Case-Smith, 2000; Esdaile,1996; Saunders, Sayer, & Goodale, 1999; Morrison & Metzger, 2001; Neville-Jan, Fazio, Kennedy, & Snyder, 1997; Parham & Primeau, 1997
Social nature of occupations and social skills	Baloueff & Cohn, 2003; Cartledge & Milburn, 1995; Cox & Schopler, 1996; Greene, 1997; Lawlor, 2003; Richardson, 2002
Importance of individual choices within occupations	Burke, 1998; Segal, Mandich, Polatajko, & Cook, 2002; Frank et al., 2001
Importance of end product, clear steps for success, and sequence simple to complex	Florey & Greene, 1997; Frank et al., 2001; Hartman, Miller, & Nelson, 2000; Murphy, Trombly, Tickle-Degnen, & Jacobs, 1999

REFERENCES

American Psychiatric Association. (2000). *Diagnostic and statistical manual of mental disorders* (4th ed.). Washington, DC: Author.

Baloueff, O., & Cohn, E. (2003). Introduction to the infant, child and adolescent population. In E. Crepeau, E. Cohen, & B. Schell (Eds.), *Willard & Spackman's occupational therapy* (pp. 691-698). Philadelphia: Lippincott, Williams & Wilkins.

Beery, K., & Beery, N. (2004). *The Beery-Buktenica developmental test of visual-motor integration. Administration, scoring, and teaching manual* (5th ed.). Minneapolis: NCS Pearson, Inc.

Burke, J. (1996). Moving occupation into treatment: Clinical interpretation of "legitimizing occupational therapy's knowledge." *American Journal of Occupational Therapy, 50*(8), 635-638.

Burke, J. (1998). Clinical interpretation of "health and the human spirit for occupation." *American Journal of Occupational Therapy, 52*(6), 419-422.

Cartledge, G., & Milburn, J. (1995). *Teaching social skills to children and youth* (3rd ed.). Boston: Allyn and Bacon.

Case-Smith, J. (2000). Effects of occupational therapy services on fine motor and functional performance in preschool children. *American Journal of Occupational Therapy, 54*(4), 372-380.

Coster, W. (1998). Occupation-centered assessment of children. *American Journal of Occupational Therapy, 52*(5), 337-344.

Cox, R., & Schopler, E. (1996). Social skills training for children. In M. Lewis (Ed.), *Child and adolescent psychiatry: A comprehensive textbook* (2nd ed., pp. 902-908). Baltimore: Williams & Wilkins.

Esdaile, S. (1996). A play-focused intervention involving mothers of preschoolers. *American Journal of Occupational Therapy, 50*(2), 113-123.

Florey, L. (2003). Psychosocial dysfunction in childhood and adolescence. In E. Crepeau, E. Cohen, and B. Schell (Eds.), *Willard & Spackman's occupational therapy* (10th ed., pp. 731-744). Philadelphia: Lippincott, Williams & Wilkins.

Florey, L., & Greene, S. (1997). Play in middle childhood: A focus on children with behavior and emotional disorders. In L. D. Parham & L. Fazio (Eds.), *Play in occupational therapy for children* (pp. 126-143). St. Louis: C.V. Mosby.

Frank, G., Fishman, M., Crowley, C., Blair, B., Murphy, S., Montoya, J., et al. (2001). The new stories/new cultures after-school enrichment program: A direct cultural intervention. *American Journal of Occupational Therapy, 55*(5), 501-508.

Greene, S. (1997). Playmates: Social interaction in early and middle childhood. In B. Chandler (Ed.), *The essence of play: A child's occupation* (pp. 131-157). Bethesda: American Occupational Therapy Association.

Hartman, B., Miller, B., & Nelson, D. (2000). The effects of hands-on occupation versus demonstration on children's recall memory. *American Journal of Occupational Therapy, 54*(5), 477-483.

Humphry, R. (2002). Young children's occupations: Explicating the dynamics of developmental processes. *American Journal of Occupational Therapy, 56*(2), 171-179.

Lawlor, M. (2003). The significance of being occupied: The social construction of childhood occupations. *American Journal of Occupational Therapy, 57*(4), 424-434.

McDonald, A. (1987). The construction of a self-report instrument to measure play activities and play styles in 7 to 11 year old children. Unpublished master's thesis, University of Southern California.

Morrison, C., & Metzger, P. (2001). Play. In J. Case-Smith (Ed.), *Occupational therapy for children* (4th ed., pp. 528-544). St. Louis: Mosby.

Murphy, S., Trombly, C., Tickle-Degnen, L., & Jacobs, K. (1999). The effect of keeping an end-product on intrinsic motivation. *American Journal of Occupational Therapy, 53*(2), 153-158.

Neville-Jan, A., Fazio, L., Kennedy, B., & Snyder, C. (1997). Elementary to middle school transition: Using multicultural play activities to develop life skills. In L. D. Parham & L. Fazio (Eds.), *Play in occupational therapy for children* (pp. 144-157). St. Louis: C. V. Mosby.

Parham, L. D., & Primeau, L. (1997). Play and occupational therapy. In L. D. Parham & L. Fazio (Eds.), *Play in occupational therapy for children* (pp. 2-21). St. Louis: C. V. Mosby.

Reilly, M. (1966). The educational process. *American Journal of Occupational Therapy, 23*, 299-307.

Richardson, P. (2002). The school as social context: Social interaction patterns of children with physical disabilities. *American Journal of Occupational Therapy, 54*(4), 296-304.

Saunders, I., Sayer, M., & Goodale, A. (1999). The relationship between playfulness and coping in preschool children: A pilot study. *American Journal of Occupational Therapy, 53*(2), 221-226.

Segal, R., Mandich, A., Polatajko, H., & Cook, J., (2002). Stigma and its management: A pilot study of parental perceptions of the experiences of children with developmental coordination disorder. *American Journal of Occupational Therapy, 56*(4), 422-428.

U.S. Department of Health and Human Services. (1999). *Mental health: A report of the surgeon general.* Rockville, MD: Author.

OCCUPATIONAL THERAPY
PATIENT INFORMATION AND TREATMENT
PLANNING NOTES

TONY

DATE OF ADMISSION _3-9-04_
DX _ODD R/O PTSD_
SHARPS STATUS _SUPERVISED_
ALLERGIES/MEDICAL
PROBLEMS _—_
ETHNICITY _LATINO / CAUCASIAN_
BIRTHDATE/AGE

CURRENT LIVING SITUATION _Biomom (6 m pregnant)_
Stepfather, Biobrother 4,
PRESENTING PROBLEM _aggression @ home and_
school - threw furniture in classroom,
punched teacher, verbal threats to
brother & mom

ADDITIONAL INFORMATION _physical abuse by bio-_
father (alcoholic) witnessed bio mom
beaten by his dad
- problems in school - poor grades,
picks on others

NOTES FROM TREATMENT PLANNING
3-10-04 - isolative and/or bossy c̄ unit
peer. Testing limits but no aggression
3-12-04 - several time outs for non
compliance. Bossy c̄ peers. Low VMI & fear
of failure - puts on bravado. Academic
difficulties - school achievement testing
ordered. Stepdad thinks behavior
"normal" and "needs" for a kid
who has been abused.
3-15-04 - bossy and non compliant
escalated to hitting peer. Unable to
take time out, ↑ in aggression - open
5R. Given Benadryl PRN for aggression to calm
down.
Below grade level (K level) in all
areas - cognitive testing ordered.

Real record 15-1A. Real record for a client with oppositional defiant disorder.

Very irritable mood – childhood depression inventory to be done by MD. Consider antidepressant

3-17-04 – In clinical range for depression on inventory – start low dose of anti-depressant.

Psych testing – verbal – 101 ⎫ 15 pt
performance – 84 ⎭ difference
potential learning disability
coordinate visual and motor subtests
X→ of VMI

Nar working ē parents re: parent training how to observe on unit and in OT, RT sessions sometime this week.

3-19-04 Continued intensive bossy on isolative ē peers but no aggression mood still irritable. Fear of failure in OT/RT activities – low frustration tolerance. Able to take time outs ē escalating. Prepare family for DC on Monday.

3-22-04 Family feedback by all disciplines 1:00. DC following feedback
School – needs IEP – ED class + potential learning disorder, 15 pt. differential in IQ. See OT testing
OT – below chronological age in both motor and visual subtests but lower in motor. Needs OT in school. Recommend some skill to learn + skills ē peers success activities / camp
RT – involve in big brother sport program
MD – continue antidepressant ē outpatient psychiatrist for follow up in 1 week.

Real record 15-1B. Real record for a client with oppositional defiant disorder.

Key Concepts

- Common behaviors of children with attention deficit disorder (ADD)/attention deficit hyperactivity disorder (ADHD): Inattention, impulsivity, emotional instability, and excessively high level of activity.
- Assessment: May involve various parent and/or teacher checklists, sensory histories, observations, and evaluation of related areas of occupation, including ADL, IADL, education, work, play, leisure, and social participation.
- Eligibility for related services: Children who are not eligible for services under the Individuals with Disabilities Education Act may be eligible under Section 504 of the Rehabilitation Act.
- Individuals with Disabilities Education Act (IDEA): A set of principles and guidelines for providing special education services to children with disabilities.
- Section 504 of the Rehabilitation Act of 1973: A federal law that guarantees reasonable accommodations to individuals attending federally-funded programs. Anyone regarded as having a disability is eligible for these accommodations.
- Environmental adaptations: In the school setting, this includes such things as preferential seating, use of a desktop easel, or special paper. Home adaptations may include the use of timers, headphones/earplugs, reminder lists, and organizational strategies.
- Home visit: Visit to the home to consult with caregivers regarding modifications for play, self-help, social interactions, routines, etc.
- Consultation: Sharing of expertise by one team member to another.
- Recommendations and strategies: Specific suggestions to assist the child, teacher, and caregiver with identified concerns.
- Follow-up: Therapist returns to the setting to offer suggestions for any new or continuing concerns.

Essential Vocabulary

distractibility: Difficulty paying attention to the task at hand while "tuning out" other less relevant information.
executive functioning: The brain's ability to organize, focus, integrate, activate, and direct information (Brown, 2000).
hyperactivity: Excessive level of activity.
impulsivity: The inability to regulate emotions or behavior, giving little consideration to the consequences of a behavior before doing it.
inattention: Lack of attention span or concentration.
level of arousal: Varying states of alertness.
organizational skills: The ability to organize materials, space, and time in order to complete a task.
reasonable accommodations: Modifications and adaptations to accommodate or provide access to activities.
social skills: Behaviors including greeting, taking turns, listening, and maintaining a topic during social interactions.

Clinical Summary

Diagnosis

Must be made by a physician according to 3 patterns of behavior.

Etiology

No exact cause; genetic factors, prenatal trauma, toxin exposure, and metabolic disorders have all been hypothesized to cause ADHD.

Prevalence

According to a 2003 report by the National Institute of Mental Health (NIMH), ADHD is the most commonly diagnosed childhood disorder. It is estimated to affect between 3% and 5% of school-age children. NIMH reports that ADHD occurs 3 times more often in boys than in girls.

Common Behaviors

Inattention, impulsivity, emotional instability, and excessively high level of activity.

Precautions

It is important to consider how the characteristic symptoms of ADHD (impulsivity, inattention, hyperactivity, and disregard for safety) impact all areas of occupational performance.

A Third-Grader With Attention Deficit Hyperactivity Disorder

Sue Gallagher, MA, OTR

Introduction

ADHD is the official term used to describe both ADD and ADHD. The DSM-IV-TR (APA, 2000) has identified 3 subtypes of ADHD:

1. Predominantly inattentive type.
2. Predominantly hyperactive and impulsive type.
3. Combined type.

ADHD is one of the most common mental health disorders among children today, occurring more often in boys than girls (NIMH, 2003). Children with ADD/ADHD are persistently more impulsive and less attentive than their same-aged peers. The DSM-IV-TR (2000) identifies several symptoms to assist the physician in making an ADHD diagnosis according to the 3 above-mentioned categories. The symptoms identified with inattention include lack of attention to detail, poor listening when spoken to directly, difficulty with following instructions and completing tasks, an avoidance of tasks requiring mental effort, distractibility, and forgetfulness. Hyperactivity can be identified from symptoms that include fidgeting; excessive running, climbing, or restlessness; excessive talking; and difficulty enjoying leisure activities quietly. The DSM-IV-TR (APA, 2000) describes impulsivity to include blurting out answers; difficulty waiting one's turn; frequently interrupting and/or intruding; demonstrating significant social, school, or work-related impairment; and impairment that can be observed in 2 or more settings.

There is no exact cause of ADD/ADHD; however, research suggests that it may be biologically and neurologically based. According to Batshaw (2002), genetic factors are the most common cause of ADHD and may account for 80% of diagnosed cases. Other conditions that may result in ADHD symptoms or increase the likelihood for related symptoms in genetically predisposed individuals include prenatal exposures to lead, cigarette smoking, alcohol, and possibly cocaine; prematurity; brain infections; and inborn errors of metabolism (Batshaw, 2002).

Many positive traits can be associated with people with ADHD. These characteristics may include high energy, creativity, perseverance, resourcefulness, high intelligence, risk taking, spontaneity, and high verbal skills. However, some symptoms of ADHD may also present challenges for many children by impacting their day-to-day functioning.

The symptoms of ADHD range from mild to severe and may be inconsistently displayed. Inattention, impulsivity, and emotional instability are among the most common issues for people with ADHD. Although children with ADHD may be able to pay attention to activities that are highly motivating to them, they often have difficulty completing tasks that are unfamiliar or that require organization and sustained focus. Impulsivity interferes with the development of age-appropriate social skills as these children often interrupt or act before thinking about the possible consequences of their words or actions. Poor safety awareness is also a common concern for families of children and adults with ADHD, as these children are not only impulsive, but also seek out novel experiences. Limited interpersonal awareness is another common trait of individuals with ADHD, as characterized by angry outbursts, blaming others for problems, and oversensitivity to criticism.

A psychiatrist, pediatrician, neurologist, or a family physician can make the diagnosis of ADHD. According to the DSM-IV-TR (APA, 2000), the following 3 patterns of behavior must be identified in order for an accurate diagnosis to be made:

1. The pattern must appear before the age of 7.
2. The pattern must continue for at least 6 months.
3. The behaviors must negatively affect at least 2 areas of the child's life, such as school, home, or social settings.

Although ADHD can be diagnosed at any age, typically only preschoolers who show extremes in temperament, activity level, and impulsive aggression toward peers will be diagnosed (Batshaw, 2002). As problems with listening, task completion, compliance, and "fitting in" often become more evident when children enter the structured environment of a school, many children are not diagnosed until this time.

Brown (2000) and Merrell & Boelter, (2001) report that identification of children with ADHD requires a multidisciplinary team and a multimethod assessment that includes the individual's academic, behavioral, and social performance and that includes medical, family, experiential, and developmental history. It is also important to consider cultural and linguistic factors when identifying students with ADHD, as students from culturally diverse backgrounds may display behaviors that can be mis-interpreted as ADD (Salend & Rohena, 2003).

Research indicates that although the primary symptoms of ADHD tend to diminish during the adolescent years, some behaviors may remain, including low self-esteem, restlessness, impulsivity, low self-confidence, and impaired social interactions. Often, as adults, these individuals show less hyperactivity but are accident prone and impulsive (Kaplan & Sadock, 1998; Sadock & Sadock, 2003). Sadock and Sadock (2003) report that many adults with ADHD also have secondary depressive disorders related to low self-esteem and impaired performance in both social and occupational functioning.

Children and adults diagnosed with ADHD often have one or more of the following associated impairments:
- Limited adaptive and social functioning (Roizen, Blondis, Irwin, & Stein, 1994).
- Deficits in executive functioning especially in the areas of working memory, sustaining and shifting attention, organizing and prioritizing information, planning, self-monitoring, and inhibiting responses (Mercugliano, Power, & Blum, 1999).
- Academic underachievement (Batshaw, 2002) particularly in processing auditory information (Mercugliano et al., 1999).
- Developmental coordination disorder (Blondis & Opacich, 1999; Hamilton, 2002). It is important to note, however, that Hamilton suggests that clumsiness in children with ADHD is caused by inattentiveness and impulsivity rather than by incoordination.
- Accidental and nonaccidental injury (DiScala, Lescohier, Barthel, & Li, 1998) due to increased risk-taking on their part as well as their difficult behavior, which may place them at risk for physical abuse from caregivers.
- Poor vestibular processing and motor planning (Mulligan, 1995).
- Difficulties related to playfulness such as entering groups, initiating play with others, sustaining cooperative interactions, negotiating, and sharing toys and space (Leipold & Bundy, 2000).

ADHD often occurs with other disorders, including learning disorders and behavioral disorders such as conduct disorder and ODD. It is important to note that although the behavioral problems associated with ADHD and the academic problems associated with learning disorders often occur together, not all children diagnosed with ADHD have learning disabilities (Wender, 2000).

Nathan is a third-grade student who has recently begun to have difficulty with social situations both at home and at school. He has shown increased impulsivity while playing at home with his sister and on the playground with classmates. His irritability and lack of judgment are of concern to both his mother and his teacher. Although Nathan continues to work at grade level, his teacher reports a high level of distractibility, immature handwriting, and disorganized work habits. Nathan's pediatrician has diagnosed him with ADHD as a result of these behaviors.

THEORY THAT FRAMES PRACTICE

Several conceptual models and theoretical foundations should be considered when working with the child with ADHD, including developmental, occupational, and SI frames of reference. The Person-Environment-Occupation (PEO) (Law et al., 1996) perspective is an overarching model that is useful when providing OT services to children with ADHD. When applying this model, the clinician recognizes that occupational performance is the result of the inter-relationship between the person and their roles; the cultural, social, and physical environment; and occupation.

Family-centered practice is critical when working with children with ADHD. This philosophy of service provision recognizes 3 important concepts:
1. Parents are the "experts" regarding their child and their child's needs.
2. All families are different and unique.
3. Families function most optimally when they have supportive families and communities.

ASSESSING THE CHILD WITH ATTENTION DEFICIT HYPERACTIVITY DISORDER

A useful tool when assessing a child with ADHD is a behavioral checklist. Nathan's pediatrician, in collaboration with Nathan's mother and teacher, completed one such checklist to assist with making the diagnosis. Several behavioral checklists are available, and these checklists provide a good starting point to gain insight into the behaviors that are interfering with the child's daily life and frequently assist the physician in making the diagnosis of ADHD. The parent or teacher can complete the Achenbach Child Behavior Checklist (Achenbach & Edelbrock, 1983). This tool is designed for children from age 4 to 16 years. The Conners' Parent Rating Scale or the Conners' Teachers Rating Scale (Conners, 1990a, 1990b) is also completed by either the teacher or the parent and is for children from 3 to 17 years of age. Both the OTA and the OT should review the checklist and keep in mind that the behavior of children with ADHD fluctuates from place to place and time to time.

Mulligan (1995) and Dunn & Bennett (2002) have found that many children with ADHD exhibit sensory-seeking behaviors in addition to inattention and distractibility. When assessing the child with ADHD who is suspected of having sensory-processing difficulties, several caregiver checklists may be useful. These tools include the Touch Inventory for Elementary School-Aged Children (Royeen & Fortune, 1990), Teacher Questionnaire of Sensorimotor Behavior (Carrasco & Lee, 1993), and the Sensory Profile (Dunn, 1999). Once caregivers have completed these questionnaires, the data should be reviewed, analyzed, and interpreted in collaboration with the OT.

Children with concomitant developmental coordination disorder and ADHD are particularly at risk for clumsiness

(Hamilton, 2002). In these instances, a motor assessment may be useful. The Peabody Developmental Motor Scale-2 (PDMS-2) (Folio & Fewell, 2000) assesses both fine and gross motor skills in children from birth to 83 months. The Bruininks-Oseretsky Test of Motor Proficiency (BOTMP) (Bruininks, 1978) assesses gross motor skills, including speed, agility, balance, bilateral coordination, strength, and upper limb coordination. The fine motor portion of the BOTMP tests response speed, visual-motor control, upper limb speed, and dexterity. Both the PDMS-2 and the BOTMP can be administered under the supervision of an OT after practicing the administration of the test on several typically developing children. The OT and OTA should collaborate to review and interpret the results of either assessment. In addition, clinical observations of muscle tone, posture, reflex development, and strength should be completed in conjunction with the OT.

Visual-motor perception has been identified as a common area of weakness in individuals with ADHD in a study by Raggio (1999) in which preadolescent children with a diagnosis of ADHD-Combined Type were required to copy geometrical designs using pen and paper. Visual-motor perception may be associated with poor handwriting performance, a common area of OT practice. Tests useful in assessing visual-motor integration skills are listed in Table 16-1. Visual perceptual assessment may also be indicated and these tools are also identified in Table 16-1. Most of these tests can be administered and scored by the OTA, with supervision from the OT as necessary. Although these scores may be useful in planning interventions, best practice in school-based therapy indicates that goals and objectives be functional and not directed at improving test scores.

When concerns are specifically directed at handwriting, it is necessary to evaluate visual perception, visual-motor integration, posture, and fine-motor skills in addition to using specific tools to evaluate handwriting. Handwriting assessments can also be administered by the OTA who has acquired experience in this testing domain. See Table 16-1 for a list of handwriting assessments commonly used by OTs. These handwriting tools evaluate speed and legibility of handwriting, and analysis of the results should be a cooperative effort between the OT, OTA, and teacher. A checklist with accompanying video entitled *Assessment of Hand Skills in the Primary Child* (Benbow, 1995) may be useful in determining specific areas of fine motor function that impact handwriting. It is recommended that the OTA view the video and observe several typically developing children perform these tasks prior to using the checklist with a child who has ADHD.

Social skills and play (Leipold & Bundy, 2000) have also been identified as problematic in many children with ADHD. A study by Leipold and Bundy (2000) reported that children with an ADHD diagnosis scored low in areas of internal control, intrinsic motivation, and framing. Framing refers to verbal and nonverbal communication regarding the intent to play. The Test of Playfulness (ToP) (Bundy, 1997) assesses 4 characteristics of play: intrinsic motivation, internal control, freedom to suspend reality, and framing through observation of the child during free play.

Williamson and Dorman (2002) identify several rating scales and questionnaires designed to gather information regarding the child's social functioning. See Table 16-1 for evaluation tools that may be useful when assessing the child with ADHD who is demonstrating problems with social skills. These questionnaires assist the practitioner in gathering information regarding prosocial skill development, problem behaviors, and academic competence through the use of parent, teacher and student-self rating forms. As mentioned previously, behavioral observations are an essential component of social skills assessment and these tools guide the practitioner to observe social and play behavior, self-regulation, communication, and social decision making. Since a child's social behavior may vary dramatically according to the social context, Williamson and Dorman (2002) urge practitioners to observe children in a variety of social settings such as the playground, cafeteria, home, and community.

Adaptive tasks, including dressing, safety awareness, and organizing personal belongings, should also be informally assessed as these skill areas may present difficulties for the child with ADHD.

DETERMINING ELIGIBILITY FOR INDIVIDUALS WITH DISABILITIES EDUCATION ACT OR SECTION 504

The Education of the Handicapped Act (EHA) was passed in 1975 and established 6 principles to guide the education of individuals with disabilities. These principles have remained unchanged although the law is now referred to as the IDEA. Under the IDEA, OT is defined as a related service that may be required to enable students with disabilities to benefit from special education. See Table 16-2 for a list of IDEA principles.

When a student with a disability is not eligible for special education services, yet has difficulty participating in and benefiting from educational programs, he or she may be eligible for OT services under Section 504 of the Rehabilitation Act of 1973. Under Section 504, anyone who is identified as having a physical or mental impairment that substantially limits a major life activity, has a record of the impairment or is regarded as having such impairment, is eligible for reasonable accommodations. Any program receiving federal funding is required by law to make reasonable accommodations. These accommodations might include menu modifications, therapy services, or environmental adaptations for these individuals.

Reid (1999) reports that approximately half of all school age children with ADHD will qualify for special education services under the IDEA, and that most children with ADHD also qualify for services under Section 504. Reid (1999) goes on to report that whether receiving services under IDEA or Section 504, most children with ADHD will spend the majority of their time in a general education classroom.

Table 16-1

Assessments Commonly Used With
Children With Attention Deficit Hyperactivity Disorder

Test	Area of Occupation or Performance Skill Addressed
Social Skills Rating System (SSRS) (Gresham & Elliot, 1990)	Social participation
Test of Playfulness (ToP) (Bundy, 1997)	Play
Self-Awareness Assessment (Dorman, 1999)	Social participation
Identification of Social Difficulties Questionnaire (Dorman & Williamson, 2000)	Social participation
Components of Social Competence Observation Scale (Williamson, 2000)	Social participation
Test of Visual-Motor Skills-Revised (TVMS-R) (Gardner, 1995)	Visual-motor integration
Developmental Test of Visual Perception-2 (DTVP-2) (Hammill, Pearson, & Voress, 1993)	Visual perception and visual-motor integration
Developmental Test of Visual Perception-Adolescent and Adult (DTVP-A) (Reynolds, Pearson, & Voress, 2002)	Visual perception and visual-motor integration
Developmental Test of Visual-Motor Integration-4th ed. (VMI-4) (Beery & Buktenica, 1997)	Visual-motor integration
Motor-Free Visual Perceptual Test-3 (MVPT-3) (Colarusso & Hammill, 2002)	Visual perception
Test of Visual-Perceptual Skills (Nonmotor)-Revised (TVPS-R) (Gardner, 1997)	Visual perception
Evaluation of Children's Handwriting (Manuscript: ETCH-M and Cursive: ETCH-C) (Amundson, 1995)	Handwriting
Minnesota Handwriting Assessment (Reisman, 1999)	Handwriting
Children's Handwriting Evaluation Scale (CHES) (Phelps, Stempel, & Speck, 1984)	Handwriting
Children's Handwriting Evaluation Scale for Manuscript Writing (CHES-M) (Phelps et al., 1984)	Handwriting
Assessment of Hand Skills in the Primary Child (Benbow, 1995)	Fine-motor handwriting

---

Table 16-2

Guiding Principles of the Individuals With Disabilities Education Act

- Free and appropriate public education for all.
- Least restrictive environment, meaning that children with disabilities are educated with children without disabilities except in specific circumstances.
- Appropriate education refers to the individualized assessment for eligibility determination, educational programming, and individualized monitoring of each child's program.
- The IEP is the document that outlines needs, services, and goals for each child receiving special education and related services. This plan is written annually.
- Parent and student participation in decision making.
- Procedural safeguards to ensure that the rights of children with disabilities and their families are protected and provided with the information they need to make informed decisions regarding their child's education.

Table 16-3

Strategies for Calming/Decreasing Arousal Level

- Dim lighting
- Soft or natural colors
- Steady visual input
- Classical music
- Rhythm
- Resistive activities: weighted vests, back packs, or lap weights; pulling on rubber bands; assisting to move classroom furniture; carrying a stack of books; and squeezing a small, rubber ball
- Slow rocking, swinging
- Use of a "fidget" such as a rubber band, squeeze ball, or other small toy

---

INTERVENTIONS

Pharmacological interventions are the most commonly reported form of intervention for children with ADHD (Purdie, Hattie, & Carroll, 2002). Other interventions include behavioral interventions, cognitive behavioral interventions, parental interventions, and educational interventions. Experts in the field of ADHD conclude that multimodal interventions (those combining medication, behavioral, cognitive behavioral, environmental, educational, and parenting interventions) are the most effective (Purdie et al., 2002).

Behavioral interventions refer to strategies such as positive or negative contingencies and positive or negative reinforcements to reduce target behaviors and replace them with more acceptable behaviors (Mulligan, 2001; Reid, 1999).

Cognitive-behavioral programs utilize self-talk, self-instruction, self-monitoring, and self-reinforcement to improve attention and impulse behavior problems (Purdie et al., 2002).

Educational interventions may include environmental adaptations such as preferential seating, noise reduction strategies, reduction of visual distracters, behavior management, token economies, peer tutoring, cooperative learning, social skill training, and self-instruction (Purdie et al., 2002). Curriculum modification is also a commonly used approach to ADHD in the classroom. Selecting topics that are of particular interest to the child and novelty may enhance the child's selective and sustained attention (Zentall, 1993). Many books and Web sites offering a variety of classroom management strategies and educationally-oriented strategies are available.

Sensorimotor strategies are often employed by the occupational therapist to improve classroom performance (Mulligan, 1995, 2001). Based on the results of the sensory history questionnaire and observations across various settings, the OT may recommend sensory modulation strategies to either calm the child or help him or her to increase his or her arousal level in order to maintain attention. See Tables 16-3 and 16-4 for specific strategies. The Alert Program (Williams & Shellenberger, 1994) is a structured program that assists children in learning to recognize how alert they are and to identify sensorimotor strategies that are useful in regulating their level of alertness. This program also helps children to learn how to self-monitor their arousal levels in a variety of settings (Parham & Mailloux, 2001).

Environmental adaptations are another strategy that OTs can offer to school personnel and parents to enhance the child's ability to sustain attention and organize personal belongings. See Table 16-5 for specific strategies.

Table 16-4

Strategies for Increasing Arousal Level

- Bright lights, colors
- Varied intensity music/sound
- Dysrhythmic movement
- Rocking, jiggling, bouncing
- Gentle, quick rubbing of skin

- Sucking on sour, salty, or citrus foods or drinks
- Drinking cold liquids
- Chewing gum or resistive snack food
- Using resistive activities (as in Table 16-3)

Table 16-5

Environmental Adaptations

- Three-ring notebooks with color-coded pocket dividers that can be labeled according to subject (e.g., math, reading, history)
- Reminder lists and checklists placed on student's desk such as "Take Home," "Math Formulas," or "Assignments Due"
- Self-adhesive hole reinforcers for torn papers
- Labeled shelves and drawers
- Calendar or daily planner with "due date warnings," special events, and due dates for assignments
- Labeled containers to organize materials and belongings in lockers, desks, closets, and bureaus
- Tape record lectures or class discussions
- Use of earplugs or headphones with environmental sounds or calming music during independent work times

---

As noted earlier, children with ADHD may have difficulty with fine- or gross-motor skills. Interventions to address these skill deficits should be functionally based and offer the child the "just-right" challenge. Activities that offer novelty and are of special interest to the child will most likely result in sustained interest and attention.

Many children with ADHD experience difficulty in making or maintaining friends and lack the ability to sustain participation in games and cooperate with peers (Cronin, 2001). The OT can provide intervention related to social skill development through a variety of group activities. Self-management training may be useful with children with ADHD as it involves modeling and instruction in productive peer relations by helping the child become aware of expectations regarding social behavior (Cronin, 2001). Dorman and Williamson (2002) also offer many ideas for structuring a social skills group that includes conversation time, a short-term activity designed to facilitate social interaction and burn energy, a project activity, and closure of the group, which may involve a snack and review time.

CASE STUDY

Nathan is a third grader in Mr. Roth's class at Dawson Elementary School. He lives at home with his mother and 13-year-old sister, Elizabeth. Nathan's mother, Mrs. L., has become increasingly concerned with Nathan's recent behavior at home. Although he has never been an "easy" child, Mrs. L. had always excused his rambunctious behavior on the fact that he was "just being a boy" and was subjected to various family stressors. When

Nathan was 5, his father moved out of the house after dropping out of a rehabilitation program for cocaine addiction. It was a very stressful time for the family, and Mrs. L. was forced to return to work a few months earlier when her husband's drug abuse had become so out of control that he was fired from his job. During this time, Nathan became even more distracted and irritable. Mrs. L. noticed that he could not seem to stay focused long enough to play a simple game with his sister or even finish a sandwich at lunch. He was always "flitting" around the house, never seeming to get engaged with a toy or activity. His arguments with his sister quickly escalated to name calling and angry outbursts. He would often throw a tantrum if he did not get his way.

As a baby, Nathan had always been fussy and had not begun sleeping through the night until he was almost 6. Now at 7.5, he seemed very immature in contrast to how Elizabeth had behaved at that age. Recently, during a visit to the pediatrician for his asthma, Nathan created a real scene in the waiting area when another child would not immediately give up the remote-controlled car with which Nathan wanted to play. When Mrs. L. mentioned her concern over Nathan's high level of activity and difficulty staying with certain tasks to the pediatrician, he asked for her input as he completed a behavioral checklist. The pediatrician also asked Mrs. L. to give another checklist to Nathan's teacher the next day. Using the information from both Mrs. L. and Mr. Roth, the pediatrician diagnosed Nathan as having ADHD.

Mr. Roth had also been concerned about Nathan's behavior in school. Nathan had begun to fall behind in classroom work, despite the fact that Mr. Roth felt that Nathan understood the material and was a bright student. Nathan's assignments were often crumpled and torn, sometimes barely legible. Nathan's personal space was often disorganized. Sometimes he did not get started on an assignment until long after the others, as he was unable to locate his pencil, workbook, scissors, etc. Math was especially difficult for Nathan; he was unable to copy equations from the board and could not consistently align numbers or letters on the lines of primary paper. Mr. Roth indicated that soon the class would be beginning cursive writing instruction, and that he was concerned this would be difficult for Nathan. He also noted that Nathan was out of his seat so often that he was disrupting the whole class. Problems on the playground were reported, too. He seemed to lack all judgment on the equipment, standing on the top rung of the jungle gym, jumping off the teeter-totter in midair, and running wildly into groups of children. Fortunately, he seemed to have excellent gross motor skill and coordination and always regained his balance and landed on his feet. Playground supervisors were concerned with Nathan's safety as well as the safety of the other children in the area.

Soon after the diagnosis was made, Mr. Roth requested permission from Mrs. L. for a meeting with the Child Study Team to identify possible services to help Nathan at school. At the meeting, Mrs. L. and the team determined that Nathan was still managing to function within the normal range for his grade and that he did not require special education services, thus making him ineligible for services under the IDEA. However, the team felt that he might benefit from some services and modifications in order to continue to meet the academic requirements of the third-grade curriculum. A referral to OT was made.

Occupational Therapy Assessment

After meeting briefly with Mr. Roth before school, the OTA reviewed the behavior checklists that Mr. Roth and Mrs. L. had filled out. She noted Nathan's high activity level, his lack of organizational skills, and problems with handwriting. Using this information, she and the OT determined that the following assessments would be useful:

- Completion of the Classroom Observation Worksheet (Figure 16-1).
- Collection of handwriting samples (Figure 16-2) and class assignments to:
  - Determine which task is more problematic—copying from the board or composing.
  - Note letter formation, alignment, orientation, spacing, and slant.
- Playground, physical education, and cafeteria observation of:
  - Social skills
  - Organizational skills
  - Distractibility/off-task behavior
  - Safety awareness
  - Use of gross motor equipment
- Observation in art room.

- Home visit or phone interview with Mrs. L. related to play and self-care skills.
- Administration of Test of Visual-Motor Integration Skills.
- Assessment of Hand Skills in the Primary Child.

The OT and OTA designed a plan for assessing and observing Nathan based on the therapy assistant's previous experience with the various tools being utilized. The OTA administered and scored the TVMS and completed the Benbow observations. The OT made classroom, gym, art, and playground observations. The OT also scheduled a consultation visit with Mr. Roth during his planning period.

Functional Impact of Attention Deficit Hyperactivity Disorder

The classroom observation provided information regarding Nathan's disorganization, distractibility, and level of activity/arousal. See Figure 16-1 for classroom observations made by the OTA. Nathan's postural control was adequate for the task of writing; however, his desk and chair height needed to be adjusted. Pencil grasp was immature. Nathan's desk and workspace were disorganized, and he had difficulty finding papers, pencils, etc. During writing tasks, Nathan found many other things to do, sometimes completely avoiding the assignment until the class was moving on to another activity. Work samples indicated that copying was more difficult than creating. Letter formation, alignment, orientation to line, and spacing were problematic. See Figure 16-2 for handwriting samples.

On the playground, social skills were a concern. Nathan was unable to successfully participate in child-directed games. This appeared due to his limited ability to take turns and stay on task. He quickly became angry and would either antagonize other kids or abandon that game and attempt entering another. Social skills were also an issue in the cafeteria. Nathan typically moved through the lunch line without waiting his turn. He had difficulty listening during conversations at the lunch table and often blurted out information not related to the conversation.

Nathan scored within 6 months of his age on the TVMS-R, and no further testing was done in this area.

When observed using the Benbow assessment, Nathan was unable to maintain a palmar arch or adequately separate the 2 sides of his hand. Precision rotation was also difficult and impaired his ability to use math manipulatives.

Intervention

Under Section 504, an accommodation plan is recommended. Formal, written goals and objectives are not required (Figure 16-3). The therapist and assistant collaborated with Mrs. L. and Mr. Roth to design Nathan's plan. Direct OT was recommended on a short-term basis to address Nathan's handwriting and organizational skills. Handwriting was an area the OTA had spent considerable time learning about. She had attended conferences and reviewed various handwriting programs. *Loops and Other Groups: A Kinesthetic Writing System* (Benbow, 1990) was determined to be an appropriate program to use with Nathan.

Dawson Elementary School
Occupational Therapy

Classroom Observation Worksheet

Student: _Nathan_   Date observed: _12/15/03_

Therapist: _Susan_   Teacher: _Roth_

Setting observed: _Classroom - 3rd_

Activity demands:
math lesson - rulers, graphs, complete indep assign
playground & cafe. observations

Posture while seated: _upright, feet on floor. fidgets constantly_

Chair and desk height appropriate fit to child: yes___ no _X_ adjusted _12/15/03_

Moves independently around room: yes _X_ no___ describe _freq out of seat_

Attention to task:

spontaneous _initially_ requires adult direction/redirection _yes_

time on task _~3 min_   number of redirections in 15 min _LHT II_

attention during group activity: _<3 min_ attention during individual activity _<3 min_

can independently return focus to work: yes___ no _✓_

Environmental distractions: _22 kids in small classroom, very_
visually stim - posters, etc.
Organizational skills: _several subjects on blackboard_

Workspace free of clutter: yes___ no _✓_

Desk contents: organized___ disorganized _✓_

Cubby/locker contents: organized___ disorganized _✓_

Backpack/book bag contents: organized___ disorganized _✓_

Readily finds necessary materials: in desk _no_ in classroom _yes, usually_

Observation worksheet
1

Figure 16-1A. Classroom observation worksheet.

Dawson Elementary School
Occupational Therapy

Organizational Skills, cont.

Papers are organized per teacher instruction: yes ✓ no___

Knows/follows classroom routine: yes ✓ no___

Comments regarding organizational skills:
no consistent place for assignments in notebook
shoves papers in desk —

Handwriting: Manuscript ✓ Cursive___

Pencil grasp: Right ✓ Left___ Switches___

Prehension pattern: *thumb wrap closed web space*

Near point copy: *legible*

Copy from board: *takes excessive time ? loses place*

Writing without visual model: *see spelling list work sample*

Worksamples collected: *spelling - workbook - creative writing*

Placement of paper on desk: *left slant*

Letter formation: *hurried, but correct*

Spacing: *inconsistent - clear spaces between words*

Placement on line: *poor — ? due to visual inattent.*

Letter size consistency: *fair → good*

Letter or number reversals: *none*

Adapts words/letters to available space: *yes*
heavy pressure
erasures → tearing, smudging, wrinkling of paper

Observation worksheet
2

Figure 16-1B. Classroom observation worksheet.

Dawson Elementary School
Occupational Therapy

Use of classroom materials:

neutral

Scissors: scissor holding hand R   paper holding hand L   *more pronated*

overflow: yes___ no X   snips *no*   accuracy *fair*   ↓ *visual attention*

Glue: uses appropriate amount ✓   places within boundaries ✓   cleans up ✓

Paperclips: can attach 2+ papers ✓ *w/difficulty*   can remove without tearing paper yes___ no ✓

Stapler: safely and effectively attaches 2+ papers - *yes, poor alignment*

Manipulatives: in-hand translation keeps pace with counting? yes___ no ✓

difficulty stabilizing ruler to draw line on graph

Pencil sharpener: electric___ manual X

Playground - kickball
cuts in line - insists on being 1st
in outfield - lost interest left game ~ 3-5min

wandered between groups - no prolonged
engagement in games
in line to re-enter building - teacher cue to
stay in line x3 coat unzipped, shoes untied

Cafeteria - forgot ticket, impatient in line
table - interrupts - poor manners →
burps, chews/talks with mouth
full of food - open

Art - doesn't wait for teacher instruction,
rushes through project - tips stool over,
spills paint
constant redirection to clean up
teacher moved to table w/ fewer kids

Observation worksheet
3

Figure 16-1C. Classroom observation worksheet.

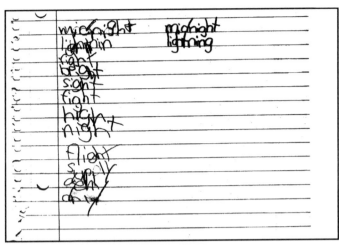

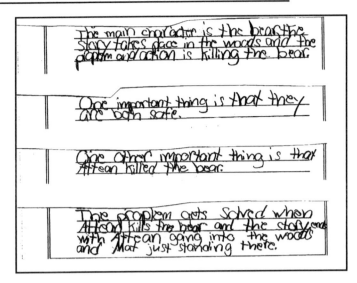

Figure 16-2. Handwriting samples.

The OTA and OT volunteered to provide in-service training to third-grade teachers who were interested in using this curriculum in their classrooms. Other interventions designed to help Nathan with handwriting included trial use of adaptive equipment such as pencil grips, clipboards, raised line paper, highlighters, and graph paper. Nathan's seat and desk height were adjusted. The OTA implemented these interventions in the classroom.

The therapy assistant designed various strategies to help Nathan with organizing his materials and workspace. She provided organizational strategies that could then be maintained and monitored by Mr. Roth. These strategies included:

- Use of a 3-ring notebook with Velcro closures.
- Use of self-adhesive hole reinforcers for torn papers.
- Pocket folders for homework marked with "Done" on one side and "To Do" on the other.
- Pocket folders that are color coded for specific subjects.
- Use of compartmental tray for art supplies, with clearly marked areas for various materials.
- Name labels on all materials.
- Use of a small pocket notebook to keep track of homework assignments.
- Checklists for Nathan to refer to materials he needs to bring home, steps to completing assignments, etc.

A "Lunch Bunch" group was recommended for improving socialization skills. This group consisted of 3 to 4 of Nathan's peers who were chosen by the teacher. The children ate lunch together for a 1-week period. Different students joined Nathan every week. Strategies for improving listening skills, turn-taking, reading facial expression, staying on topic, and manners were introduced, modeled, and reinforced by more socially mature students and the intermittent attendance of the OTA.

The OTA and OT created activities for developing palmar arches, improving precision rotation, and separating the 2 sides of the hands. These activities included various manipulatives, age-appropriate games, and crafts that could be used during math, cooperative learning activities, and "down time" in the classroom. Activities and materials were changed often, as novelty is a key factor in maintaining interest and attention. In addition, the OTA offered suggestions for crafts and games that corresponded to the general curriculum during monthly consultations with Mr. Roth.

The therapy assistant and OT collaborated in designing a "sensory diet" for Nathan, using activities that could be integrated into his daily classroom routine or used at home when necessary. These activities were discussed with Mr. Roth and were adapted in order to be implemented on a regular basis.

Once adaptations and materials were in place within the classroom, the OTs continued to meet on a regular basis with various school personnel and Mrs. L. to brainstorm and plan further modifications, as needed.

Home Visit

A home visit was requested by Mrs. L. to address several issues. Mrs. L.'s priority was for Nathan to become more independent in his morning routine. It was very difficult to constantly monitor him, as she also had to get herself and Elizabeth ready for work and school each morning. Nathan required constant redirection to continue getting dressed, eat breakfast, and pack his backpack. He often got to school without his homework or with inadequate clothes for the season. The OTA recommended that brief, colorful lists be designed and placed in strategic places to serve as a reminder of the things he needed to do while he was in that particular place. She also recommended that Nathan be required to pack his backpack and lay out appropriate clothes for the weather the night before, again utilizing the brief checklists. A timer was suggested to help Nathan stay on task for each segment of his morning routine. Mrs. L. would set the timer for the appropriate amount of time needed for a particular task and this would allow her to quickly check in on his progress.

Another idea the team came up with was to involve Nathan in an extracurricular activity. This would provide opportunities outside of school to practice his newly acquired social skills and to enhance his self-confidence and self-esteem. Knowing

Student: _____ DOB: _____ District: _____   Meeting Date: _____
          Last Name, First Name   mm/dd/yyyy   mm/dd/yyyy

PROGRAM MODIFICATIONS/ADAPTATIONS - INCLUDING NONACADEMIC AND EXTRACURRICULAR ACTIVITIES / COLLABORATION/SUPPORTS FOR SCHOOL PERSONNEL

Modifications/Adaptations - including Nonacademic and Extracurricular Activities	Sites/Activities Where Required and Duration	
Materials/Books/Equipment: ☐ Alternative Text ☐ Consumable Workbook ☐ Modified Worksheets ☐ Manipulatives ☐ Access to Computer ☐ Tape Recorder ☐ Supplementary Visuals ☐ Large Print Text ☐ Spell Check ☐ Calculator ☐ Assistive Technology: (specify) _____ ☐ Other: (specify) _____		**Assistive Technology Devices:** _____ _____ _____ _____
Tests/Quizzes/Time: ☐ Prior Notice of Tests ☐ Preview Test Procedures ☐ Test Study Guide ☐ Simplify Test Wording ☐ Oral Testing ☐ Limited Multiple Choice ☐ Student Write on Test ☐ Shortened Tasks ☐ Hands-on Projects ☐ Reduced Reading ☐ Alternative Tests ☐ Objective Tests ☐ Extra Credit Options ☐ Extra Time–Written Work ☐ Extra Time–Tests ☐ Extra Time–Projects ☐ Extra Response Time ☐ Modified Tests ☐ Test Read ☐ Pace Long Term Projects ☐ Rephrase Test Questions/Directions ☐ Other: (specify) _____		_____ _____ _____ _____ _____
Grading: ☐ No Spelling Penalty ☐ No Handwriting Penalty ☐ Grade Effort + Work ☐ Grade Improvement ☐ Course Credit ☐ Base Grade on IEP ☐ Base Grade on Ability ☐ Modified Grades ☐ Pass/Fail ☐ Audit Course ☐ Other: (specify)		**Frequency and Duration of Supports Required for School Personnel to Implement this IEP.**
Organization: ☐ Provide Study Outlines ☐ Desktop List of Tasks ☐ List Sequential Steps ☐ Post Routines ☐ Post Assignments ☐ Give One Paper at a Time ☐ Folders to Hold Work ☐ Pencil Box for Tools ☐ Pocket Folder for Work ☐ Assignment Pad ☐ Daily Assignment List ☐ Daily Homework List ☐ Worksheet Formats ☐ Extra Space for Work ☐ Assign Partner ☐ Other: (specify)		_____ _____
Environment: ☐ Preferential Seating ☐ Clear Work Area ☐ Study Carrel ☐ Other: (specify) _____		_____ _____
Behavior Management/Support: ☐ Daily Feedback to Student ☐ Chart Progress ☐ Behavior Contracts ☐ Parent/Guardian Sign Homework ☐ Positive Reinforcement ☐ Collect Baseline Data ☐ Set/Post Class Rules ☐ Parent/Guardian Sign Behavioral Chart ☐ Cue Expected Behavior ☐ Structure Transitions ☐ Break Between Tasks ☐ Time Out from Positive Reinforcement ☐ Proximity/Touch Control ☐ Contingency Plan ☐ Other: (specify)		_____ _____ _____
Instructional Strategies: ☐ Check Work in Progress ☐ Immediate Feedback ☐ Pre-teach Content ☐ Have Student Restate Information ☐ Extra Drill/Practice ☐ Review Sessions ☐ Review Directions ☐ Provide Lecture Notes/Outline to Student ☐ Use Manipulatives ☐ Modified Content ☐ Assign Study Partner ☐ Computer Assisted Instruction ☐ Monitor Assignments ☐ Provide Models ☐ Repeat Instructions ☐ Support Auditory Presentations with Visuals ☐ Multi-Sensory Approach ☐ Highlight Key Words ☐ Oral Reminders ☐ Display Key Vocabulary ☐ Visual Reinforcement ☐ Pictures/Charts ☐ Visual Reminders ☐ Provide Student With Vocabulary Word Bank ☐ Mimed Clues/Gestures ☐ Concrete Examples ☐ Use Mnemonics ☐ Personalized Examples ☐ Number Line ☐ Other: (specify) _____		_____ _____ _____

Note: When specifying required supports for personnel to implement this IEP, include the specific supports required, how often they are to be provided (frequency) and for how long (duration).

August, 2002   **Page 8 of 8**   **State of Connecticut**

Figure 16-3. Page 8 of the Connecticut State Individualized Education Program. Program modifications/adaptations in regular education including nonacademic and extracurricular activities/collaboration/supports for school personnel. August, 2002.

Nathan's love of the water, Mrs. L. enrolled him in the town's recreational swimming program for 1 night each week. Not only did Nathan have the opportunity to learn new strokes and gain skills, he also seemed to come home very relaxed and proud of his new accomplishments.

Follow-Up

The OTA made several visits to the classroom over the next 6 months. She and Mr. Roth utilized a form they referred to as an "Input Sheet" (Figure 16-4), which proved to be very helpful. Mr. Roth and various other teachers involved with Nathan were encouraged to leave Input Sheets in the OTA's school mailbox regarding tasks that were causing problems for Nathan at school. The OTA could observe Nathan and discuss the concerns with the OT before offering suggestions in writing on the bottom half of the Input Sheet. The sheet would then be returned to the teacher. These sheets were also helpful for communicating with Mrs. L. so that she might utilize some of the strategies at home. Input Sheets were kept in a notebook as a method of documenting problems, progress, and plans on a regular basis.

Program Discontinuation

Consultation continued throughout the school year. Nathan's fine-motor skills improved through the use of toys, games, and manipulatives that were highly motivating. Nathan's handwriting also improved; however, he continued to require cueing to slow down and more carefully orient his letters. Nathan was also able to more effectively organize his time and space. Initially, he relied heavily on environmental adaptations such as lists and pocket folders, but within a few months had memorized many of the simple checklists and could organize his materials for most projects. Mrs. L. also noticed changes at home. She had become aware of how important structure was for Nathan. She felt that many of the strategies offered had been instrumental in his increasing independence with self-help skills.

Socially, Nathan continued to have some difficulty, although he remained very popular among the more outgoing kids in his class. His impulsivity caused him to say hurtful things, but he had become more aware of other's feelings and would be quick to apologize upon recognizing his insults. The "Lunch Bunch"

INPUT SHEET

To: _____

From: _____

Date: _____

Student: _____

Activity	Comments
Activity	Comments
Activity	Comments
Activity	Comments

Special Notes:

Next Week/Session:

Figure 16-4. Input sheet. (Reprinted with permission from Sanderson, C. [1999]. *Input sheet for classroom consultation.* Therapist developed unpublished worksheet.)

club continued, and various resource room, classroom, and special education staff participated on a rotating basis.

A meeting was held prior to school starting the following year to discuss strategies that were helpful with Nathan's new teacher. The Input Sheets provided a review of both successful and unsuccessful interventions. The OTA assisted the teacher in designing new "cue cards" and other organizational strategies appropriate to the fourth-grade curriculum. The OTA made 2 visits to the classroom in the first month of school to help problem solve any issues related to handwriting, organization of materials, etc. A phone call was also made to Mrs. L., who felt that things were going well, thus far. At this point, OT was discontinued with the understanding that if further issues arose, additional consultative visits might be requested.

ADULTS WITH ATTENTION DEFICIT HYPERACTIVITY DISORDER

For many adults with ADHD, the hyperactivity they experienced in their childhood will have diminished; however, other symptoms of ADHD may persist.

Often considered only a childhood disorder, ADHD affects an estimated 9 million adults, with approximately 85% of adults with ADHD remaining undiagnosed and untreated. It is estimated that 60% of children with ADHD continue to be significantly impaired as adults (*Health and Medicine Week*, 2003).

Hallowell and Ratey (1994) have compiled a list of common symptoms reported by adults with ADHD. These symptoms include the following:

- A sense of underachievement
- Difficulty getting organized
- Chronic procrastination
- Many ongoing and simultaneous projects
- A tendency to worry needlessly
- Low frustration tolerance and/or lack of patience
- Lack of verbal inhibition
- Need for high stimulation
- Trouble with following "proper" procedures
- Mood swings
- Restlessness

In addition, the authors report that these individuals are often highly intelligent, intuitive, and creative.

There are many adults with ADHD who have developed strategies for staying on task, attending to things not intrinsically interesting, and organizing their time. Strategies such as the use of tape recorders to record important meetings and colored files for organizing written materials are effective. The use of bill-paying software, oversized calendars placed in prominent locations, and daily planners may also be effective for the adult with ADHD.

CLINICAL PROBLEM SOLVING

1. Clarissa is an 8-year-old girl recently diagnosed with ADHD. Clarissa has great difficulty tuning out noise or activity in the classroom. She is constantly moving about the room, unable to sit still for more than 1 or 2 minutes. Her high level of activity has significantly impacted her performance at school. She has been identified as in need of special education services secondary to her ADHD. Clarissa has been referred for OT. Completion of a Sensory Profile indicates that she has problems in the area of sensory processing, in particular, with regulating her overall state of arousal. The OT observed Clarissa in the classroom and noted that Clarissa was so busy it was impossible for her to engage in classroom assignments and discussions, despite the fact that she had a lot to contribute. OT was recommended by the team to address her sensory-processing skills and her ability to modulate her level of arousal. The OT and OTA designed an intervention plan that included use of a "sensory diet" for use in the school environment. What strategies might be implemented in the classroom for helping Clarissa to calm herself down? What strategies could be useful in teaching her to modulate her level of arousal and alertness? The OT and OTA offered strategies that could be easily incorporated into her daily routine such as listening to calming music through headphones during silent reading or while completing written work. Other strategies included the use of heavy work activities interspersed throughout the day. The Alert Program (Williams & Shellenberger, 1994) was also implemented for use in individual and

group sessions with the OTA. The therapy assistant taught visual imagery and relaxation techniques to the class once each week. What type of data collection could be done to document Clarissa's progress in the area of sensory modulation? The therapists met periodically to discuss Clarrisa's progress. They also met with the classroom teacher to brainstorm additional approaches to address self-regulation issues in the classroom.

2. Uri, a second-grader, was referred to OT due to his clumsiness at school. His teachers noted problems with organization and with sequencing of tasks. Upon evaluation by the OT, it was determined that Uri had poor balance, immature bilateral hand skills, motor planning problems, and poor visual-motor integration. Physical education was especially difficult for Uri. His self-esteem was suffering due to poor performance during team sports. The team recommended therapy and the therapists worked together to design an intervention plan. Handwriting, ball handling, and balance skills were targeted. The OTA provided direct weekly therapy for 6 months to concentrate on these skills. The OTA also provided consultation to school staff to address classroom performance in the area of handwriting. Can you think of activities that would address his self-esteem issues? Handwriting? Balance? Ball handling skills? How could these issues be addressed within the context of a physical education class?

3. Ray is a 22-year-old man who has been referred to OT by his psychologist. He has recently taken a job as a traveling sales representative and is having difficulty preparing for trips and sales calls. Recently, he has forgotten important information presented at sales meetings and frequently misses meetings and appointments. What suggestions can you make to help Ray become more prepared and organized for his new job?

LEARNING ACTIVITIES

1. Search the Internet for information related to ADHD. Identify sites that may be useful for parents, teachers, or therapists. Create an annotated list of sites to distribute to parents.

2. Compile a list of after-school recreational activities that would be appropriate for children with ADHD in your community. Discuss ways in which OT might become involved within these contexts.

3. Create a handout for teachers. Include strategies for helping students organize their workspace, assignments, personal belongings, and information.

4. Check your local library for books about ADHD. These books often include ideas for use in the classroom and at home. Make a poster to display in the library about ADHD.

5. Ask school personnel for a copy of the Connors' Teacher Rating Scale or the Connors' Parent Rating Scale. Try to identify items that might indicate a problem with sensory processing.

REFERENCES

Achenbach, T. M., & Edelbrock, C. (1983). *Manual for the child behavior checklist and revised child behavior profile.* Burlington: University of Vermont, Department of Psychology.

American Psychiatric Association. (2000). *Diagnostic and statistical manual of mental disorders* (4th ed., text revision). Washington, DC: Author.

Amundson, S. J. (1995). *Evaluation tool of children's handwriting: Manuscript and cursive examiner's manual.* Homer, AK: O.T. KIDS.

Batshaw, M. L., (2002). *Children with disabilities* (5th ed.). Baltimore, MD: Brookes Publishing Co.

Beery, K. E., & Buktenica, N. A. (1997). *Beery-Buktenica developmental test of visual-motor integration* (4th ed., revised). Parsippany, NJ: Modern Curriculum Press.

Benbow, M. (1990). *Loops and other groups: A kinesthetic writing system.* San Antonio, TX: The Psychological Corporation.

Benbow, M. (1995). *Assessment of hand skills in the primary child.* Video. Albuquerque, NM: Clinician's View.

Blondis, T., & Opacich, K. (1999). Developmental coordination disorder and ADHD. In P. J. Accardo, T. A. Blondis, B. Y. Whitman, & M. A. Stein (Eds.), *Pediatric habilitations series: Vol. 10. Attention deficits and hyperactivity in children and adults: Diagnosis, treatment, management* (2nd rev. ed., pp. 265-288). New York: Marcel Dekker.

Brown, T. E. (2000). *Attention-deficit disorders and comorbidities in children, adolescents, and adults.* Washington, DC: American Psychiatric Press.

Bruininks, R. (1978). *Bruininks-Oseretsky test of motor proficiency examiner's manual.* Circle Pines, MN: American Guidance Service.

Bundy, A. C. (1997). Play and playfulness: What to look for. In L. D. Parham & L. S. Fazio (Eds.), *Play in occupational therapy for children* (pp. 52-66). St. Louis: Mosby.

Carrasco, R. C., & Lee, C. E. (1993). Development of a teacher questionnaire on sensorimotor behavior. *Sensory Integration Special Interest Newsletter, 16*(3), 5-6.

Colarusso, R. P., & Hammill, D. D. (2002). *Motor-free visual perception test-3.* Novato, CA: Academic Therapy Publications.

Conners, C. K. (1990a). *Conners' Teacher Rating Scales.* North Tonawanda, NY: Multi-Health Systems, Inc.

Conners, C. K. (1990b). *Conners' Parent Rating Scales.* North Tonawanda, NY: Multi-Health Systems, Inc.

Cronin, A. F. (2001). Psychosocial and emotional domains. In J. Case-Smith (Ed.), *Occupational therapy for children* (4th ed., pp. 413-452). St. Louis, MO: Mosby.

DiScala, C., Lescohier, I., Barthel, M., & Li, G. (1998). Injuries to children with attention deficit hyperactivity disorder. *Pediatrics, 102*(6), 1415-1421.

Dorman, W. J. (1999). Self-awareness assessment. In G. G. Williamson & W. J. Dorman (Eds.), *Promoting social competence.* San Antonio, TX: Therapy Skill Builders.

Dorman, W. J., & Williamson, G. G. (2000). Identification of social difficulties questionnaire. In G. G. Williamson & W. J. Dorman (Eds.), *Promoting social competence.* San Antonio, TX: Therapy Skill Builders.

Dunn, W. (1999). *The sensory profile user's manual.* San Antonio, TX: The Psychological Corporation.

EVIDENCE-BASED TREATMENT STRATEGIES

Treatment Strategies	Authors
Interactive metronome	Koomar et al., 2001; Shaffer et al., 2000
Environmental modifications	Mulligan, 2001
Providing routine and structure	Mulligan, 2001
Use of motor breaks	Mulligan, 2001
Assistance during transitions	Mulligan, 2001
Sensory modulation techniques	Mulligan, 2001
Weighted vest	VandenBerg, 2001
Allow nondisruptive, directed movement in classroom	Stormont & Stebbins, 2001
Identify student's interest	Stormont & Stebbins, 2001
Point out cause and effect of behavior	Stormont & Stebbins, 2001
Verbal compliments for improved behavior	Stormont & Stebbins, 2001
Instruct and reinforce social routines	Stormont & Stebbins, 2001
Organize locker/cubby with labels and places for items	Stormont & Stebbins, 2001
Encourage parents to establish places for things at home	Stormont & Stebbins, 2001

Dunn, W., & Bennett, D. (2002). Patterns of sensory processing in children with attention deficit hyperactivity disorder. *Occupational Therapy Journal of Research, 22*(1), 4-15.

Folio, M. R., & Fewell, R. R. (2000). *Peabody developmental motor scales examiner's manual* (PDMS-2). Austin, TX: Pro-ed.

Gardner, M. F. (1995). *Test of visual-motor skills—Revised and test of visual-motor skills: Upper level adolescents and adults.* Hydesville, CA: Psychological and Educational Publications, Inc.

Gardner, M. F. (1997). *Test of visual-perceptual skills (non-motor)—Revised.* Hydesville, CA: Psychological and Educational Publications, Inc.

Gresham, F. M., & Elliot, S. N. (1990). *Social skills rating system.* Circle Pines, MN: American Guidance Service.

Hallowell, E. M., & Ratey, J. J. (1994). *Driven to distraction.* New York: Pantheon.

Hamilton, S. S. (2002). Evaluation of clumsiness in children (problem-oriented diagnosis). *American Family Physician, 66*(8), 1435.

Hammill, D. D., Pearson, N. A., & Voress, J. K. (1993). *Developmental test of visual perception: Examiner's manual* (2nd ed.). Los Angeles, CA: Western Psychological Services.

Health and Medicine Week. (2003). Attention deficit hyperactivity disorder. June 30, 2003. Author. Retrieved July 2, 2003 from http://www.newsrx.com.

Kaplan, H. I., & Sadock, B. J. (1998). *Synopsis of psychiatry: Behavioral sciences/clinical psychiatry* (8th ed., p. 1197). Baltimore, MD: Williams & Wilkins.

Koomar, J., Burpee, J. D., DeJean, V., Frick, S., Kawar, M. J., & Fischer D. M. (2001). Theoretical and clinical perspectives on the interactive metronome: A view from occupational therapy practice. *American Journal of Occupational Therapy, 55*(2), 163-166.

Law, M., Cooper, B., Strong, S., Steward, D., Rigby, P., & Letts, L. (1996). The person-environment-occupation model: A transactive approach to occupational performance. *Canadian Journal of Occupational Therapy, 63*(1), 9-23.

Leipold, E. E., & Bundy, A. C. (2000). Playfulness in children with attention deficit hyperactivity disorder. *Occupational Therapy Journal of Research, 20*(1), 61-82.

Mercugliano, M., Power, T. J., & Blum, N. J. (1999). *The clinician's practical guide to attention-deficit/hyperactivity disorder.* Baltimore: Paul H. Brookes Publishing Co.

Merrell, K. W., & Boelter, E. (2001). An investigation of relationships between social behavior and ADHD in children and youth. *Journal of Emotional and Behavioral Disorders, 9*(4), 260-269.

Mulligan, S. (1995). An analysis of score patterns of children with attention disorders on the sensory integration and praxis tests. *American Journal of Occupational Therapy, 50*(8), 647-654.

Mulligan, S. (2001). Classroom strategies used by teachers of students with attention deficit hyperactivity disorder. *Physical and Occupational Therapy in Pediatrics, 20*(4), 25-44.

National Institute of Mental Health. (2003). Attention deficit hyperactivity disorder—Questions and answers. Retrieved July 2, 2003, from http://www.nimh.nih.gov/publicat/adhdqa.cfm.

Parham, L. D., & Mailloux, Z. (2001). Sensory integration. In J. Case-Smith (Ed.), *Occupational therapy for children* (4th ed., pp. 329-379). St. Louis, MO: Mosby.

Phelps, J., Stempel, L., & Speck, G. (1984). *Children's handwriting evaluation scale and children's handwriting scale for manuscript writing.* Dallas, TX: CHES.

Purdie, N., Hattie, J., & Carroll, A. (2002). A review of the research on intervention for attention deficit hyperactivity disorder: What works best? *Review of Educational Research, 72*(1), 61-99.

Raggio, D. J. (1999). Visuomotor perception in children with attention deficit hyperactivity disorder-combined type. *Perceptual and Motor Skills, 88,* 448-450.

Reid, R. (1999). Attention deficit hyperactivity disorder: Effective methods for the classroom. *Focus on Exceptional Children, 33*(4), 1-20.

Reisman, J. E. (1999). *Minnesota handwriting assessment.* San Antonio, TX: The Psychological Corporation.

Reynolds, C. R., Pearson, N. A., & Voress, J. K. (2002). *Developmental test of visual perception—Adolescent and adult.* Los Angeles, CA: Western Psychological Services.

Roizen, N. J., Blondis, T. A., Irwin, M., & Stein, M. (1994). Adaptive functioning in children with attention-deficit hyperactivity disorder. *Archives of Pediatric and Adolescent Medicine, 148,* 1137-1142.

Royeen, C. B., & Fortune, J. C. (1990). TIE: Touch inventory for school aged children. *American Journal of Occupational Therapy, 44,* 165-170.

Sadock, B. J., & Sadock, V. A. (2003). *Kaplan and Sadock's synopsis of psychiatry: Behavioral sciences/clinical psychiatry* (9th ed.). Philadelphia, PA: Lippincott, Williams and Wilkins.

Salend, S. J., & Rohena, E. (2003). Students with attention deficit disorders: An overview. *Intervention in School and Clinic, 38*(5), 259-266.

Shaffer, R. J., Jacokes, L. E., Cassily, J. F., Greenspan, S. I., Tuchman, R. F., & Stemmer, P. J. (2000). Effect of interactive metronome training on children with ADHD. *American Journal of Occupational Therapy, 55*(2), 155-162.

Stormont, M., & Stebbins, M. S. (2001). Teachers' comfort and importance ratings for interventions for preschoolers with ADHD. *Psychology in the Schools, 38*(3), 259-267.

VandenBerg, N. L. (2001). The use of a weighted vest to increase on-task behavior in children with attention difficulties. *American Journal of Occupational Therapy, 55*(6), 621-628.

Wender, P. H. (2000). *ADHD: Attention deficit hyperactivity disorder in children and adults.* New York: Oxford Press.

Williams, M. S., & Shellenberger, S. (1994). *How does your engine run? A leader's guide to the Alert program for self-regulation.* Albuquerque, NM: Therapy Works.

Williamson, G. G. (2000). Components of social competence observation scale. In G. G. Williamson & W. J. Dorman (Eds.), *Promoting social competence.* San Antonio, TX: Therapy Skill Builders.

Williamson, G. G., & Dorman, W. J. (2002). *Promoting social competence.* San Antonio, TX: Therapy Skill Builders.

Zentall, S. S. (1993). Research on the educational implications of attention deficit hyperactivity disorder. *Exceptional Children, 60*(2), 143-153.

Key Concepts

- Mood disorder: A psychiatric disorder characterized by disturbance of mood involving either elation or depression.
- Asperger's syndrome: A psychiatric disorder characterized by severe and pervasive impairment in social interaction and restricted and stereotypic patterns of behavior and activities.
- Occupational behavior: A frame of reference that targets the broad parameters of play, student role, and socialization as the primary concern of OT practitioners working with individuals of this age.
- Task performance: An assessment of attention span, ability to make decisions, follow directions, sequence steps, use tools and materials, and solve problems using a craft or activity.
- Pervasive developmental disorders (PDDs): Psychiatric disorders characterized by severe and pervasive impairment in social interaction, communication, and other areas of development in addition to the presence of stereotypic behavior, interests, and activities.
- Individual Educational Plan (IEP): A plan aimed at improving the child's educational performance. It contains specific instructional objectives, including specific services and modifications needed to achieve the objectives.

Essential Vocabulary

Allen cognitive levels: Six levels of cognitive ability with corresponding expectations for functional capabilities for daily living.

depression: A psychiatric disorder characterized by disturbance in mood in which there is diminished interest and loss of pleasure in most activities.

psychomotor agitation: Irregular action, unrest, or disquiet.

role dysfunction: Inability to perform and adjust adaptively to social expectations associated with roles of player, student, worker, homemaker, volunteer, or retiree.

social skills: One of the skills of social competence that refers to the ability to produce mutually reciprocal interactions with others.

somatic complaints: Complaints focused on bodily functions such as loss of energy and reduced sleep.

visual motor integration: Ability of the eyes and hands to work together effectively and efficiently.

Clinical Summary

Etiology

Genetic, biological, psychosocial, and environmental factors may lead to the expression of depressive symptoms. Prominent risk factors include family disharmony, learning difficulties, and parental psychiatric disorder (Harrington, 1994; Weller, Weller, & Svadjian, 1996).

Prevalence

Prevalence of depression increases with age. The prevalence of major depressive disorder in children is approximately 2% and in adolescents, 4% to 8% (American Academy of Child and Adolescent Psychiatry [AACAP], 1998).

Classic Signs

Depression is a disorder of mood in which mood is either depressed or irritable. There is a diminished interest and loss of pleasure in most activities. Somatic complaints, social withdrawal, disturbances in sleep, appetite, psychomotor agitation, or retardation are common (Weller et al., 1996).

Precautions

The most serious complication of depression is suicidal thoughts, including recurrent thoughts of death, or actual attempts at suicide (Weller et al., 1996).

A Teenager With Depression

Linda Florey, PhD, OTR, FAOTA

Introduction

Depression is a disorder of mood in which mood is either depressed or irritable. There is diminished interest and loss of pleasure in most activities, and somatic complaints and social withdrawal are common. Associated symptoms include disturbances in sleep and appetite, psychomotor agitation (irregular action, or unrest) or retardation, and decreased concentration. Adolescents experience hopelessness and feelings that things will never change for the better. The most serious complication of depression is suicidal thoughts, including recurrent thoughts of death, or actual attempts at suicide (Weller et al., 1996). Suicide is the third leading cause of death for the adolescent population (DHHS, 1999).

Michael is a thin, poorly groomed, 17-year-old boy admitted to an adolescent inpatient unit of a psychiatric hospital because of self-mutilation of his arms and legs with a razor blade. He said that he was not trying to commit suicide, but that he had made the deep cuts to his body to see how his "body worked." He was not on any drugs when he made the cuts although he admitted to using pot in the past as it helped him relax. He wore green nail polish and dressed in black. Michael said that he dressed this way and was unshaven because he was "Gothic."

Michael is an only child and grew up with his mother in a rural community near the coast in central California. His mother and father divorced when he was young, and he had not had any contact with his father since the divorce, which occurred when he was 3. Michael's mother reported that his father had been diagnosed with bipolar disorder. His mother worked during the day, and she felt that he was somewhat of a "latch key" kid. His mother reported that he never had many friends that he played with as a child because they lived in an isolated area. She assumed that he had friends in school. He had always received good grades until 2 years ago when his grades slipped from As and Bs to Cs and Ds. He was also spending a lot of time on the weekends on the Internet. His mother was concerned with his change in grades and the increase in isolative behavior and took him to a physician who placed him on an antidepressant.

Michael's grades improved in the next few years, but his mother continued to be concerned with his general physical appearance of dressing "Gothic" and his increasing time spent on the Internet. His mother learned that *Gothic* was a term used to represent a particular style of dress and detached demeanor in which dressing in black was prevalent and a cynical view of life dominated. Michael had not withdrawn from friends as is typical with youth with depression, as his teachers reported to his mother that he did not have friends at school and had been a "loner" in high school. His mother was concerned that he was spending most of his time on the Internet and engaging in computer games. When he was not on the Internet, he read scary novels. His hygiene was poor, and she had to remind him to bathe and to shave. He picked at his food and often roamed the house at night. His mood was not irritable as is typical of many with depressive disorder. His mother described him as "empty."

The night prior to admission, his mother found him bleeding in the bathroom from cuts he had made on his arms and legs with a razor blade.

Theory That Frames Practice

The frame of reference used in this chapter is occupational behavior. It is the same one used in the chapter on the child with ODD, and theoretical considerations are addressed in that section (see Chapter 15). This frame of reference targets the broad parameters of play, student role, and socialization as the primary concern of OTs in working with children and adolescents (Florey, 2003). In adolescence, work, play, and major daily activities focus on the role of student, which includes concerns with mastery of social learning and expectations as well as academic learning. A major clinical focus for OTs is to determine the extent to which mental illness has disrupted or impoverished occupational behavior and to identify steps to ameliorate dysfunction and to foster new learning (Reilly, 1966).

Assessments and treatment techniques drawn from additional frames of reference may be used to better understand and ameliorate dysfunction in occupational role and socialization. The cognitive disability frame of reference is very useful in uncovering cognitive deficits and their impact on daily activities. This frame of reference targets deficits in functional capabilities as a result of biological and chemical changes in the brain. There are 6 levels of cognitive ability and corresponding expectations for functional capabilities for daily living. Identifying the cognitive level is helpful in guiding the team in developing behavioral expectations and goals that are realistic for the patient (Grant, 2003).

ASSESSMENT

The overall focus of inpatient hospitalization for adolescents is to stabilize behavior, identify major problems, clarify diagnosis, and initiate medication trials if indicated. The treatment of long-term psychiatric problems is not done at the inpatient level, but rather at a less expensive level of care such as in a partial hospital program or as an outpatient.

The length of stay on the inpatient adolescent service of the hospital to which Michael was admitted is 10 to 14 days. The OT assessment is documented in the chart within 48 hours of admission and the focus is on determining direction for intervention both as an inpatient and at discharge. Additional evaluations may be performed following 48 hours to probe deficit areas first identified.

The typical OT assessment includes several separate evaluations. These include an interview regarding patterns of daily activity, observation of task performance, observation of social interaction, the Allen Cognitive Level, and an assessment of visual motor integration. The specific format, purpose, the responsible OT personnel, and the results or findings follow.

The Daily Living Interview is a semistructured interview designed to determine patterns of function in daily living, school, and leisure activities. The OT found that Michael was difficult to interview. His response to open-ended questions regarding time use was that he did not know exactly what he did or when he did it. He did not volunteer any information and the OT had to probe each area. The OT obtained a skeleton of his typical day as one of arising in the morning, taking the bus to and from school, and then getting on the Internet once he reached home. He said that he did not have any friends at school, but that he had one friend on the Internet. He was unable to identify any parts of school that he liked or disliked but said that he liked to read and write on his own. He particularly liked reading Stephen King novels. Aside from the Internet, he played games on the computer. He said he did not like sports, did not have any hobbies, and hated crafts. When asked about his self-care routine, he said he did not have a regular time when he did anything. Michael was asked if he helped out around the house, and he replied that he used to and that sometimes he did if his mother made him. He replied that he could fix himself a meal and that he had made spaghetti and quesadillas on his own. When asked what kind of work he might like to do, he said that he wanted to go to college and be a writer. On the weekends, he said that he liked to go to the beach by himself, watch the waves, and smoke.

The OT noted that Michael had a restricted and rigid pattern of interests, no regular or meaningful social contacts, and that he did not assume responsibility for his self-care or helping around the house. He also did not do well with open-ended

questions but needed categories identified for him such as, "What hobbies do you have?" and then he could answer.

A task performance checklist to determine decision making, ability to follow directions, attention span, ability to sequence steps, and ability to solve problems was used by the OTA. Michael was given the choice of 2 board games to play with the therapist or making a craft project. He said that he didn't want to do anything, but the OTA selected a board game and he agreed to play with her. They played Parcheesi and the OTA observed that he demonstrated more animation than she had seen with him on prior meetings. He quickly learned the game and he seemed to like the strategy involved. The OTA noted that he was not able to make a decision from choices given, but was able to respond and participate once a decision was made for him. He attended well to the game and was able to concentrate and plot game moves.

The OTA used a semistructured guide in observation of socialization in the OT area, recreation deck, and on the inpatient unit. The purpose was to determine frequency and content of interactions with peers and adults.

Michael was observed during structured activities such as a community meeting, recreation activities, and informal activities on the unit including mealtime. The OTA observed that his pattern of interaction with others was consistent in all settings. He isolated himself from his peers and if forced to sit next to a peer at meals or in a meeting, he did not initiate any contact. The other adolescents on the unit "gave him space" and did not talk with him because he did not respond to their questions or comments. His eye contact was generally poor and sporadic but was better when he was with an adult rather than peers. He would respond to questions from adults, and he would engage in board games with them. He refused to play shuffleboard, volleyball, ping-pong, or any physical games.

The OT used the Allen Cognitive Level test (Allen, Earhart, & Blue, 1992), which involves demonstrating a variety of leather lacing stitches. The purpose is to determine an initial estimate of Michael's ability to function and to master new learning. Michael said that he did not want to do this lacing and reminded the therapist that he hated crafts. She told him that this was perfect for him as it was not a craft at all but rather a way to check out his ability to solve problems on something he had not done a million times. He participated in the process and achieved a score of 5.6, indicating that he was at the level of exploratory actions and could problem solve by trial and error but had difficulty anticipating the results of his actions. He was able to learn new activities but needed assistance with activities requiring him to plan ahead. The therapist concluded that this cognitive level was typical of many adolescents and that many needed assistance in planning and structuring their time.

Lastly, the OTA administered the Beery-Buktenica Developmental Test of Visual-Motor Integration (VMI) (Beery & Beery, 2004), which is a structured test involving form copying. Michael achieved an age equivalent score of 12 years 3 months, indicating some impairment in this area. This did not seem to interfere with his daily functioning as in handwriting and his ability to handle small objects on board games, but it may have contributed to his dislike of crafts, which typically require visual-motor skill.

The OT and OTA decided that additional assessments such as vocational surveys were not warranted until deficits in social and daily functioning were addressed. They speculated that remediation of his functional pattern would require a significant period of time.

FUNCTIONAL IMPACT AND GOAL SETTING

The functional impact of a disorder is the extent to which the disorder interrupts or impoverishes current and future occupational behavior. For an adolescent, this includes the extent to which a disorder is interrupting normal learning in school, play, and daily living skills within many environments. The OT and OTA summarized their findings and presented them to the treatment team. A psychiatrist headed the team and other members included a nurse, psychologist, recreation therapist, social worker, speech and language specialist, and a school consultant. The primary concerns of the OT practitioners were his disorganized daily routine, his poor eye contact, poor grooming, lack of identified friendships or social contacts, lack of observed ability to initiate social contact or to initiate activities on his own, and his restricted and rigid pattern of interests. His strengths included his ability to learn new activities and to participate in social and activity situations if they were expected of and set up for him.

The treatment team as a whole was concerned not only with his knife cuts, disorganized routine, sleep and appetite disturbances, and social isolation, which were all part of the syndrome of depression, but they were also concerned with his prolonged history of poor social interactions and his restricted and rigid pattern of interests. The team considered that they may be dealing with an adolescent with 2 disorders: depression and Asperger's syndrome, which is one of the PDD characterized by severe and pervasive impairment in social interaction and restricted and stereotypic patterns of behavior and activities. His physician planned a more extensive history of his social functioning gained by interviewing Michael's mother in more depth in this area. Michael was placed on a trial of new antidepressant medication, and the team was asked to observe for increasing signs of social interaction and increase in interests as the depression lifted.

General OT goals for Michael included participation in a pattern of adolescent occupations within the hospital, enhancing social interaction with others by including him in groups and having him initiate contact with others, improving his self-care and sense of responsibility in keeping his room and area clean, and improving his time management by having him engage in purposeful activities during free time periods.

TREATMENT ACTIVITIES/TECHNIQUES

Treatment activities focus on constructing a pattern of daily occupations that provide interest and challenge for the adolescents. The OT practitioners work closely with other disciplines in developing a variety of occupations throughout the day and week. The program is designed to simulate selected social and task expectations that adolescents encounter in the community to gain a sense of how they function in these situations. In short-term hospitalization, there is no clear cut demarcation between assessment and treatment. OT practitioners are always assessing the performance of individuals.

The OT program assumes an occupation-based approach in that the focus is on providing a variety of occupations and inserting treatment goals within those occupations. The OT program is broadly designed to meet the needs of most adolescents. The goals for individual patients are implemented individually and within small group programs. The specific needs of each adolescent are addressed within these occupations. Specific features of the occupations within a program for adolescents follow.

- A variety of adolescent occupations should be provided. These may include occupations focusing on arts and crafts, games, sports, music, cooking, and grooming. These occupations should be graded to the skill level of each adolescent and should allow individual choice. The functional level of an activity is one of the most difficult to determine, so the start point is to present from simple to complex. Any activity can be made more challenging, but it is difficult to simplify a complex activity once engaged. There should be individual choices within occupations so that adolescents may learn skills that interest them.

- Social skills learning should be part of all occupations. There is a social nature to occupations, and occupations are a natural arena for the learning and relearning of social skills. It is critical to have adolescents work in small groups with others, since it is in the social domain that the functional impact of a psychiatric disorder is most obvious. The OT practitioners help model and frame social interactions in these contexts.

Program planning is also accomplished within the context of the interdisciplinary team in order that there are individualized, yet consistent, expectations for all adolescents.

Throughout his 14-day hospitalization, Michael was included in a boy's grooming group co-led with nursing, a room check program, a cooking group, and a craft/recreation groups co-led with recreation therapy. The OTA and OT worked separately and together depending on the needs of the group. Michael's participation in these groups and his specific goals in each one are briefly reviewed.

Boy's Grooming Group

The purpose of this group was to engage adolescents in performing routine self-care habits. This group of 6 adolescents met daily with nursing staff and the OTA. Expectations for self-care were given, but there were choices the adolescents had within those expectations and they were also able to set a special goal for themselves. General expectations included bathing or showering daily, shaving if necessary, combing hair, and brushing teeth. Michael selected showering in the evening each day, combing hair daily, and shaving every other day. He could not think of any special goals so the OTs suggested removing his green nail polish and cleaning his nails. Michael instead selected flossing his teeth but toward the end of the second week, he finally removed the green nail polish. His overall self-care improved; he bathed and combed his hair daily and his body odor was no longer offensive.

Room Check Program

The purpose of this group was to instill a sense of responsibility in maintaining personal space. The OT led this group. The OT gave points for clean and organized rooms and the adolescents then used the earned points for extra privileges, which included such activities as selecting the music on the radio during some OT groups or going on special outings. Michael was to have his bed made, shirts and jeans hung in the closet, other clothing folded and placed in drawers, counter tops clean, and books and games orderly. He had only one book that he brought with him and was responsive to keeping his clothing organized. He earned points and privileges but could not decide what privilege to select and said that he really did not care about that.

Cooking Group

The purpose of this group was to teach basic cooking skills and to enhance social interaction. Both the OT and OTA worked together in the weekly lunch and snack groups of 4 to 6 adolescents, as 2 individuals were needed to assess functional and social behavior and to direct the tasks. Both groups were held in the OT kitchen, which is a small space with no opportunity to isolate one's self. In the first lunch group, Michael and another male peer were asked to make the salad together. His peer was friendly and outgoing and asked Michael a number of questions regarding the task at hand to which he had to respond. In the second lunch group and in the snack groups, he continued to respond to peer questions and even initiated some communication with his peers regarding the task. He would also respond to questions during these mealtimes but he seemed awkward and unable to initiate casual mealtime talk with others. The OT practitioners routinely modeled casual talk and asked him questions so that he had to respond.

Craft/Recreation Groups

The purpose of these groups is to engage adolescents in productive and meaningful activities, to teach new skills, to promote decision making and problem solving, and to promote social engagement with others. Michael did not wish to participate, but the OTA told him that he had to attend this group with the other adolescents and that he had to select something to do with his time. A computer was not made available to him because he would further isolate himself from others. Initially, he was unable to spontaneously select anything and this pattern persisted throughout his hospital stay. He demonstrated no ability to initiate activities on his own, but would engage if an activity was selected for him. He was able to select a craft project from 2 choices and worked on 2 craft projects to completion. His mood seemed better because his face was less "mask like."

He was responsive to selecting among choices of board games or outdoor activities that did not involve sports (e.g., shuffleboard); however, he was participating in volleyball by discharge.

DISCHARGE PLANNING

At discharge, there was a meeting that included the mother and all the disciplines, in which each discipline presented their findings and recommendations. The team explained to the mother that Michael had 2 psychiatric disorders: mood disorder (depression) and Asperger's syndrome. Asperger's syndrome is one of the disorders in the PDD spectrum characterized by severe and sustained impairment in social interaction and the development of restricted and repetitive patterns of behavior, interests, and activities. Unlike autistic disorder, which is also in the PDD spectrum, there are no significant delays in areas other than social interaction such as language and adaptive skills (APA, 2000). Asperger's syndrome explained the long history of social isolation, lack of friendships, and his restricted pattern of interest and behavior centered around isolative activities such as the Internet and computer in general. Michael was uneasy in the company of others, especially peers. He was more responsive to adults and even initiated contact with adults toward the end of hospitalization. His cutting himself to "see how his body worked" was not a typical suicide threat.

Michael was also depressed, which accounted for his decreasing concentration in his studies and his changing grades; his mask-like face and generally depressed mood; his cutting himself for any reason; and his deterioration in self-care, including sleeping and eating patterns. His inability to initiate and plan activities on his own other than the computer was probably attributable to both disorders.

The OTs were concerned that Michael maintain his self-care responsibilities and that he receive some social skill training to learn some of the rudiments of working with others that he had never learned. The OT explained to the mother that Michael had difficulty initiating tasks but that he had been responsive to specific expectations and directions and that he would probably need her or someone to organize his time and expectations. The OTA gave the mother a list of standards for self-care he had accomplished in the hospital and discussed with the mother specific expectations for caring for his room and for assisting her with preparation of the evening meal and other chores. The mother was very responsive to this and said that she had done this when he was younger and he had done well. She had stopped as she assumed he knew how to organize his time and tasks. The OT also recommended that Michael have an IEP to address his social awkwardness and to learn social skills. There was such a program in his school system.

The OT told the mother that Michael had seemed to enjoy low key recreation activities such as shuffleboard and board games and that a few of these activities could be expectations for him to engage in on the weekends. He would also be in the company of others on these occasions. This would represent an expansion of his interests and behavior beyond the computer. She suggested that the mother determine if any such programs were offered through YMCA or youth groups in their commu-

EVIDENCE-BASED TREATMENT STRATEGIES

Treatment Strategies	Authors
Occupation-based treatment approach	Burke, 1996; Henry & Costner, 1997; Holm, Santangelo, Fromuth, Brown, & Walter, 2000; Legault & Rebeiro, 2001
Social nature of occupations and social skills training	Baloueff & Cohn, 2003; Cartledge & Milburn, 1995; Cox & Schopler, 1996; Lawlor, 2003; Richardson, 2002
Importance of individual choices within occupations	Burke, 1998; Frank et al., 2001; Legault & Reberio, 2001
Importance of end product, clear steps for success, and sequence of steps simple to complex	Frank et al., 2001; Florey & Greene, 1997; Murphy, Trombly, Tickle-Degnen, & Jacobs, 1999

nity with the eventual goal of having Michael participate on his own on a regular basis. The OT and OTA both advised an approach of gradualism in that expecting too much of him at once would be too uncomfortable for him. They suggested that the mother initially play board games with him and at the same time introduce him to one other setting to which he was expected to go one time on the weekend. His mood was improving, and although his social awkwardness persisted, this was the time to introduce gradual changes in his daily pattern.

CLINICAL PROBLEM SOLVING

Michael as an Adult

Imagine Michael at age 27. Do you think he would be able to respond to questions about his daily routine and elaborate on answers? Does he identify any friends other than ones on the Internet? Has he developed any more interests? Do you think he went to college and that he is now a writer? What type of work might he be doing? Would living in a rural or urban setting make any difference? Will he still need someone to organize his time and his tasks for him? Has his social communication improved? What kinds of issues might be arising and might need to be addressed?

Ann

Ann is an attractive, 15-year-old, African American girl admitted to the adolescent inpatient service for threatening to kill herself with her stepfather's gun. She had recently given birth to a baby whose father was her stepbrother. The stepbrother had sexually abused her for years and Ann had become pregnant. The department of family and social services had become involved and the stepbrother had been arrested and removed from the home. The stepfather was furious with Ann as he blamed her for ruining the family and said she had probably done something provocative to lead his son on. The admitting diagnosis was depression secondary to PTSD due to sexual abuse.

What are the major concerns of the OT and OTA with Ann? How would the evaluations differ from those used with Michael? Are there some cultural stereotypes concerning women operating here? What might discharge concerns and recommendations center on?

LEARNING ACTIVITIES

1. Discuss ways of simulating activities that are part of the daily pattern of adolescents within the hospital setting.
2. If adolescents have several different disorders, how does one prioritize treatment intervention?
3. What types of skills and patterns are deficit in Michael's case? What impact would these deficits have on vocational planning?
4. If Michael had a cognitive level in the 4 range, would this alter his treatment in any way?
5. Describe the role of the OT working in an acute psychiatric facility and discuss the possible factors contributing to multiple disorders seen in this setting.

REFERENCES

Allen, C., Earhart, C., & Blue, T. (1992). *Occupational therapy treatment goals for the physically and cognitively disabled*. Bethesda, MD: American Occupational Therapy Association.

American Academy of Child and Adolescent Psychiatry. (1998). Practice parameters for the assessment and treatment of children and adolescents with depressive disorders. *Journal of the American Academy of Child and Adolescent Psychiatry, 73*(10 Suppl.), 63S-83S.

American Psychiatric Association. (2000). *Diagnostic and statistical manual of mental disorders* (4th ed tr.). Washington, DC: Author.

Baloueff, O., & Cohn, E. (2003). Introduction to the infant, child and adolescent population. In E. Crepeau, E. Cohn, & B. Schell (Eds.), *Willard & Spackman's occupational therapy* (10th ed., pp. 691-698). Philadelphia: Lippincott, Williams & Wilkins.

Beery, K., & Beery, N. (2004). *The Beery-Buktenica developmental test of visual-motor integration. Administration, scoring, and teaching manual* (5th ed.). Minneapolis: NCS Pearson, Inc.

Burke, J. (1996). Moving occupation into treatment: Clinical interpretation of "legitimizing occupational therapy's knowledge." *American Journal of Occupational Therapy, 50*(8), 635-638.

Burke, J. (1998). Clinical interpretation of "health and the human spirit for occupation." *American Journal of Occupational Therapy, 52*(6), 419-422.

Cartledge, G., & Milburn, J. (1995). *Teaching social skills to children and youth* (3rd ed.). Boston: Allyn & Bacon.

Cox, R., & Schopler, E. (1996). Social skills training for children. In M. Lewis (Ed.), *Child and adolescent psychiatry: A comprehensive textbook* (2nd ed., pp. 902-908). Baltimore: Williams & Wilkins.

Florey, L. (2003). Psychosocial dysfunction in childhood and adolescence. In E. Crepeau, E. Cohn, and B. Schell (Eds.), *Willard & Spackman's occupational therapy* (10th ed., pp. 731-744). Philadelphia: Lippincott, Williams & Wilkins.

Florey, L., & Greene, S. (1997). Play in middle childhood: A focus on children with behavior and emotional disorders. In L. D. Parham & L. Fazio (Eds.), *Play in occupational therapy for children* (pp. 126-143). St Louis:, MO C. V. Mosby.

Frank, G., Fishman, M., Crowley, C., Blair, B., Murphy, S., Montoya, J., et al. (2001). The new stories/new cultures after-school enrichment program: A direct cultural intervention. *American Journal of Occupational Therapy, 55*(5), 501-508.

Grant, S. (2003). Cognitive disability frame of reference. In E. Crepeau, E. Cohn, & B. Schell (Eds.), *Willard & Spackman's occupational therapy* (10th ed., pp. 261-264). Philadelphia: Lippincott, Williams & Wilkins.

Harrington, R. (1994). Affective disorders. In M. Rutter, E. Taylor, & L. Hersov (Eds.), *Child and adolescent psychiatry modern approaches* (3rd ed.). Oxford: Blackwell Scientific.

Henry, A., & Costner, W. (1997). Competency beliefs and occupational role behavior among adolescents: Explication of the personal causation construct. *American Journal of Occupational Therapy, 51*(4), 267-276.

Holm, M., Santangelo, M., Fromuth, D., Brown, S., & Walter, H. (2000). Effectiveness of everyday occupations for changing client behaviors in a community living arrangement. *American Journal of Occupational Therapy, 54*(4), 361-371.

Lawlor, M. (2003). The significance of being occupied: The social construction of childhood occupations. *American Journal of Occupational Therapy, 57*(4), 424-434.

Legault, E., & Rebeiro, K. (2001). Case report—Occupation as means to mental health: A single-case study. *American Journal of Occupational Therapy, 55*(1), 90-96.

Murphy, S., Trombly, C., Tickle-Degnen, L., & Jacobs, K. (1999). The effect of keeping an end-product on intrinsic motivation. *American Journal of Occupational Therapy, 53*(2), 153-158.

Reilly, M. (1966). The educational process. *American Journal of Occupational Therapy, 23,* 299-307.

Richardson, P. (2002). The school as social context: Social interaction patterns of children with physical disabilities. *American Journal of Occupational Therapy, 54*(4), 296-304.

U.S. Department of Health and Human Services. (1999). *Mental health: A report of the surgeon general.* Rockville, MD: Author.

Weller, E., Weller, R., & Svadjian, H. (1996). Mood disorders. In M. Lewis (Ed.), *Child and adolescent psychiatry: A comprehensive textbook* (2nd ed.). Baltimore: Williams & Wilkins.

OCCUPATIONAL THERAPY INTERVIEW

Name *Michael*   Age *17*   Date *2-19-04*

FREE TIME AND FRIENDSHIPS
What kinds of things do you do for fun? *Internet, Stephen King novels, no hobbies, into anime*

Do you prefer to engage in activities inside or outside? *into sports*

Do you feel you have enough free time? *OK*

What do you do in your free time? *go to beach, watch waves, smoke*

Do you like to spend your free time alone or with others? *alone*

Do you have any friends? What are their names? *one friend James - or internet*

Do you have home friends? School friends? *no*

Do you have as many friends as you want or would you like more? *OK*

What do you look for in a friend? ___ *did not respond to question*

What does it mean to be a friend? ___

What do you do with your friends? ___

SCHOOL AND WORK
Do you like school? ___

What do you like most about school? ___ *did not respond to question*

Any favorite subjects/classes? Why? ___

What do you like least about school? ___

Any least favorite subjects/classes? Why? ___

How do you do in school? How are your grades? ___

Do you belong to any school groups/clubs? ___

Have you had any paid jobs? *no*

- poor eye contact
- green nail polish
- very vague about everything

Real record 17-1A. Real record for a client with depression.

Do you know what type of job you would like to have? _writer_

FAMILY AND HOME RESPONSIBILITIES
Who do you live with? _mom_

Do you have any pets? Do you help care for them? _no_

Do you have any chores? _"not really" - helps if mom makes him_

Do you receive an allowance? _no - gets $ from mom when he needs to_

Do you need any help caring for yourself? _says no but does not bathe or groom regularly per mom's report - unable_

Do you need any help in dressing? _____ In grooming? _to specify a care routine_

Can you fix a meal for yourself? _spaghetti, quesadillas_

Who cares for your clothes? _mom_ Do you know how to do your laundry? _no_

Iron your clothes? _no_

Can you handle money? _yes_

HOSPITAL AND GOALS
Why did you come to the hospital? _"cut myself to see how my body works"_

Do you have any goals while you are in the hospital? _no_

TYPICAL DAY
Describe a typical school day - a typical weekend day.

get up 6:30
take bus to school 7:30
take bus home 3:00 (?) - vague about time

go on internet, maybe do homework

— unable to describe day in detail. Very vague response

Real record 17-1B. Real record for a client with depression.

Key Concepts

- Traumatic brain injury (TBI): Deformation of the brain's soft tissue as a result of an external, traumatic force.
- Patterns of recovery: The Rancho Levels of Cognitive Functioning and the Glasgow Coma Scale are used to identify injury to the client and measure progress.
- Interdisciplinary approach: Professionals from multiple disciplines address common concerns. The client and his or her family are at the core of this approach.
- Continuum of care: OT services begin with coma level of functioning in an acute hospital setting and continue to community re-entry.

Essential Vocabulary

community re-entry: Simulated or actual activities used to prepare a client for discharge into the public community.

coup/contrecoup: Refers to the points of actual contact made between the brain and the skull encasement in the event of a trauma.

executive functions: An umbrella term to describe higher level, multi-step, cognitive functions or abilities requiring skill/precision, such as flexibility, planning, organization, and problem solving.

memory notebook: An external compensatory strategy to provide cues to increase initiation of tasks and retention of information.

metacognition: Insight, self-awareness, and self-regulatory capacity.

neural plasticity: Innate healing ability of the brain via rerouting neural pathways in an effort to compensate for areas of tissue damage.

Clinical Summary

Etiology

Traumatic or acquired brain injury is caused by sudden trauma to the head in which damage occurs at time of impact. Damage may include hematoma, contusion, or hemorrhage. Secondary injury may result due to swelling and cellular changes. The skull may be intact (closed head injury) or fractured or displaced (open head injury). Severity of the injury may be mild to severe.

Prevalence

Approximately 1.5 million Americans sustain a TBI each year. Males are twice as likely as females. Ages 15 to 24 years and over 75 years are at highest risk. The leading causes are motor vehicle crashes, firearm use, and falls.

Classic Signs

Physical, cognitive, and behavioral impairments with both short- and long-term impact to daily life functioning. This may include movement, coordination, balance, memory, judgment, attention span, impulsivity, mood changes, and instability.

Precautions

In the acute stage, intracranial pressure (ICP) must be monitored as well as other body regulatory systems. In later stages, fall precautions to avoid further injury, supervision to assist in daily tasks, or one-to-one precautions to monitor behavior changes may be instituted.

A Car Mechanic With Traumatic Brain Injury

Deanna Proulz-Sepelak, OTR and Paula Jo Belice, MS, OTR

INTRODUCTION

TBI is a term commonly used throughout the medical profession to describe an event that physically alters the composition of the skull cavity and, more importantly, its contents. This term is often interchanged with others such as head injury, which is formally defined by *Mosby's Medical, Nursing, and Allied Health Dictionary* (2002) as "any traumatic damage to the head resulting from blunt or penetrating trauma of the skull. Blood vessels, nerves, and meninges can be torn; bleeding, edema and ischemia may result." This definition has been analyzed more specifically to include several separate subcategories:

- Primary injury—Damage to the brain that occurs at the time of impact. Examples would be hematomas, axonal shearing, and contusions. These may be diffuse or focal injuries.
- Secondary injury—Damage that occurs as a result of the body's response to the injury and is influenced by medical intervention. Examples would be swelling and cellular changes in the brain.
- Focal brain injury—Specific, observable brain lesions such as contusions, hemorrhage, or hematoma. These account for more than two-thirds of head injury deaths (Boss, 2002). Examples include penetrating injuries such as gunshot wounds and stabbings.
- Diffuse axonal injury (DAI)—Injury occurs as a result of inertial forces (high levels of acceleration and deceleration) that deform the white matter, causing axonal disruption. Often invisible to current imaging techniques. This accounts for the greatest number of severely disabled survivors (Boss, 2002). Examples include motor vehicle crashes (MVC), falls, and assaults.
- Closed head injury—Skull is intact.
- Open head injury—Inner or outer skull is fractured or displaced, causing compression or laceration directly to the brain.

TBI may result in problems with cognition, movement abilities, sensation, and emotion (Thurman, Alverson, Dunn, Guerrero, & Sniezek, 1999). The effects of these types of injuries are life altering not only to the client but to his or her family members, loved ones, friends, and the caregivers who nurture the often slow recovery process.

TBI is among the leading cause of death and long-term disability in the United States. The Centers for Disease Control and Prevention (National Center for Injury Prevention and Control [National Center], 2001) estimates that approximately 1.5 million Americans sustain a TBI each year. Fifty thousand persons die from a TBI and 80,000 to 90,000 people experience the onset of long-term disability. Males are about twice as likely as females to sustain a TBI (National Center, 2001). Thurman et al. (1999) report persons ages 15 to 24 years and those over age 75 are the 2 age groups at highest risk for TBI. The leading causes of TBI are MVCs, firearm use, and falls (Thurman et al., 1999). TBI-related deaths have overall decreased since 1980. This is due in part to a decline in transportation-related deaths with the improved use of safety seats, seat belts, and vehicle safety features as well as improved emergency medicine practices. Firearms, however, have surpassed MVC as the leading cause of death from TBI. They cause about 10% of all TBIs, but account for 44% of TBI-related deaths, with nearly two-thirds of those classified as suicidal intent. The findings of a study developed by the Centers of Disease Control and Prevention reports that of those that survive their TBI, 1 of every 6 people is unable to return to work or school when discharged from the hospital (Langlois et al., 2003). In 1996, Congress passed Public Law 104-166, the Traumatic Brain Injury Act. This act is an amendment to the Public Health Service Act and provides for the conduct of expanded studies and the establishment of innovative programs related to TBI, including those involving rehabilitation. The support for skilled personnel to provide assistance to all who have been touched by a TBI is evident.

NEUROANATOMY OF HEAD INJURY

The brain itself can be likened to several different analogies in order to describe the mechanisms of injury to which it is susceptible. The preferred analogy is that of a gelatinous mold sus-

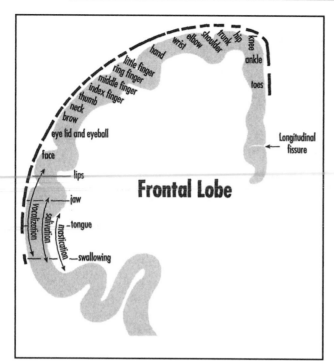

Figure 18-1. The homunculi of the primary motor cortex: frontal lobe. (Adapted from Hole, J. W., Jr. [1984]. *Human anatomy and physiology*. Dubuque, IA: Wm. C. Brown Publishers.)

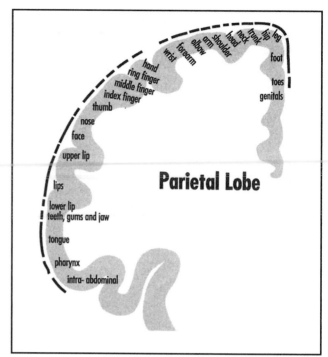

Figure 18-2. The homunculi of the sensory areas: parietal lobe. (Adapted from Hole, J. W., Jr. [1984]. *Human anatomy and physiology*. Dubuque, IA: Wm. C. Brown Publishers.)

pended in a fluid-like substance that is entirely encased within a roughly lined cavity. With this analogy, the gelatin mold represents the brain, the fluid is cerebrospinal in nature, and the roughly lined cavity represents the inner surface of the skull. In normal stasis, the brain remains relatively protected. Its primary role is to direct all conscious and unconscious functions of the body via the CNS. These functions are classically "mapped" within the brain itself and vary in degree of complexity from heart rate, respiration, and arousal to concept formation, generalization, and overall executive function. One specific type of map is commonly referred to in the realm of neurology as a homunculus of the brain (Figures 18-1 and 18-2).

This homunculus, Latin for "a little man," represents a cortical mapping of functions specific to primary motor and sensory cortices (Afifi & Bergman, 1998). By understanding the normal neuroanatomical structures and functions of an intact brain, one can better understand and analyze the effects of injury specific to its location within the skull.

In the event of an injury, the brain is jarred from its normal stasis and makes direct contact with the roughly lined skull encasement. A diffuse axonal injury is caused by rotational or angular acceleration and deceleration of the brain, causing a coup and contrecoup effect. These terms are used to describe the actual points of the brain that make direct contact with the skull. Coup injuries are those directly at or below the point of impact, whereas contrecoup injuries are the polar opposite to the site of impact (Boss, 2002). Therefore, with one external force or injury to the head, 2 areas of the brain are injured. In comparing this type of injury to that of a single area or focal injury, such as seen with a CVA, we can more clearly under-

stand why the latter manifests itself on only one half of the body, while with head injury, it is much more common to see bilateral disabilities.

As indicated earlier, understanding the neuroanatomy and mechanisms of injury to that anatomy, the OTA and OT are at an advantage in their ability to accurately treat a client's strengths and weaknesses. For example, a client has sustained a head injury to the frontal lobe in a motor vehicle accident and has a tracheostomy, which is inhibiting his or her ability to communicate. Based on the understanding of neuroanatomy, even without means of communication, the therapist can be suspicious of a degree of memory deficit from the frontal lobe and possible visual deficit from the occipital lobe as a result of the coup and contrecoup. This small bit of information regarding the possible areas of weakness can have a very large impact on the degree of success you will have during your initial interaction with a client who has sustained a TBI.

THE RECOVERY PROCESS

It is true that everyone is individual in his or her response to an injury. It is uncommon to see any 2 injuries to the brain that present exactly alike, though similarities do exist. These similarities are frequently referred to stages of recovery after a brain injury. So similar, in fact, that 2 separate objective methods have been adopted to assess and measure an injury to the brain: the Rancho Levels of Cognitive Functioning-Revised (RLA) (Hagen, 1998) and the Glasgow Coma Scale (Teasdale & Jennett, 1974).

Rancho Levels of Cognitive Functioning-Revised

Level I

No Response
Total Assistance

Level II

Generalized Response
Total Assistance

Level III

Localized Response
Total Assistance

Level IV

Confused-Agitated
Maximal Assistance

Level V

Confused-Inappropriate-Nonagitated
Maximal Assistance

Level VI

Confused-Appropriate
Moderate Assistance

Level VII

Automatic-Appropriate
Minimal Assistance for Routine Daily Living Skills

Level VIII

Purposeful and Appropriate
Stand-By Assistance

Level IX

Purposeful and Appropriate
Stand-By Assistance on Request

Level X

Purposeful and Appropriate
Modified Independent

Figure 18-3. The Rancho Levels of Cognitive Functioning. (Adapted from Hagen, C. [1998]. *The Rancho levels of cognitive functioning*. Downey, CA: Rancho Los Amigos Medical Center.)

The RLA was first introduced at the Rancho Los Amigos Hospital in Downey, CA, and formally developed into an objective evaluation tool via the outlining of similarities in behaviors observed at each stage. In 1998, it was revised to include 2 new levels to the original 8, to better depict the later phases of recovery. This evaluation, specific to cognitive awareness, is outlined at 10 different levels and graded along a continuum from most primitive and basic reflexes up to higher level executive functioning. These levels are indicative of the more commonly observed behaviors expected from a client at any particular time in the recovery process (Figure 18-3).

The Glasgow Coma Scale is the evaluative measure of choice for physicians presented with a client who has sustained an acute TBI. This measure determines severity of injury by numerically identifying a person's abilities for speaking, eye opening, and motor abilities. Points are accrued based on the quality of responses and an overall rating is applied.

The patterns of recovery within the brain and the appropriate utilization of OT intervention collaboratively are designed to facilitate healing and promote function.

Although the RLA and the Glasgow Coma Scale outline generalizations of behaviors or expectations, each presents clinicians with a much clearer outline of the treatment for a client with a brain injury. In theory, the brain remains a relatively mysterious organ affixed at the very center of our being. We are aware of its capacity to heal and compensate for weakness through neural plasticity; we also have become rather skilled at saving the lives of those with brain injuries who may not have previously been saved. Yet we as the clinicians continue to struggle with its management over the entire duration of recovery. Some clients progress much quicker than others. Some will skip a level or two; some will remain stationary in any one particular level for an extended period of time. Some become fixed at any one point and no longer progress.

It is crucial for OTAs and OTs to develop a familiarity with both the RLA and the Glasgow Coma Scale in order to best maximize the choice of treatment techniques available. Too often clients are asked to perform tasks that are not congruent with the current level of function, and this results in a sense of failure to both the caregiver and the client. Although each client has been objectively judged to be at a particular Rancho level or Glasgow level, we are constantly reminded of the individual and the dynamics behind his or her specific injury through his or her level of success with a particular task or ADL. These subtle differences often create the complexity associated with the success, or lack thereof, in treating a client with a brain injury.

FRAMES OF REFERENCE

It would be a fallacy to say that any one particular frame of reference is applied to OT assessment and intervention with the client who has sustained a head injury. Rather, diverse spectrums of frames available are used at various levels of recovery appropriate to the behaviors and motor skills manifested by each individual. In translation, this simply indicates the ongoing need for re-evaluation and restructuring of the environment necessary to progress to the next recovery level, while also attending to all the deficits presented at any given time. For example, you may be treating a client following a brain injury at the RLA IV who requires a memory notebook applying the dynamic interactional model (Toglia, 1998), a token system for using the notebook appropriately in the cognitive behavioral model (Duncombe, 1998), and an overall endurance training program within the biomechanical frame (Dutton, 1995). All of these may be used together to address the client's needs specific to that particular point of recovery.

INTERDISCIPLINARY APPROACH

The model in which treatment is most often delivered to clients who have sustained a brain injury is the interdisciplinary model. Within this model, professionals of different backgrounds with varying perspectives are brought together to plan and execute a designed approach to the care of the client. Team meetings provide a formal structure to listen and to interpret the contributions of each member relative to the concerns of the client. The result is a meaningful plan of intervention. A secondary result is often a reduction in the duplication of services or gaps in the client's care. Decisions regarding treatment and discharge can be made in a timely manner.

For example, an interdisciplinary team working within a brain injury division may include, but is not limited to, the following: the medical doctor, the primary nurse, the social worker or discharge planner, the physical therapist, the OT, the speech pathologist, the neuropsychologist, and the dietitian. This routine collaboration of specialists allows for the continuous planning of the most optimal treatment in accordance with all strengths or weaknesses, while allowing for a forum of support and structure so often necessary to the treating members working with this population. The OT and OTA are unique members of this team and need to articulate their role and their contributions to the care of the client. Central to any interdisciplinary team is the client and family. It is only through the inclusion of their voices that a meaningful plan is followed.

EVALUATION, GOALS, AND TREATMENT: CASE APPLICATIONS

Physical impairments often accompany the cognitive impairments. Motor approaches to treatment would be implemented in conjunction with the cognitive approach. For the purpose of this case, focus will be placed on the cognitive approach. The complexity of the injury itself is very important to remember at this particular point of the text. Each individual presents differently, having his or her own set of specific strengths and weaknesses that can change frequently throughout the duration of treatment. This treatment is also provided along a continuum of care based on the client's changing needs, including a combination of the following: acute hospitals, rehabilitative hospitals, subacute care facilities, transitional living facilities, day treatment programs, outpatient care centers, and home care agencies. It is due to this fact that the presentation of evaluative procedures, goal setting, and actual treatment intervention strategies are best outlined according to the RLA.

CASE STUDY

Client

Michael is a 24-year-old, single man living independently in a second floor apartment. His parents and a younger sister live nearby, and he enjoys going home for traditional Sunday gatherings.

Socially, he likes to get together with his buddies to play pool and darts, listen to music, and have a good time. He graduated from high school and took some coursework toward an automotive service technology degree. Prior to the accident, Michael worked at an automotive service center as an assistant mechanic.

Diagnostic History

Michael was an unbelted passenger in a head-on motor vehicle accident. He was thrown from the vehicle, resulting in a compound skull fracture and TBI. He sustained no other injuries other than general bruising and muscle soreness. The driver, a close friend, survived but is hospitalized with multiple fractures.

Service Delivery

It is important to note here that with Michael's case, both the OT and the OTA worked collaboratively to address his needs. The OTA cared for much of Michael's direct therapeutic intervention with supervision from the OT and handled much of the family education. This working relationship acted as a means of support and clarification for the OTA based on having already succeeded in demonstration of competency skills specific to the treatment facility.

RLA I—No Response

Complete absence of observable change in behavior when presented with any stimuli.

Setting

Acute care hospital: The acute care hospital routinely refers all clients with TBI to OT and physical therapy as soon as the individual is medically stable.

Evaluation

Michael is currently in a coma state and unresponsive. Assessment of tone, PROM, and positioning are conducted. Other formalized assessments requiring patient response are inappropriate and not implemented.

Goals

The general goal at this stage of recovery is to elicit any response to external stimulation while preventing long-term deformities, such as contractures.

Intervention

Intervention at this stage of recovery is focused on prevention. The OTA or OT will provide the following:
- PROM to all joints to prevent contractures and provide proprioceptive and tactile input.
- Proper positioning to assist in normalizing tone and to prevent contractures and decubitus formation. Pillows, dense foam bolsters, and splints may be used. Bilateral resting hand splints were fabricated and issued.
- Create an immediate environment that is familiar. Michael's family members were asked to bring many items from his apartment that were part of his regular routine, including familiar music, pillows, blankets, and photographs.

- An individualized sensory kit was developed and utilized routinely to attempt to promote a response from Michael to external stimulation. The purpose of a sensory stimulation program is to increase the unconscious patient's responsiveness to the environment via multisensory stimulation. Institution of a sensory stimulation program is an organized, coordinated effort by all team members. It is conducted in 15-minute sessions with rest in between administration of the therapy.
- Education is very important to both the family and other team members. Michael's family required training regarding the role of OT, proper positioning, PROM techniques, use and application of splints, and the importance of eliciting a response. It is also important here to consider the need for support systems available to the family, make necessary referrals, and act as a resource when necessary.

RLA II—Generalized Response

Demonstrates generalized response through reflex, gross body movement, or sound when presented with any stimuli. Response may be nonpurposeful, delayed, or random.

Setting

Acute care hospital and subacute care facility.

Evaluation

Michael has progressed to the next level of recovery based on his ability to produce a reflexive response to noxious stimuli. Assessments are not formalized and are concentrated on level of alertness, recognition, attention/concentration, and ability to follow commands. Assessment of positioning, tone, and PROM continue. Objective documentation by the OTA or OT reflects Michael's motor and sensory responses to stimuli via touch, taste, smell, sound, and light.

Goals

The general goal of this stage of recovery is to increase arousal based on responses to sensory stimulation as measured by the frequency, duration, and quality.

Intervention

Intervention at this stage is similar to that of RLA I. The OTA or OT will provide the following:
- Continuation and revision of the positioning techniques that have been implemented, including splinting.
- Emphasis on familiar surroundings remains very important and is a vital piece of treatment of which the family is an integral part. Continue to explore and generate ideas directly with the family members.
- Continuation of the sensory stimulation program to promote response to external stimuli on a routine basis. For example, reading from a favorite magazine creates a sound stimulus. Responses to look for are blinking of the eyes, turning of the head, or change in facial expression. Olfactory stimulation may be Michael's cologne or coffee. Changes to his heart rate and blood pressure are also positive responses. Caution should be taken, however, to prevent sensory overload.

- Education and reinforcement of the carryover in techniques with Michael's family and caregivers continues to be a focus of treatment. Family members should be performing PROM to all joints independently as instructed by the OTA or OT. Structure is important in the management of all stages of recovery, and here it is emphasized through consistency in the sensory techniques used to elicit the responses for all who are in contact with Michael.

RLA III—Localized Response

Responses become more specific to stimuli presented. May turn toward auditory stimuli, blink in response to light, pull tubes in response to discomfort, and may respond to familiar persons (e.g., family, friends).

Setting

Subacute care facility or rehabilitation hospital. A standard referral from the medical doctor overseeing Michael's care is issued.

Evaluation

At this level, the therapist can expect to be able to establish a means of simple communication with the patient in order to progress toward more formal evaluation procedures. In Michael's case, he is now able to respond with simple head nodding of "yes" or "no." With this skill established, the OTA and/or OT will need to determine the accuracy of those responses prior to implementing a more formal evaluation, such as sensation. This determination was achieved through asking simple yes/no questions of Michael in which the answers were already known, such as: "Are you married?" or "Are you a man?" Functional skills can also begin to be assessed by the OT, including basic ADL such as washing his face or brushing his teeth. Ongoing assessments for joint ROM, motor control, orientation, recognition, attention, following commands, and behavioral factors are also conducted.

Goals

Goals are focused on directing the patient's response to stimulation and elicit specific responses. Orientation to person and place, attend to an activity, use of common objects, and increase ability for simple self-care skills are important at this level. A sample of a documented goal may be: Patient will attend to task for 5 minutes in preparation for completion of ADL in 5 sessions.

Intervention

- A highly structured environment is key for success in therapy. For Michael, a memory notebook was compiled including personal information such as his name, age, where he was, why he was there; photos of people to remember; names of common caregivers and significant others; and most importantly, the schedule he would need to follow on a daily basis. This notebook was referred to routinely by the family and therapy team as a means of directing Michael's thinking and to provide him with a source of information. At this stage of recovery, Michael's level of arousal and insight continue to be considerably deficient. With this in mind, the memory notebook was initiated with a heavy emphasis on family and caregivers to carryover throughout Michael's day and make its use more routine. This responsibility will shift to Michael at a later stage of recovery and is implemented here to promote a smooth transition at that time.

- Focus is also placed on Michael's ability to perform ADL. On a routine basis, the therapist would work closely with Michael in an early morning session to provide the tactile and auditory cues necessary to facilitate independence in his ability to perform his morning routine. The OTA uses a cloth to wash his face and hands (tactile stimulation) while providing orientation to body parts (auditory stimulation). In later sessions, the OTA can progress to utilizing a hand-over-hand method to have Michael begin to sense the movement necessary to complete the task on his own (kinesthetic input).

- Education is important at every stage of recovery. At this stage, it is common for significant others to have a lot of questions based on how their loved one is functioning. Once awake from a coma state, families are often frightened by what is observed and confused about what to expect. The role of the therapist here is to provide resources and information regarding support groups, make the necessary referrals as appropriate, and educate about the recovery process following a brain injury. It is crucial for family members to receive accurate information regarding realistic expectations for recovery. The most successful forum for this type of discussion is in a family conference. This is an opportunity for all immediate caregivers, including the OT and OTA, to discuss with family members all matters at hand so as not to have inconsistencies in information provided.

RLA IV—Confused-Agitated

Response is heightened, but the person possesses a severe inability to process information. The patient may show aggressive behavior. Verbalizations may be frequently inappropriate to the activity or situation.

Setting

Rehabilitation hospital. Patients at RLA IV can present with significant agitation, rehabilitation hospitals are often equipped with special units or programs specific to those needs. The team may recommend a referral for these types of special services at this level of recovery.

Evaluation

At this level, the therapist can expect agitated, inappropriate behaviors with confusion. The patient is unable to process all the sensory stimuli and filter out the nonessential information in order to participate in a formal evaluation process. Assessments should be provided in a quiet, calming environment rather than a busy, noisy environment to minimize distraction and possible agitation. Allowing the person to pace, move about freely, or propel the wheelchair may produce a calm state and allow for assessments to take place in short time periods. Evaluation of functional skills may be possible, however, safety must always be considered for both the client and caregivers. The Comprehensive Occupational Therapy Evaluation Scale (COTE) (Brayman & Kirby, 1976) or the Routine Task Inventory-2 (RTI-2) (Allen, 1992) can be implemented and scored by the OTA under the supervision of the OT for a more measurable evaluation of functional abilities at this level. The OT and OTA will need to utilize objective documentation of behaviors observed and possible precursors to that behavior. Again, emphasis is on brief sessions to prevent adverse reactions and increased agitation.

Goals

The following general goals are established in consideration of the client's degree of confusion and agitation:

- Increase the duration of time that the client is able to attend to a task without an agitated outburst.
- Increase appropriateness of interactions with others and participation in therapy sessions.
- Increase client's overall orientation to person, place, and time.
- Ensure safety of the client, the therapist, and all others in the immediate area in the event of an agitated outburst.
- Promote participation in all areas of occupation.

Intervention

- Safety is of utmost importance during this stage of recovery. Michael would often have agitated outbursts throughout the day as a result of his current level of confusion. Aggressive posturing; verbal harassment; and the throwing of objects at the therapists, family members, and other caregivers characterized these outbursts. These outbursts often occurred following any attempt to orient Michael to the accident and his injuries. His comments reflected his lack of insight and were commonly associated with his perception of being locked up for no apparent reason.
- Michael is now able to come down to the OT clinic in a wheelchair. All of the highly structured treatment sessions were planned for Michael based on his interests and conducted in the least distracting environment (corner of the clinic area). Numerous alternatives were prepared to account for his low frustration tolerance and impatience. Activities involving concentration and cognitive skills were alternated with those allowing for free, motoric movement. At this stage, it is not appropriate to offer Michael choices; rather a single task is presented for participation. In the event that Michael would disengage from any one particular task, the therapist would attempt to re-engage with a different task. Introducing tasks that were meaningful and focused on identified occupations were key in engaging him during treatment sessions. Providing Michael with a pool stick or darts is too dangerous at this juncture, but engaging him in a soft foam target ball toss would be more appropriate. This could be accomplished in sitting or standing to work on motoric issues such as decreased postural control.
- All members of the treatment team and the family were informed of the importance in the uniform use of the

memory notebook. Michael was encouraged to begin to participate in the use of this notebook. The contents were expanded to include a token economy system as a means of modifying Michael's behavioral outbursts. With a given number of tokens achieved through actively participating in therapeutic sessions, Michael's family agreed to provide him with positive reinforcements such as video games and short, supervised outings approved by the doctor.

- The utilization of bilateral upper extremity splints for positioning at night was discontinued at this stage due to his increased ability to use his hands and upper extremities.
- Education is again a critical piece at this level of recovery. Emotional outbursts and inappropriate acts or comments occur not only in the presence of family but directed at the family members themselves. Family must be educated regarding the fact that these behaviors are a result of the injury. It is important to continue to emphasize the need for support and the benefits of that support. With Michael, education was provided to the family regarding the catalysts for the emotional outbursts, how to manage outbursts, the use of the memory notebook for reorientation, need for constant and direct supervision due to the lack of insight as well as the degree of confusion, and the importance of carryover with the token economy system devised.

RLA V—Confused, Inappropriate, Nonagitated

Appears alert and responds appropriately to simple commands. Responses become nonpurposeful and random with increased complexity of directions or unstructured environment. Lacks initiation of functional tasks, but may perform previously learned tasks when structure and cues given. Unable to integrate new information. Not oriented to person, place, time, or situation. Severely impaired recent memory, with problem-solving and self-monitoring behavior absent.

Setting

Rehabilitation hospital.

Evaluation

Formal assessment procedures can be attempted by the OTA who has either demonstrated service competency for the specific assessment or is under the supervision of the OT. These include, but are not limited to motor assessments, such as tone; AROM/PROM; strength; and functional assessments, such as Assessment of Motor and Process Skills (AMPS) (Fischer, 1994), COTE (Brayman & Kirby, 1976), or the Kohlman Evaluation of Living Skills (KELS) (Kohlman Thomson, 1992). As with RLA IV, assessments should be conducted in short time intervals and in a quiet environment.

Goals

Goals focus on guidance and direction for sustained attention to tasks, increased short-term memory, and promote initiation in areas of occupation.

- Facilitate use of memory notebook for orientation and daily routine.

- Increase awareness into strengths and weaknesses via repetition.
- Increase attention span and ability to problem solve in functional situations.
- Maximize level of independence with ADL using compensatory strategies for initiation.
- Promote the use of appropriate social skills within interactive group environments.
- Facilitate the use of visual-motor skills based on repetition of simple commands.

An example of a documented goal may be: Patient will perform grooming task with 2 to 3 verbal cues for redirection in 5 sessions.

Intervention

- At this point of recovery, Michael was able to participate with the therapist in the clinic for a 30-minute session involving simple tabletop tasks when given moderate redirection. He also responded to short breaks every 10 minutes. During this break, Michael would walk with the therapist one lap around the department and return to the table as a means of managing his irritability and decreased attention span.
- A focus of Michael's treatment at this stage was on cognitive skills. Although puzzles and paper-pencil tasks were available, Michael responded best to activities that were meaningful for him. For example, Michael played cards with his buddies prior to his accident. Using a deck of cards, the therapist would devise a memory game beginning with a minimal number of choices to insure success. This activity impacted Michael's memory, attention span, and motoric capabilities. Michael would attend to this activity for 10 minutes at a time.
- Michael began to work in a small group based on the development of orientation skills on a daily basis. Here, the therapist expected Michael to remain for the 20 minute duration of the group and conduct himself appropriately to both the other group members and the group leader. At first, the primary therapist supervised these group meetings in the event that Michael would leave the group and the group leader was not able to follow. Within 2 weeks, Michael was performing this function appropriately with moderate supervision.
- The development of insight regarding Michael's strengths and weaknesses was a crucial component at this stage of recovery. This was addressed through the use of functional activities, such as dressing. For example, Michael would commonly arrive to therapy in the clothes he had worn the previous day. If approached, Michael would defend himself and state that the therapist must be mistaken. To address this area, repetition was used. The therapist created a section of the memory notebook that was added to at the beginning of each session and included what Michael was wearing. Michael required maximal assistance to refer to his memory book.

RLA VI—Confused-Appropriate

Inconsistently oriented to person and place. Demonstrates goal-directed behavior, but requires external input for direction. Shows carryover for relearned familiar tasks, but new learning requires maximal assistance with little to no carryover. Lacks awareness of disability and safety risks. May be able to attend to a 30-minute task in a nondistracting environment with moderate redirection. Consistently follows 1- to 2-step directions.

Setting

Rehabilitation hospital or transitional living facility.

Referral

As Michael became prepared for discharge from inpatient services, the OTA and OT spoke with the case manager to arrange for the continuation of appropriate OT intervention on an outpatient basis.

Evaluation

At this stage of recovery, the client will present with an increased attention span and will better able to participate in standardized evaluation procedures. As some were indicated previously in RLA V, these assessments include, but are not limited to, the following: KELS (Kohlman Thomson, 1992), COTE (Brayman & Kirby, 1976), Lowenstein Occupational Therapy Cognitive Assessment (LOTCA) (Itzkovich, Elazar, Averbuch, & Katz, 1990), and the Test of Everyday Attention (TEA) (Robertson, Ward, Ridgeway, & Nimmo-Smith, 1994). A home assessment prior to discharge may be deemed appropriate. Each formal assessment can be provided by the OTA who has demonstrated service competency or with the OT.

Goals

Goals continue to focus on guidance and direction for sustained attention to tasks. In addition, safety awareness, promotion of independence in ADL, and increasing carryover for learning are essential components to intervention.

- Increase ability to independently manage a daily schedule.
- Perform IADL with moderate supervision.
- Improve higher level cognitive skill ability, including associations, categorization, generalizations, and problem solving in familiar situations.
- Increase overall safety awareness through carryover of compensation techniques for memory and judgment with moderate supervision.

A sample of a documented goal is: Patient will identify potential hazards in the environment (obstacles, untied shoelaces) with moderate cues for safety within 5 sessions.

Intervention

- The underlying basis of all treatment at this level is based on principles of repetition and the creation of a highly structured environment to promote success. Emphasis has been removed on the use of the token economy as a form of behavior modification and reinforcement of expected outcomes.

- The focus of Michael's current treatment became based in the awareness of the external environment and his daily routine. The therapist took on a more passive role, allowing for the "control" to be decided upon by Michael. These steps were made to facilitate the adjustment to a transitional living facility where Michael would be responsible for his self-care and getting to all scheduled appointments with appropriate requests for assistance if necessary. It was important to introduce Michael to these expectations. Using his notebook as a memory aid, he became responsible for getting himself to and from all of his scheduled therapy appointments without the assistance of a transportation staff member. It was also important to reinforce time management principles for eventual preparation to independent living. The responsibility for maintaining the notebook was transferred to Michael, with the therapist providing structure as needed.

- The complexity of all tasks that were addressed in the clinic were graded in order to provide the optimal amount of challenge, including such tasks as supervised cooking, actual hospital navigation using maps and signs, and money management.

- Education at this point was provided to the family regarding compensation techniques that are successful in promoting Michael's independence, with emphasis placed on the importance of carryover. A family conference was again conducted where all members of the team, including the OT and OTA, discussed with the family Michael's discharge plan to the transitional living facility. Here, he would be expected to care for his own needs between Monday and Friday with only occasional supervision, then transition to home with weekend overnight visits.

RLA VII—Automatic-Appropriate

Consistently oriented to person and place. Able to use memory devices with minimal assistance. Will initiate and carry out daily routine automatically but often cannot recall what has been done. Requires minimal supervision for new learning. Shows superficial awareness of condition, but lacks insight and realistic planning for the future. Often overestimates ability to perform tasks. Unaware of other's needs or feelings, and displays inappropriate social interaction.

Setting

Transitional living facility or day treatment program.

Referral

The outpatient OT/OTA team began services after speaking with the case manager and family members. The transition is made smoother if the previous OT/OTA team is able to communicate with the current team to discuss current status in detail and any particular intervention strategies that were successful specific to Michael.

Evaluation

Michael's residual weaknesses include his executive functioning skills, including initiation, flexibility, planning, organization, and problem solving. Specific assessments can be conducted that may include the following: Comprehensive Trail Making Test (CTMT) (Reynolds, 2002), Executive Function Route Finding Task (EFRT) (Boyd & Sautter, 1993), or the Test of Functional Executive Abilities (TOFEA) (Barndad, Ryan, & Warden, 2003). In addition, assessments identifying physical abilities for eventual return to work may include Minnesota Rate of Manipulation Test (University of Minnesota Employment Stabilization Research Institute, 1969), Purdue Pegboard Test (Tiffin, 1960), Jebsen Test of Hand Function (Jebsen, Taylor, Trieschmann, Trotter, & Howard, 1969), and the Box and Block Test (Mathiowetz, Volland, Kashman, & Weber, 1985). Again, these assessment procedures can be provided by either the OT or the OT and OTA collaboratively.

Goals

Goals begin to focus on cognitive flexibility strategies, problem solving for novel situations, and awareness of situation and actions.

- Independence with daily routine with cues for memory device use.

- Integration of cognitive ability into community re-entry skills.

- Identify return to work status and address performance skills of difficulty.

Intervention

- At this point in Michael's treatment, the focus became community re-entry and return to work. On a routine basis, Michael joined a small group of other clients who had sustained head injuries. In this group, members were responsible for planning and implementing a community outing on a weekly basis. Clients were given a goal sheet that had been contributed to by each member of the treating team and required Michael to complete certain tasks while in the community. These tasks included asking for assistance, following directions, or identifying means of transportation. Michael was given the freedom of navigation within the community on these trips with supervision; however, he was responsible for completing the task at hand within the time frame allotted.

- The therapist contacted Michael's employer to request a copy of his previous job description. The long-term plan is for Michael to return to this capacity of work and, therefore, it is necessary to incorporate these functions into his therapy sessions. The job description was broken down into components and performed individually. Items such as appropriate tool selection, identification of work hazards, and identification of engine parts become activities utilized in treatment.

- Education at this stage of recovery included both Michael and his family. It is often at this stage that clients begin to experience grief over their loss based on the development of insight. This grief is often very difficult for families to manage as a result of their own grieving process over their loss of who their loved one previously was and who he or she is now evolving into. Education regarding coping skills, role adjustment, and support services is very important, making sure to refer to other professionals as necessary.

RLA VIII—Purposeful, Appropriate–Stand-By Assistance

Consistently oriented to person, place, and time. Attends to and completes tasks for 1 hour in a distracting environment. Utilizes memory devices with occasional assistance. Demonstrates initiation of routine tasks and will modify the plan with minimal assistance. Although awareness of impairments and disabilities is emerging, at times they may interfere with task performance and require assistance to take appropriate action. Depressed, irritable, low frustration tolerance.

Setting

Day treatment program or outpatient rehabilitation.

Evaluation

Some clients will not regain this level of functioning dependent on the severity of their injury. Mild brain injuries have a higher capacity to reach this level, however, Michael has not. Assessments continue to focus on executive functions and target specific return to productive living. Assessment for vocational testing is common and a vocational counselor may be added to the team as a specialist at this point of recovery.

Goals

Goals continue to focus on cognitive flexibility strategies, problem solving for novel situations, and awareness of situation and actions with less assistance. Appropriate communication/interaction skills in social situations are also targeted.

- Increase tolerance in stressful situations.
- Implement the independent use of compensatory strategies to address residual memory, social, and IADL skills.
- Participation in a support group therapy environment.
- Maximize automatic reactions to environmental stimuli.
- Successful return to a productive living situation, including work or school.

Intervention

- The focus of treatment would address residual deficit areas and implementation of compensatory strategies. Tasks that include work roles or IADL tasks are often addressed.
- Community reintegration is continued at this stage with higher expectations and a greater level of independence.
- Ideally, the client will return to work in a smaller capacity while continuing therapy intervention in order to overlap in skills necessary to master.
- Education continues for both clients and families in the form of support groups as a means of addressing loss and grief.

RLA IX—Purposeful, Appropriate–Stand-By Assistance on Request

Increased ability to shift between tasks for up to 2 hours. Initiates and carries out daily routine with assistance only when requested. Acknowledging others' needs and feelings appropriately with assistance. Self-monitors appropriateness of social interaction with assistance.

Setting

Outpatient or home with supervision.

Evaluation

Assessments continue to focus on executive functions and target specific return to productive living. Additional assessments to perform may include Behavioral Assessment of Dysexecutive Syndrome (BADS) (Wilson, Evans, Emslie, Alderman, & Burgess, 1998), Toglia Categorization Assessment (TCA) (Toglia, 1994), and Observed Tasks of Daily Living (OTDL) (Diehl, Willis, & Schaie, 1995). Informal function assessment tasks could also be performed such as planning a day, running an errand at a store, seeking information, and planning a meal.

Goals

Goals continue to refine cognitive flexibility strategies, problem solving, and self-regulation and self-control with ability to identify when to request assistance.

- Self-monitor attention and memory lapses.
- Monitor reactions to situations that cause feelings of frustration and irritability.
- Perform tasks with specified time restraints and under stressful conditions.

Intervention

- Focus of treatment at this stage is on changing the task or environment to present appropriate level challenges. The client may be taught common external strategies, such as use of timers; use of checklists; and when reading, cover information that is not necessary and circle or highlight important information.
- Educate the client on internal strategies, such as self-questioning, self-evaluation, and brainstorming for problem-solving situations.

RLA X—Purposeful, Appropriate–Modified Independent

Able to assume multiple tasks simultaneously but may need breaks. Independently functions at home and community but may require more time or use of compensatory strategies to complete tasks. Social interaction is appropriate. Low frustration and irritability occurs only when fatigued or under emotional or physical stress. Recognizes the needs and feelings of others and responds appropriately.

Intervention

At this stage, OT is involved on an as-needed basis. The client has developed performance patterns that allow for independent living. He or she may continue to work on metacognitive issues.

SUMMARY

TBI remains in a league of its own. It is an extremely complex diagnosis requiring a multitude of professional intervention and skill. Brain injury robs a person of him- or herself; the person prior to the injury often disappears and in his or her place evolves a different person who may only resemble the first. The mechanism of brain injury has changed over time, yet its prevalence remains stable and the need for intensive, precise, and individualized treatment continues. It is thought that these are the very same reasons that OTAs, OTs, and many other disciplines find this subspecialty area extremely rewarding. It is not often that a therapist is granted the privilege to work this closely with his or her client for weeks or months at a time, influencing each stage of recovery. It is becoming an even more rare occasion in the event of managed care service delivery models. As therapists within this practice domain, we are given a true opportunity to help those who are in need. We are able to guide their recovery and become part of an experience that no one is likely to soon forget.

CLINICAL PROBLEM SOLVING

Although Michael's recovery process has not reached RLA X, he is a success story for others who have sustained a brain injury. After 18 months of intensive therapeutic intervention, Michael was able to return to a supervised living situation, independently manipulate his immediate environment for use of public transportation, and return to his place of work but with less responsibility. He was now 26 years old and the better portion of 2 long years had passed. Not all clients who sustain brain injuries are able to attain these goals. A key function of Michael's recovery was the supportive investment of his family and his employer, who together enabled his success alongside the treatment team. Michael will continue to learn following his injury and demonstrate further progress over time; the capacity of the brain to heal does not have a time limit. He may continue with outpatient therapy, group therapy, and even one day return to living independently. However, until then, he is proud of what he has achieved, and those around him know he worked harder than many of us are ever asked to in order to achieve what he has at this point in his life.

Important to reinforce here are the compounding effects of the individual when treating a brain injury. For example, what if Michael's recovery had reached its highest stage at RLA V? What if Michael was married and the provider for his 2-year-old son? Would these factors influence the previously outlined OT intervention? Yes, the treatment plan would be considerably different to accommodate for these factors had they occurred.

Had Michael reached recovery RLA V and had ceased to make gains characteristic of RLA VI, treatment and discharge plans as outlined previously would be changed dramatically. At this level, Michael would require direct supervision 24 hours per day. More than likely he would need cueing to complete his ADL efficiently. He would be unable to conduct necessary IADL without assistance and may pose a significant safety risk if responsible for any cooking. His insight would continue to be compromised and, therefore, he may be highly resistive to any limits placed on him. Michael's family would require extensive education prior to discharge to consider factors such as hiding car keys and unplugging the stove in order to limit safety risks associated with limited insight. The family would also require more of a support system than described earlier to address psychosocial issues around Michael's injury, his need for constant supervision, and the possibility of external services to assist with his care.

Had Michael been married and the father of a 2 year old, other factors would need to be integrated into the treatment plan. Considerations would be made vocationally and financially regarding the impact of his inability to work during his recovery. Attention would need to be paid to his wife's capacity to handle all tasks required of a household and associated with providing sole care of a 2 year old. Encouragement would be provided to the wife by the entire treatment team regarding possible support systems and need for assistance from various other family members if possible. Often it is very difficult to include the spouse in treatment and provide necessary education due to the time constraints associated with being a sole child caregiver while also working to accommodate for any loss of income. These types of scenarios present with very difficult and individualized issues that arise continuously throughout the recovery process and require specific integration into the treatment plan.

LEARNING ACTIVITIES

1. Develop a comprehensive resource guide that you will use to refer the families of your clients with TBI. Include topics such as recent publications, research centers, and support groups or services available.

2. Using the Web site of the National Recovery Center for TBI as a guide, discuss what changes can be expected by the managed care environment on the treatment of clients with brain injury.

3. Research and create a generalized listing of the most common functions specific to the frontal, parietal, occipital, and temporal lobes.

4. Create a pamphlet to present to your fellow clinicians outlining safety precautions to observe while treating a client at the RLA level IV of recovery. This should include the "Dos and Don'ts" for maintaining the safety of the client, the therapist, and others in the immediate area. For example, the therapist should never sit him- or herself between an agitated client and the exit of the room in which he or she is providing treatment.

REFERENCES

Afifi, A., &. Bergman, R. (1998). Gross topography. In A. Afifi & R. Bergman (Eds.), *Functional neuroanatomy* (pp. 43). New York: McGraw-Hill.

Allen, C. K. (1992). Routine Task Inventory-2. In C. K. Allen, C. A. Earhart, & T. Blue (Eds.), *Occupational therapy treatment goals for the physically and cognitively disabled* (pp. 54-68). Bethesda, MD: American Occupational Therapy Association.

EVIDENCE-BASED TREATMENT STRATEGIES

Treatment Strategies	Authors
Remedial/restorative approach	Beardmore, Tate, & Liddle, 1999; Dirette, Hinojosa, & Carnevale, 1999; Neistadt, 1992, 1994; Novack, Caldwell, Duke, Bergquist, & Gage, 1996; Page, 2003; Rath, Simon, Langenbahn, Sherr, & Diller, 2003; Thomas-Stonell, Johnson, Schuller, Jutai, & Psych, 1994
Compensatory/adaptive approach	Dirette, 2002; Dirette et al., 1999; Dirette & Hinojosa, 1999; Neistadt, 1992; Schmitter-Edgecombe, Fahy, Whelan, & Long, 1995; Wilson, Emslie, Quirk, & Evans, 2001
Cognitive rehabilitation training	Carney et al., 1999; Chesnut et al., 1999; Cicerone et al., 2000; Ruff & Niemann, 1990; Salazar et al., 2000
Goal attainment	Prigatano & Wong, 1999; Trombly, Radomski, & Davis, 1998; Zhang et al., 2003
Community re-entry	Huebner, Johnson, Bennett, & Schneck, 2003; Landa-Gonzalez, 2001; Willer, Button, & Rempel, 1999
Treatment intensity	Heinemann, Hamilton, Linacre, Wright, & Granger, 1995; Slade, Tennant, & Chamberlain, 2002

Barndad, M. J., Ryan, L. M., & Warden, D. L. (2003). Functional assessment of executive abilities following traumatic brain injury. *Brain Injury, 17*, 1011-1020.

Beardmore, S., Tate, R., & Liddle, B. (1999). Does information and feedback improve children's knowledge and awareness of deficits after traumatic brain injury? *Neuropsychological Rehabilitation, 9*(1), 45-62.

Boss, B. (2002). Alterations of neurologic function. In K. H. S. McCance (Ed.), *Pathophysiology: The basis for disease in adults and children* (4th ed., pp. 487-495). St. Louis, MO: Mosby.

Boyd, T. M., & Sautter, S. W. (1993). Route-finding: A measure of everyday executive functioning in the head-injured adult. *Applied Cognitive Psychology, 7*, 171-181.

Brayman, S. J., & Kirby, T. (1976). Comprehensive occupational therapy evaluation. *American Journal of Occupational Therapy, 30*(2), 94-100.

Carney, N., Chesnut, R. M., Maynard, H., Mann, N. C., Patterson, P., & Helfand, M. (1999). Special article—Effect of cognitive rehabilitation on outcomes for persons with traumatic brain injury: A systematic review. *Journal of Head Trauma Rehabilitation, 14*(3), 277-307.

Chesnut, R. M., Carney, N., Maynard, H., Mann, N. C., Patterson, P., & Helfand, M. (1999). Special report—Summary report: Evidence for the effectiveness of rehabilitation for persons with traumatic brain injury. *Journal of Head Trauma Rehabilitation, 14*(2), 176-188.

Cicerone, K., Dahlberg, C., Kalmar, K., Langenbahn, D., Malec, J., Bergquist, T., et al. (2000). Evidence-based cognitive rehabilitation: Recommendations for clinical practice. *Archives of Physical Medicine and Rehabilitation, 81*(12), 1596-1615.

Diehl, M., Willis, S. L., & Schaie, K. W. (1995). Everyday problem solving in older adults: Observational assessment and cognitive correlates. *Psychology of Aging, 10*(3), 478-491.

Dirette, D. (2002). The development of awareness and the use of compensatory strategies for cognitive deficits. *Brain Injury, 16*(10), 861-871.

Dirette, D. K., & Hinojosa, J. (1999). The effects of a compensatory intervention on processing deficits of adults with acquired brain injuries. *Occupational Therapy Journal of Research, 19*(4), 223-240.

Dirette, D. K., Hinojosa, J., & Carnevale, G. J. (1999). Comparison of remedial and compensatory interventions for adults with acquired brain injuries. *Journal of Head Trauma Rehabilitation, 14*(6), 595-601.

Duncombe, L. (1998). The cognitive-behavioral model in mental health. In N. Katz (Ed.), *Cognition and occupation in rehabilitation: Cognitive models for intervention in occupational therapy* (pp. 165-191). Bethesda, MD: American Occupational Therapy Association.

Dutton, R. (1995). Biomechanical postulates regarding intervention. In R. Dutton (Ed.), *Clinical reasoning in physical disabilities* (pp. 44-57). Baltimore: Williams & Wilkins.

Fischer, A. G. (1994). *Assessment of motor and process skills.* Fort Collins, CO: Colorado State University.

Hagen, C. (1998). *The Rancho levels of cognitive functioning.* Downey, CA: Rancho Los Amigos Medical Center.

Heinemann, A. W., Hamilton, B., Linacre, J. M., Wright, B. D., & Granger, C. (1995). Functional status and therapeutic intensity during inpatient rehabilitation. *American Journal of Physical Medicine & Rehabilitation, 74*(4), 315-326.

Huebner, R. A., Johnson, K., Bennett, C. M., & Schneck, C. (2003). Adult brain injury—Community participation and quality of life outcomes after adult traumatic brain injury. *American Journal of Occupational Therapy, 57*(2), 177-185.

Itzkovich, M., Elazar, B., Averbuch, S., & Katz, N. (1990). *Lowenstein occupational therapy cognitive assessment.* Pequannock, NJ: Maddak, Inc.

Jebsen, R. H., Taylor, N., Trieschmann, R. B., Trotter, M., & Howard, L. A. (1969). An objective and standardized test of hand function. *Archives of Physical Medicine & Rehabilitation, (June)*, 311-319.

Kohlman Thomson, L. (1992). *Kohlman evaluation of living skills* (3rd ed.). Bethesda, MD: American Occupational Therapy Association.

Landa-Gonzalez, B. (2001). Multicontextual occupational therapy intervention: A case study of traumatic brain injury. *Occupational Therapy International, 8*(1), 49-62.

Langlois, J., Kegler, S., Butler, J., Gotsch, K., Johnson, R., Reichard, A., et al. (2003). *Traumatic brain injury-related hospital discharges: Results from a 14-state surveillance system, 1997. MMWR, 52*(No. SS-4), 1-10.

Mathiowetz, A., Volland, G., Kashman, N., & Weber, K. (1985). Adult norms for the box and block test of manual dexterity. *American Journal of Occupational Therapy, 39*, 386-391.

Mosby's medical, nursing, & allied health dictionary (6th ed.). (2002). St. Louis, MO: Mosby.

National Center for Injury Prevention and Control. (2001). *Injury fact book 2001-2002*. Atlanta, GA: Centers for Disease Control and Prevention.

Neistadt, M. E. (1992). Occupational therapy treatments for constructional deficits. *American Journal of Occupational Therapy, 46*(2), 141-148.

Neistadt, M. E. (1994). The effects of different treatment activities on functional fine motor coordination in adults with brain injury. *American Journal of Occupational Therapy, 48*(10), 877-882.

Novack, T. A., Caldwell, S. G., Duke, L. W., Bergquist, T. F., & Gage, R. J. (1996). Focused versus unstructured intervention for attention deficits after traumatic brain injury. *Journal of Head Trauma Rehabilitation, 11*(3), 52-60.

Page, S. (2003). Forced use after TBI: Promoting plasticity and function through practice. *Brain Injury, 17*(8), 675-684.

Prigatano, G. P., & Wong, J. L. (1999). Cognitive and affective improvement in brain dysfunctional patients who achieve inpatient rehabilitation goals. *Archives of Physical Medicine and Rehabilitation, 80*(1), 77-84.

Rath, J. F., Simon, D., Langenbahn, D. M., Sherr, R. L., & Diller, L. (2003). Group treatment of problem-solving deficits in outpatients with traumatic brain injury: A randomized outcome study. *Neuropsychological Rehabilitation, 13*(4), 461-488.

Reynolds, C. (2002). *Comprehensive trail making test*. Austin, TX: Pro-Ed, Inc.

Robertson, I., Ward, T., Ridgeway, V., & Nimmo-Smith, I. (1994). *Test of everyday attention*. Gaylord, MI: National Rehabilitation Services.

Ruff, R. M., & Niemann, H. (1990). Cognitive rehabilitation versus day treatment in head-injured adults: Is there an impact on emotional and psychosocial adjustment? *Brain Injury, 4*(4), 339-347.

Salazar, A., Warden, D. L., Schwab, K., Spector, J., Braverman, S., Walter, J., et al. (2000). Cognitive rehabilitation for traumatic brain injury: A randomized trial. *Journal of the American Medical Association, 283*, 3075-3081.

Schmitter-Edgecombe, M., Fahy, J. F., Whelan, J. P., & Long, C. J. (1995). Memory remediation after severe closed head injury: Notebook training versus supportive therapy. *Journal of Consulting and Clinical Psychology, 63*(3), 484-489.

Slade, A., Tennant, A., & Chamberlain, M. A. (2002). A randomized controlled trial to determine the effect of intensity of therapy upon length of stay in a neurological rehabilitation setting. *Journal of Rehabilitation Medicine, 34*(6), 260-266.

Teasdale, G., & Jennett, B. (1974). Assessment of coma and impaired consciousness. A practical scale. *Lancet, 7872*(2), 81-84.

Thomas-Stonell, N., Johnson, P., Schuller, R., Jutai, J., & Psych, C. (1994). Evaluation of a computer-based program for remediation of cognitive-communication skills. *Journal of Head Trauma Rehabilitation, 9*(4), 25-37.

Thurman, D., Alverson, C., Dunn, K., Guerrero, J., & Sniezek, J. (1999). Traumatic brain injury in the united states: A public health perspective. *Journal of Head Trauma Rehabilitation, 14*(6), 602-615.

Tiffin, J. (1960). *Purdue pegboard*. Lafayette, IN: Lafayette Instrument Company.

Toglia, J. P. (1994). *Dynamic assessment of categorization skills: The Toglia category assessment*. Pequannock, NJ: Maddak.

Toglia, J. P. (1998). A dynamic interactional model to cognitive rehabilitation. In N. Katz (Ed.), *Cognition and occupation in rehabilitation: Cognitive models for intervention in occupational therapy* (pp. 5-50). Bethesda, MD: American Occupational Therapy Association.

Trombly, C. A., Radomski, M. V., & Davis, E. S. (1998). Achievement of self-identified goals by adults with traumatic brain injury: Phase I. *American Journal of Occupational Therapy, 52*(10), 810-818.

University of Minnesota Employment Stabilization Research Institute. (1969). *Minnesota rate of manipulation tests*. Circle Pines, MN: American Guidance Service, Inc.

Willer, B., Button, J., & Rempel, R. (1999). Residential and home-based postacute rehabilitation of individuals with traumatic brain injury: A case control study. *Archives of Physical Medicine and Rehabilitation, 80*(4), 399-406.

Wilson, B. A., Evans, J. J., Emslie, H., Alderman, N., & Burgess, P. W. (1998). The development of an ecologically valid test for assessing patient with a dysexecutive syndrome. *Neuropsychological Rehabilitation, 8*(3), 213-228.

Wilson, B. A., Emslie, H. C., Quirk, K., & Evans, J. J. (2001). Reducing everyday memory and planning problems by means of a paging system: A randomized control crossover study. *Journal of Neurology, Neurosurgery and Psychiatry, 70*(Part 4), 477-482.

Zhang, L., Abreu, B. C., Seale, G. S., Masel, B., Christiansen, C. H., & Ottenbacher, K. J. (2003). A virtual reality environment for evaluation of a daily living skill in brain injury rehabilitation: Reliability and validity. *Archives of Physical Medicine and Rehabilitation, 84*(8), 1118-1124.

Michael's Notebook

DATE: AUGUST 2 DAY: THURSDAY

A.M. ROUTINE

- ☑ Wash face
- ☑ Brush teeth
- ☑ Shave
- ☐ Comb hair
- ☑ Get dressed

What I am wearing:

JEANS

RED T.SHIRT

SHOES

- ☑ Eat breakfast

What I ate:

EGG

TOAST

CORN FLAKES

DAILY SCHEDULE

PEOPLE

THINGS TO DO

Real record 18-1. Real record for a client with traumatic brain injury.

Metropolitan City Hospital

SIGN ALL NOTES AND INCLUDE PROFESSIONAL TITLE
(M.D., R.N., R.I.)

| DATE /
TIME | FOCUS / PROBLEM # /
CONSULT | PROGRESS NOTE |
|---|---|---|
| 8/12/04
6:45a | | Nursing
Pt turned q4° per report. no redness or areas of breakdown noted. Splints & positioners in place. Vitals BP 130/74 P 68 RR 16 O₂ Sat 98%. Report dictated. Ann Waxner, RN |
| 8/12/04
8:30 a.m.
10 min
97530 | | Occupational Therapy
S: Ø
O: Pt. seen bedside for stimulation program. Conducted 15 mins. of alternating olfactory and auditory stimulus. Coffee aroma presented in short intervals. Noted slight ↑ to pulse rate ~ 5 bpm. On calling his name, pt. responded 75% of the time c̄ turning his head in the direction of sound. ↑ in UE tone noted c̄ both stimuli.
A: Pt. exhibits responses consistent c̄ Rancho Level 2. Documented in team binder. Progress seen c̄ ↑ in frequency of responses.
P: Continue OT services to work toward goal of accurate response in preparation for participation in ADL. ————— Sally Greenhover, OTR/L
pgr # 55-6001 |

Real record 18-2. Real record for a client with traumatic brain injury.

PROGRESS NOTES

NAME: Michael _____ PATIENT # _____

MEDICARE # _____ SOCIAL SECURITY # _____

DATE & TIME	
Sept. 10/04	S/ "I'm ready to go back to work." O/ Pt. seen daily for OT. Total sessions: 8. Focus on memory training, IADL, & social interactions. Michael participated in a cooking group where menu development, shopping & preparation of food was completed over the course of the week. He required Mod. cues for redirection to task. Mod. assistance c̄ money management when purchasing items in the store. In the kitchen, he required (S) c̄ Mod. cues for safety. Pt. conts. to use memory notebook c̄ occasional reminders. His is consistently oriented to person & place. A/ Pt. continues to require (S) in all tasks for safety & completion. Interactions in public require monitoring for appropriateness. Difficulty c̄ money management persists. Recommend continued inpt. rehab stay for 2-3 weeks to insure smooth transition to home & day treatment. P/ Continue OT daily. Next week to focus on goals of safety awareness & problem-solving situations. Dottie C. Hall, OTA/L

Real record 18-3. Real record for a client with traumatic brain injury.

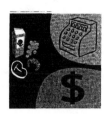

MONEY MANAGEMENT

WORKSHEET # 4

Complete each of the problems below. Show your work.

1.   At the local burger stand, you order a cheeseburger deluxe, large fries and a large root beer. The cheeseburger deluxe is $3.00, the fries are $1.49 and it is $1.25 for the drink. How much will you need to pay?

$ 5.64

3.00
1.49
1.25
5.64

2.   To pay for your meal, you give the cashier a ten dollar bill. How much change will you get back?

$4.36

10.00
5.64
4.36

3.   You run into a buddy on your way home and decide to treat him to some ice cream. Banana splits are $3.25. Single dip cones are $1.50. What can you order?

2 cones

3.25 , 1.50
3.25   1.50
6.50   3.00

Real record 18-4. Real record for a client with traumatic brain injury.

Key Concepts

- Levels of spinal cord injury (SCI): The level at which the spinal cord is injured determines which peripheral sensory and motor nerves are affected (quick method of estimating the remaining functional abilities of the patient).
- Complications: In addition to loss of feeling and movement, SCI results in a variety of secondary complications, including blood pressure problems, breathing difficulties, incontinence/other bladder problems, and loss of skin integrity. These complications increase the complexity of treatment planning and intervention.
- Precautions: Because of the various complex problems with SCI, therapists must observe precautions in bringing the patient to an upright position, ROM activities of the neck and shoulders, length of sitting time, and environmental temperature.
- Intervention strategies: Treatment for patients with SCIs involves increasing endurance and strength in remaining performance components (biomechanical approach) and the provision of and training in the use of techniques and equipment that substitute for lost functions (rehabilitative approach).
- Adaptive equipment: A manual and/or power wheelchair for mobility is the most common type of equipment prescribed for use by patients with SCI. Other types of equipment include wrist-hand orthoses, mouth sticks, hand controls in cars, and environmental control systems.
- Community reintegration: Comprehensive treatment programs for patients with SCI include helping them develop methods or plans for public or private transportation, home assessment and adaptation, and return to school or work.

Essential Vocabulary

autonomic dysreflexia: Nervous system disorder triggered by a variety of stimuli. May result in dangerously high blood pressure.

decubitus ulcers: Skin breakdown from unrelieved pressure on the skin, frequently over bony prominences.

heterotrophic ossification: Abnormal calcifications at shoulder, elbow, hip, or knee joints, resulting in redness, swelling, limitations in ROM, and pain.

orthostatic hypotension: Sudden drop in blood pressure upon changing from supine to sitting or sitting to standing, resulting in dizziness and fainting.

paraplegia: Loss of movement in lower body and legs.

self-catheterization: Insertion of a flexible plastic tube into the urethra by the patient, permitting the bladder to be emptied and controlled.

tenodesis: Fingers naturally flex when the wrist is extended and extend when the wrist is flexed. When combined with a splint holding the thumb and fingers rigid, this permits patients with SCI to have finger grasp and release functions.

tetraplegia: Loss of movement in both arms and legs.

Clinical Summary

Etiology

Motor vehicle accidents (MVAs), sports injuries, acts of violence, diving injuries, falls, others (tumors, infection, and vascular accidents).

Prevalence

Mean age is 34.5 years. The male vs. female ratio is 4:1. Ethnicity is as follows: Caucasian (56.2%), African American (28.7%), and Hispanic (10.5%).

Classic Signs

There are 2 types: incomplete (some function below primary level of injury, may be able to move one limb or more, may feel body parts that cannot be moved) and complete (no function below injury level, no sensation, and no voluntary movement).

Level

C-1 to C-4	May be ventilator dependent, tetraplegia
C-5	Shoulder and bicep control, no wrist or hand function
C-6	Wrist control, no hand function
C-7 to T-1	Dexterity problems, can move upper extremities
T-1 to T-8	Poor trunk control, good UE function
T-9-T-12	Good trunk and abdominal muscle control

Precautions

Autonomic dysreflexia, thermal regulation, ROM restrictions, sensory losses, orthostatic hypotension, heterotrophic ossification, respiratory complications, spinal shock, and spasticity.

Chapter 19

A Telephone Repairman With Spinal Cord Injury

M. Laurita (Lita) Fike, MA, OTR; Karen Pendleton, MA, OTR;
and Liane Hewitt, MPH, OTR

Introduction

There are between 230,000 and 450,000 people living with SCI, or spinal cord injury, in the United States, and each year one-third to one-half of these people are hospitalized (Woodruff & Baron, 1994). Nearly 10,000 new SCIs occur every year, and while 10% to 15% of these patients are admitted to specialty SCI hospitals, the rest are treated at community rehabilitation facilities or general hospitals. Because of the complexity of this health condition, OT practitioners are highly likely to be involved in the care of people with SCI on both initial admission and subsequent readmissions (National Spinal Cord Injury Association [NSCIA], 1998).

Definition

The spinal cord, which is part of the CNS, is a band of motor and sensory nerves that travels through the vertebral canal, extending from the base of the brain to just below the waist. The nerves that exit from and return to the spinal cord through the spinal vertebrae carry neuronal information to and from the brain and various parts of the body. SCI refers to damage to the spinal cord that stops the information flow and results in a functional deficit (i.e., a loss of ability to move, to control bodily processes [such as respiration and control of bladder or bowel], or to feel sensation) (NSCIA, 1998).

Etiology

The National Spinal Cord Injury Statistical Center (NSCISC) (1998) reported that since 1991, the majority (35%) of SCIs result from MVAs. Acts of violence (gunshot or stabbing wounds) account for another 30.4%. The percentage due to violence has been steadily increasing, while the percentage due to MVAs is decreasing. Falls rank third in cause at 19.5%, although after age 45, falls account for nearly half of all SCIs. Sports injuries cause 8.9% of SCIs, and two-thirds of these are from diving injuries. Various other causes, including vascular accidents, tumors, and infectious diseases, account for 6.9% (Go, DeVivo, & Richards, 1995).

The specific SCIs derived from the causes include compression and hyperextension (stretch) cord injuries, fractures and dislocations of the vertebrae that crush or transect the cord, and penetration of the cord.

Prevalence

Data from the NSCISC (1998) suggest that, in addition to the numbers noted above, another 5,000 people suffer SCIs but die before they can be treated. SCI primarily affects young adults, with the mean age increasing since 1973, when it was 28.6 years. Since 1990, the mean age has been 34.5 years. Males outnumber females 4 to 1, and this has remained the same during the time such statistics have been collected (DeVivo, Richards, & Stover, 1991; Go et al., 1995).

Over the past 25 years, there has been a significant change in the ethnic distribution. In 1973, Caucasians accounted for 77.5% of SCI, African-Americans 13.5%, Hispanics 6%, and other ethnic minorities were 3%. But since 1990, the incidence of injuries among African-Americans has increased to 28.7%, and among Hispanics to 10.5%, while that among Caucasians has fallen to 56.2% (NSCISC, 1998).

Levels of Injury

SCIs are initially classified as complete or incomplete. In a complete injury, the damage prevents the passing of any neuronal information between the brain and various parts of the body. This indicates a total loss of movement and sensation. In an incomplete injury, some nerve pathways, either sensory or motor, may be preserved. However, incomplete injuries can also result in devastating functional losses. Three types of incomplete injuries are:

1. Central cord lesion—This occurs when the central portions of the cervical spinal cord are damaged; the patient usually has less functional return in the arms and upper body than in the legs.

2. Brown-Sequard lesion—In this type of injury, one-half of the cord is transected (hemisection); the patient loses postural stability, motor function on the same side as the lesion, and the ability to feel pain and temperature changes on the opposite side.

3. Anterior cord lesion—The anterior structures of the cord are injured, and the patient loses the ability to move below the level of the lesion. The patient also loses the ability to feel pain or temperature changes, but the senses of touch, proprioception, and vibration are preserved.

When the injury occurs to the spinal cord as it passes through spinal vertebrae in the neck, known as the cervical (C-1 to C-8) vertebrae, loss of function generally involves the respiratory system, the trunk, bowel, bladder, sexual function, and both the arms and the legs. This type of SCI has traditionally been called quadriplegia, but in the newer, international classification, it is termed tetraplegia, referring to involvement of all 4 limbs.

SCIs that occur through the thoracic (T-1 to T-12) vertebrae usually affect the chest and the legs. Damage to the spinal cord at the level of lumbar vertebrae causes loss of control of the legs, bowel, bladder, and sexual function. At the sacral level, there is some functional loss involving the legs, bowel, bladder, and sexual function. Injuries at the thoracic, lumbar, and sacral level are generally termed paraplegia, meaning involvement of the lower half of the body.

The SCI is normally described by referring to the first letter of the skeletal level (cervical, thoracic, lumbar, sacral) and the number of the most distal uninvolved segment of the spinal nerve segment with full function, for example, C-4 or T-3 (American Spinal Injury Association [ASIA], 1992).

Historically, the incidence of tetraplegia has been slightly higher than that of paraplegia, but current trends indicate that incomplete paraplegia is increasing, while complete tetraplegia is decreasing. Since 1991, the incidence of SCI by neurological category is as follows:

- Complete paraplegia—28.9%
- Incomplete tetraplegia—28.6%
- Incomplete paraplegia—21.8%
- Complete tetraplegia—18.4%

Approximately half of all SCI result in tetraplegia, but the proportion of tetraplegics increases dramatically after age 45, accounting for 66% of all injuries after age 60 and nearly 90% of all injuries after age 75. Further, 92% of all sports injuries result in tetraplegia. Most people who suffer SCI at or above C-3 still die at the time of the accident, and those who survive are usually ventilator dependent for life (DeVivo et al., 1991).

INITIAL MEDICAL AND REHABILITATIVE TREATMENT

Patients are generally admitted to the emergency room, where physical examination is followed by neurological examinations to determine the level of injury. Medications such as methylprednisolone, a steroid, are frequently given to reduce

swelling at the site of the injury; this is believed to reduce the severity of the damage to the spinal cord, particularly in cases of incomplete injury. The injured spine must be immediately stabilized, either surgically, with internal fixation, or with traction on bed frames designed to immobilize the patient. Patients with cervical injuries may require halo traction, which involves a metal band attached to the skull, held in place with metal rods affixed to a plastic body jacket. Patients with paraplegia may require only a plastic jacket or brace (Yarkony, 1994).

Patients with tetraplegia must also receive respiratory assistance; those with C-1 to C-3 lesions will require a ventilator. Patients are also catheterized. At least one-half of patients admitted to emergency rooms with SCIs also have other injuries, including brain injuries, and these injuries will be treated as well, with the patient usually moving to the intensive care unit. If the patient's spine is stabilized, rehabilitation generally starts within 48 hours of admission. After the patient's medical condition has normalized, the patient with SCI transfers to a rehabilitation unit or hospital, where inpatient treatment will last 1 to 3 months (Yarkony, 1994). In 1992, patients with tetraplegia averaged 95 hospital days, while those with paraplegia stayed an average 67 days. This is a significant reduction in hospital stay from 1973, when on average, tetraplegia treatment lasted 6 months, and paraplegia treatment lasted 3 months (NSCISC, 1998).

PROGNOSIS

According to the National Spinal Cord Injury Database (NSCISC, 1998), overall, 85% of SCI patients who survive the first 24 hours are still alive 10 years later. This is compared with the 10-year survival of 98% of the non-SCI population, given similar age and sex. Historically, the most frequent cause of death among people with SCI was renal failure. However, medical advances in urologic management have reduced the number of deaths due to this cause. The current most common causes of death include pneumonia, pulmonary emboli, and septicemia. An increasing number of people with SCI are now dying of unrelated causes, such as cancer or cardiovascular disease, which is similar to the general population.

Life expectancies for persons with SCI are increasing, but are still somewhat below those for people with no SCI. Mortality rates are significantly higher in the first year following injury than in subsequent years.

Almost all people with SCI return to private residences after rehabilitation; less than 6% go into nursing homes or to other hospitals. Those who go into nursing homes tend to be elderly or have very high cervical injuries with no resources for home care.

At the time of injury, more than half of patients age 16 to 59 are employed, while the rest are students, homemakers, or unemployed. Eight years after injury, about one-third of persons with paraplegia and one-fourth of persons with tetraplegia are employed. People who return to work within the first year of injury tend to return to work at the same job, for the same employer. Those who return to work after the first year either work for different employers or were students who found work.

The National Spinal Cord Injury Database has not yet evaluated the impact of the Americans with Disabilities Act on the reemployment of persons with SCI.

PRECAUTIONS AND COMPLICATIONS

SCI is a complex health problem because of the multiple systems affected. The OT practitioner must be aware of a large number of potential medical problems and must observe many precautions, during both the evaluation and the treatment stages of the patient's care.

Autonomic Dysreflexia

Autonomic dysreflexia is an autonomic nervous system disorder that can be triggered by a variety of stimuli and may result in dangerously high blood pressure. The patient may complain of a sudden headache; he or she may exhibit sudden sweating and reddening of the face, restless behavior, increased spasticity, or a sudden drop in pulse rate. This is a medical emergency and immediate intervention is required. The OT practitioner should bring the patient to a sitting position if he or she has been prone or supine in order to lower the cranial blood pressure. The urinary catheter and drainage bag should be checked to make sure that urine is flowing. If the catheter is clamped, it should be released. If the drainage bag is full, it should be emptied. Tight clothing should be loosened, and the OT practitioner should check for other sources of skin irritation, such as a clothing gather or cushion roughness. In the hospital, nursing personnel should be notified as quickly as possible; in community or home care, the home care nurse or the patient's physician should be contacted by phone for further directions in patient care (Jones, 1986; Hollar, 1989).

Range of Motion Restrictions

Patients with PROM past 90 degrees at the shoulder, nor should manual muscle testing or strengthening exercises be provided to the shoulder muscles until advised by the physician. The shoulder muscles affect movement of the cervical and thoracic spine, and this must be avoided until the spine is fully stabilized (Schneider, 2001).

Patients with lower tetraplegia are potentially able to use their arms and wrists for tasks requiring manual dexterity by taking advantage of natural tenodesis. When the wrist is extended, the fingers and thumbs assume a flexed position. When the wrist is flexed, the fingers extend. This motion can be used, with or without the assistance of a splint, to substitute for hand grasp and finger pinch tasks. It is important that wrist extensors and finger flexors be allowed to tighten in order to provide as much power as possible to the tenodesis grasp. Therefore, the OT practitioner must never extend the wrist and fingers at the same time, nor flex the wrist and fingers at the same time. ROM exercises for full flexion of the fingers should only be done with the wrist in extension, and for full extension of the fingers, with the wrist in flexion (Hill & Presperin, 1986).

Orthostatic Hypotension

An SCI not only affects the motor and sensory spinal nerves, but also the autonomic nervous system, which is responsible for regulating blood pressure in response to position changes. Patients with SCI usually have been immobilized in a supine or prone position to stabilize the spine, and when they first attempt to sit up, will experience sudden drops in blood pressure that may result in dizziness, nausea, and fainting. If the patient experiences these symptoms during treatment, the OT practitioner should recline the patient in bed or tip the wheelchair back to allow for increased cerebral blood flow. The OT practitioner should work with the patient and other health care providers to provide a consistent and slow introduction of moving the patient from bed-lying to sitting, until the patient develops adequate sitting tolerance (Kovich, 1986).

Respiratory Impairment

Patients with tetraplegia will experience respiratory difficulties due to paralysis of the phrenic nerve and diaphragm, and often require tracheostomy with assisted ventilation. Patients with C-1 to C-3 require permanent assisted respiration. Patients with tracheostomies often have difficulty in coughing to clear their respiratory passageways and will need suctioning at various times, including during OT treatment. The OT practitioner must be alert to signs of need for suctioning (such as an unproductive cough or rasping, congested sounds during respiration) and must either learn to perform suctioning as required or must contact the appropriate personnel in a timely manner (Daniel & Strickland, 1988).

Hypothermia and Hyperthermia

As in the case of orthostatic hypotension, patients with SCI may have impaired thermal control due to damage to the autonomic nervous system. They may have difficulty maintaining an even body temperature and must avoid prolonged exposure to heat and humidity and to moderate to severe cold. The OT environment should be mild, and exercise must be discontinued if air-conditioning is unavailable during hot and humid months. The OT practitioner must be alert for signs that the patient is suffering subnormal body temperature or is overheating, and contact nursing as appropriate for intervention (Hollar, 1989).

Sensory Losses

Patients with SCI will have sensory loss below the level of the lesion and are in danger of suffering pressure ulcers (decubiti) as well as other injuries to the skin. OT practitioners should observe standard precautions for sensory loss and should encourage patients to use vision to compensate for sensory loss.

During transfers and bed mobility, patients as well as their caregivers must avoid shearing stress or friction injuries to the skin by lifting the body away from surfaces, rather than sliding.

Patients should use a wheelchair cushion whenever seated for long periods of time, including when out of the wheelchair.

They should also perform weight shifts every 15 to 20 minutes throughout the day in order to relieve pressure.

While in bed, patients should reposition every 2 hours, unless on an alternating pressure mattress or other pressure reduction device.

Patients should also inspect their skin daily for evidence of pressure injuries, using a curved handle mirror to inspect the buttocks. The stages of pressure injury development are as follows:

- Stage I—The skin is intact but stays reddened for over 20 minutes after the pressure is relieved. The reddened area is often warm to touch. At this level of injury, the treatment is primarily prevention of further injury by increasing the amount of cushioning, by removing the irritant causing the pressure, or by increasing the number of weight shifts and repositioning periods.
- Stage II—The skin is broken, but the injury is confined to superficial areas. Treatment consists of removing the pressure until the skin heals completely. This means if the buttocks area is involved, the patient must not sit, and must be positioned in prone or side-lying at all times.
- Stage III—The pressure wound has extended into deeper levels of the skin.
- Stage IV—The wound area has extended into the level of muscles.

Treatment at stages III and IV typically requires surgical debridement and may require grafting. Again, until the area has healed, the patient must not put any pressure on the wound site. Decubitus ulcers can be life threatening if infection develops, and the cost of surgical care and hospitalization is staggering (Garber, 1985; Garber & Krouskop, 1982).

Heterotopic Ossification

This condition involves abnormal calcification around joints, usually the elbows or knees, but may also involve hips and shoulders. Symptoms include swelling and redness, as well as limitations in joint ROM. Above the level of the lesion, the patient may also experience pain or tenderness. OT practitioners should report the symptoms to the patient's physician (Kovich, 1986).

Spinal Shock and Spasticity

Immediately after the SCI, the patient experiences flaccid paralysis, which may last for days, weeks, or months. However, once the spinal shock is reduced, the patient at T-12 or above may experience mild to moderate spasticity caused by the reflexive motor synapse through the spinal cord. Muscle relaxing medications are often very effective in relieving spasticity. However, the OT practitioner must assist the patient in managing spasticity to increase the patient's functional independence. Spasticity in the hips and legs, for example, can be triggered deliberately by patients to assist in lower extremity dressing. However, it can also cause problems during transfers. The OT practitioner must teach the patient to use positioning and other techniques to inhibit spasticity. In addition, the patient must do regular ROM exercises to prevent contractures (Hollar, 1995).

EVALUATION

After initial stabilization, all members of the treatment team will evaluate the patient. Initial OT evaluations could include observation, interview, and a variety of assessments that are generally based on areas of occupation and performance skills. These tests are most often completed by the OT. Qualified OTAs may contribute to the evaluation by gathering data, particularly in such areas as dynamometer and pinch strength tests and dexterity tests such as the 9-hole-peg test (Daniel & Strickland, 1988).

The OT practitioner also evaluates occupational performance to the extent that is possible with patients who have suffered such catastrophic functional losses. Patients with paraplegia will be evaluated regarding their ability to perform BADL. Some tasks, such as washing the face, brushing teeth, combing hair, shaving, and self-feeding, will be accomplished by these patients with little difficulty once they are able to assume a full sitting position. While prone or supine for spinal stabilization, however, patients with paraplegia may need equipment positioned for them in order to be independent in these tasks. Other BADL, such as toileting, bathing, and lower extremity dressing, will require both adaptive techniques and special equipment in order for the patient to become independent. Training in these areas will begin once the patient is able to tolerate sitting for 2 to 4 hours.

Patients with tetraplegia will be unable to do most BADL without training in the use of special equipment or adaptive techniques. For lower level tetraplegia, the use of a universal cuff around the palm of the hand may permit self-feeding and facial hygiene after equipment set-up. High-level tetraplegics will be dependent in most BADL, even with adaptive equipment. Therefore, evaluation of BADL is generally deferred until sitting tolerance is achieved and initial treatment for strengthening has begun. Either OTs or OTAs may conduct BADL evaluations.

After the patient with SCI has achieved sitting tolerance and initial treatment has begun, OT practitioners will also gather information regarding the patient's education and vocational history, avocational interests, psychological adaptation to the injury, and personal goals. OTAs will often conduct these assessments in consultation with their supervising therapist.

During ongoing treatment and prior to discharge, patients will participate in assessment of their IADL. These usually involve assessments regarding mobility needs, including manual and/or powered wheelchairs, home care and safety, environmental accessibility, and driving assessments. OTAs may contribute to these assessments by gathering measurement data and by specific communication with the patient and the patient's family, such as filling out questionnaires and drawing floor plans with them. Patients are often referred to community resources for driving assessments and training.

OTs and OTAs should work together with the patient to develop an individualized treatment plan based on the patient's goals and the results of the various evaluations (Daniel & Strickland, 1988; Farmer, 1986; Hollar, 1995).

CASE STUDY

Assessments

John R. is a 24-year-old, right-dominant Mexican-American who was working for the local telephone company when he fell and sustained a C-6 fracture. He was admitted to the county general hospital, where his medical condition was stabilized and he was placed in head tongs with traction in a suspension bed for 2 weeks. In the suspension bed, John's position was changed from supine to prone every 2 hours to relieve skin pressure. During this time, he was referred to the general rehabilitation services in the acute care wing of the hospital. His OT team consisted of an OT and an OTA. Because John was in traction and confined to bed, the initial activities of assessment of sitting tolerance and skin integrity and prescription of wheelchair were deferred. Instead, while John was in the supine position, the OT assessed John's hand, wrist, and elbow ROM and sensation. She then fitted John with a universal cuff for his right hand, which had good wrist extension and pronation. She also adapted and applied a wrist-driven orthosis to his left hand, which was weaker than his right.

At the next session, John was in the prone position, and he was able to move his arms freely below the bed. The OTA was then able to assess his ability to wash his face, brush his teeth with a toothbrush in the universal cuff, and feed himself a snack of finger foods using both hands. The OTA also took an occupational history, helped John fill out a leisure interest list, and discussed his goals for therapy. Based on these initial assessments, and a review of the assessments by the physician and the rest of the team, the 2 OT practitioners felt they had enough information to design an early intervention program for John.

Frames of Reference

The CNS, of which the spinal cord is a part, does not regenerate, and although many scientists are engaged in research to develop methods to encourage regeneration, at this time there is no cure for SCI. This means that health care providers have no methods to directly restore the motor and sensory functions that are lost when the spinal cord is transected. Treatment therefore consists of methods to enhance and increase remaining functions, which is considered a biomechanical treatment approach, and methods to provide substitutions for abilities that have been permanently lost, known as the rehabilitative treatment approach (Hollar, 1989).

In the OT intervention for SCI, the OT practitioner focuses on occupational performance and generally utilizes the biomechanical and rehabilitative approaches simultaneously. However, to simplify discussion, these methods will be presented separately.

The biomechanical approach (remedial/restorative) includes activities and exercises that target occupational performance subcomponents. For example, intervention may involve training or instructions designed to increase muscle strength, improve or prevent loss of joint ROM, increase endurance for daily activities, enhance dexterity and manipulative skills, and

prevent loss of skin integrity. In most instances, the therapeutic goal will only be achieved through repetition and practice. The skill of the OT practitioner is required to provide intervention that will motivate and satisfy the patient despite the occasional monotony of repetition (Hollar, 1989).

The rehabilitative approach (compensatory/modify) consists of teaching alternative methods for achieving satisfactory occupational performance (e.g., teaching a patient to transfer to the toilet from a wheelchair) and providing equipment that will assist the patient in accomplishing tasks that he or she can no longer do without assistance (e.g., a wheelchair may provide the patient with mobility). Although most of the compensatory techniques and equipment provided to people with SCI are readily identified, the OT practitioner may need to be creative in obtaining equipment and modifying techniques to benefit the specific needs of the patient (Hollar, 1989). Table 19-1 presents intervention strategies based on occupational performance and performance components at the various levels of SCI and has been compiled using information from Daniel and Strickland (1988); Hill (1986a); Adler (2001); Hollar (1989); and Wilson, McKenzie, Barber, and Watson (1984).

Intervention Programming

Intervention for patients with SCI can be effectively carried out in both individual and group settings. During individual treatment, the OT practitioner usually works on goal setting and goal revision, personal hygiene and dressing skills, equipment measurement and fabrication, and patient and family teaching. An early morning care program is particularly useful for practicing BADL skills, such as bathing, dressing, and bowel and bladder care, at realistic times. Some hospitals have also developed late evening care programs, often involving family members, focus on undressing, personal hygiene, and preparation for bed, including positioning and padding to prevent pressure sores. These programs are often organized and staffed by OTAs (Hollar, 1995).

Early Intervention Programming

John is a young, single male diagnosed with a C-6 lesion resulting from an injury at work. John had told the OTA he wanted to be as independent as possible in taking care of himself. The OT and OTA decided to use both the biomechanical and rehabilitative approaches, working to increase John's endurance and upper extremity strength while providing him with the adaptive equipment he needed to substitute for weak hand function. The OTA worked with John on early morning self-care and self-feeding, using the universal cuff, wrist orthosis, and utensils with built-up handles. Because John had also expressed an interest in woodworking, the OTA also started John on a small bird house kit, which required sanding and painting; she increased the length of time John worked on his project as his endurance improved. At the end of the 2 weeks, when the traction was removed and he was placed in a body jacket with a head brace, John was able to feed himself independently in the prone position after set-up. He was also able to wash his face, brush his teeth, comb his hair, and work at his

Table 19-1

Intervention Approaches for Patients With Spinal Cord Injury, Based on Level of Injury

SCI Level with Muscles and Movements Available	Areas of Occupation	Biomechanical Intervention (Remedial/Restorative)	Rehabilitative Intervention and Equipment Needed (Compensatory/Modify)
C-1 to C-3 Head and neck muscles innervated by cranial nerves Patient can talk, chew, swallow, blow	Dependent for respiration BADL: Directs others for all self-care IADL: Can use environmental control unit to move bed, turn on TV, answer phone, open doors Directs others for all other IADL Mobility: Can use power wheelchair control led by sip and puff or head motion Communication: Word processing by electronic typewriter or computer Can use speakerphone with automatic dial Leisure: Can play computer and electronic games, use mouth stick for art activities, read using page turner Work: Operate computer, phone services by voice only	Joint ROM to all joints once spine is stabilized Increase sitting tolerance and increase general endurance by increasing length of time patient sits and engages in activities. Monitor for fatigue; observe precautions for hypotension and skin pressure Identify available muscles; provide manual resistance to help strengthen head, neck, and facial muscles Work to improve strength in blowing, in rhythm with respirator Provide activities involving use of mouth stick and/or head pointer to increase strength and endurance	Requires ventilator at all times Head support needed during prolonged sitting Education must be provided to patient regarding directing own care, including the selection and training of own attendants in future The involvement of family and friends in the educational process is also important Patient must receive training in use of all equipment, including instructing others in set-up Environmental control unit (ECU) operated by computer, mouth stick, head pointer, head switch, or tongue switch Power wheelchair with tilt and recline for pressure control, for inside use. Requires supervision for outside use Computer or word processor with switches operated by mouth stick (requires maximal assistance) or head pointer, head switch, or tongue switch (requires set-up and minimal assist)
C-4 Diaphragm and trapezius Patient often has independent respiration; has scapular elevation	BADL: Can drink independently after set-up with long straw Directs others for all self-care IADL: Can use environmental control unit to move bed, turn on TV, answer phone, open doors	All interventions as for C-1 to C-3 Provide manual resistance to trapezius, to increase strength/mobility of neck Provide respiratory exercises in conjunction with respiratory and physical therapy to increase strength and endurance of diaphragm	May increase level of independence similar to C-5 if using externally powered flexor hinge splint and electric mobile arm support, but this is expensive and uncommon Equipment needs similar to C-1 to C-3, but can operate chin controls, has better neck

(continued)

Table 19-1 (continued)

Intervention Approaches for Patients with Spinal Cord Injury, Based on Level of Injury

SCI Level with Muscles and Movements Available	Areas of Occupation	Biomechanical Intervention (Remedial/Restorative)	Rehabilitative Intervention and Equipment Needed (Compensatory/Modify)
C-4	Directs others for all other IADL Mobility: Can use power wheelchair control led by sip and puff, chin control, or head switch Communication: Word processing by electronic typewriter or computer Can use speakerphone with automatic dial Leisure: Can play computer and electronic games, use mouth stick for art activities, read using page-turner Work: Operate computer, phone services; can use mouth stick to operate other equipment, such as tape recorder, adding machine		control and endurance, and can use mouth stick for long periods Needs mouth stick holder As for C-1 to C-3, education must be provided to patient regarding directing own care, including the selection and training of own attendants in future Patient must receive training in use of all equipment, including instructing others in set-up Office or school equipment may need minor modifications to operate by mouth stick
C-5 Infraspinatus and deltoid, biceps brachialis, brachioradialis, supinator Patient has shoulder abduction to 80 to 90 degrees, external rotation; elbow flexion and supination; use of gravity can substitute for shoulder adduction, internal rotation, and pronation	BADL: Patient can feed self, do facial hygiene and make-up, and can assist with dressing and bathing after set-up, with use of adaptive equipment IADL: Can use hand controls to move bed, turn on TV, answer phone, open doors, and operate other equipment such as electric lifts. Directs others for all other IADL Mobility: Need power wheelchair for long distances. Can use manual chair with quad pegs for short distances Communication: Word processing by electronic typewriter or computer and phone using typing stick or orthosis	Joint ROM to all joints once spine is stabilized Increase sitting tolerance and increase general endurance, increasing length of time patient sits up and engages in activities. Monitor for fatigue; observe precautions for hypotension and skin pressure Provide activities and exercises that will increase strength of shoulder and elbow muscles in all available ranges. Practice activities in which patient uses gravity to accomplish full range Provide activities that will increase patient's dexterity in use of orthosis and typing sticks, particularly to increase typing speed	Equipment needs for BADL include mobile arm support, wrist orthosis, and universal cuff for utensils, toothbrush, comb; plate guard; long drinking straw; Dycem to stabilize plate and glass; long-handled bath sponge Requires joystick-controlled power wheelchair with tilt and recline for pressure relief Needs manual wheelchair, can operate for short distances using quad pegs on wheels Requires gel or air cushion Needs adaptation for orthosis or cuff to utilize typing stick May need adaptations to operate equipment if it requires holding down several keys at one time

(continued)

Table 19-1 (continued)

Intervention Approaches for Patients with Spinal Cord Injury, Based on Level of Injury

SCI Level with Muscles and Movements Available	Areas of Occupation	Biomechanical Intervention (Remedial/Restorative)	Rehabilitative Intervention and Equipment Needed (Compensatory/Modify)
C-5	Leisure: Can play computer and electronic games, use orthosis for art activities, read using page-turner Work: Operate computer, phone services; can use orthosis to operate other equipment, such as tape recorder, adding machine		As for the above SCI patients, education must be provided to patient regarding directing own care, including the selection and training of own attendants in future Patient must receive training in use of all equipment, including instructing others in set-up
C-6 Pectoralis major, serratus anterior, lattisimus dorsi, pronator teres, radial wrist extensors Patient can flex shoulder and reach forward; additional movements include shoulder internal rotation, extension, and adduction, and pronation and extension of the wrist—this provides the patient with tenodesis grasp, a major increase in function	BADL: Can feed self, do facial and hair grooming using tenodesis grasp, although may also use universal cuff for some activities. Wrist-driven hinge orthosis (WHO) is also used at this level, giving more power and control to the tenodesis grasp. Can bathe self using tub bench and long shower hose. Dressing can be done independently with modified techniques Bowel and Bladder Care: Can insert suppositories for bowel program using adaptive device. Can transfer independently to toilet. Can empty own catheter bag and clamp. Requires assistance for intermittent catheterization IADL: Can operate TV, radio, phone, typewriter, computer using tenodesis grasp, or orthosis, and typing stick. Can do light housekeeping and cooking. Needs wheelchair accessible kitchen Mobility: Can use manual wheelchair for short distances. May need power wheelchair for long distances. Can drive car using hand controls and adapted steering wheel	Joint ROM to all joints once spine is stabilized. Major precaution: preserve tenodesis grasp as noted before Increase sitting tolerance and increase general endurance by increasing length of time patient sits up and engages in activities. Monitor for fatigue; observe precautions for hypotension and skin pressure Provide activities and exercises that will increase the strength of shoulder, elbow, and wrist muscles in all available ranges, noting particularly the position of fingers during tenodesis. Will need to increase endurance for operating manual wheelchair Provide activities to increase patient's dexterity in donning and doffing clothing, any orthosis, and use of typing sticks, particularly to increase typing speed and ease of equipment operation	May use universal cuff, or WHO for BADL and IADL Some equipment may need enlarged handles. Rocker knife may be useful. Will need tub bench and long shower hose, and equipment for bowel and bladder programs Will need training in adapted techniques for dressing Can use manual wheelchair, but may need power wheelchair for long distances. Will need training in independent side-to-side weight shifts for pressure relief, and use of sliding board for transfers Will need special driver's education for operating an adapted motor vehicle May need assistance in acquiring car adaptations

(continued)

Table 19-1 (continued)

Intervention Approaches for Patients with Spinal Cord Injury, Based on Level of Injury

SCI Level with Muscles and Movements Available	Areas of Occupation	Biomechanical Intervention (Remedial/Restorative)	Rehabilitative Intervention and Equipment Needed (Compensatory/Modify)
C-6	Leisure: Can play table games, such as cards, table tennis with some adaptations. Can participate in some wheelchair sports Work: Can operate very light-weight hand tools, computers, office equipment; can perform desk and phone jobs		
C-7 Triceps, extrinsic finger extensors, flexor carpi radialis Patient can now do elbow extension and can actively extend fingers, as well as flex wrist	In general, the patient with C-7 SCI functions much as the C-6, except most occupational performances are easier. At the C-7 level the patient can do a push-up transfer and weight shift because of the triceps. Primary mobility is with a manual wheelchair	Biomechanical intervention is much the same as for C-6, with emphasis on strengthening the additional muscles and increasing endurance of operation of manual wheelchair	May need wrist splint for self-feeding or no adaptations. Will need training as above for dressing. Needs equipment for management of bowel and bladder Requires manual wheelchair and training in push-up weight shifts for pressure relief and push-up transfers Will need special driver's education for operating an adapted motor vehicle. May need assistance in acquiring car adaptations
C-8, T-1 (T-2,3,4) Intrinsics, including thumb, extrinsic finger flexors and thumb flexors, extrinsic thumb extensor, ulnar wrist flexors and extensors Patients at this level have upper extremity control with fine motor and prehension	BADL and IADL are similar to C-7, but are easier. Patient is able to dress from a sitting position	Similar to C-7	Independent in upper extremity tasks without orthosis, including management of bowel and bladder. Requires manual wheelchair and needs special driver's education for operating an adapted motor vehicle. May need assistance in acquiring car adaptations
T-5 to T-11 Intercostals begin to come in, as well as long muscles of the back Patients at these levels are beginning to establish functional trunk control in sitting; they are able to lean forward without using upper extremity. Limited ambulation with long leg braces may be possible	Independent in most BADL and IADL. Can stand with assistance and do moderately heavy work while seated. Endurance is increased due to better respiratory reserve	Aggressive strengthening to upper extremities and trunk. Work at standing table with leg braces to increase overall endurance	Independent in self-care and home-care from wheelchair. Requires manual wheelchair since ambulation is still difficult. Will need hand controls for motor vehicle

(continued)

Table 19-1 (continued)

Intervention Approaches for Patients with Spinal Cord Injury, Based on Level of Injury

SCI Level with Muscles and Movements Available	Areas of Occupation	Biomechanical Intervention (Remedial/Restorative)	Rehabilitative Intervention and Equipment Needed (Compensatory/Modify)
T-12, and lower Full function of intercostals and abdominal muscles At L-4, low back muscles, hip flexors, and quadriceps come in Patients at these levels have full trunk control, more endurance, and increasingly easier ambulation with long leg braces and crutches	Similar to T-5, 6. Has better endurance, can use outdoor lawn and recreation equipment, such as rider mower or snow mobile with hand controls	Aggressive strengthening for all available muscle groups. At L-4, standing and ambulating during IADL will be useful in increasing both leg strength and endurance	At the higher levels, patients will still need manual wheelchair for long distances and for convenience. May or may not need hand controls in motor vehicle at L-4. Still lacks voluntary control of bowel and bladder

project for 2 hours daily without fatigue. At this time, his OT team measured him for a hospital wheelchair and cushion and started his sitting program. Within 2 days, John was able to sit up in the wheelchair for 2 hours without symptoms. He was then transferred to the rehabilitation unit, where he was reassessed by his new OT treatment team.

In spinal injury rehabilitation settings, group treatment can be very effective because patients are able to see each other at various stages of rehabilitation. Patients can help one another problem solve and provide emotional support for each other (Fike, 1984). Typical groups might include a leisure interest group, in which crafts and games are used not only to develop avocational interests, but also to develop strength and endurance. For example, mouth stick drawing, painting, ceramic glazing, and computer games help develop strength of head and neck muscles and sitting endurance, as well as manipulative skills of the mouth and tongue. For patients with paraplegia, leatherwork and light woodworking can help develop upper extremity strength, as well as provide opportunities for the patient to work on weight shifting and trunk balance (Hollar, 1995).

Lunch groups offer patients the opportunity to practice self-feeding skills, including the use of adapted equipment. Home skills groups involve cooking and other light housekeeping skills; for patients with tetraplegia, these groups offer the opportunity for decision making and supervision of others in carrying out tasks for them. Some institutions offer "mat classes," in which patients with C-6 and lower level injuries can practice putting on outer clothing, such as slacks, shirts, and shoes. Community integration groups assist patients in making the transition from hospital to home, including the use of public transportation and management of architectural barriers (Hill, 1986a).

Transitional Intervention Programming

Upon transfer to the rehabilitation unit, John found himself surrounded by other patients with SCIs, amputations, strokes, and head injuries. This was initially surprising to John, but he continued to state he wanted to be as independent as possible. The physical therapy department, with consultation from the OT team, had ordered a wheelchair for John, but he would use the hospital chair until his own arrived. The OT team fitted his chair with a tray and worked with him until he could remove and attach it himself. He was expected to join other patients in the lounge for meals, where he became increasingly independent, working with the OTA to apply his own adaptive equipment, select his food from the cafeteria line, and bring it to the table using a wheelchair tray. He also joined 2 groups run by OTAs, one in the morning, a mat class that worked on self-dressing skills with 3 other patients who had SCIs, and an afternoon home-care group, that worked on meal preparation, laundry, and housekeeping tasks as they would need to be done from a wheelchair. Since John lived by himself in an apartment, he needed to learn to use standard equipment as much as possible, so he had his treatment program in an unmodified kitchen area. Fortunately for John, his incomplete injury was proving to have spared some peripheral neurons; his right hand functioned at the C-7 to C-8 level, while his left remained at the original diagnostic level of C-6. John was therefore able to develop more independence than might be expected for a complete C-6 injury. For example, he proved to have good trunk balance and was able to completely dress himself, transfer to his wheelchair, and manually push his wheelchair using regular rims rather than quad-pegs. Two nights a week John also participated in community reintegration groups supervised by OTAs, in which the patients arranged for their own public transportation with modified vans and attended local community events such as baseball games.

Even in community hospitals, it is effective to work with patients who have spinal injuries in mixed diagnosis groups and not just from the necessity imposed by pressures from health maintenance organizations. The motivation, psychological support, and assistance in problem-solving that group members offer each other should not be underestimated (Fike, 1984).

From the beginning of the patient's admission to rehabilitation services, intervention must be coordinated with the treatment team members. This includes not only the doctor, nurses, physical therapists, and others involved in the patient's care, but also the patient and the patient's designated family members. Care must be taken to schedule services so that the patient is challenged, but not overwhelmed or overfatigued. The patient and family must be involved in setting goals and should be kept informed at all times of changes in program or treatment.

When the team anticipates discharge, a plan should be established to help the patient make the transition, including short-term visits to the anticipated home setting. This provides the patient with opportunities to try his or her new skills in a realistic setting and to build self-confidence. When the patient returns to the hospital, any encountered difficulties can be the focus of the final sessions of treatment. It may also be important to assist the patient in contacting the state department of vocational services for possible assistance in returning to school, occupational training, or previous work settings (Hill, 1986b).

Planning for Discharge

Since John had been injured on the job, his medical and rehabilitation expenses were being covered by workers' compensation. The representative from the workers' compensation board met with the treatment team and John early in his intervention program to begin planning for discharge. John's apartment was on the third floor, but his building had an elevator and was wheelchair accessible. John was given a weekend pass, in which he returned to his apartment, accompanied by a friend. There John tried out the skills he had been working on in the hospital and returned on Monday with a list of accomplishments and challenges. The OT team worked with John to overcome the problems he had found at home by suggesting ways he could modify his environment and by helping him select adaptive equipment for his home. The workers' compensation representative also met with John's employer, the public telephone company. John would not be able to return as a lineman, but other jobs were available within the company that involved deskwork, including customer representative and operator. The OT met with the personnel director of the telephone company to obtain various job descriptions. Then she, the OTA, and John established prevocational goals, including increasing fine motor skills and more efficient operation of computers and calculators. John was able to use departmental equipment to work on his goals while hospitalized.

Psychological and Cognitive Implications

Throughout the treatment program, the cognitive and emotional needs of the patient must be considered and addressed.

SCI is a massive trauma to the neurological system, and a certain percentage have simultaneous brain injuries. These dual injuries may cause changes in the cognitive status of the patient, necessitating modifications in training and rehabilitation, similar to programs developed for patients with TBIs (Brown, 1992; Hollar, 1995).

Paralysis, dependence on ventilators, loss of mobility, loss of bowel and bladder control, and changes in sexual function can all result in massive disturbances to the patient's self-image, to self-esteem, and to occupational role effectiveness. The intervention program must be designed to incorporate methods that will address these needs, as well as the physical and functional problems (Jordan, Wellborn, Kovnick, & Salzstein, 1991). The use of group treatment to provide group support and the OT practitioner's skillful use of active listening and interpersonal skills may be effective in designing a holistic treatment program for patients with SCI (Fike, 1984).

Providing Group Support

Early in John's rehabilitation program, he had difficulty discussing personal or private issues with either of his 2 female OT practitioners. He avoided eye contact when discussing bowel and bladder concerns and became extremely embarrassed when the topic of sexuality was discussed. John had broken up with his long-time girlfriend just 2 weeks before his injury. He had one brother who visited him regularly, but the rest of his family was in Mexico. Several friends also visited and attended his therapy and some of the recreational events with him. The OTA in charge of the evening recreational program decided to ask a male social worker to be a guest speaker one evening to discuss sexuality following SCI or other traumatic injuries. John's brother and a friend attended, as did several other patients and their family members. As the group began to ask questions and discuss their concerns, John gradually joined the discussion. At the following OT sessions, John was then able to ask for specific information regarding sexual activity, which the OTA was able to provide in a matter-of-fact manner using materials from the departmental resource library. While nursing had taken care of his bowel program and catheterization, John also wanted to be more independent in this area. Since these topics had come up during the group discussion, John now felt comfortable asking the OTA about equipment for these personal needs. He was able to use the equipment in the privacy of his room and report back on his progress. John was discharged at the end of 4 weeks on the rehabilitation unit, approximately 6 weeks after his injury. His plans included on-the-job training as a service representative at the phone company. He was independent in his BADL and IADL and in using public transportation. His one, unmet goal was driver education, and this was to be arranged on an outpatient basis.

Follow-Up and Chronic Care Needs

Patients with SCI may be followed as outpatients for several months to 2 years, and some may continue to show improvements in strength, endurance, and self-care skills during this time (Yarkony, Roth, Heinemann, Lovell, & Wu, 1988). Other patients may be involved in prevocational or vocational training or may return for additional training in orthotics use or use of other equipment. Some research has suggested that OTs tend to supply patients with more equipment than is actually used by patients after discharge. Therefore, equipment needs should periodically reassessed (Garber & Gregorio, 1985).

Some patients will return for tendon transfers to improve grasp, although this surgery is not as common as it has been in the past. Those patients who do choose to have tendon transfers will need training to learn to use the transferred muscles in new ways (Hollar, 1995).

Despite maintaining appropriate routines in self-care, patients with SCI are susceptible to respiratory infections, urinary tract and kidney infections, and the development of skin breakdown. Patients with SCI may also develop contractures and may lose function due to increases in spasticity. Rehospitalization is common (NSCISC, 1998). On these occasions, the OT practitioner may take advantage of the opportunity to make modifications in equipment or self-care techniques or to provide other intervention as indicated by evaluation.

As improvements in medical care have increased the survival rate of patients with SCI, there has also been an increase in the numbers of elderly people with SCI. As this population ages, they will experience the normal decrease in strength, endurance, and physical fitness, as well as such age-associated problems as joint degeneration and skin fragility (Yarkony, Roth, Heinemann, & Lovell, 1988). During rehospitalization, changes in status due to aging should be considered at these times, with appropriate modifications in equipment and adaptive techniques.

CASE STUDY: FOLLOW-UP CARE

John returned for driver education and driver training using a modified sedan, which he accomplished in 1 month. John owned a relatively new car, a 4-door Ford. Since he already had a job lined up, the Department of Vocational Services was willing to modify the vehicle by purchasing and fitting the car with hand controls. The department also modified the car to accommodate a roof-based lift system that electrically lifted John's wheelchair to the roof of his car and stored it under a plastic cover. John returned to the rehabilitation unit every 6 months for 2 years. During that time he had no incidences of skin breakdown, no respiratory problems, and he remained independent in his self-care. After 2 years, John returned to Mexico to be closer to his family and was lost to further follow-up.

CLINICAL PROBLEM SOLVING

1. Review the real records section and consider a mother of 2 young children who has an injury similar to John's, or an elderly man with a T1 injury.
2. How might group treatment enhance the therapy program for patients with SCI?
3. What problems may these patients with SCI experience after discharge?

LEARNING ACTIVITIES

1. Interview a person with SCI and ask about community mobility issues that are frustrating for the person. Visit these areas to assess for barriers. Write a letter to the landowner to advocate for changes.
2. Interview an OT or OTA who specializes in SCI. Ask probing questions on how they manage the psychosocial and sexual issues of SCI.
3. Make a summary sheet or study cards for the different levels of SCI and the functional impairments. Use this study tool before the NBCOT exam.

REFERENCES

Adler, C. (2001). Spinal cord injury. In L. W. Pedretti (Ed.), OT: Practice skills for physical dysfunction (5th ed.). St. Louis, MO: Mosby-Year Book.

American Spinal Injury Association. (1992). Standards for neurologic classification of spinal injury patients. Atlanta, GA: Author.

Ballinger, D. A., Rintala, D. H., & Hart, K. A. (2000). The relation of shoulder pain and range of motion problems to functional limitations, disability and perceived health of men with spinal cord injury: A multifaceted longitudinal study. Archives of Physical Medicine and Rehabilitation, 81(12), 1575-1581.

Boschen, K., Tonack, M., & Gargaro, J. (2003). Long-term adjustment and community reintegration following spinal cord injury. International Journal of Rehabilitation Research, 26(3), 157-164.

Brown, D. J. (1992). Spinal cord injury: The last decade and the next. Paraplegia, 30, 77-82.

Bushnik, T. (2002). Access to equipment, participation, and quality of life in aging individuals with high tetraplegia (C1-C4). Topics in Spinal Cord Rehabilitation, 7(3), 17-27.

Craig, A., Moses, P., Tran, Y., Kirkup, L., & McIsaac, P. (2002). The effectiveness of a hands-free environmental control system for the profoundly disabled. Archives of Physical Medicine and Rehabilitation, 83(10), 1455-1458.

Daniel, M. S., & Strickland, R. L. (1988). OT protocol: Management in adult physical dysfunction. Rockville, MD: Aspen Publishers.

DeVivo, M. J., Richards, J. S., & Stover, S. L. (1991). Spinal cord injury: Rehabilitation adds life to years. Western Journal of Medicine, 154, 602-606.

Farmer, A. R. (1986). Evaluation. In J. P. Hill (Ed.), Spinal cord injury: A guide to functional outcomes in OT (pp. 7-18). Rockville, MD: Aspen Publishers.

Fike, M. L. (1984). The role of OT in psychological rehabilitation of the physically disabled. In D. W. Kruger (Ed.), Rehabilitation psychology (p. 221). Rockville, MD: Aspen Publishers.

Garber, S. (1985). Wheelchair cushions for spinal cord individuals. American Journal of Occupational Therapy, 39, 722-725.

Garber, S., & Gregorio, T. (1985). Upper extremity assistive devices: Assessment of use by spinal-cord injured patients with quadriplegia. American Journal of Occupational Therapy, 44(2), 126-131.

Garber, S., & Krouskop, T. (1982). Body build and its relationship to pressure distribution in the seated wheelchair patient. Archives of Physical Medicine & Rehabilitation, 63, 17-20.

EVIDENCE-BASED TREATMENT STRATEGIES

Treatment Strategies	Authors
Upper extremity function	Ballinger, Rintala, & Hart, 2000; Gronley et al., 2000; James, Khapchik, & O'Dell, 2000; Wise, Ellis, & Trunnell, 2002
Technology	Bushnik, 2002; Craig, Moses, Tran, Kirkup, & McIsaac, 2002; Garber & Gregorio, 1985; Pell, Gillies, & Carss, 1999
ADL	Boschen, Tonack, & Gargaro, 2003; Bushnik, 2002; Pentland, Harvey, & Walker, 1998; Schönherr, Groothoff, Mulder, & Eisma, 2000; Scivoletto, Morganti, Ditunno, Ditunno, & Molinari, 2003; Sumida et al., 2001
Environment	Bushnik, 2002; Noreau, Fougeyrollas, & Boschen, 2002; Pentland et al., 2003; Thapar et al., 2004
Collaboration in treatment	Leary & Mardirossian, 2000; Ray, 1998; Schönherr et al., 2000; Toto & Hill, 2001
Psychosocial considerations	Boschen et al., 2003; Mulcahey, 1992; Murphy, Young, Brown, & King, 2003; Noreau et al., 2002

Go, B. K., DeVivo, M. J., & Richards, J. S. (1995). The epidemiology of spinal card injury. In S. L. Stover, J. A. DeLisa, & G. G. Whiteneck (Eds.), *Spinal cord injury: Clinical outcomes from the model systems* (pp. 21-55). Gaithersburg, MD: Aspen Publishers.

Gronley, J., Newsam, C., Mulroy, S., Rao, S., Perry, J., & Helm, M. (2000). Electromyographic and kinematic analysis of the shoulder during four activities of daily living in men with C6 tetraplegia. *Journal of Rehabilitation Research and Development, 37*(4), 423.

Hill, J. P. (1986b). Putting it all together: Discharge planning. In J. P. Hill (Ed.), *Spinal cord injury: A guide to functional outcomes in OT* (pp. 225-228). Rockville, MD: Aspen Publishers.

Hill, J. P. (1986a). *Spinal cord injury: A guide to functional outcomes in OT* (pp. 225-228). Rockville, MD: Aspen Publishers.

Hill, J. P., & Presperin, J. (1986). Deformity control. In J. P. Hill (Ed.), *Spinal cord injury: A guide to functional outcomes in OT* (pp. 49-86). Rockville, MD: Aspen Publishers.

Hollar, L. D. (1995.) Spinal cord injury. In C. A. Trombly (Ed.), *OT for physical dysfunction* (4th ed.). Baltimore, MD: Williams & Wilkins.

James, M., Khapchik, V., & O'Dell, M. (2000). Restoration of elbow extension in tetraplegia: Posterior deltoid to triceps transfer when the deltoid is partially paralyzed. *Topics in Spinal Cord Injury Rehabilitation, 6*(Suppl.), 213-214.

Jones, R. (1986). Bladder and bowel management. In J. P. Hill (Ed.), *Spinal cord injury: A guide to functional outcomes in OT* (pp. 145-168). Rockville, MD: Aspen Publishers.

Jordan, S. A., Wellborn, W. R. III, Kovnick, J., & Salzstein, R. (1991). Understanding and treating motivation difficulties in ventilator-dependent SCI patients. *Paraplegia, 29*(7), 431-442.

Kovich, K. (1986). Related disorders. In J. P. Hill (Ed.), *Spinal cord injury: A guide to functional outcomes in OT*. Rockville, MD: Aspen Publishers.

Leary, D. A., & Mardirossian, J. (2000). Ethical knowledge = collaborative power: AOTA's Code of Ethics provides key guidelines for OT/OTA role delineation. *OT Practice, 5*(18), 19-22.

Mulcahey, M. J. (1992). Returning to school after a spinal cord injury: Perspectives from four adolescents. *American Journal of Occupational Therapy, 46*, 305-312.

Murphy, G., Young, A., Brown, D., & King, N. (2003). Explaining labor force status following spinal cord injury: The contribution of psychological variables. *Journal of Rehabilitation Medicine, 35*(6), 276-283.

National Spinal Cord Injury Association. (1998). Fact Sheet #1. Retrieved January 8, 1999, from http://www.erols.com/nscia/resource/factshts/fact02.html.

National Spinal Cord Injury Statistical Center (1998). Spinal Cord Injury FAQ. Retrieved January 8, 1999 from, http://www.sci.rehabm.uab.edu/shared/faq.data.html.

Noreau, L., Fougeyrollas, P., & Boschen, K. (2002). Perceived influence of the environment on social participation among individuals with spinal cord injury. *Topics in Spinal Cord Injury Rehabilitation, 7*(3), 56-72.

Pell, S., Gillies, R., & Carss, M. (1999). Use of technology by people with physical disabilities in Australia. *Disability and Rehabilitation, 21*(2), 56.

Pentland, W., Harvey, A., & Walker, J. (1998). The relationships between time use and health and well-being in men with spinal cord injuries. *Journal of Occupational Science, 5*(1), 14-25.

Pentland, W., Walker, J., Minnes, P., Tremblay, M., Brouwer, B., & Gould, M. (2003). Occupational responses to mid life and aging in women with disabilities. *Journal of Occupational Science, 10*(1), 21-30.

Ray, M. D. (1998). Shared borders. Achieving the goals of interdisciplinary patient care. *American Journal of Health Syst Pharm, 55*, 1369-1374.

Schneider, F. S. (2001). Traumatic spinal cord injury. In D. S. Umphred (Ed.), *Neurological rehabilitation* (4th ed., pp. 423-484). St. Louis: C.V. Mosby.

Schönherr, M. C., Groothoff, J. W., Mulder, G. A., & Eisma, W. (2000). Prediction of functional outcome after spinal cord injury: A task for the rehabilitation team and the patient. *Spinal Cord, 38*(3), 185-191.

Scivoletto, G., Morganti, B., Ditunno, P., Ditunno, J. F., & Molinari, M. (2003). Effects of age on spinal cord lesion patients' rehabilitation. *Spinal Cord, 41*(8), 457-464.

Sumida, M., Fujimoto, M., Tokuhiro, A., Tominaga, T., Magara, A., & Uchida, R. (2001). Early rehabilitation effect for traumatic spinal cord injury. *Archives of Physical Medicine and Rehabilitation, 82*(3), 391-395.

Thapar, N., Warner, G., Drainoni, M., Williams, S., Ditchfield, H., Wierbicky, J., et al. (2004). A pilot study of functional access to public buildings and facilities for persons with impairments. *Disability and Rehabilitation, 26*(5), 280.

Toto, P., & Hill, D. M. (2001). OT/OTA teambuilding in the SNF environment: Meeting the challenge. *Gerontology Special Interest Section Quarterly, 24*(2), 1-4.

Hollar, L. D. (Ed.). (1989). Spinal cord injury. In C. A. Trombly (Ed.), *Occupational therapy for physical dysfunction* (4th ed., pp. 795-813). Baltimore: Williams & Wilkins.

Wilson, D. J., McKenzie, M. W., Barber, L. M., and Watson, K. L. (1984.) *Spinal cord injury: A treatment guide for occupational therapists* (rev. ed.). Thorofare, NJ: SLACK Incorporated.

Wise, J., Ellis, G., & Trunnell, E. (2002). Effects of a curriculum designed to generalize self efficacy from weight training exercises to activities of daily living among adults with spinal injuries. *Journal of Applied Social Psychology, 32*(3), 500-521.

Woodruff, B. A., & Baron, R. C. (1994). A description of nonfatal spinal cord injury using a hospital-based registry. *Am J Prev Med, 10*(1), 10-14.

Yarkony, G. M. (1994). *Spinal cord injury: Medical management and rehabilitation.* Gaithersburg, MD: Aspen.

Yarkony, G. M., Roth, E. J., Heinemann, A. W., & Lovell, L, (1988). Spinal cord injury rehabilitation outcome: The impact of age. *Journal of Clinical Epidemiology, 41*(2), 173-177.

Yarkony, G. M., Roth, E. J., Heinemann, A. W., Lovell, L., & Wu, Y. (1988). Functional skills after spinal cord injury rehabilitation: Three-year longitudinal follow-up. *Archives of Physical Medicine & Rehabilitation, 69,* 111-114.

TEAM: *Spinal Cord Injury*   INITIAL EVAL. DATE: *1-1-04*

DIAGNOSIS: *C4 quadriplegia, S/P fusion*   PRIMARY THERAPIST: _____

HX OF PRESENT ILLNESS: *Forty two year old male. Involved in a MVA. He was not wearing a seat belt, ejected form vehicle. No movement in LE's + majority of UE's following MVA. In ER noted complete subluxation of C6-C7. S/P fusion, instrumentation, open reduction*

PRECAUTIONS: *Trach, scapular fx, sacral ulcer. Shoulder, elbow + forearm contractures. MRSA*

_____

_____

_____

DISCHARGE DATE: *TBD*

DISCHARGE PLANS: *TBD*

_____

_____

_____

_____

DISCHARGE DESTINATION: *TBD*

PRIOR LEVEL OF FUNCTION: *Living c̄ parents, in a trailer, had two children. Independent in ADL's*

_____

_____

CONTACT PERSON AND #: _____

ASSESSMENTS PERFORMED (check):

☒ UPPER EXTREMITY EVALUATION: ☐ FUNCTIONAL   ☒ ISOLATED

☐ SENSATION PERCEPTION

☐ TONE/POSTURING

☐ REFLEXES

☒ ACTIVITIES OF DAILY LIVING   ☒ SELF CARE   ☒ COMMUNITY/HOME MANAGEMENT

☐ DYSPHAGIA

☐ PERCEPTION/COGNITIVE STATUS

☐ STIMULUS RESPONSE LEVEL

THERAPIST SIGNATURE   DATE

LOMA LINDA UNIVERSITY MEDICAL CENTER
OCCUPATIONAL THERAPY EVALUATION
OCCUPATIONAL THERAPY

PATIENT IDENTIFICATION

White — Chart   Yellow — Therapy   n/s 29-1158 (9-92)

Real record 19-1A. Real record for a client with spinal cord injury. (Reprinted with permission of Loma Linda University Medical Center, Loma Linda, CA.)

PATIENT GOALS: _"To be able to care for myself."_

Key: ADL = Activities of Daily Living, DME = Durable Medical Equipment

Problems: (check)

✓ Impaired ROM	✓ Abnormal tone	___ Limited stimulation tolerance
✓ Decreased strength	✓ Impaired sensation	___ Edema
✓ Decreased endurance	___ Impaired visual perception	✓ Contracture/fracture
✓ Impaired coordination	___ Neglect: left or right	___ Abnormal reflex/movement patterns
✓ Impaired task tolerance	___ Decreased reaction time	___ Apraxia
✓ Impaired trunk control	___ Impaired attention	___ Ataxia
✓ Impaired balance	___ Impaired cognition	✓ Impaired ADL's
✓ Decreased upright tolerance	___ Impaired safety/judgment	___ Other: _____
___ Impaired oral motor skills		

Goals: (check)

✓ Increase ROM	___ Integrate abnormal reflex response	___ Dysphagia Evaluation
✓ Normalize tone		___ Improve direction following
✓ Prevent contractures	✓ Increase upright sitting tolerance	___ Community reentry
✓ Increase upper extremity strength/endurance	___ Improve cognitive skills	✓ ADL's/self care
	___ Increase appropriate responses to stimulation	☐ Independent
___ Decrease edema		☐ Supervised
✓ Patient/family education	___ Improve coordination	☑ Assisted
✓ Assess adaptive equipment needs	___ fine ___ gross	___ Driving evaluation
	___ Improve Visual discrimination	✓ Home program
✓ Home evaluation	___ Other: _____	✓ Other: _Self direct cath_

PROGNOSIS: _Fair_

Plan: (check)

✓ ROM	___ Weight bearing tasks	___ Multi sensory stimulation
✓ Tone reduction/facilitation	✓ Graded therapeutic activities	___ Cognitive retraining
✓ Functional strengthening/endurance	✓ Splinting/positioning needs	___ Dysphagia program
✓ Coordination tasks	✓ Muscle reeducation	✓ Self care tasks
✓ Balance activities	___ Edema control	___ Household task
	___ Therapeutic group activities	___ Community activities

Frequency: _M-F, BID   1x on weekend_

Comments:

Pt is motivated. H.O. in shoulders, elbows c̄ limited movements. C/o pain on movement. Parents may be caregivers.

Discharge Comments:

Parents have been trained. Pt will need to wear elbow splints several hours/day + at night. Parents instructed to assess for pressure areas c̄ return demo.

Recommendations: (check)

✓ No driving	___ Community agency referral	✓ Home program
___ 1:1 supervision	✓ Home Health	___ Other _____
___ Outpatient therapy	✓ Adaptive Equipment/DME	___

INITIAL: DATE	SIGNATURE	DISCHARGE: DATE	SIGNATURE

LOMA LINDA UNIVERSITY MEDICAL CENTER

SUMMATION SHEET

OCCUPATIONAL THERAPY

White — Chart   Yellow — Therapy

n/s 29-1165 (9-92)

PATIENT IDENTIFICATION

Real record 19-1B. Real record for a client with spinal cord injury. (Reprinted with permission of Loma Linda University Medical Center, Loma Linda, CA.)

KEY: D = Dependent / A = Physical Assist Required / S = Independent after Setup or Equipment / IO = Independent with orthosis /
I = Independent / * = Indicates activity performed at standing/ambulating level / N/A = Not applicable / ECU = Environmental Control Unit

	INITIAL	DISCHARGE			INITIAL	DISCHARGE
COMMUNICATION:				Change sheets	D	D
Writing	P	D		Change pillowcases		
Typing				Reach shelves		
Telephone				Drawers		
Turn Pages				Hang clothes		
Tape recorder				Household chores		
Open mail						
Communication board	NA	NA		**LEISURE:**		
Computer skills	D	D		Table Games	D	D
				Crafts		
MOBILITY:				Table Tennis		
Bed controls	D	D		Pool		
Turn in bed				Bowling		
Transfers				Badminton		
Wheelchair				Basketball		
Ambulation with assistive device	NA	NA		Community outing		
Ambulation	I	I		Spectator sports		
				Gardening		
HOME MANAGEMENT:				ECU for TV, radio, tape recorder		
Food preparation — hot	Dep	Dep		Wood working		
Food preparation — cold				Leather work		
Sink (reach top)				Other: _____		
Stove use						
Oven use				**COMMUNITY SKILLS:**		
Set table				Money Management	D	D
Clean up				Shopping		
Plan menus/budget				Driving		
Food shopping				Mobility		
Laundry				Mapping		
Make beds						

COMMENTS: *Needs instruction on how to self direct cath.*
Technology will provide some indep in function, household
needs.

DAILY LIVING SKILLS EVALUATION

	INITIAL	DISCHARGE			INITIAL	DISCHARGE
				Denture care		
FEEDING:				Nail care	D	D
Drink/straw	D	D		Set hair	NA	NA
Drink/cup						
Finger feed				**DRESSING:**		
Utensil feed				Bra	NA	NA
Cut food				Shirt/blouse	D	D
Poor liquids				Pullover garment		
Open containers				Buttons		
				Hooks/snaps/etc.		
SIMPLE GROOMING:				Zippers		
Wash face	D	D		Slacks/trousers		
Brush teeth				Underpants		
Apply toothpaste				Socks/stockings		
Shave				Corset/jacket		
Make-up				Shoes		
Dry hair				Shoelaces		
Don glasses						
Floss teeth				**GENERAL HYGIENE:**		
Comb hair				Bathing upper extremities	D	D
Wash hands				Bathing trunk		
Clean glasses				Bathing lower extremities		
Apply deodorant				Wash hair		
Insert contacts				Perineum		
Ear care						

COMMENTS: *Dependent in all areas of ADL's. Equipment for*
bathing + toileting is needed. Is able to verbally direct care

INITIAL: _____		DISCHARGE: _____	
DATE	THERAPIST SIGNATURE	DATE	SIGNATURE

LOMA LINDA UNIVERSITY MEDICAL CENTER

HOME/COMMUNITY SKILLS
OCCUPATIONAL THERAPY

White – Chart   Yellow – Therapy   n/s 29-1109 (9-92)

PATIENT IDENTIFICATION

Real record 19-1C. Real record for a client with spinal cord injury. (Reprinted with permission of Loma Linda University Medical Center, Loma Linda, CA.)

KEY: Grade: 5 = Normal; 4 = Good; 3+ = Fair Plus; 3 = Fair; 2+ = Poor Plus; 2 = Poor; 1 = Trace; 0 = Zero
R = Right, L = Left, EDC = Extensor Digity Communus, Opponens D.M. = Opponens Digity Minimi

		INITIAL		DISCHARGE	
	LEVEL	R	L	R	L
SHOULDER GIRDLE:					
Upper trapezius	C2-4	3+	3+	3+	3+
Middle trapezius	C2-4	3-	3+	2+	3+
Lower trapezius	C2-4	3-	3+	2+	3+
Anterior deltoid	C5-6	2-	2+	2+	2+
Middle deltoid	C5-6	2+	2+	2+	2+
Posterior deltoid	C5-6	2+	2+	2+	2+
Rhomboids	C5-6	2-	2+	2-	2+
Internal rotators	C5-T1	2-	2-	2-	2-
External rotators	C5-6	2-	2-	2-	2-
Serratus anterior	C6-7	2-	2-	2-	2-
Pectoralis major —					
Sternal	C7-T1	0	0	0'	0'
Clavicular	C5-7	1	2-	1	2-
Latissimus Dorsi	C7-8	0	1	0	1
ELBOW/FOREARM:					
Biceps	C5-6	3-	3-	3-	3-
Brachioradialis	C5-6	3-	3-	3-	3-
Triceps	C7-8	1	1	1	1
Supinators	C5-6	2-	2-	2-	2-
Pronators	C6-7	0'	0'	0'	0'
WRIST:					
Flexor Carpi —					
Ulnaris	C5-6	1	1	1	1
Radialis	C5-6	1	1	1	1
Extensor Carpi Radialis					
Longus	C6-7	2+	2+	2+	2+
Brevis	C6-7	2+	2+	2+	2+
Extensor Carpi Ulnaris	C7-8	0	2-	0	2-
HAND:					
FDP - 1	C8-T1	0	0	0	0
- 2	C8-T1				
- 3	C8-T1				
- 4	C8-T1				
FDS - 1	C8-T1	0	0	0	0
- 2	C8-T1				
- 3	C8-T1				
- 4	C8-T1				
EDC - 1	C7-8	0	0	0	0
- 2	C7-8				
- 3	C7-8				
- 4	C7-8				
Lumbricales -		0	0	0	0
1	C8-T1				
2	C8-T1				
3	C8-T1				
4	C8-T1				
Dorsal Interossei -		0	0	0	0
1	C8-T1				
2	C8-T1				
3	C8-T1				
4	C8-T1				
Palmer Interossei -		0	0	0	0
1	C8-T1				
2	C8-T1				
3	C8-T1				
4	C8-T1				
Abductor pollices longus	C7-8	0	0	0	0
Abductor pollices bevis	C8-T1				
Adductor pollices	C8-T1				
Flexor pollices longus	C8-T1				
Opponens pollices	C8-T1				
Extensor pollices longus	C7-8				
Extensor pollices brevis	C7-8				
Opponens D.M.	C8-T1				

(handwritten note at Discharge, shoulder girdle: "Disp due to scapular pain.")

Real record 19-1D. Real record for a client with spinal cord injury. (Reprinted with permission of Loma Linda University Medical Center, Loma Linda, CA.)

ACTIVE / PASSIVE RANGE

Key: R = Right, L = Left, MP = Metacarple Phalangial Joint, IP = Interphalangial Joint, PIP = Proximal Interphalangial Joint, DIP = Distal Interphalangial Joint.

		NORMAL RANGE	INITIAL R	INITIAL L	DISCHARGE R	DISCHARGE L
Neck protraction		0 - 4°	3°	—	3°	—
Head:	flexion	0 - 45°	25°	—	35°	—
	extension	0 - 45°	15°	—	15°	—
	rotation	0 - 60°	35°	30°	39°	30°
	lateral flexion	0 - 45°	10°	15°	10°	15°
Shoulder:	flexion	0 - 180°	20°	56°	20°	60°
	extension	0 - 40°	15°	15°	10°	15°
	abduction	0 - 180°	65°	55°	20°	60°
	internal rotation	0 - 80°	15°	15°	15°	15°
	external rotation	0 - 80°	15°	15°	5°	15°
Elbow:	flexion	0 - 150°	140°	145°	140°	145°
	extension	0 - °	75°	75°	75°	65°
Forearm:	supination	0 - 90°] contracted	90°	90°	90°	90°
	pronation	0 - 90°] in supine	0°	0°	0	0
Wrist:	flexion	0 - 80°	5°	5°	5°	5°
	extension	0 - 70°	60°	50°	50°	40°
	radial deviation	0 - 20°	15°	20°	10°	10°
	ulnar deviation	0 - 30°	0	10°	0	5°
Digits:	1: MP flexion (Thumb)	0 - 50°	0	0	0	0
	IP flexion	0 - 90°	0	0	0	0
	radial abduction	0 - 50°	0	0	0	0
	palmer abduction	0 - 50°	0	0	0	0
	opposition to 5th finger) (measure distance between pads)					
	2: MP flexion	0 - 90°	0	0	0	0
	MP extension	0 - 15°				
	PIP flexion	0 - 110°				
	DIP flexion	0 - 90°				
	3: MP flexion		0	0	0	0
	MP extension					
	PIP flexion					
	DIP flexion					
	4: MP flexion		0	0	0	0
	MP extension					
	PIP flexion					
	DIP flexion					
	5: MP flexion		0	0	0	0
	MP extension					
	PIP flexion					
	DIP flexion		1	1	1	1

DOMINANCE:

Premorbid: **L**

Present: **L**

Grip Strength

3 point pinch/palmer pinch **unable to participate**

Lateral pinch

COMMENTS: *Elbow & FA contractures prevent tenodesis. Scapular fx remains painful*

INITIAL: DATE ___   THERAPIST SIGNATURE ___   DISCHARGE: ___ DATE ___ SIGNATURE ___

LOMA LINDA UNIVERSITY MEDICAL CENTER

ISOLATED UPPER EXTREMITY EVALUATION

OCCUPATIONAL THERAPY

White — Chart   Yellow — Therapy   n/s 29-1195 (9-92)

PATIENT IDENTIFICATION

Real record 19-1E. Real record for a client with spinal cord injury. (Reprinted with permission of Loma Linda University Medical Center, Loma Linda, CA.)

Key Concepts

- Brain disease: The neurological system of the person with schizophrenia is different from the general population. There are structural differences, blood-flow differences, and chemical differences.
- Schizophrenia affects the individual, the family, and society.
- Stigma: The name "schizophrenia" has had a stigma associated with it for many decades.
- Positive symptoms: These include hallucinations, disorganized speech, loosened associations, and bizarre behavior. Positive implies that these features are an excess added unto the patient's existing personality.
- Negative symptoms: These features represent a loss of normal function, such as decreased emotional response, loss of enjoyment in life, decreased cognition interfering with meaningful communication, and little interest in activities or in socializing.

Essential Vocabulary

delusion: A firmly held, false belief for which there is no basis in fact. Common delusions are paranoid, grandiose, religious, or feeling everything, including TV stories, refers to him or her.

disorganized speech: Phrases and ideas expressed follow no theme or line of thought and may include preservation, which is involuntary repetition of words or phrases; neologisms, which are newly coined words; or clanging, in which words are made to rhyme despite their meaning in the sentence.

flattened affect: Incongruous absence of appropriate emotional response.

hallucination: A false sensory perception. Can occur in all sensory systems; however, the most common are auditory hallucinations.

illusion: A misinterpretation of a real experience, such as a mirage in which it appears water is on a road that is known to be dry.

loose associations: Ideas switch from one subject to another unrelated topic.

psychosis: Out of touch with reality, disorganized thinking resulting in loss of functional capacity.

Clinical Summary

Etiology

While some kinds of schizophrenia have been found to be associated with particular genetic markers, others have no such familial identification. Individuals with family members with schizophrenia are more likely to have the disease.

Prevalence

Approximately 1% of the population worldwide will develop schizophrenia during their lifetime. Equally as many males as females have the disease; however, females have a later onset.

Classic Signs

The individual displays a combination of positive and negative symptoms. The onset may be gradual or abrupt. Hallucinations, delusions, and disorganized behavior or speech are the most recognizable symptoms.

Precautions

Keep track of all sharp tools such as knives and scissors as frequent auditory hallucinations often instruct the patient to hurt him- or herself. A further precaution is to avoid supporting any delusional ideas such as delusions of grandeur.

A Teacher's Aide With Schizophrenia

Margaret Drake, PhD, OTR, FAOTA and Tonia Taylor, BS, COTA

Introduction

Schizophrenia is a brain disease. This disorder has been found in all cultures (Ninan, Mance, & Lewine, 1998; Torrey, 2001). While symptoms of the disease have been recognized for centuries, schizophrenia was not given this name until the beginning of the 20th century (Kaplan & Sadock, 2000; Stoudemire, Fogel, & Greenberg, 2000). In the classification used in the United States, a person must have experienced the general symptoms of schizophrenia for 6 months and strong symptoms for at least 1 month, before the diagnosis becomes official (APA, 2000). Approximately 1% of the population develops schizophrenia, though only half of this group gets treatment. Equally as many women as men develop schizophrenia (Kaplan & Sadock, 2000). The onset of schizophrenia for males usually happens earlier than for females (Kaplan & Sadock, 1998; Lewine, Haden, Caudle, & Shurett, 1998). Males often have their first episode in their teens while females are more likely to experience the disease after age 25. This debilitating mental disorder affects 1% of the population worldwide. Almost half of homeless Americans have this diagnosis (Kaplan & Sadock, 2000).

There are 5 types of schizophrenia. When the person is unresponsive to the environment, either from being overexcited or in a stupor, this is called catatonia. In disorganized schizophrenia, the person appears to have no system of thought or communication pattern for appropriately interacting with others. A person who has paranoid type schizophrenia is usually preoccupied with delusions, auditory hallucinations, and feelings of persecution. Undifferentiated refers to a type of schizophrenia in which a person may have symptoms of schizophrenia but not paranoia, catatonia, or disorganization. Residual schizophrenia is typically comprised of remaining chronic symptoms, which are usually negative ones, after the major dysfunctional aspects of the disease have disappeared (APA, 2000).

Frames of Reference

Theories, or frames of reference, commonly used with persons diagnosed as schizophrenic are the Person-Environment-Occupation Model, the Neuromotor Behavior Model, and the Cognitive Disabilities Model.

- The Person-Environment-Occupation Model includes ideas from anthropology, environmental-behavioral studies, social science, architecture, human geography, psychology, and OT to explain mental illness. The basic assumption is that a person's environment is integral to the way a person behaves. The environment includes the time when something occurs and how it affects a person's psychology. Environments are constantly in the process of change, and they change more easily than people change. The environment can either help or hinder a person's ability to perform tasks (Stewart, Letts, Law, Cooper, Strong, & Rigby, 2003).

- Neuromotor Behavior Model includes ideas such as SI, the biochemistry of medication, and neurodevelopmental treatment. These theories focus on the necessity of biological balance for proper neurological function. The neurological system is considered the basis of mental dysfunction (Crepeau, Cohn, & Schell, 2003).

- Cognitive Disabilities Model focuses on discovering what cognitive capabilities a client has and providing the person with appropriate activities for his or her level of function. How information is processed in the neurological system indicates whether or not the person has cognitive dysfunction. This can be determined by his or her performance. The cognitive performance level achieved is often used as a predictor of future function (Allen, Earhart, & Blue, 1992; Grant, 2003).

Case Story

Lindy comes from a loving, well-educated family. She is a white female born and raised in a large metropolitan area. From birth she was a loving child but was considered somewhat slow in reaching developmental milestones. Despite the fact that her mother was a healthcare professional, when Lindy had a high fever at age 6, her mother was unable to prevent convulsions on the way to the hospital. Following this episode, Lindy was noticed by her teacher, as well as her 2 sisters and parents, to have more behavioral problems. Within a few months after this episode, her father, who was a community college teacher, died of a heart attack. This unexpected event put a great deal of stress on all family members. By the time Lindy was 12, her emotional outbursts and frequent shoplifting episodes persuaded her family to place her in a residential treatment facility run by a religious order. Lindy functioned well in this structured setting, which provided special education, recreation, and religious instruction. When she came of age, she was no longer eligible for this placement. She hovered on the borderline diagnostically between moderately mentally retarded and merely somewhat slow. She continued to have intermittent seizures that could be controlled with medication adjustment. During the next 5 years, Lindy moved back and forth from living with her mother to living in a group home for the mentally handicapped. She attended a day treatment program in a center that prepared clients for employment. At the center, she met a male who was a little more disabled than her and with the reluctant permission of their 2 families, they married. This union lasted a little over a year. Both families had been supportive, but the new husband and wife needed even more daily assistance and supervision as a couple than they had as individuals. After the divorce, Lindy returned to the treatment center and re-established her residence in a group home. Eventually at age 28, Lindy was employed as a teacher's aide in a public school special education class for people with severe and profound retardation. Lindy was physically tall and strong and well-suited to the work of lifting the immobile, severely and profoundly retarded students with whom she worked. Near the beginning of the second year in this class, Lindy began to experience episodes of crying and frequent arguments with her supervising teacher. Her coworkers found her sitting on a bench near the playground during a noon recess talking to herself. Her mother learned of this incident and took Lindy to see the family doctor. The family doctor thought she needed to see a psychiatrist. The psychiatrist to whom she was referred thought Lindy needed to reduce her stress. With the support of her sisters and mother, Lindy requested and was given a leave of absence from her job as teacher's aide. During this leave, she was hospitalized at a private psychiatric hospital and diagnosed with schizophrenia.

Referral

This hospital was a 60-bed facility. There were 3 20-bed units: one for substance abusers, one for newly admitted acute care psychiatric patients, and one for those being treated in more specialized programs such as eating disorders, obsessive compulsive disorders, dissociative disorders, depression, and schizophrenia.

In this particular hospital, the psychiatrist wanted all her newly admitted patients to receive OT if possible. Lindy received a referral to OT. Notices of new referrals were placed in the OT message box. The OTA picked up all the referrals each morning. She and the OT decided together how to go about screening and evaluating the new clients. They used a variety of evaluation tools depending upon which they thought fit the client. Eclecticism, using whichever theory seemed to fit

the individual patient, was the basis for evaluation and treatment choices in this setting. This meant that sometimes they used the Person-Environment-Occupation Model and sometimes they used the Cognitive Disabilities or Neuromotor Behavior Model. Sometimes patients had the benefit of being evaluated by assessments from more than one model.

Lindy had been put on a regimen of a new antipsychotic medication.

Assessment and Evaluation Process

It was decided to assess Lindy using the Canadian Occupational Performance Measure (COPM) (Law et al., 1998) and the Allen Cognitive Levels (ACL) test. The OT administered the COPM first. During the identification of occupational performance issues, the OT learned about Lindy's recent job and that she thought her best asset was her physical strength and capability to do heavy lifting. She felt badly about her recent problems communicating with her supervising teacher. She had enjoyed the socialization she shared in the teachers' lounge and with the other aides while loading and unloading students from vans and buses. Lindy had also enjoyed the approval from her family while she had been employed. The aide position was the only gainful employment she had ever had. The most difficult part of this job was the boredom with the simple curricula used in the classroom for the students. Lindy tired of the feeding routines that took up so much of the school day. She was able to discuss the classes she had enjoyed in the residential school from which she had graduated. Because the school had been so structured with little time for leisure, Lindy had not developed any particular leisure preferences other than swimming. She had won swimming medals in the Special Olympics. Aside from references to her work, Lindy was unable to summarize any of her activities for a typical week. The 5 occupational performance problems identified and prioritized from the evaluation were as follows:

1. Keeping a job.
2. Not enough money.
3. Difficult to participate in swimming due to work.
4. Transportation.
5. Socialization.

She scored her performance level with "keeping a job" as 2 out of 10 since she was on sick leave. Her satisfaction with that performance was 1. Lindy scored "not enough money" on performance as 5 out of 10 and satisfaction with this problem was also 5. Lindy reported running out of money before each payday. Her difficulty "getting to swimming" was 3 out of 10 on the performance scale with satisfaction at 1. The problem with "transportation" was that she had to be driven to work. She had been able to ride her bicycle on the familiar route from the group home to the school until she began to have seizures. The doctor told her to discontinue riding to avoid injury from falling. This situation made her very unhappy, and she scored her performance at 1 and her satisfaction also at level 1. "Socialization" performance was scored by Lindy at level 4 with a satisfaction level of 6.

The OTA and the OT discussed this information. Then the OTA administered the ACL. Lindy scored 4.2 as she was able to do the 3 whip stitches but could not figure out how to fix the mistake made by the OTA. The OT verified these findings by doing the Routine Task Inventory (Allen et al., 1992). Lindy was able to dress herself appropriately but left the label hanging out of her t-shirt. When combing her hair, she missed part of the back of her head. Nursing reported that she did not need supervision when bathing but she needed to be reminded to do it at the scheduled time. She needed 3 reminders to clean up after herself in the bathroom she shared with a roommate. Unfortunately, the hospital had no swimming pool, so aerobic exercise was agreed upon as a substitute. Lindy was excited about joining the daily exercise group and promised to be there on time. She had no trouble at mealtime apart from eating too quickly and interacting only when others spoke to her. The medication nurse reported that Lindy required explanations each time she took her medication. Housekeeping was not a routine she could manage without assistance and supervision. She could heat a can of soup for herself but left the dishes on the table and the dirty pot in the sink until reminded to clean up. However, she was satisfied with this behavior. It only bothered those around her.

General Goals

From the 3 assessments, the following 5 goals were designed when Lindy sat down with the OT and OTA:

1. Practice initiating conversation with others during mealtime.
2. Make a daily budget to spread her 2 weeks' salary to last until the next payday.
3. Increase her tolerance for aerobic exercise from 5 minutes to 10 minutes.
4. Complete at least one dish for the weekly meal prepared by the cooking group.
5. Decrease the reminders about cleaning up after herself to one reminder per day.

It was felt that all of these goals would enhance her chances of resuming her job. Transportation solutions would have to wait until she was discharged.

Treatment Activities/Techniques

To accomplish goal #1, a game was devised in which patients were to ask another patient a question during mealtime. This became a round robin exercise in which the person to whom the question was asked would respond to each of the questions asked by previous participants at the table, as well as responding to his or her own question. After each had responded to all the questions, a new round would start. The psychiatric technicians were instructed in how the game was played and took over supervision during mealtime.

To accomplish goal #2, Lindy was given play money in the amount of her regular paycheck. She was then asked to divide the money into 14 equal piles and put them into separate envelopes. She then took one envelope and divided it into the cost of breakfast at a fast-food restaurant; lunch in the school cafeteria; $20 for the group home operator where she usually had her evening meal; and $2 for other needs such as toothpaste, sanitary pads, etc.

To accomplish goal #3, Lindy was included in the aerobic exercise group, which met daily in the dayroom for 30 minutes before lunch. Initially, she did the low impact aerobics with several older patients; however, by the end of the first week, she was spontaneously joining in the regular aerobic exercises.

To accomplish goal #4, on Friday, the regular cooking group session planned a spaghetti luncheon. Lindy chopped enough carrots, radishes, green peppers, and green onions to mix nicely with the 2 heads of lettuce, which she tore into bite-sized pieces. She then mixed 2 envelopes of ranch dressing mix with a pint of no-fat yogurt to complete the salad. The other patients declared it a tasty, crisp salad.

To accomplish goal #5, Lindy was enlisted in a pact with her roommate, in which they would remind each other and record how many reminders it took. The one who achieved the fewest reminders, as verified by nursing, would be taken by the OTA to the gift shop to look around or out onto the grounds for a walk on the marked exercise trail.

Lindy and her roommate chose these rewards.

Discharge Planning

After the second week, the treatment team met to discuss Lindy's future. The medication appeared to be decreasing Lindy's auditory hallucinations. She was less argumentative. The OT reported that her cognitive level had improved to 4.4 on the ACL test. This meant that she was able to follow a routine as long as nothing unusual happened. It was decided by the psychiatrist, in consultation with the OT, nurse, and social worker, that Lindy could return to the group home and to the treatment center but not to her aide job until her cognitive level had improved to level 4.8. This would require that she return every 2 weeks for an evaluation by the OT and other treatment team members. This was felt to be a good solution so that Lindy could continue to work on problems like the transportation and swimming since she had been unable to address these problems mentioned in the COPM as an inpatient. Her satisfaction level with keeping a job had improved from a 1 to a 3 as Lindy had become more used to the idea that it might be some time before she could return to employment. Transportation continued as a deeply felt problem with both performance and satisfaction remaining at number 1 out of a possible 10.

CLINICAL PROBLEM SOLVING

Often other factors, especially performances contexts, change the focus of the OT treatment. The following stories are intended to stimulate clinical problem solving.

Lindy was able to maintain her independence while living in a group home for up to 6 months at a time. She appeared to have the type of schizophrenia in which stability on one medication could not be maintained for more than 6 months.

Episodes of psychotic behavior reoccurred regularly. These reoccurrences, were sometimes linked with Lindy's involvement with a series of boyfriends whom she met in the group home or at the activity center where she eventually went for daytime supervision. She was never able to return to her teacher's aide job. What activity could the OTA in the activity center provide to engage Lindy's interest and distract her from inappropriate come-ons to male clients? Review the progress notes in the records section; what issues might effect OT treatment?

A 35-year-old, Caucasian male patient named Tom, whom Lindy met at the activity center, was diagnosed as a paranoid schizophrenic when he was 18 years old. He had been in many treatment facilities since that time. At the time he met Lindy, he was living at home with his parents because the last group home where he had lived had evicted him when he attacked another male patient. He and Lindy had a short intimate relationship. He functioned at a higher cognitive level than Lindy and was able to persuade her to join him in evading the rules. The two of them would meet at the bus stop and ride the metropolitan transit bus together to the activity center. They would touch and arouse each other while sitting in the rear seat. Sometimes, they would get off the bus at a bus-stop short of their final destination and go into the public park restroom to have sexual relations. When Tom began to demonstrate jealousy by threatening to hurt other male clients in the activity center when they spoke to Lindy, the staff told him that they must discontinue their relationship. The case managers for both Tom and Lindy were informed. What activities could the OTA use to engage him and distract him from his involvement with Lindy? How could she arrange the scheduling or the environment to keep the two of them apart?

In the activity center, there was a 46-year-old African-American female named Millie with a dual diagnosis of schizophrenia and alcoholism. During an exercise class at the center, she began to become friends with Lindy. The 2 women lived in group homes only 2 blocks apart. The OTA and other staff members thought that by encouraging this relationship, they would be protecting Lindy from Tom. One morning, the group home operator called the activity center to notify them that the previous evening Lindy had returned late and was drunk. Neither Lindy nor Millie was supposed to drink alcohol while taking the antipsychotic medication prescribed. What other information should the OTA find out before talking to Lindy and Millie? How could Lindy be protected from repeating the drinking episode with Millie?

Lindy's roommate in the group home was a 40-year-old Hispanic female with schizophrenia named Helena who sometimes had catatonic episodes. These episodes usually occurred after she had been on a holiday visit to her family home in a rural area more than 100 miles from the group home. Her large family would fail to supervise her medication regime because there were so many people visiting. In the confusion, Helena's medication would be forgotten. When the family realized that Helena had not had her previous doses of medication, they would have her just double the dose. This erratic medication regimen would throw Helena into a catatonic stupor. By the time she returned to the group home, she often could not be aroused. At this time, the group home operator would ask Lindy to awaken her roommate for meals. Lindy would be unable to do this and would become upset and fearful that she would have to adapt to a new roommate. Helena did not attend the activity center. How could the OTA assist Lindy in solving this problem?

LEARNING ACTIVITIES

1. Contact a community clubhouse program for people with chronic mental health issues. Organize a basic interest needs assessment and lead groups in addressing their needs.
2. Investigate the National Alliance for the Mentally Ill (NAMI). What services do they provide and who can access the services?
3. Invite a person with schizophrenia or the parent of a person with schizophrenia to speak to the class.
4. Have each person in class develop a worksheet to address a specific need for a person with schizophrenia. Photocopy the worksheets to form a class resource book.

REFERENCES

Ahmed, M., & Goldman, J. A. (1994). Cognitive rehabilitation of adults with severe and persistent mental illness: A group model. *Community Mental Health, 30,* 385-394.

Allen, C. K., Earhart, C. A., & Blue, T. (1992). *Occupational therapy treatment goals for the physically and cognitively disabled.* Rockville, MD: American Occupational Therapy Association.

American Psychiatric Association. (2000). *Diagnostic and statistical manual of mental disorders: DSM-IVTR.* Washington, DC: American Psychiatric Association.

Bustillo, J. R., Lauriello, J., Horan, W. P., & Keith, S. J. (2001). The psychosocial treatment of schizophrenia: An update. *American Journal of Psychiatry, 158,* 163-175.

Creegan, S., & Williams, F. L. R. (1997). Supportive employment for individuals with chronic schizophrenia: The case for a National Health Service community-based sheltered workshop. *Occupational Therapy International, 4,* 99-115.

Crepeau, E. B., Cohn, E. S., & Schell, B. A. B. (2003). *Willard & Spackman's occupational therapy.* Philadelphia: Lippincott, Williams & Wilkins.

Dobson, D. J. G., McDougall, G., Busheikin, J., & Aldous, J. (1995). Effects of social skills training and social milieu treatment on symptoms of schizophrenia. *Psychiatric Services, 46,* 376-380.

Goodman, L. A. (1997). Physical and sexual assault history in women with serious mental illness: Prevalence, correlates, treatments, and future research directions. *Schizophrenia Bulletin, 23,* 685-696.

Grant, S. (2003). Cognitive disability frame of reference. In E. B. Crepeau, E. S. Cohn, & B. A. B. Schell (Eds.), *Willard and Spackman's occupational therapy* (10th ed.). Philadelphia: Lippincott, Williams & Wilkins.

Hayes, R. L., Halford, W. K., & Varghese, F. N. (1991). Generalizations of the effects of activity therapy and social skills training on the social behavior of low functioning schizophrenic patients. *Occupational Therapy in Mental Health, 11,* 3-20.

EVIDENCE-BASED TREATMENT STRATEGIES

Treatment Strategies	Authors
Social skills training	Bustillo, Lauriello, Horan, & Keith, 2001; Dobson, McDougall, Busheikin, & Aldous, 1995; Hodgkinson, Evans, O'Donnell, Nicholson, & Walsh, 1999; Landeen, 2001; Liberman et al., 1993; Mann et al., 1993; Salo-Chydenius, 1996
Activity therapy	Hayes, Halford, & Varghese, 1991; Hodgkinson et al., 1999
Sexual behavior	Goodman, 1997; Herman, Kaplan, Satriano, Cournos, & McKinnon, 1994; Howden, Zipple, & Tyrrell, 1994; Miller, 1997; Miller & Finnerty, 1996
Supported employment	Bustillo et al., 2001; Creegan & Williams, 1997; Iraurgi, Bombin, & Imaz, 1999; Landeen, 2001
Cognitive rehabilitation	Ahmed & Goldman, 1994; Liberman, Eckman, & Marder, 2001; Roder, Zorn, Muller, & Brenner, 2001
Goal setting	Roder et al., 2001

Herman, R., Kaplan, M., Satriano, J., Cournos, F., & McKinnon, K. (1994). HIV prevention with people with serious mental illness: Staff training and institutional attitudes. *Psychiatric Rehabilitation Journal, 17,* 97-103.

Hodgkinson, B., Evans, D., O'Donnell, A., Nicholson, J., & Walsh, K. (1999). The effectiveness of individual therapy and group therapy in treatment of schizophrenia. *Best Practice: Evidence-Based Practice Information Sheets for Health Professionals, 3,* 1-6.

Howden, M., Zipple, A. M., & Tyrrell, W. F. (1994). Dating skills for residential consumers. *Psychiatric Rehabilitation Journal, 18,* 67-76.

Iraurgi, I., Bombin, I., & Imaz, I. (1999). Professional training in the rehabilitation of people with psychiatric disability. *Psychiatric Rehabilitation Journal, 23,* 75-180.

Kaplan, H. I., & Sadock, B. J. (1998). *Kaplan and Sadock's synopsis of psychiatry* (8th ed.). Baltimore, MD: Williams & Wilkins.

Kaplan, B. J., & Sadock, V. A. (2000). *Kaplan & Sadock's comprehensive textbook of psychiatry* (7th ed.) Philadelphia: Lippincott, Williams & Wilkins.

Landeen, J. (2001). Review: Social skills training, supported employment programmes, and cognitive behaviour therapy improve some outcomes in schizophrenia. *Evidence-Based Nursing, 4,* 115.

Law, M., Baptiste, S., Carswell, A., McColl, M. A., Polatajko, H., & Pollock, N. (1998). *Canadian occupational performance measure* (3rd ed.). Ottawa, Ontario: Canadian Association of Occupational Therapists.

Lewine, R., Haden, C., Caudle, J., & Shurett, R. (1998). Sex-onset effects on neuropsychological function in schizophrenia. *Schizophrenia Bulletin, 23,* 51-61.

Liberman, R. P., Wallace, C. J., Blackwell, G., Eckman, T. A., Vaccaro, J. V., & Kuehnel, T. G. (1993). Innovations in skills training for the seriously mentally ill: The UCLA social and independent living skills module. *Innovations & Research, 2,* 43-59.

Liberman, R. P., Eckman, T. A., & Marder, S. R. (2001). Training in social problem solving among persons with schizophrenia. *Psychiatric Services, 52,* 31-34.

Mann, N. A., Tandon, R., Butler, J., Boyd, M., Eisner, W. H., & Lewis, M. (1993). Psychosocial rehabilitation in schizophrenia: Beginnings in acute hospitalization. *Archives of Psychiatric Nursing, 7,* 154-162.

Miller, L. J. (1997). Sexuality, reproduction, and family planning in women with schizophrenia. *Schizophrenia Bulletin, 23,* 623-635.

Miller, L. J., & Finnerty, M. (1996). Sexuality, pregnancy, and child-bearing among women with schizophrenia-spectrum disorders. *Psychiatric Services, 47,* 502-506.

Ninan, P. T., Mance, R. M., & Lewine, R. R. J. (1998). Schizophrenia and other psychotic disorders. In A. Stoudemire (Ed.), *Clinical psychiatry for medical students* (3rd ed., pp. 153-185). Philadelphia: Lippincott-Raven Publishers.

Roder, V., Zorn, P., Muller, D., & Brenner, H. D. (2001). Rehab rounds: Improving recreational, residential, and vocational outcomes for patients with schizophrenia. *Psychiatric Services, 52,* 1439-1441.

Salo-Chydenius, S. (1996). Changing helplessness to coping: An exploratory study of social skills training with individuals with long-term mental illness. *Occupational Therapy International, 3,* 174-189.

Stewart, D., Letts, L., Law, M., Cooper, B. A., Strong, S., & Rigby, P. J. (2003) The person-environment-occupation model. In E. B. Crepeau, E. S. Cohn, & B. A. B. Schell (Eds.), *Willard and Spackman's occupational therapy* (10th ed.). Philadelphia: Lippincott, Williams & Wilkins.

Stoudemire, A., Fogel, B. S., & Greenberg, D. (Eds.). (2000). *Psychiatric care of the medical patient.* New York: Oxford University Press.

Torrey, E. F. (2001). *Surviving schizophrenia: A manual for families, and providers.* New York: Quill.

THE UNIVERSITY HOSPITALS AND CLINICS	Lindy
	Patient number
	Room number **Bed**
	Admit Date _____

3/16/03: 2:30 PM Pt. saw Dr. and attended St. Pat's Party on unit. Asked to take nap after. Slept X one hour.
— E. Merton, RN

3/16/03 4:30 p.m; Administered ACL in afternoon. Scored 4.2.
— M Crawford COTA

3/16/03 10:30 PM Dr. increased Loxitane to 70 mg. Pt. eats well and asked for 2nds. Will discuss weight control
V Ewen RN

3/17/03 6:30am Pt. had a restful night and awoke at 6am. Sat through community meeting and volunteered to help clean up day room. Is OK with roommate. — S. Brumfield RN

3/17/03 Occupational Therapy: Met c̄ Lindy and OTA to make treatment goals 1) increase conversation during meal times 2) make a budget, 3) aerobic exercise 4) cooking group, 5) cleaning up after self. She attended exercise group and was able to keep up with others 4/4 min. Will start on conversation during mealtime with OTA and technician this noon. — R. Stone OTR/L

3/17/03 2:30 PM: Pt attended exercise group and group therapy with SW. No evidence of active hallucinations.
— E. Merton, RN

3/17/03 4:30 Worked with group of patients and psych tech Phillips to play the round robin socialization game during lunch. Lindy was able to remember all the questions and her answers were appropriate. — M Crawford COTA

FORM 1724
REPLACES UMC 345

Real record 20-1A. Real record for a client with schizophrenia.

THE UNIVERSITY HOSPITALS AND CLINICS

Lindy

Patient Number

Room number   Bed

Admit Date _____

3/15/03: 2 PM 30 y/o white female admitted to Rm C325 c/o auditory hallucinations. Accompanied to unit by mother and sister. Medical hx obtained from pt's mother. Pt. given 50 mg. Loxitane p.o. per MD order. Lunch tray ordered for pt. ——————— E. Merton, RN

3-15-03 Social Work Interviewed pt + mother who is very involved. Pt. lives in Wesley's Group home and attends Case Activity Ctr. Pt. seems "calm" enough now but mom described recent outbursts and hallucinations. Mom also indicated possible MR. Pt. was employed as a teacher's-aide at Swiss School until she went on sick leave last week. Pt. is used to taking direction and is cooperative enough though emotionally fragile. Dr. has referred her to OT + RT. Will start tomorrow. A Hull LSW

3/13/03 10:30 PM Pt. went to bed at 8PM and is still asleep. Ate all her supper. Had to be encouraged to bathe. Obvious BO. V Ewem RN

3/16/03; 6:30 am. Pt awoke at 4am and got up and paced alone in the hallway. She appears to be responding to internal stimuli– gesturing and talking as if someone else was present. B Brunfield RN

3/16/03 Occupational Therapy. Interviewed pt. as part of the COPM. Pt. sat passively and waited to be asked questions. She had some difficulty choosing five occupational therapy performance problems to focus on but she finally prioritized them; 1) Job 2) Money 3) Swimming 4) Transportation 5.) Socialization. OTR will administer ACL. Treatment planning session tomorrow ——————— R. Stone, OTR/L

FORM 1724
REPLACES UMC 345

Real record 20-1B. Real record for a client with schizophrenia.

Key Concepts

- Multiple sclerosis (MS): Chronic, disabling disease of the CNS.
- Occupation: Daily activities that provide meaning and/or purpose.
- Canadian Model of Occupational Performance: A conceptual framework that looks at the interaction between person, environment, and occupation.
- Canadian Occupational Performance Measure (COPM): An assessment that emphasizes a client-centered approach by determining client's valued occupations and goals.

Essential Vocabulary

autoimmune: Condition in which the body attacks itself.
diplopia: Double vision.
lassitude: Fatigue or tiredness.
myelin sheath: Covering of nerve fibers.
nystagmus: Rhythmic jerkiness of the eye(s).
relapse: Exacerbation or increase in symptoms.
remission: Lessening of symptoms.

Clinical Summary

Etiology

Unknown. Possible etiologies include allergies, viruses, infections, genetics, and environment.

Prevalence

MS occurs in 250,000 to 350,000 individuals and occurs 2 to 3 times more often in women than men.

Classic Signs

Fatigue, difficulty walking, balance problems, coordination problems, sensory deficits, visual problems, cognitive deficits, emotional lability, depression, pain, sexual dysfunction, and bowel and bladder dysfunction.

Precautions

Avoid fatigue, overheating, and extreme cold temperatures.

Chapter 21

A MOTHER AND CATERER WITH MULTIPLE SCLEROSIS

Lori T. Andersen, EdD, OTR, FAOTA and Barbara L. Kornblau, JD, OT/L, FAOTA

INTRODUCTION

MS, a chronic and often disabling disease of the CNS (National Multiple Sclerosis Society, 2003a), involves the myelin sheaths that surround the brain and spinal nerves. When the myelin sheath functions properly, it serves to insulate the nerve cells, facilitating the speed of transmissions along the nerves. In an individual with MS, the myelin sheath, normally a soft or fatty material, becomes sclerotic or hardened, thus slowing the transmissions. No one knows exactly why this happens.

ETIOLOGY

Although many scientists studying the cause of MS look to allergies, viruses, infections, genetics, environment, and other agents as possible causes, its etiology remains a mystery. Most evidence, however, points to the generally accepted theory of MS as an autoimmune or body-attacking-itself response (National Multiple Sclerosis Society, 2003b).

Another popular theory looks at environment as a cause of MS. Studies show individuals residing in northern areas of the United States report a higher incidence of MS than among those residing in southern states. Those who change regions prior to the age of 15 take on the same risk as those residing in their new home region. Those who move after age 15 show the same incidence as their previous home. This suggests exposure to an environmental factor in childhood may trigger MS later in life (National Multiple Sclerosis Society, 2003b).

A third theory, as yet unproven, looks at a variety of viruses as a cause of MS, since viruses often cause demyelination and inflammation. Though not contagious to others, the virus theory examines the idea that a virus could cause the immune system to attack the body. Finally, genetic factors, another yet unproven theory, show one's chances of contracting MS increases several fold if a family member contracts the disease. While scientists cannot pinpoint a specific genetic cause of MS, some studies suggest genetic material of individuals with MS contains some common genetic markers that, with future advances in genetic techniques, may show an increased suscep-

tibility to MS (Adams, Victor, & Ropper, 1997; National Multiple Sclerosis Society, 2003b).

EPIDEMIOLOGY

The Multiple Sclerosis Society, the organization dedicated to ending the devastating effects of MS, estimates that in the United States MS affects between 250,000 and 350,000 or more individuals. MS occurs more in women than men at a ratio of approximately 2 to 3. The frequency is greater in whites of northern European ancestry than in African Americans and Asian Americans (National Multiple Sclerosis Society, 2003f; Smith & Schapiro, 2000). MS virtually never occurs in some populations, such as Eskimos. MS often strikes individuals in the prime of life, during young adulthood, with two-thirds of the cases of MS showing an onset between ages 20 to 50 (National Multiple Sclerosis Society, 2003c).

CLINICAL SIGNS AND SYMPTOMS

When one speaks of MS, one speaks of a disease of unknown origin whose unpredictable symptoms, both visible and hidden, vary in severity from individual to individual. The variability of symptoms and the similarity of its symptoms with other neurological disorders often trick physicians into confusing MS with other conditions, such as systemic lupus erythematosus or vertigo. Physicians often make the diagnosis of MS as a last resort, after the other possible diagnostic labels prove incorrect. This sometimes takes 5 to 10 years. Though magnetic resonance imaging (MRI) can confirm the diagnosis in most cases, pressure to curb high-priced diagnostic tests often influences physicians to look for alternative methods of diagnosis.

In order to make a formal diagnosis of MS, physicians must find 2 basic signs in their patients. One must show a history of at least 2 attacks separated in time where the symptoms come and go, commonly referred to as relapses (exacerbations) and remissions. One must also show signs of damage to 2 or more parts of the myelin sheaths of the CNS (Hall, Rohaly, & Shneider, 1995; Martin & Dhib-Jalbut, 2000).

Table 21-1

Signs and Symptoms That Individuals With Multiple Sclerosis May Experience

Sensory Functions	Movement-Related Functions	Mental Functions
Blurred vision	Spasticity	Short-term memory difficulties
Diplopia (double vision)	Gait and balance difficulties	Shortened attention span
Blank spots in the visual field	Paralysis of some degree	Difficulty concentrating
Nystagmus	Intention tremor	Emotional lability
Paresthesia or numbness	Ataxia	Depression
Vertigo	Incoordination	
Auditory disturbances (rare)	Fatigue	
	Incontinence	

Individuals with MS may experience symptoms that affect sensory, movement-related, and mental functions (Table 21-1) (National Multiple Sclerosis Society, 2003e). Problems with sensory functions usually include visual difficulties such as blurred vision, diplopia or double vision, nystagmus, and blank spots. Other sensory symptoms may include paresthesia and/or numbness, vertigo, and auditory disturbances. Movement-related symptoms may include spasticity, gait and balance difficulties, paralysis of some degree, weakness, intention tremor, ataxia, bladder dysfunction, bowel problems, and sexual dysfunction. Impaired mental functions may include problems with short-term memory and attention span (National Multiple Sclerosis Society, 2003b; Paty, 2000; Smith & Schapiro, 2000). Fatigue or lassitude is one of the most common symptoms of MS. This fatigue usually occurs in the late afternoon or early evening. Fatigue in individuals with MS may be due to the disease process itself, or from difficulty sleeping, depression, muscle weakness, deconditioning, motor control difficulties, and/or medication side effects (Smith & Schapiro, 2000). Many individuals report feeling slightly more energized after a brief rest (National Multiple Sclerosis Society, 2003d; Smith & Schapiro, 2000).

Not all individuals diagnosed with MS will find themselves with the same symptoms. Following diagnosis, MS generally follows 1 of 4 patterns:

1. Relapsing-remitting
2. Primary-progressive
3. Secondary-progressive
4. Progressive-relapsing

The relapsing-remitting pattern causes those affected to experience a sudden onset of symptoms or attacks followed by partial or total recovery over time. A slow progressive decline characterizes the primary-progressive pattern. In some cases, there are occasional plateaus and/or minimal improvements. The secondary-progressive pattern initially starts as a relapsing-remitting pattern that changes to a progressive decline with few, if any, remissions or plateaus. The rare progressive-relapsing pattern is characterized by a progressive decline with evident relapses or exacerbations. There are no remissions between periods of relapses/exacerbations, just continual worsening of symp-

toms (National Multiple Sclerosis Society, 2003a; Smith & Schapiro, 2000).

Other conditions can cause pseudoexacerbations, or worsening of symptoms that are not caused by the disease process itself. An increase in body temperature, caused by infection, fever, or overexertion, can cause a flare-up in symptoms (Smith & Schapiro, 2000). Others also claim stress serves to exacerbate symptoms (Hall et al., 1995; National Multiple Sclerosis Society, 2003c).

MEDICAL TREATMENT

Physicians use a variety of medications to treat the symptoms of MS. Those people with MS who have increased muscle tone, spasticity, or "stiffness" may be treated with antispasticity medications such as baclofen. These medications may cause side effects, such as increased fatigue, for the individuals taking them. In some cases, injections of botulinum toxin or a nerve block may be given to reduce spasticity and improve functional movement. Lassitude may be treated with medications such as Prozac (Eli Lilly and Company, Indianapolis, IN). Depression can be treated with antidepressive medications and psychotherapy (Smith & Schapiro, 2000).

OT intervention can minimize the effects of MS on one's occupation—those activities and tasks of everyday life given value and meaning by the individual performing them—and one's roles (Finlayson, Imprey, Nicolle, & Edwards, 1998). The person with MS may also be seen by other health care professionals such as speech therapy for improving communication, physical therapy for improving mobility, and nursing.

REFERRAL SOURCES

Individuals with MS may receive referrals for OT services from case managers, the state vocational rehabilitation services, certified rehabilitation counselors, the National Multiple Sclerosis Society, primary care physicians, physiatrists, neurologists, rehabilitation nurses, and others.

Table 21-2

Mrs. Simon's Signs and Symptoms

- Balance difficulties
- Difficulty walking
- Incoordination
- Numbness in right upper extremity

- Impaired sensation for light touch and stereognosis
- Decreased strength in the right hand
- Fatigue

IMPACT ON OCCUPATION

Symptoms of MS may impair the ability to perform one's occupations (i.e., the meaningful and purposeful activities in one's life) (Finlayson et al., 1998). MS symptoms can interfere with or change one's role as worker, parent, spouse, homemaker, and others. For example, a mother may find she can no longer care for her baby or a husband may find that his wife now needs to bathe him, thus altering their previous roles.

Decreased endurance, a common symptom in individuals with MS, may interfere with independent performance in daily living activities. The severity of the endurance problem will vary from individual to individual. For example, one individual may fatigue while participating in homemaking activities such as cooking and cleaning. Another individual may fatigue during less strenuous activities such as taking a shower or getting dressed. For others, participation in a single activity may not be so fatiguing, but the combination of all activities they must participate in during the day may be beyond their endurance level.

Motor problems are also symptoms of MS, although they may not occur in every person with MS and the degree of severity varies. These problems include a) difficulty with balance, b) paralysis or paresis, c) ataxia, d) intention tremors, and e) incoordination. Difficulty with balance will often compromise a person's functional mobility such as walking around one's kitchen to cook or prepare simple meals, transferring in and out of a shower or bathtub, and getting in and out of a car. A person with balance problems would also experience difficulty moving in community settings such as a shopping mall or grocery store in which an unexpected "bump" from another person may cause a fall. Paralysis or paresis, ataxia, intention tremors, and incoordination in the upper extremities will hamper a person's ability to put on clothes, fasten buttons, use utensils to eat, write, or otherwise pick up and manipulate tools used in daily living tasks.

Sensory problems, numbness, or parethesias may also cause difficulty with manipulating tools and objects. The person with sensory problems also needs to take extra precautions to avoid injury from burning him- or herself on hot objects or cutting him- or herself on sharp objects.

The cognitive symptoms acting alone or in concert with motor and sensory symptoms can contribute to difficulties in the workplace. An individual may lack the ability to remember details required for work or may find it difficult or impossible to concentrate on job responsibilities. Some symptoms may interfere with safe task performance or the person's safety in general. For example, short-term memory problems may cause an individual working in a restaurant to leave the stove on.

CASE STUDY

Mrs. Ryeman Simon, 31 years old, is married and has 2 children, one boy age 9 and one girl age 7. She works as a catering manager at a large resort hotel on the grounds of Rocky Raccoon's Fantasy World. She lives with her family in a 3-bedroom house. The house has a basement where the laundry room is located.

Mrs. Simon was recently diagnosed with MS (Table 21-2). Two weeks ago, Mrs. Simon had numerous symptoms, particularly constant fatigue, incoordination, and numbness in her dominant right hand. She experienced these types of symptoms before, but they went away after a week of rest. This time she was admitted to the hospital where the diagnosis of relapsing-remitting MS was finally made. She continues on sick leave following her discharge from the hospital.

Prior to this hospitalization, Mrs. Simon was independent in all ADL and IADL. Mrs. Simon considers herself a good wife and mother, taking good care of her husband and children. Since the exacerbation, she tires easily when participating in self-care activities. Her husband assists her with bathing and dressing. While she always assumed responsibility for all the cooking, laundry, and housecleaning activities, her family has now taken over these duties. Mrs. Simon enjoys working in her flower beds and garden in the backyard. However, she stopped gardening because she lacks energy and cannot get down to the ground or up from the ground without help.

Mrs. Simon has worked for Rocky Raccoon's Fantasy World for 7 years and is a well-liked employee, winning employee of the month awards 12 times. As catering manager, she is responsible for all arrangements for catered events at the Bandit Hotel. This includes coordinating events with resorts' sales managers and their clients, ordering all food, and coordinating outside vendors who provide decorations or entertainment. Her job requires her to schedule and supervise 12 employees. These employees need direction in arranging the room set-up for specific events, setting tables, and serving food. She knows she will have to regain her strength and energy before she can return to work.

Mrs. Simon's doctor has a note for her to give to her boss. It reads as follows: "Mrs. Simon is able to return to her job with the following restrictions: no work around steam and/or heat, no prolonged standing, no work over 40 hours per week, no lifting over 20 pounds. Mrs. Simon fatigues easily. Recommend an on-site assessment by OT to evaluate the need for further workplace accommodations to facilitate return to work to fullest extent possible."

She is concerned she will be unable to return to her job. She is having so much difficulty just caring for herself and her family. She knows some things must change in order for her to continue to care for herself and her children, manage her home, and do her job again, but she does not know what changes need to be made.

Mrs. Simon was referred to an outpatient clinic by her health maintenance organization (HMO) physician for an evaluation. This HMO authorized the evaluation but requires the OT to phone in with the recommended plan of treatment to obtain authorization for additional visits.

THEORY THAT FRAMES PRACTICE

The Person-Environment-Occupation Model provides a framework for OT practice. This model, which emphasizes client-centered practice, looks at the interaction among the person, environments, and occupations (Law et al., 1996; Stewart et al., 2003). The interplay between the person, the environment, and occupation leads to occupational performance. In the client-centered approach, the client plays a central role setting goals and prioritizing treatment to enable occupational performance. A client-centered approach will be used with Mrs. Simon.

Because MS is a chronic progressive disease, the rehabilitation frame of reference is often used. When motor, sensory, and/or cognitive impairments cannot be remediated, clients are educated in compensatory methods, given adaptive devices/equipment, and/or the environment is adapted to enable occupation (Trombly, 2002).

Assessment and Evaluation Process

Prior to Mrs. Simon's first visit, the OT reviewed the medical evaluation that the referring physician sent and the prescription ordering OT. With knowledge of the MS disease process, knowledge about specific deficits documented by the referring physician, and some background information on Mrs. Simon's occupational roles, the OT gathered several assessment tools in preparation for Mrs. Simon's first visit to the outpatient clinic. The OT assessment looked at how Mrs. Simon functions, the different environments in which Mrs. Simon functions, and the occupations in which she participates. The simulated apartment in the outpatient clinic was the setting for the OT evaluation.

As Mrs. Simon walked into the outpatient facility, the OT noted she was using a straight cane to assist her with ambulation. The OT introduced herself and the OTA. The OT

described how OT might help Mrs. Simon resume her roles—wife, mother, and caterer—and help her participate in her occupations. Mrs. Simon displayed a positive attitude and appeared receptive to making necessary modifications to her lifestyle in order to resume her roles.

To start the evaluation process, the OT asked about Mrs. Simon's past medical history and recent medical problems that resulted in her hospitalization. The OT continued to interview Mrs. Simon to obtain an occupational profile. The OT wanted to determine Mrs. Simon's occupational roles and related tasks, her interests, and her priorities.

The OT administered the COPM. The COPM determines which occupations are most important to the client and the client's perception of performance in these occupations. Mrs. Simon's priorities included a) managing her own self-care, b) caring for her family (cooking, cleaning, and laundering), c) returning to her job as a catering manager, and d) tending to her flower gardens.

As part of the evaluation to determine her daily occupations, the OTA helped Mrs. Simon fill out an activity configuration to illustrate a typical day prior to her hospitalization. Figure 21-1 shows the activity configuration. A typical weekday includes helping the children get ready for school before going to work, picking the children up at an after school program before going home to prepare dinner, cleaning up after dinner, and fixing everyone's lunch for the next day. Her typical weekend consists of housecleaning, laundry, driving the children to and from various activities, and preparing meals.

Mrs. Simon explained that her work requires a great deal of walking, especially in and out of the kitchen area as she coordinates schedules of employees and catered events. Other job functions include using the computer to maintain schedules, write reports, place orders, and complete Internet searches for special services and supplies. Although not an essential function of her job, she often assists food services employees with the set up of decorations and food, including lifting and carrying items that weigh up to 30 pounds.

The OTA assessed Mrs. Simon's ability to dress and undress herself. Mrs. Simon needed assistance to button and unbutton her shirt, as well as assistance to manage the zipper and snap for her jeans due to decreased strength in her right hand. She needed contact guard assist to maintain her standing balance while standing to pull up her pants. She also needed assistance to tie her running shoes because of the incoordination in her right hand.

Mrs. Simon told the OT she loves to soak in a hot bath but now is unable to sit down in and get up from the bottom of the bathtub. She needs Mr. Simon's assistance to step in and out of the bathtub. She says she stands and braces herself by placing a hand on the wall so she does not lose her balance, while Mr. Simon helps her to bathe. She tries to help bathe herself but has difficulty holding onto the wet bar of soap in her free hand. Asking Mrs. Simon to transfer in and out of the bathtub in the simulated apartment, the OT found that Mrs. Simon requires moderate physical assistance to maintain her standing balance while stepping in and out of the bathtub.

The OT assessed Mrs. Simon's ability in home management activities. Mrs. Simon required minimal assistance to maintain

Time	Monday	Tuesday	Wednesday	Thursday	Friday	Saturday	Sunday
6-7 am	Bathe, dress	Bathe, dress	Bathe, dress	Bathe, dress	Bathe, dress	Sleep	Sleep
7-8 am	Make breakfast, wash dishes, get children off to school	Make breakfast, wash dishes, get children off to school	Make breakfast, wash dishes, get children off to school	Make breakfast, wash dishes, get children off to school	Make breakfast, wash dishes, get children off to school	Bathe, dress, make breakfast, wash dishes	Bathe, dress, make breakfast, wash dishes
8-9 am	Make beds, drive to work	Make beds, drive to work	Make beds, drive to work	Make beds, drive to work	Make beds, drive to work	Make beds	Make beds
9-10 am	Work	Work	Work	Work	Work	Drive children to activities	Church
10-11 am	Work	Work	Work	Work	Work	Laundry	Church
11-Noon	Work	Work	Work	Work	Work	Cleaning	Change clothes
12-1 pm	Work	Work	Work	Work	Work	Make lunch, wash dishes	Make lunch, wash dishes
1-2 pm	Work	Work	Work	Work	Work	Drive children to activities	Drive children to activities
2-3 pm	Work	Work	Work	Work	Work	Laundry	Gardening
3-4 pm	Work	Work	Work	Work	Work	Cleaning	Gardening
4-5 pm	Work	Work	Work	Work	Work	Gardening	Gardening
5-6 pm	Pick up children, make dinner	Pick up children, make dinner	Pick up children, make dinner	Pick up children, make dinner	Pick up children, make dinner	Pick up children, make dinner	Pick up children, make dinner
6-7 pm	Eat dinner	Eat dinner	Eat dinner	Eat dinner	Eat dinner	Eat dinner	Eat dinner
7-8 pm	Wash dishes	Wash dishes	Wash dishes	Wash dishes	Wash dishes	Wash dishes	Wash dishes
8-9 pm	Other chores, such as laundry, grocery shopping, clothes shopping, etc.					Family activity	Family activity
9-10 pm	Make lunches	Make lunches	Make lunches	Make lunches	Family activity	Family activity	Make lunches
10-11 pm	TV	TV	TV	TV	TV	TV	TV

Figure 21-1. Activity configuration.

her standing balance when bending to the lower cabinet to get out pots and pans and when reaching into the lower part of the refrigerator to get food items. Since she fatigues quickly, Mrs. Simon told the OT she is unable to complete simple meal preparation tasks. As part of the evaluation of her environments, the OT discovered that currently, Mrs. Simon does not do the laundry at home because she is unable to go up and down the stairs and has difficulty carrying the laundry. In the simulated apartment, Mrs. Simon was able to place laundry into the washer and dryer, but needed contact guard assist with balance when attempting to take laundry out of the washer and dryer. When making the queen-sized bed in the simulated apartment, Mrs. Simon was only able to complete half of the task before tiring.

The OTA used a dynamometer and a pinch meter to assess Mrs. Simon's grip and pinch strengths. Mrs. Simon's right grip strength measured 26 pounds compared to the left side of 42 pounds. Her 3-point pinch strength in her right hand measured 7 pounds compared to 10 pounds in her left hand. The OTA used the 9-hole peg test to assess fine motor coordination. Results of this assessment showed a mild deficit in finger dexterity. Sensory tests completed by the OT revealed diminished sensation for light touch and stereognosis in Mrs. Simon's right hand. This deficit was evident in functional tasks as Mrs. Simon had difficulty manipulating buttons, tying her shoes, and difficulty holding a pen to write. Mrs. Simon's writing was shaky, letters were poorly formed, and she tired quickly.

Treatment Planning

Problem List

- Mrs. Simon requires minimal assistance in self-care activities, grooming, bathing, and dressing.
- Mrs. Simon requires minimal assistance to safely transfer in and out of bathtub.
- Mrs. Simon requires maximal assistance with meal preparation tasks.
- Mrs. Simon requires maximal assistance in light household cleaning activities and laundering activities.
- Mrs. Simon is unable to participate in gardening activities.
- Mrs. Simon is unable to perform work tasks of catering manager.

Treatment Goals

- Mrs. Simon will be independent in self-care activities (grooming, bathing, and dressing) using adaptive aids and energy conservation techniques as needed.
- Mrs. Simon will independently and safely transfer in and out of bathtub using safety grab bars.
- Mrs. Simon will be independent in meal preparation tasks using energy conservation techniques, work simplification techniques, and adaptive aids as needed.
- Mrs. Simon will be independent in light household cleaning activities and laundering activities using energy conservation techniques, work simplification techniques, and adaptive equipment as needed.
- Mrs. Simon will be independent in maintaining her table top flower garden and flower window boxes using energy conservation techniques and adaptive equipment as needed.
- Mrs. Simon will be independent in performing her job of catering manager using energy conservation techniques, work simplification techniques, and adaptive equipment as needed.

Treatment Interventions

- Provide education in principles of energy conservation and work simplification techniques and incorporation of principles into daily living tasks.
- Provide assistance to obtain a safety bath bench and education in care and use of safety bath bench.
- Provide safety education.
- Provide transfer training.
- Provide education and assistance in modifying various environments such as the bathroom, bedroom, kitchen, and work area to promote safety and independent performance.
- Provide education in the disease process of MS and precautions.

Treatment Implementation

The OT contacted and received approval from the HMO to provide OT services 3 times a week for 3 weeks. The OT and OTA worked together closely as a team, providing intervention strategies to help Mrs. Simon return to her roles.

Typical in clients with MS, endurance is a major limiting factor in Mrs. Simon's daily life that interferes with occupational performance. The OT discusses Mrs. Simon's daily routine and makes several recommendations to modify this routine. This will enable Mrs. Simon to complete all priority tasks within her endurance level with less fatigue. Avoiding fatigue is a precaution for people with MS. The OT also educates Mrs. Simon in other energy conservation and work simplification techniques to promote occupational performance (Table 21-3). The OT and OTA make recommendations on how to incorporate energy conservation and work simplification techniques in all daily living tasks so that new habits and routines are developed. These techniques (Fasoli, 2002) include:

- Participate in activities while seated.
- Organizing the work area and obtaining all supplies, tools, and equipment prior to starting the task.
- Minimize energy expenditure by combining tasks and eliminating unnecessary tasks.
- Use lightweight tools that do not require as much energy to lift.
- Use electrical appliances to do work.
- Use equipment that will eliminate need to bend (e.g., reacher) or to lift and carry heavy items (e.g., rolling cart).
- Arrange materials so that gravity assists with task completion.
- Pace self when participating in an activity and take rest breaks.
- Have others do the task for you.
- Plan daily/weekly schedule to pace self, distributing tasks requiring more energy throughout the day/week.

Intervention Strategies to Promote Independence in Personal Activities of Daily Living (Self-Care Activities)

To facilitate independence in dressing, the OT discussed the arrangement of Mrs. Simon's bedroom with her. The OT suggested the easy chair in the bedroom become the center of Mrs. Simon's "dressing station." She suggested Mrs. Simon choose her clothing for the next day and lay the items out next to her "dressing" chair each night before work.

She also suggested that Mrs. Simon consider bathing in the evening. This would spread out the tasks of bathing and dressing. A good night's rest after bathing would enable Mrs. Simon to regain her energy for the morning dressing routine. The OTA provided Mrs. Simon with a button hook that has a zipper pull on one end. The OTA showed Mrs. Simon how to use this adaptive aid and had her practice using the button hook and zipper pull. Mrs. Simon was able to manage buttons and zippers with this adaptive device.

For grooming activities, the OTA suggested Mrs. Simon place a stool in her bathroom vanity area so that she could sit and conserve energy while brushing her teeth, fixing her hair,

Table 21-3

Treatment Strategies

Treatment Strategy	Research
Aerobic exercise	Petajan et al., 1996
Aquatics programs	Broach, Groff, Dattilo, Yaffe, & Gast, 1997/1998; Vanage, Gilbertson, & Mathiowetz, 2003
Compensatory techniques to cope with cognitive changes in the workplace	Gulick, 1992; Yorkston et al., 2003
Setting priorities and other compensatory strategies to address fatigue in the workplace	Gulick, 1992; Yorkston et al., 2003
Assistive technology and environmental adaptations	Mann, Ottenbacher, Fraas, Tomita, & Granger, 1999
Fatigue management program, including energy conservation techniques	Bowcher & May, 1998; Veenstra, Brasile, & Stewart, 2003; Ward & Winters, 2003
Tai chi	Mills, Allen, & Morgan, 2000

and putting on make-up. If she is sitting while doing these activities, Mrs. Simon does not have to worry about losing her balance while standing.

To ensure safety and independence in bathtub transfers, the OT explained to Mrs. Simon the necessity to obtain safety grab bars for the bathtub. She provided Mrs. Simon with the names of several hardware stores where she could purchase the safety grab bars. Mr. Simon knew a reliable handyman who could install them. The OT provided directions on the placement and angle of the safety grab bars in Mrs. Simon's bathtub. The OT also recommended that Mrs. Simon obtain a safety tub seat to sit on while bathing. This will help her save energy while bathing. The OT informed Mrs. Simon that the Multiple Sclerosis Society provides durable medical equipment to people with MS who have the need for such equipment.

A hand-held showerhead was also recommended. This showerhead eliminates the need for someone to stand and turn to rinse off in the bathtub. Mrs. Simon was cautioned not to shower with very hot water, as this would contribute to fatigue. To save energy, it was recommended that Mrs. Simon wrap herself in a full terry cloth robe to dry. The robe will absorb the water, eliminating the need for reaching and rubbing to dry off. The OT also recommended soap on a rope or soap in a pump bottle so that Mrs. Simon would not have difficulty with dropping the soap while bathing.

Intervention Strategies to Promote Independence in Meal Preparation and Home Management

The OT asked Mrs. Simon to outline her kitchen set up. The OT made several recommendations to Mrs. Simon on how to put needed tools and items in easily accessible areas or areas where it was easier to obtain and restore tools and items. Those items Mrs. Simon uses less frequently for meal preparation should be placed on the higher cabinet shelves and further back in the cabinets. Those items most often used should be placed in areas where Mrs. Simon can reach them without excessive bending or having to move other items to access them. Items in the refrigerator that are used most often should be placed on the higher shelves in the front. If the family buys items in larger containers, these items may be split up into smaller containers. For example, a gallon of milk can be poured into 2 half gallon containers so that Mrs. Simon can lift them more easily. Electrical appliances such as food processors and electrical mixers can help with food preparation while saving energy. With a little planning ahead, Mrs. Simon can gather all needed supplies and use a rolling cart to help transport those supplies to the designated work area. Mrs. Simon can also use the rolling cart to transport items to the dining room, or other area in the house, eliminating the need to lift and carry.

A kitchen stool placed near a kitchen counter can enable Mrs. Simon to sit while preparing foods. The OT also suggested Mrs. Simon consider enlisting family assistance on the weekend to make larger amounts of food that can be frozen or refrigerated for use throughout the week. In this way, Mrs. Simon will not have to prepare a meal each weekday evening; she can merely heat a meal. The children were encouraged to assume such chores as setting and clearing the table and loading and unloading the dishwasher to help Mrs. Simon save energy. She also suggested Mrs. Simon assign her husband and children to prepare their own lunches for work and school, respectively.

The OTA discussed ways to enable Mrs. Simon to do some light housekeeping activities. She recommended Mrs. Simon use a lightweight vacuum throughout the house, including the kitchen area. She further recommended that Mrs. Simon sit while vacuuming and dusting, moving to another seat when unable to easily reach another area of the room. She had Mrs. Simon practice this in the simulated ADL apartment, demonstrating how Mrs. Simon can move her body while seated in order to reach much of the surrounding area with the vacuum. The OTA showed Mrs. Simon a way to make the bed while saving energy. She had Mrs. Simon sit at various places on the edge of the bed while making one trip around the bed to straighten the sheets, blankets, and bedspread.

Discussion revealed Mr. Simon is "handy" and he previously considered installing a laundry chute. He will do this to eliminate the need to carry dirty laundry to the basement. Mrs. Simon can make one trip to the basement to sort the clothing and start the laundry. Other family members can take responsibility to place laundry in the dryer, and when dry, carry it upstairs to a work area where Mrs. Simon will iron and fold clothing. Family members can then take their own clothes to their rooms.

Intervention Strategies to Promote Independence in Leisure Participation

It was noted that Mr. Simon already started construction of a gardening table and several window flower boxes. Mrs. Simon can now sit at the table and tend to her window boxes. The rolling utility cart can transport flower boxes to and from desired locations, as well as to transport a watering can to water flowers. These compensatory techniques and adaptive equipment will help her save energy.

Intervention Strategies to Facilitate Return to Work

To facilitate Mrs. Simon's return to work, the OT and OTA will review with Mrs. Simon the specific functions involved in her job. Reviewing the specific tasks and comparing them to the work restrictions outlined by Mrs. Simon's physician will help determine which tasks Mrs. Simon is able to do, which tasks may require reasonable accommodations, and which tasks she shouldn't do.

Reasonable accommodations Mrs. Simon may require to perform her job include a) rearrangement of her work station to eliminate the need to retrieve items from other areas by extended reach or bending, b) using voice activation software for the computer at work, c) having a shortened workday, d) having a flexible work schedule, e) having an area and time to rest during the day, and f) having a power scooter for transportation in the facility.

The OT and OTA will work with Mrs. Simon to develop the skills she needs to advocate for needed accommodations from her employer. The OT, with the assistance of the OTA, offered to provide consultation to the employer to facilitate the reasonable accommodation process and Mrs. Simon's smooth transition back into the workplace. This consultation could include an on-site workplace evaluation to further explore essential job tasks and how they can be modified or accommodated to enable Mrs. Simon to perform her job.

Discharge Planning

The Simon family was also invited to the clinic for an educational session on how Mrs. Simon has redesigned her lifestyle, how she uses adaptive equipment and compensatory techniques to manage her daily living tasks, and how they can help. The OT and the OTA plan to make a visit to Mrs. Simon's home to help Mrs. Simon implement and carryover ideas and concepts learned in the clinic. Mrs. Simon was also given information on how to contact the National Multiple Sclerosis Society and the local chapter for support and information on discharge.

CLINICAL PROBLEM SOLVING

In OT, treatment plans are individualized for each patient/client. Patient/client goals, stage in life, roles, and the context in which he or she lives are some of the factors that guide the treatment planning process. How will you change your treatment plan for each change listed below?

1. Mrs. Simon tells her employer about her diagnosis. Her employer would like her to come back to work and contacts you to do a site visit to determine whether or not reasonable accommodations could enable Mrs. Simon to return to work.

   You visit the work site with Mrs. Simon and interview her employer and supervisor. You look at how Mrs. Simon functions in the workplace and try to determine the essential functions of the job. (See Real Record 21-1)

2. Mrs. Simon tells you that while she was out on sick leave she received notice that she was "let go" from her job. What can you do to facilitate her return to competitive employment?

   OTs and OTAs should consider referring Mrs. Simon to her state's Department of Vocational Rehabilitation for assistance with job searching and retraining. OTs and OTAs can also help Mrs. Simon look at her skills and abilities and help determine which strengths can transfer to opportunities for other types of jobs. Suggest part-time employment as an option and discuss coping strategies for the workplace.

   OTs and OTAs can also help Mrs. Simon advocate for herself if she feels she was terminated for a discriminatory reason and wishes to pursue that avenue. OT input into the determination of one's functional abilities in everyday activities can play a key role in this area (Williams v. Toyota Motor Mf, 534 U.S. 184, 2002).

3. Mrs. Simon explains to you that in her culture it is expected that she perform all housekeeping tasks. Housekeeping work is considered woman's work; men do not help with these activities. What can you do to help Mrs. Simon develop alternative strategies?

Can certain tasks be eliminated or performed another way to enable Mrs. Simon's to perform them? If not, consider whether Mrs. Simon has support systems in the community through her church, synagogue, or mosque who might help her with housekeeping, and individuals from the same cultural background who understand the situation might be willing to help.

Can the National Multiple Sclerosis Society help with referrals to community agencies? Are there community agencies that provide housekeeping services? Can the family afford to pay for these services if the community cannot provide them?

4. During the initial interview, you find out that Mrs. Simon is employed as a short order cook at one of the resort restaurants. Her job requires her to cook over a hot stove and stand on her feet all day long. How can you accommodate Mrs. Simon's job?

Together with Mrs. Simon, look at whether there are alternative ways that Mrs. Simon can perform her job. Can she do her job sitting on a bar stool-height chair? Are there other strategies Mrs. Simon can use to enable her to work at her job? If not, are there other jobs Mrs. Simon can do for her same employer? If not for the same employer, can Mrs. Simon work for another employer doing similar work?

5. Mrs. Simon is a 70-year-old retired nurse. Her grown children live more than 500 miles away in another state. She is the primary caretaker of her elderly husband. Her husband requires maximal assist with all his self-care, bed mobility, and transfers. How can we enable Mrs. Simon to manage her situation? What does she need?

Mrs. Simon needs to process what she will need to manage her situation. The OT and OTA can help Mrs. Simon evaluate what she can and can't do, what she will need assistance with, and what support systems she has in the community. Can her husband acquire a higher level of independence in self-care through OT intervention to make his care easier?

Mrs. Simon may need referral to community agencies that can provide support for her husband. She may benefit from support groups sponsored by the National Multiple Sclerosis Society and other supportive literature it provides.

The OT and OTA may want to encourage Mrs. Simon to consult with her adult children to help evaluate alternatives for their parents as a family. Financial matters may become an issue should Mrs. Simon need to hire a caretaker.

LEARNING ACTIVITIES

1. Go to the National Multiple Sclerosis Society Web site and download information about the latest research and treatment of MS.

2. List specific activities Mrs. Simon can assign to her children to assist her in the home as a form of energy conservation.

3. Go to a grocery store and make a list of energy conservation ideas for Mrs. Simon to use during her grocery shopping.

4. List 5 things Mrs. Simon can do each day to lower her stress level.

5. List 2 other things the handy Mr. Simon can construct around the house to enable his wife to participate more in meaningful activities with less fatigue.

REFERENCES

Adams, R. D., Victor, M., & Ropper, A. H. (1997). *Principles of neurology* (6th ed.). New York, NY: McGraw Hill.

Bowcher, H., & May, M. (1998). Occupational therapy for the management of fatigue in multiple sclerosis. *British Journal of Occupational Therapy, 16*(1), 488-492.

Broach, E., Groff, D., Dattilo, J., Yaffe, R., & Gast, D. (1997/98). Effects of aquatic therapy on adults with multiple sclerosis. Annual in Therapeutic Recreation, Volume 7; abstract available on line at http://www.indiana.edu/~lrs/lrs95/ebroach95.html.

Fasoli, S. E. (2002). Restoring competence for homemaker and parent roles. In C. A. Trombly & M. V. Radomski (Eds.), *OT for physical dysfunction* (5th ed., pp. 695-713). Baltimore, MD: Williams & Wilkins.

Finlayson, M., Imprey, M. W., Nicolle, C., & Edwards, J. (1998). Self-care, productivity and leisure limitations of people with multiple sclerosis in Manitoba. *Canadian Journal of Occupational Therapy, 65*(5), 299-308.

Gulick, E. (1992). Model for predicting work performance among persons with multiple sclerosis. *Nursing Research, 41,* 266-272.

Hall, H. L., Rohaly, S. M., & Shneider, M. A. (1995). Multiple sclerosis. In M. G. Brodwin, F. Tellez, & S. K. Brodwin, (Eds.), *Medical, psychological, and vocational aspects of disability* (pp. 455-471). Athens, GA: Elliot & Fitzpatrick, Inc.

Law, M., Cooper, B., Strong, S., Stewart, D., Rigby, P., & Letts, L. (1996). The person-environment-occupational model: A transactive approach to occupational performance. *Canadian Journal of Occupational Therapy, 63*(1), 9-23.

Mann, W. C., Ottenbacher, K. J., Fraas, L., Tomita, M., & Granger, C. V. (1999). Effectiveness of assistive technology and environmental interventions in maintaining independence and reducing home costs for the frail elderly: A randomized controlled trial. *Archives of Family Medicine, 8*(3), 210-217.

Martin, R., & Dhib-Jalbut, S. (2000). Immunology and etiologic concepts. In J. S. Burks and K. P. Johnson (Eds.), *Multiple sclerosis: Diagnosis, medical management, and rehabilitation* (pp. 75-79). New York: Demos Medical Publishing, Inc.

Mills, N., Allen, J., & Morgan, S. C. (2000). Does Tai Chi/Qi Gong help patients with multiple sclerosis? *Journal of Bodywork and Movement Therapies, 4*(1), 39-48.

National Multiple Sclerosis Society. (2003a). What is multiple sclerosis? Retrieved January 2, 2004, from http://www.nationalmssociety.org/What is MS.asp.

National Multiple Sclerosis Society. (2003b). Causes of MS (Etiology). Retrieved January 2, 2004, from http://www.nationalmssociety.org/Sourcebook-Etiology.asp.

National Multiple Sclerosis Society. (2003c). Emotional aspects. Retrieved January 2, 2004, from http://www.nationalmssociety.org/Sourcebook-Emotional.asp.

National Multiple Sclerosis Society. (2003d). Symptoms. Retrieved January 2, 2004, from http://www.nationalmssociety.org/Symptoms.asp.

National Multiple Sclerosis Society. (2003e). Visual symptoms. Retrieved January 2, 2004, from: http://www.nationalmssociety.org/Sourcebook-Visual Symptom.asp.

National Multiple Sclerosis Society. (2003f). Who gets MS? Retrieved January 2, 2004, from http://www.nationalmssociety.org/Who gets MS.asp.

Paty, D. W. (2000). Initial symptoms. In J. S. Burks and K. P. Johnson (Eds.), *Multiple sclerosis: Diagnosis, medical management, and rehabilitation* (pp. 75-79). New York: Demos Medical Publishing, Inc.

Petajan, J. H., Gappmaier, E., White, A. T., Spencer, M. K., Mino, L., & Hicks, R. W. (1996). Impact of aerobic training on fitness and quality of life in multiple sclerosis. *Annals of Neurology, 39*, 432-441.

Smith, C. R., & Schapiro, R. T. (2000). Neurology. In R. C. Kalb (Ed.), Multiple sclerosis: *The questions you have—The answers you need* (pp. 7-41). New York: Demos Medical Publishing, Inc.

Stewart, S., Letts, L., Law, M., Cooper, B. A., Strong, S., & Rigby, P. J., (2003). The person-environment-occupation model. In E. B. Crepeau, E. S. Cohn, and B. A. Shell (Eds.), *Willard & Spackman's occupational therapy* (pp. 227-231). Philadelphia: Lippincott, Williams & Wilkins.

Trombly, C. A. (2002). Conceptual foundations for practice. In C. A. Trombly & M. V. Radomski (Eds.), *Occupational therapy for physical dysfunction* (pp. 1- 15). Philadelphia: Lippincott, Williams & Wilkins.

Vanage, S. M., Gilbertson, K. K., & Mathiowetz, V. (2003). Effects of an energy conservation course on fatigue impact for persons with progressive multiple sclerosis. *American Journal of Occupational Therapy, 57*, 315-323.

Veenstra, J., Brasile, F., & Stewart, M. (2003). Perceived benefits of aquatic therapy for multiple sclerosis participants. *American Journal of Recreation Therapy, 2*(1), 33-48.

Ward, N., & Winters, S. (2003). Results of a fatigue management program in multiple sclerosis. *British Journal of Nursing, 12*(18), 1075-1080.

Williams v. Toyota Motor Mf, 534 U.S. 184, (2002).

Yorkston, K. M., Johnson, K., Klasner, E. R., Amtmann, D., Kuehn, C. M., & Dudgeon, B. (2003). Getting the work done: A qualitative study of individuals with multiple sclerosis. *Disability and Rehabilitation, 25*(8), 369–379.

Creative Clinical Resources

Occupational Therapy Services for the Community

Susan Skunk
Human Resource Director
Rocky Raccoon's Fantasy World
2222 Fantasy Drive
Fantasy World, USA

Re: Ryeman Simon

Dear Ms. Skunk;

Last week I made a site visit to the Bandit Hotel, Fantasy World to review the Catering Manager position held by Mrs. Simon to see whether or not reasonable accommodations would enable Mrs. Simon's safe performance of the essential functions of this position. Her physician recommended this OT evaluation.

I have reviewed the relevant information in Mrs. Simon's files, including medical reports, and I interviewed you, the Executive Chef ,and Mrs. Simon. I examined the premises and Mrs. Simon's kitchen work area and office. I observed Mrs. Simon's gait and balance in the workplace. However, I did not perform a complete job analysis at this time. Based upon this information, I have found the following:

1. Mrs. Simon was recently diagnosed with MS. At this time, when Mrs. Simon fatigues, her gait becomes unsteady. She currently uses no assistive devices for walking. Mrs. Simon explained that towards the end of the workday, she often uses the wall or equipment she may be moving (ie. carts) for support as she moves about the kitchen. She has never fallen in the kitchen but towards the end of her shift, she does fear falling.

2. Mrs. Simon has the following work restrictions according to her physician's statements:

   a. No work around steam or heat.

   b. No prolonged standing.

   c. No lifting over 20 lbs.

   d. No more than 40 hour work weeks.

   e. Mrs. Simon fatigues easily.

3. After discussing Mrs. Simon's situation with you and the Executive Chef, it is obvious that you both desire to do whatever you can to accommodate Mrs. Simon's job so she may stay in your employ. It is also obvious Mrs. Simon is well liked by both supervisors and fellow employees. Mrs. Simon indicated to me that she wants to remain working for the Bandit Hotel as long as she can. According to both you and the Executive Chef, even before my involvement, the subject of reasonable accommodations for Mrs. Simon had been discussed extensively. From our discussions, it is obvious you have made a concerted effort to accommodate Mrs. Simon. It is my understanding Mrs. Simon has been asked to provide specific reasonable accommodations suggestions but has provided only her restrictions and lists of tasks she cannot perform. Your comprehensive efforts to make the appropriate reasonable accommodations for Mrs. Simon has led you to seek outside technical assistance from me.

4. One problem I see is that Mrs. Simon as an employee, and you and the Executive Chef as employer see Mrs. Simon's job responsibilities very differently. Specifically, you each have different concepts of the essential functions of the position.

   Mrs. Simon listed the following as essential functions:

   a. Ordering all food for catered events.

   b. Coordinating with outside vendors providing decorations and entertainment.

   c. Scheduling and supervising 12 regular employees and casual labor as needed.

   d. Pulling equipment for banquets (silver, plates, coffee cups, etc.).

   e. Organizing and arranging banquet room setup, table setup, and food service for all events.

   f. Assuring the dirty dishes and equipment are returned to the kitchen following events.

The Executive Chef has provided me with checklists of tasks that he considers essential to Mrs. Simon's position as catering manager. The job description lists still a different set of essential functions. After reading the three different versions of the essen-

Real record 21-1. Real record for a client with multiple sclerosis.

tial functions, it seems clear the Executive Chef's checklists and the job description contain the same basic elements, with an emphasis on the catering manager's responsibility to assure that the kitchen is clean following the completion of catered events.

5. The kitchen has not been returned to a clean condition following catered events. This has been discussed with Mrs. Simon and she has indicated that she is very tired at the end of events and fears she will be unable to see this function carried out unless she has subordinate workers perform this task. Mrs. Simon has also reported that she has dropped dishes and other equipment due to numbness in her hand.

6. At this time Mrs. Simon is not performing the essential functions as they exist on all of the three essential function lists. Mrs. Simon is not able to do some functions, due to restrictions imposed by her disability and other functions just don't get done for unknown reasons. His lack of performance does not appear related solely to her disability. There are two issues here. First, there are essential functions Mrs. Simon physically cannot do. Second, there are job tasks, specifically the cleaning functions that Mrs. Simon and her subordinates are not getting done. Mrs. Simon has been disciplined for this insufficiency, which is not disability related. It seems a large part of Mrs. Simon's problem may be ineffective management style, or lack of management and/or supervisory skills. However, her inability to perform certain tasks due to her disability imposed restrictions, seems to be creating a situation where the resort lacks of enough staff to do all of the required work because Mrs. Simon is not able to do her part. I do want to stress that Mrs. Simon has been disciplined for her failure to insure the cleanliness of the kitchen at the end of catering events, although she doesn't list this as an essential function of her job, though it is stated in the job description.

7. Mrs. Simon and I explored accommodations, you, the chef, and I also explored various reasonable accommodations. Mrs. Simon would like to get a scooter type mobility device and keep it outside the kitchen in a cage for security, where she could plug it in to keep the battery charged. You agreed that this accommodation would not be a problem for the resort. I made other suggestions such as splitting Mrs. Simon's shift so she could rest in between but Mrs. Simon did not feel this was feasible. Mrs. Simon also suggested eliminating certain tasks she cannot do and looking at other tasks she might be able to do for the resort.

8. Mrs. Simon and I reviewed other open positions but unfortunately, none of the positions open at that time fit within her work restrictions. I would recommend that you review all openings as they are posted to see if any of the openings are suited to Mrs. Simon.

9. I must mention safety concerns. You cannot overlook Mrs. Simon's fear of falling in the kitchen. The kitchen tends to be a wet place with much activity. Mrs. Simon's unsteady gait presents a genuine risk of falls. The kitchen has a hard floor and heavy metal equipment that will cause serious injury should Mrs. Simon hit these areas during a fall.

10. Mrs. Simon is a client of vocational rehabilitation and she has been in touch with the rehabilitation engineers about making reasonable accommodations in the kitchen. It is my understanding the rehabilitation engineer has visited the job site. It is my understanding the rehabilitation engineer has discussed motorizing some of the equipment. When I met with Mrs. Simon, I told him I would be glad to discuss the situation with vocational rehabilitation if they call me but to date they have not.

11. Finally, a complete job analysis may be beneficial to identify the actual essential functions so we can determine whether Mrs. Simon is able to perform her job and whether the any of the suggested accommodations will have a positive impact on her job performance. The job analysis may help further separate Mrs. Simon's failure to perform from her physical inability to perform.

Please feel free to contact me should you wish me to perform the job analysis or if I can assist you in any other way.

Sincerely,

Octavia Occupational Therapist, OTR/L
Creative Clinical Resources

Real record 21-1 (continued). Real record for a client with multiple sclerosis.

Key Concepts

- Fight or flight reaction: Although people may not need to physically flee from danger, they may feel the need to do so while being unable to identify the direct source of their fear.
- Stress reaction: A stress cycle is (1) initial surprise at an event, (2) getting used to the situation followed by (3) exhaustion. If the individual does not allow (4) the resting phase of the cycle to occur, eventually dysfunction sets in (Selye, 1976).
- Disturbance of attention: An individual focused on internal feelings from the autonomic system is less able to focus on the external environment and therefore becomes inattentive (Rapee & Barlow, 1991).
- Information processing disturbance: Anxiety interferes with the normal transfer of the biochemical impulses carrying information in the CNS (Rapee & Barlow, 1991).

Essential Vocabulary

agoraphobia: Fear of being out in the open or being unable to escape a situation.

compulsion: Uncontrollable impulse to perform an act one would not normally feel the need to do. It relieves anxiety produced by an obsession.

obsession: Tendency to have a recurrent unwanted thought.

panic: Sudden acute fear or anxiety.

phobia: An irrational fear of places, situations, or things.

post traumatic stress: The state of tension some time after a stressful event in which the individual belatedly experiences the stressful event again and feels the feelings as though it were still happening.

Clinical Summary

Etiology

Panic results from environmental conditions rather than a physiological state. Something in the individual's life causes the panic response.

Prevalence

Approximately 2% of individuals worldwide have panic disorder. One in three of those have agoraphobia with the condition.

Classic Signs

The individual feels intense fear, has shortness of breath, heart palpitations, chest pains, sweating or chills, numbness or a feeling of choking or dying. The panic attacks are unexpected, followed by continual worry that another attack is imminent. The individual worries about having a heart attack or losing control.

Precautions

Give constant reassurance that the patient does not have a life-threatening illness. The individual may be reluctant to take some medication, fearing the side effects are symptoms of a terminal illness. OTAs need to be able to distinguish between a "real" heart attack that needs immediate medical attention and a panic attack.

A SELF-HELP GROUP LEADER WITH ANXIETY

Margaret Drake, PhD, OTR, FAOTA and Tonia Taylor, BS, COTA

INTRODUCTION

Anxiety disorders are among the most common disorders experienced by people who live outside the hospital. They affect approximately 7% of the US population (Granoff, 1996). These same people with anxiety often overuse the healthcare system because of the physical symptoms of their distress (Melmed, 2001; Nagy, Riggs, Krystal, & Charney, 1998; Rush, 1998). Symptoms can include afflictions of the circulatory system such as heart palpitations, chest pain, chills, hot flashes, sweating, or faintness. Symptoms of gastrointestinal distress such as nausea or diarrhea are also common (APA, 2000). Anxiety often blends with other emotions such as guilt and anger so that it is difficult to delineate it from other basic emotions of fear, love, and hate. Anxiety encompasses a future-oriented attitude in which one expects negative events and hopes to be prepared for them. Depressed people are almost always anxious, but anxious people are not necessarily always depressed. One way in which many students experience this emotion is test anxiety (Rapee & Barlow, 1991).

FRAMES OF REFERENCE

- Neuromotor behavior model: This model assumes that biology is at the foundation of all human behavior as demonstrated through the responses of the neurological system. Manipulation of the neurobiological system will change the person's experience and response to anxiety. This theory includes such ideas as those in sensory integration, the biochemistry of medication, and neurodevelopmental treatment.
- Cognitive behavioral model: This model assumes that behavioral responses are learned and can be unlearned (Fontaine, Mollard, Yao, & Cottraux, 2001). Psychiatric units adhering to this model often think of the entire psychiatric unit as a teaching situation (Sanderson & Wetzler, 1995). Some of the ideas are consistent with Maxwell Anderson's milieu therapy in which all doctors, staff, and patients are considered teachers and students

learning together. The patient is expected to respond to rewards, such as privileges to leave the psychiatric unit, or punishments, such as loss of telephone privileges.
- Person-Environment-Occupation Model: Assumes that the way a person behaves mirrors what a person has learned in his or her environment. The environment includes the concept of timing of events and what effect it has on a person's thought processes. Change is constant in environments and environments change more readily than people. An environment can either enhance or put barriers in the way of a person's performance (Stewart et al., 2003).

CASE STUDY

Ella Mae was born in a rural area of the South. She was the youngest of 8 children born to a Scotch-Irish miner and his Cajun wife in a village owned by the mining company. The family was always in poverty due to low wages and no union benefits for miners in that region. Ella Mae was a good student compared to her brothers and sisters; however, schooling was not emphasized as the parents did not make the connection between education and wages. Consequently, at age 16, when she could legally drop out of high school, Ella Mae did so. She took a factory job in a nearby crossroads village. At this small factory, she met a man nearly 10 years older and was soon pregnant. The Vietnam War was beginning to escalate. Her new husband realized he could have a living wage and home for his family if he joined the army. After boot camp, Ella Mae was able to join her husband at his station in Texas. Her 2 children were born there on the army base. Compared to the poverty stricken life of a miner's daughter, the army life felt rich. After his first stint in the service, he re-enlisted. Though Ella Mae realized her husband was drinking more, she had no thought of what to do as her own father had frequently been drunk on payday. Eventually, when her husband took discharge rather than be shipped to Asia, the family moved back to the city near where they had met. At a family reunion shortly after their return, Ella Mae had a sinking sensation when she saw her father begin to fondle her 3-year-old daughter. This episode stimulated her memory of her father fondling her at that same age. This distressing memory was denigrated and denied by her mother. After a discussion with her older sister, Ella Mae was convinced that indeed her memory was correct as her sister had also caught the grandfather fondling her 3-year-old daughter. This situation caused much family distress as the 2 factions disbelieved each other.

Ella Mae soon became aware that her husband was not able to function without the structure of the army base. He had not found a job after their return home. After a year of conflict, she left him despite the fact that she knew he would be unable to provide child support. She began to work at a variety of low paying jobs and took evening classes at the local community college in order to achieve her general education diploma (GED). Her low wages caused her to be unable to pay for the upkeep on her car. When the car broke down, she was unable to get to her job as it was not on the bus line. Consequently, she lost the job. The apartment she and the 2 children were living in had the heat and lights turned off during winter. Eventually, she was evicted for nonpayment of rent. She then persuaded her older sister to allow her and the 2 children to live in one of the bedrooms for the remainder of the winter months. She withdrew from night school at the community college. Her sister's home was only a block from the bus line so Ella Mae was able, through some concerned friends, to find a job in a church office also near the bus line. This job did not pay well, but Ella Mae got her first opportunity to learn some computer skills. She began to meet church members who accepted her into their midst. A few months later, she joined the church, saved enough money to repair her car, and began to feel like a citizen again. She began to make friends with some other women in the church. These women were exploring ideas of feminist theology. These ideas appealed to Ella Mae who had never felt particularly valued for her thoughts.

Ella Mae had always been somewhat plump but now she began to gain weight at a rapid pace. She smoked and generally had some unhealthy habits. One evening, she and one of her new friends attended a special class in a home about earth-based spirituality. There she met a rather obese man and these 2 found many things in common. Within a few weeks, they were living together, finding an acceptance as a fat couple that neither had experienced before as a single person. His job as an electronic engineer, which had seemed secure, suddenly came to an end as his company closed their local operation. Within a few weeks, his computer electronic expertise secured him a job in the Washington, DC area. Ella Mae decided to move with him.

After arriving in Washington, DC, Ella Mae found a job in a bookstore, which suited her well since she liked to read; however, the other parts of the job—record keeping, stocking the shelves, and standing for hours at the cash register—were too demanding. She failed to go to work one day after an evening of smoking marijuana with her engineer housemate. She lost the job. Her housemate had not put her on his health insurance plan, so she had no health insurance. She began to have panic attacks. She was far from family and friends. She found a women's health clinic that would give her a reduced rate for a doctor's visit. The doctor prescribed Valium (Roche Products,

Inc., Nutley, NJ) for her panic attacks. The combination of addictive Valium and recreational marijuana soon made her feel unable to exist without some sort of drug-induced state. As she spiraled into depression, the relationship with her housemate began to deteriorate. When he became physically abusive, she decided to leave. She had enough money to take the bus home where her now-married daughter lived with her newborn son and husband. After a frantic weekend, in which the daughter no longer felt able to cope with her own family and her weeping, panicky mother, she took her mother to the emergency room at a local private hospital. Ella Mae was furious with her daughter for "dumping her" at the emergency room. Nonetheless, she was able to get evaluated for medication and stopped experiencing the muscle cramping that occurred when she did not take the Valium to which she had become addicted.

Referral

The psychiatric unit in the private hospital had 20 beds for general psychiatry and a 10-bed gero-psychiatric wing as well. By this time in her life, Ella Mae was 37 years old. On her third day in the psychiatric unit, the doctor wrote an order for an OT evaluation. Ella Mae had become calm enough to be able to participate in the group activities on the unit.

The OT arrived at 8 a.m. and attended the therapeutic milieu community meeting in the day room. This was the OT's first introduction to most of the patients as she had no time to read their charts before the meeting. Ella Mae was sitting sullenly in the corner of the day room. She did not participate in the group's discussion about smoking privileges. The OTA was unable to attend these early morning community meetings because she arrived at 11:00 a.m. and carried on the OT activities program until 8 p.m.

Assessment and Evaluation Process

The OT and OTA used a treatment theory mixture of the Cognitive Behavioral Model, which matched the milieu therapy approach used by the entire psychiatric staff, and the Person-Environment-Occupation Model. Every patient referred to OT was scored on the Comprehensive Occupational Therapy Evaluation Scale (COTE), an assessment of 25 different behaviors (Brayman, Kirby, Misenheimer, & Short, 1976; Early, 2000). The OT would evaluate each new patient during a morning task group using the COTE Scale scoring form and later with the Canadian Occupational Performance Measure (COPM). Initially, Ella Mae just sat in the task group and declined to participate in the available crafts. She would jiggle one leg, then the other, then drum her fingers on the table. After the 90-minute session was about half through, she began to ask another woman patient named Ruth about the small doily she was embroidering. When the OT asked Ella Mae if she would like to try embroidery, Ella Mae responded by turning her face away and continuing to talk to Ruth, ignoring the OT. After the session was over, the OT asked Ruth if she thought Ella Mae might like to embroider and if she might be willing to teach her. Ruth, a depressed patient, protested that she didn't feel she was good enough to teach Ella Mae. With the OT's encouragement, she agreed to teach her at the next session if Ella Mae agreed. Ella Mae's initial score on the COTE Scale was 65 out of a possible 100. The higher the score, the sicker the patient is. Her greatest difficulty was in the Task Behavior areas of engagement, interest in activities, and interest in accomplishment.

Immediately after the task group, the OT used the COPM to finish her evaluation of Ella Mae. They sat together at the corner of the long work table in the OT clinic. Ella Mae continued her unsociable mien during the discussion of her situation. In the self-care portion, the only occupational performance problems were finances and transportation, which were intertwined in their source. The importance she gave to each was number 9 on a scale, with 1 being "not at all important" and 10 being "extremely important." In the productivity section, she named keeping a job as her most important problem, assigning it a number 8. The leisure problem was most important to socialization, as she had no telephone she could call her own as well as the inability to attend events where she might socialize. She gave each of these issues a 7. She felt if she solved her finances and job problem, the telephone and socialization would be solved also. The numbers she gave to each of these areas on performance and satisfaction with her performance, with 1 being poor and 10 being very good, were as follows:

Finances	performance 3	satisfaction 1
Transportation	performance 4	satisfaction 2
Keeping a job	performance 3	satisfaction 2
No telephone	performance 5	satisfaction 5
No social life	performance 4	satisfaction 5

General Goals

The OT and OTA met with Ella Mae later that afternoon, and the OT reported her findings on the COTE Scale and the COPM. Ella Mae's passive-aggressive attitude from the morning session remained during most of the 15-minute goal-setting session. The OT explained the assessment/goal-setting process as Ella Mae sat looking away from the 2 therapists. Finally, the OT said that it was mandatory for them to have Ella Mae's input into her goals. Ella Mae burst out, "I just want to get out of this loony bin!" The OTA calmly responded, "The quickest way for that to happen is for you to help us make your treatment goals." Then, the OT explained that the 3 areas that were most problematic for Ella Mae were in the task behavior areas of engagement, interest in activities, and interest in accomplishment. She asked Ella Mae to share whether she saw these as a problem and how she might be helped. Ella Mae asked for an explanation of the 3 terms. The OT explained that engagement meant to become involved in activity and how Ella Mae had just sat during the morning session. Ella Mae responded, "How is that supposed to help me get out of here?" The OT explained that occupations such as embroidery and sanding wood helped calm some people and since anxiety was the type problem with which Ella Mae was dealing, her doctor had thought she could benefit from such activities and had referred her to OT for that reason. Ella Mae then agreed that perhaps she would try this new approach to her panic attacks and chronic anxiety. After more

discussion, the patient, OTA, and OT agreed on the following goals:

- To join the stress management group to learn:
  - ○ Time management.
  - ○ Relaxation techniques such as guided imagery.
  - ○ The benefits of group discussions.
  - ○ Stress-reducing exercises.
- To explore money management techniques and referral to a social worker.
- To begin a job possibilities exploration.
- To engage in daily activity in a small group of people to achieve calmness.
- To work to complete at least one different craft every 2 weeks.

Since caffeine is associated with greater anxiety (Nagy et al., 1998), Ella Mae additionally agreed to decrease her caffeine intake, which had often been 6 cola drinks per day.

Treatment Activities/Techniques

The following morning, the depressed patient, Ruth, patiently showed Ella Mae how to separate the embroidery threads, how to use the needle threader to thread the needle, and how to slide the embroidery hoop over the cloth. Ella Mae's initial stitches were irregular and loose but as she practiced, the quality of her stitching improved quickly.

In the afternoon stress management group, the whole group filled out an activity configuration in which each day's schedule for a week is shown in 2 block segments from 7:00 a.m. until 1:00 a.m. the next morning (Early, 2000). Ella Mae's activity configuration sheet showed that she stayed in bed until 11 a.m. most days and spent the afternoon doing errands such as buying cigarettes, calling her sister on the telephone, baby sitting for her daughter, or reading novels. These were things she wanted to do. Social interaction was an area where she confessed she did almost nothing with other people. Ella Mae protested that she felt she did not socialize very well, and it always made her anxious to be with a group of people she did not know well. The other patients in the group discussed having similar feelings though they agreed they always felt a little better after spending time with others. Ella Mae's evening schedule was mostly watching TV, smoking cigarettes, drinking colas, and trying to get to sleep. After all the patients had shared their schedules and told how much of it they felt they really wanted to do, a discussion ensued in which they agreed to support each other in trying to regulate their sleep/wake schedules. They spontaneously made a telephone list and put the hours in which they would be willing to accept calls from the other patients in the group. They hoped that they could help each other by talking on the phone when they could not sleep. They also planned an exercise session for the following morning before lunch. Ella Mae was not eager to exercise but did not become a barrier to the other patients' wishes.

The following day after the OT session, Ella Mae asked to take her embroidery with her to the dayroom to work on outside of OT. The OT agreed to this and informed the nurses and psychiatric technicians that Ella Mae had a needle and embroidery scissors that she would have to return to the nurse's station after she finished using them. This was to prevent patients from attempting to inflict injury on themselves with the needle or scissors.

The afternoon of that second day of treatment for Ella Mae, the OTA asked the patients to fill out the NPI Interest Checklist (Rogers, 1988). The NPI Interest Checklist lists 80 different activities and has places for the user to mark whether he or she has a casual, strong, or no-interest for each. There were only 3 patients in the afternoon class: a teenager with an eating disorder; Ruth, the depressed woman; and Ella Mae. Other patients who had grounds passes had gone on an outing with the psychiatric technician to the walking trail and exercise stations on property in the front of the hospital building. Ella Mae listed only a casual interest in needlework though she continued to work on her embroidered doily. She marked strong interest in just 5 areas: writing, reading, television, religion, and conversation. She had no interest in most activities; however, she had casual interest in needlework, lectures, traveling, history, and photography.

The OTA obtained a blank book for Ella Mae that afternoon so she could start a journal. The following morning, the OT showed her how to use nature print paper to experience the photography process. They went into the dayroom and clipped some leaves off the potted plants and took a daisy from a flower arrangement Ella Mae had received from the women in the church. She expressed real enjoyment at this printing process. The next day, Ella Mae had grounds pass privileges, so she, the OTA, and 2 patients with similar pass privileges took the insta-matic camera outside to take some photographs around the hospital.

Discharge Planning

The social worker had arranged for Ella Mae to be designated as an occupant of one of the indigent beds that the hospital was obliged to provide for the community. She was allowed to stay in the hospital 5 days. On the morning of the day in which she was to be discharged, she finished the embroidered doily. In the treatment team meeting, Ella Mae told the whole staff about her plans:

- To live at her sister's rather than her daughter's,
- To meeting with the psychiatrist biweekly for medication management,
- To go to the state employment office and get the necessary forms to start looking for a job,
- To attend the stress management group in OT as an outpatient, 1 time per week for 1 month,
- To keep her list of other patient's telephone numbers by her telephone,

CLINICAL PROBLEM SOLVING

The first evening at home in her sister's house, Ella Mae was unable to calm herself for sleep. First, she tried a relaxation exercise she had learned in the stress management group. She felt calm only while she was lying down doing the conscious breathing and the guided imagery. The moment she stopped the conscious breathing, she felt her anxiety return. Then, she remembered to go to her suitcase and find the telephone list she had agreed to keep by her bedside until she had a place of her own. She did not feel she could put it up by the telephone in the kitchen of her sister's home, which always seemed so clean and rigidly arranged. Her sister filed papers with phone numbers rather than tacking them up around her telephone. Ella Mae was now feeling anxious because she was not meeting her last discharge goal of keeping the list by the telephone. How could the treatment team have better stated the last discharge goal?

The first number on the list was Rosie, a 30-year-old, Hispanic woman who had also been discharged that same day. Rosie had shared in group therapy that she was married and that her husband worked at night as a weather technician at the local TV station. Ella Mae expected to hear Rosie's voice but when the phone was answered, it was her husband and he sounded irritated. Ella Mae asked to speak to Rosie. Her husband asked who she was and why she was calling so late. Ella Mae explained that Rosie had agreed to be available to talk if someone on the phone list needed to talk. Rosie's husband said gruffly, "Well, I'll see if she's stopped this crying jag she's on." After several minutes in which Ella Mae could hear a muffled conversation, she heard Rosie's querulous voice. Rosie explained that when her husband had started to leave for his night shift, she had felt panicky. When she tried to persuade him to call in sick, he got angry with her. The telephone call turned into a counseling session in which Ella Mae listened to Rosie who had been diagnosed with panic disorder with agoraphobia. Rosie and her husband had recently moved to the city from a smaller city after he took the job at the TV station. Rosie developed the panic and agoraphobia as she attempted to deal with the complexities of living in a new larger city far from her relatives and friends. As they talked, Ella Mae was able to persuade Rosie to meet the next day at a restaurant on the bus line, halfway between their 2 homes. She explained the bus system as Rosie had never had the opportunity or need to use public transportation. After several minutes, Rosie asked Ella Mae to wait while she told her husband goodbye. Then Ella Mae and Rosie spent an hour on the phone before they hung up and went to bed. What might have been an appropriate discharge goal for the staff to discuss with Rosie?

The 2 women met the following day and began to discuss ways to help each other. Ella Mae had the 4 remaining outpatient OT sessions to assist her, but Rosie had no such luxury on her husband's rather skimpy health insurance plan. They talked about starting a support group. Ella Mae said she would tell the OTA and OT about their conversation and ask for their advice. Review the progress notes in the records section; what issues might effect OT treatment?

Two days later when Ella Mae had the opportunity to discuss this plan with the OTA in the stress management group, the OTA suggested setting a regular time, arranging a place, and sending an announcement to the calendar section of the local newspaper. They brainstormed the idea with others in the OT session. The first issue was to find a public meeting place that would not cost money. As the group members offered ideas, it occurred to Ella Mae that the church in which she had former-ly worked and eventually joined might be a possibility. She agreed to call a church board member and ask before the next meeting. What other places offer public meeting space? How would the OTA go about helping Ella Mae identify these?

The board member whom Ella Mae called was a woman who had at one time been hospitalized for obsessive compulsive dis-order. Ella Mae did not know this information until the woman shared it during their telephone conversation. She was a school-teacher who had become incapacitated because she would go over and over the grades of her high school students for fear of making a mistake. Medication and some behavioral coping skills had eventually solved this problem for her. The woman was enthusiastic and agreed to bring it up at the next board meeting. She felt that since Ella Mae was still listed as a church member there would be no rental fee. Ella Mae went on to explain that since she no longer had access to a computer, if the board agreed to allow them to meet in the church, would it be possible for her to come to the church and type an announce-ment for the newspaper? The board member agreed to ask the board of trustees about this issue as well. Ella Mae felt so pleased with herself for handling all these problems associated with set-ting up a support group. What goals should such a support group have?

That evening, when Ella Mae called Rosie to report, Rosie replied that another member on the original telephone list had called her the night before. This caller was a young Caucasian man named Boyd who had been depressed as well as suffering from social phobia. His medication seemed to help his depres-sion, but his social phobia had not diminished. Boyd's state gov-ernment job required him to make frequent presentations of projects he developed. His social phobia incapacitated him so that he had called in sick the last 3 times rather than embarrass himself by being unable to successfully present his ideas. His supervisor was becoming quite irritated. Boyd had responded with enthusiasm when Rosie told him of their support group plan. What could the OTA have done in the OT clinic to assist Boyd in conquering his fear?

By the last of the 4 stress management group sessions, with the encouragement of the OTA, Ella Mae had done all the nec-essary work for the first session of the support group. The OTA had encouraged Ella Mae when she asked if she could please be allowed to lead the guided imagery session during the group. The OTA agreed that this was an excellent opportunity to prac-tice a skill she might be able to use in the support group. The church board members had agreed to allow the new group to meet in one of the smaller religious education classrooms as Alcoholics Anonymous had the use of the social hall on that night of the week. The current church secretary had allowed Ella Mae to use the computer to prepare an announcement for the calendar section of the newspaper. Additionally, she had included the same announcement in the church newsletter and put it on the e-mail list to the congregation.

At the first session of the support group, there were 6 people in attendance: Ella Mae, Rosie, Boyd, a woman church member who had gotten the e-mail announcement, a male church mem-ber who had learned about it from the newsletter, and a woman who had seen the listing in the calendar section of the newspa-per. Ella Mae started the meeting by asking each of the people present to introduce themselves and say why they were there. A discussion followed about the need for such a group. The next order of business was to discuss the time and place to see if it suited everyone. Lastly, they discussed a name for their new sup-port group. After making a list of possible choices, the group voted to call it "Don't Panic." Ella Mae was praised for her lead-ership in arranging the meeting. The group agreed to pass the leadership around the group for future meetings. Ella Mae prom-ised to keep sending the announcements to the newspaper as there was an obvious need for this service to others with anxi-ety disorders.

If a patient is not able to start his or her own support group, what other community groups might offer some support?

LEARNING ACTIVITIES

1. Develop a brochure for students who face anxiety over test taking. Provide copies to the academic learning cen-ter at your school.

2. Design stand-up posters about anxiety disorders that explain the disorder and how to get help. Leave the posters in an area that has walk-by traffic, such as the stu-dent union or local grocery store.

3. Interview a person with agoraphobia by speakerphone. Have students prepare questions well in advance and ask the person to share his or her story with the class.

4. Make a list of support groups from those listed in the local newspaper.

5. Start a support group for fellow students concerned about upcoming tests.

REFERENCES

Ackerman, C. J., & Turkoski, B. (2000). Using guided imagery to reduce pain and anxiety. *Home Healthcare Nurse, 18,* 524-530.

American Psychiatric Association. (2000). *Diagnostic and statistical manual of mental disorders: DSM-IV-TR.* Washington, DC: American Psychiatric Association.

Brayman, S. J., Kirby, T. F., Misenheimer, A. M., & Short, M. J. (1976). Comprehensive occupational therapy evaluation scale. *American Journal of Occupational Therapy, 30,* 94-100.

Cramer, S. R., Nieman, D. C., & Lee, J. W. (1991). The effects of mod-erate exercise training on psychological well-being and mood state in women. *Journal of Psychosomatic Research, 35,* 437-449.

Dossey, B. (1995). Using imagery to help your patient heal. *American Journal of Nursing, 95,* 40-47.

Early, M. B. (2000). *Mental health concepts and techniques for the occupa-tional therapy assistant* (3rd ed.). New York: Raven Press.

Epply, K. R., & Abrams, A. I. (1989). Differential effects of relation techniques on trait anxiety: A meta-analysis. *Journal of Clinical Psychology, 45,* 957-974.

Fontaine, P., Mollard, E., Yao, S. N., & Cottraux, J. (2001). Current trends in cognitive behavior therapy for anxiety disorders. In E. J. L. Griez, C. Favarelli, D. Nutt, & J. Zohar (Eds.), *Anxiety disorders: An introduction to clinical management and research.* Chichester, UK: John Wiley & Sons, Ltd.

EVIDENCE-BASED TREATMENT STRATEGIES

Treatment Strategies	Authors
Self-help groups	Humphreys, Mankowski, Moos, & Finney, 1999; Humphreys & Moos, 2001; Hyde, 2001; Myrick & Brady, 2003;
Stress management/coping strategies	Epply & Abrams, 1989; Gaab et al., 2003; Hyde, 2001; Marer, 2002; McCarty, Atkinson, & Tomasino, 2003; McClanahan & Antonuccio, 2003; Murphy, 1984; Titlebaum, 1998
Activity-based treatment	Griffiths, 2002; Haiman, 1989; Marer, 2002; Stein & Tallant, 1988
Goal setting	Haiman, 1989
Exercise and well-being	Cramer, Nieman, & Lee, 1991
Guided imagery	Ackerman & Turkoski, 2000; Dossey, 1995; Epply & Abrams, 1989; Titlebaum, 1998; Vines, 1988

Gaab, J., Blattler, N., Meni, T., Pabst, B., Stroyer, S., & Ehlert, U. (2003). Randomized controlled evaluation of the effects of cognitive-behavioral stress management on cortisol responses to acute stress in healthy subjects. *Psychoneuroendocrinology, 28,* 767-779.

Granoff, A. L. (1996). *Help! I think I'm dying: Panic attacks & phobias.* Virginia Beach, VA: Eco Images.

Griffiths, S. (2002). Focus on research... The clinical utility of creative activities used as an occupational therapy treatment medium for people with mental health problems. *British Journal of Occupational Therapy, 65,* 226.

Haiman, S. (1989). Preface: Selecting group protocols: Recipe or reasoning. *Occupational Therapy in Mental Health, 9,* 1-14.

Humphreys, K., Mankowski, E., Moos, R. H., & Finney, J. W. (1999). Do enhanced friendship networks and active coping mediate the effect of self-help groups on substance abuse? *Annals Behavioral Medicine, 25,* 54-60.

Humphreys, K., & Moos, R. (2001). Can encouraging substance abuse patients to participate in self-help groups reduce demand for healthcare? A quasi-experimental study. *Alcoholism: Clinical & Experimental Research, 25,* 711-716.

Hyde, P. (2001). Support groups for people who have experienced psychosis. *British Journal of Occupational Therapy, 64,* 169-174.

Marer, E. (2002). Knitting: The new yoga. *Health, 16,* 76-80.

McClanahan, T. M., & Antonuccio, D. O. (2003). Cognitive-behavioral treatment of panic attacks. *Clinical Case Studies, 1,* 211-223.

McCarty, R., Atkinson, M., & Tomasino, D. (2003). Impact of a workplace stress reduction program on blood pressure and emotional health in hypertensive employees. *Journal of Alternative and Complementary Medicine, 9,* 355-369.

Melmed, R. N. (2001). *Mind, body, and medicine: An integrative text.* New York: Oxford University Press.

Murphy, L. (1984). Stress management in highway maintenance workers. *Journal of Occupational Medicine, 26,* 436-442.

Myrick, H., & Brady, K. (2003). Current review of the comorbidity of affective, anxiety, and substance abuse disorders: Editorial review. *Current Opinion in Psychiatry, 16,* 261-270.

Nagy, L. M., Riggs, M. R., Krystal, J. H., & Charney, D. S. (1998). Anxiety disorders. In A. Stoudemire (Ed.), *Clinical psychiatry for medical students.* Philadelphia: Lippincott-Raven.

Rapee, R. M., & Barlow, D. H. (1991). *Chronic anxiety; Generalized anxiety disorder and mixed anxiety—Depression.* New York: The Guilford Press.

Rogers, J. (1988). The NPI interest checklist. In B. Hemphill (Ed.), *Mental health assessment in occupational therapy.* Thorofare, NJ: SLACK Incorporated.

Rush, A. J. (1998). *Mood & anxiety disorders.* Baltimore: Williams & Wilkins.

Sanderson, W. C., & Wetzler, S. (1995). Cognitive behavioral treatment of panic disorder. In G. M. Asnis & H. M. van Praag (Eds.), *Panic disorder: Clinical, biological, and treatment aspects.* New York: John Wiley & Sons, Inc.

Selye, H. (1976). *The stress of life.* New York: McGraw-Hill.

Stein, F., & Tallant, B. K. (1988). Applying the group process to psychiatric occupational therapy part 1: Historical and current use. *Occupational Therapy in Mental Health, 8,* 9-28.

Stewart, D., Letts, L., Law, M., Cooper, B. A., Strong, S., & Rigby, P. J. (2003). The Person-Environment-Occupation Model. In E. B. Crepeau, E. S. Cohn, & B. A. B. Schell (Eds.), *Willard & Spackman's occupational therapy.* Philadelphia: Lippincott, Williams & Wilkins.

Titlebaum, H. M. (1998). Relaxation. *Holistic Nursing Practice, 2,* 17-25.

Vines, S. (1988). The therapeutics of guided imagery. *Holistic Nursing Practice, 2,* 34-44.

THE UNIVERSITY HOSPITALS AND CLINICS

Ella Mae

5/5/03 1:00p Nursing Admission note—   37 y/o white female admitted for panic attacks & anxiety. Addicted to valium. Pt. is quite obese and confesses to calming herself c̄ food. Otherwise quite belligerent and resentful of being in the hospital. Given Valium 2 mg ↓ cramping. Dr. prescribed 20 mg Paxil ———————————— P. Wells, RN

5-5-03 Social Work Admission Note: Pt has hx of sexual abuse, prescription drug addiction and other family problems. She is a survivor though. Her belligerent attitude is a barrier to rehab. But she may become more tractable c̄ treatment. I am referring her to the dietitian to discuss obesity. ———————————— V. Sanchez LCSW

5/5/03 OT Note — Performed COTA & COPM evals. Pt's OT goals are to attend to stress management, employment, ↑ socialization & to learn new leisure crafts. Pt. was less belligerent after goal setting. She also agreed to drink fewer colas. Cola and valium incompatibility discussed. A. Johnson OTR/L

5/6/03 — 6:30 AM — Nursing — Pt. had a restless night. Encouraged her to walk in the hall and to work on embroidery rather than Valium. Finally slept about 2:30 AM. Difficulty arousing her for the AM program. ———————————— J. Bienvenu, RN —

5/6/03 — 2:30 PM Nursing — Pt. has marked mood change for the better. Is participating in activities s̄ reminders. Continues to overeat, finishing other patient's untouched food. Got approval for indigent bed. Cont. med. regime ——— P. Wells, RN

FORM 1724
REPLACES UMC 345

Real record 22-1A. Real record for a client with anxiety.

Ella Mae

THE UNIVERSITY HOSPITALS AND CLINICS

5/6/03 O.T. Note — Pt. filled out interest checklist in O.T. group. Pt's interests are mostly intellectual rather than physical. She promised to write in journal 2x daily. Participated well with 7 other pts. in activities. ——————————— P. Jackson, COTA

5/6/03 - 10:30 PM Nursing Note — Pt. sleeping though snoring annoys roommate. Participated actively in evening current events discussion led by tech. M Heller RN

5/7/03 - 6:30 AM — Nursing — Quiet night. Only wakeful twice. Was able to calm self, prn Valium. J. Bienvenu, RN

FORM 1724
REPLACES UMC 345

Real record 22-1B. Real record for a client with anxiety.

Key Concepts

- Energy conservation: Principles taught to individuals incorporating efficient techniques to conserve energy while performing occupations.
- Joint protection: Principles taught to individuals to protect joints and assist in preventing deformities.

Essential Vocabulary

arthritis: An inflammatory process of a joint or a noninflammatory degenerative process involving a joint.
juvenile rheumatoid arthritis (JRA): A form of arthritis that affects children.
osteoarthritis (OA): A degenerative disease of the joints.
pauciarticular: A form of JRA that involves 4 joints or less and is generally asymmetrical.
polyarticular: A form of JRA that involves 5 joints or more.
rheumatoid arthritis (RA): A chronic, systemic, autoimmune disorder.

Clinical Summary

Osteoarthritis

Etiology

At present, no known cause.

Prevalence

- Affects approximately 16 million people in the United States.
- Up to age 45, more common in men Beyond age 55, more common in women

Classic Signs

Pain, stiffness, and limited ROM.

Juvenile Rheumatoid Arthritis

Etiology

At present, no known cause

Prevalence

Affects approximately 71,000 children in the U.S.

Classic Signs

Vary with each child. May include joint inflammation, pain, heat, altered growth, and decreased ROM. Systemic form may include high fever, rash on the chest and thighs, and joint inflammation.

Rheumatoid Arthritis

Etiology

At present, no known cause.

Prevalence

Affects approximately 2.1 million people in the United States (1 in 100).

Classic Signs

Pain, swelling, stiffness, heat at the site, symmetrical pattern.

Chapter 23

THREE PEOPLE ACROSS THE AGE SPAN WITH ARTHRITIS

Lynda Bishop, MS, OTR

INTRODUCTION

Arthritis is an inflammatory process of a joint or joints or a noninflammatory degenerative process involving a joint or joints. Arthritis may be an acute or chronic condition, and there are over 100 types of arthritis. Arthritis affects approximately 38 million people and is one of the most prevalent chronic conditions in the United States (Cook, 1999). It has been reported that women age 45 and older cite arthritis as the leading cause of activity limitation (Cook, 1999). Among the elderly population (65 years or older), the prevalence of arthritis is almost 100% (Lohman, Padilla, & Connon, 1998). The etiology of most forms of arthritis remains unclear, however, researchers believe that genetics, environment, and hormones are factors in the cause of many types of arthritis. This chapter will focus on OA, JRA, and RA, as these types of arthritis are the diagnoses that are most likely to be seen for OT intervention.

FRAME OF REFERENCE

The Model of Human Occupation (MOHO) is a frame of reference that can guide the OTA in treating individuals with arthritis. In addition, the biomechanical and rehabilitation approaches fit well. The biomechanical approach focuses on ROM, strength, and endurance, while the rehabilitative approach concentrates on compensatory measures to achieve maximal levels of function.

OCCUPATIONAL THERAPY INTERVENTION

OT intervention for the individual with arthritis should be client centered and occupation based. It is important for people with arthritis to maintain and/or increase the performance skills and client factors of ROM, strength, and endurance. Therefore, in collaboration with the client, OT intervention should incorporate the daily occupations (ADL, IADL, leisure, work) the client engages in to maximize performance skills and client factors.

It is important for the person with arthritis to realize that he or she can continue to engage in occupations that are important and meaningful to him or her. However, it is paramount that pain is respected throughout the OT program. If the client experiences pain in the affected joints while engaged in an activity, the OTA must assess the cause and adapt the activity accordingly. Many times, it is the way in which the activity is performed that causes pain. For example, the client might be utilizing the small joints of the fingers while operating a hand held can opener, which can result in pain. Use of an electric can opener would eliminate this problem.

Positioning and rest are important issues in reducing pain. A client with arthritic knees should be encouraged to stand on a regular basis if engaged in activities in the sitting position. For example, recommend to home care clients that they stand during every other commercial break while watching TV for a prolonged period of time. Better yet, have the client do an activity during the breaks such as dusting, watering plants, or household chores. Prolonged sitting can result in stiffness and pain in the affected lower extremity (LE) joints.

The use of purposeful activities in OT is an excellent fit for the individual with arthritis. Apart from the fact that following a routine exercise program for upper extremity (UE) AROM and strengthening can be very tedious and boring to many individuals, exercise also gives the arthritic individual time to focus on his or her pain. However, not all individuals find exercise programs boring; to some, exercise is purposeful and enjoyable. Engaging the individual in a variety of functional activities, purposeful activity addresses AROM, strength, and endurance without the person realizing that he or she is engaged in a therapeutic program. For example, an elderly female with arthritis in both hands complained of pain in her fingers and wrists when the therapist engaged her in an exercise program using TheraPutty (North Coast Medical Inc, San Jose, CA). The patient stated that she found this activity "boring and juvenile" and "my hands hurt for ages when I'm done." This patient had been a homemaker for years. She has 6 children, all of whom are now married with children of their own. She has 10 grandchildren and looks forward to visits from them for Sunday dinner and large family gatherings during the holidays. She always enjoyed cooking for the family. A therapeutic program specifically designed for the occupations of this woman involved cooking, washing dishes, putting them away, and cleaning the kitchen area. This addressed areas of AROM, strength, and endurance. This program enabled this woman to perform activities that she enjoyed and were meaningful to her.

JOINT PROTECTION

Education of joint protection is an essential part of a therapy program (Pedretti & Early, 2001). Joint protection strategies are as follows:

- Use large joints instead of small joints whenever possible. For example, hold a coffee cup with palms of both hands, carry a handbag on the elbow or over the shoulder instead of grasping with fingers. When rising from a chair, do not push up with fists; rather, use the palms of the hand.
- Avoid frequent sustained grasps.
- Do not stand or sit for long periods of time. Change positions to avoid prolonged stress of joints.
- When performing tasks that require repetitive motions, take frequent rest periods.
- Always respect pain. If pain is experienced, stop the activity, change position, and rest.
- Do not lift heavy items. Use a wheeled cart.
- Slide pots and pans on the kitchen counter rather than carry them to the stove.

In the case example above, this patient may be provided with utensils with built-up handles, shown a device for opening jars, and informed of the need to rest during prolonged activity.

An OTA may feel the urge to order adapted equipment to assist in joint protection, as there are hundreds of assistive devices sold commercially. Many of these are costly, and the assistant should not be too hasty in recommending these items. In many instances, homemade devices will work just as well at a fraction of the cost. For example, cutting a washcloth in small strips and wrapping the material around a spoon handle will enlarge the size of the spoon handle. A built-up handle eliminates a tight grasp.

ENERGY CONSERVATION

Because of the need for regular rest periods, energy conservation should be incorporated into the OT program. Principles of energy conservation are as follows (Lohman et al., 1998):

- When performing activities, sit whenever possible.
- Take frequent rest periods.
- Organize the home environment to avoid extra lifting, carrying, reaching, and bending. For example, place dishes, utensils, pots, and pans used for meals all in one spot on the countertop or first shelf in cupboard. Place fre-

quently used items on the front, top shelf of the refrigerator. Arrange clothing on a chair the evening before for the next morning.

- Plan to do chores at the time of day when stiffness and pain is least. Many people feel stiff upon arising in the morning. Therefore, chores might best be completed early in the afternoon.
- A cart with wheels is an excellent means of transporting several items at once. For example, all cleaning supplies could be placed on the cart and wheeled to various rooms. All food items could be placed on the cart along with the proper bowls, pans, and utensils. It is also wise to prepare large quantities of food at one time and then freeze small portions.
- Maintain correct posture and use correct body mechanics. Use leg muscles when lifting; always keep the back straight and bend at the hips and knees.

OSTEOARTHRITIS

OA affects approximately 16 million people in the United States, with increasing age contributing to the susceptibility to develop OA (Cook, 1999). "Up to age 45, OA is more common in men; beyond age 55, it is more common in women" (Cook, 1999, p. 63). OA is a degenerative disease of the joints and is caused by a breakdown in cartilage and bone. It progresses slowly and is the most common form of arthritis. OA typically involves the weightbearing joints such as the hips, knees, proximal interphalangeal joints (PIPs), distal interphalangeal joints (DIPs), and carpometacarpal joint (CMC) and can range from mild to severe. While there is no known cause for OA, risk factors include obesity, sport injuries involving joints, and repetitive use of joints.

Symptoms and Management

The symptoms of OA are pain, stiffness, and limited ROM. Swelling of joints and redness may also be present (DeLisa & Gans, 1998). Medications are used to control pain; aspirin is frequently prescribed for the management of symptoms of OA. Nonsteroidal anti-inflammatory drugs (NSAIDs) are also prescribed. Weight management is indicated in the cases of obesity. In severe cases of bone degeneration, surgery might be indicated. Surgery may result in a total hip replacement or total knee replacement (DeLisa & Gans, 1998). ROM exercises and strengthening programs are also included in the management of OA.

Evaluation

The OT evaluation for the person with OA will include ROM, strength, endurance, fine motor, and observation of performance during ADL, work, and leisure. When measuring AROM and testing strength, pain must be considered with appropriate adjustments for each made during the testing process.

Case Study 1

Mrs. Surgte is a 65-year-old married female admitted with a right total hip replacement secondary to OA. Mrs. Surgte presents as a pleasant, obese female with many complaints of pain in her right knee. She states that once she recovers from the surgery on her hip, she will have her knee done. She worries that her left hip will eventually be affected by OA, as she feels "occasional twinges" at the site. Prior to the right total hip replacement, Mrs. Surgte was independent in ADL. She reports that she does not have any hobbies. She and her husband spend much of their day watching TV. They did go to the shopping mall once or twice a week for "something to do," but Mrs. Surgte reports that she would get tired walking any distance. She had not gone to the mall for the past 2 months because "it hurt too much to walk." Mr. and Mrs. Surgte have a family dinner every Sunday for their daughter, her husband, and 2 young grandchildren. Mrs. Surgte enjoys cooking and looks forward to the family gathering on Sunday.

The Surgtes live in a 2-story home with the bedrooms and bathroom upstairs. For the past 2 months, Mrs Surgte has been spending most of her day upstairs, stating, "I did not want to go up and down the stairs much because of the pain." Her husband has been bringing breakfast and lunch upstairs, but she reports that she would come downstairs for dinner. Mr. Surgte does not like to cook and has been buying fast food. Both he and his wife have gained weight in the past 2 months.

Referral

Mrs. Surgte has been admitted to a rehabilitation unit with an estimated length of stay of 2 weeks. Orders from the physiatrist for OT are to evaluate and treat.

Assessment and Evaluation Process

The supervising OT has asked the OTA to review the medical record and introduce herself to the patient. The OTA explains OT to the patient and informs her that she is scheduled for the initial evaluation later that afternoon. Through conversation with the patient, the OTA learns that the patient would like her therapies scheduled around the soap operas she watches faithfully each day. The patient has many complaints of pain in her hip during the conversation in spite of the fact that she is lying in bed and not moving. While she is pleasant and friendly with the OTA, she states that she does not like to exercise and hopes she will not have to do too much in OT.

Mrs. Surgte arrives in OT at her scheduled time of 3:00 p.m. She immediately complains to the OT and OTA that she is missing her soap opera and hopes this will not take too long. The OT assesses the patient's AROM and strength in the bilateral upper extremities. The OT evaluates sensation. The OTA assesses the patient's transfers and functional mobility.

The OTA, through review of the medical record, conversation, and observation of the patient, felt that Mrs. Surgte was cognitively and perceptually intact. The OTA discussed this with the OT and the OT concurred. The OT had found cognition and perception to be intact through observation of the patient, conversation with the patient, and information from the OTA. Therefore, the OT did not deem it necessary to conduct a formal cognitive/perceptual assessment.

The patient is able to dress her upper body independently. She is unable to dress the lower body secondary to hip precautions. Nursing reports that the patient is able to independently bathe her upper body except her back. She is dependent for lower body bathing. She is independent to brush her teeth and comb her hair. Toileting is with minimal assist to pull up pants over buttocks.

The evaluation results are as follows: bilateral upper extremities AROM is within functional limits. Strength is 3+/5 throughout the bilateral upper extremities. Sensation is intact as is perceptual and cognitive status. Transfers to all raised surfaces except tub are with minimal assist. Patient is dependent to transfer to tub. Functional mobility is with contact guard and verbal cues for safety. Dressing upper body is independent; lower body dependent. Bathing upper body is with minimal assist; lower body is dependent. Patient is independent to comb hair and brush teeth after set-up. Patient requires minimal assist for toileting.

The OT and OTA collaborate to develop the treatment plan for Mrs. Surgte. The OTA has contacted the PT, who will be working with this patient to determine what ambulatory device she will be discharged with. The PT feels that the patient will need a standard walker (extra wide) for ambulation at home. At the conclusion of the evaluation process, the OTA asked Mrs. Surgte what her goals were. Mrs. Surgte stated that she would like to be able to go up and down the stairs without any pain, cook for the family, go out shopping again, and be independent so that she did not have to rely on her husband for help anymore. She also stated that she realized that she should lose weight. The OTA asked Mrs. Surgte if she had any interests other than cooking and shopping. Mrs. Surgte admitted that in the past few years she has not been as active as she had been in the past and realized that she has fallen into a daily routine that is "not very exciting." She stated that when her children were young she enjoyed doing school projects and holiday crafts with them.

The OTA and OT design a treatment plan that will address the goals important to Mrs. Surgte. Through the interview process, Mrs. Surgte's interests were learned. These interests will be incorporated through functional activities in all OT treatment sessions with Mrs. Surgte. The treatment plan includes transfer training, dressing program, functional mobility training, home and food management, and safety training. Because the bedrooms and bathroom are upstairs, and also because Mrs. Surgte will be going home with an extra wide walker, a home visit will be planned to assess the patient in her home environment.

Long-term goals set by the OT for this patient state that by discharge, the patient will:

- Be independent in transfers to all surfaces.
- Be independent in LE dressing.
- Be independent in functional mobility.
- Be independent in home and food management.
- Practice safe techniques when moving about her home environment.
- Engage in leisure activities that will promote health and wellness both physically and psychosocially.

Treatment Activities

The OTA considers the fact that this patient does not have many interests except preparing the family dinners on Sunday. The OTA, therefore, has the patient perform functional activities in the OT kitchen, dining room, and living room such as setting the table, preparing a simple lunch, and washing the dishes. Each session will include transfers to different surfaces such as kitchen chair with arms, living room couch, and overstuffed chair with extra cushions in the dining room area.

Education on energy conservation and safe transportation of items from the kitchen to living room will be addressed. These activities address all above stated goals except dressing and bathing. The dressing and bathing program will take place in the patient's room on the unit. Note that because this patient is cognitively intact, once she is instructed in the use of assistive equipment for dressing and bathing the lower extremities, she will likely be independent in these areas after set-up. Instruction in transfers to a tub seat will be included in the OT program.

Clinical Problem Solving

A home visit was conducted 1 week prior to discharge. Mrs. Surgte states that she is not going to attempt to go upstairs for awhile. She states she will sleep downstairs in her recliner. The house is extremely cluttered with scatter rugs throughout. There is a lot of furniture in the living room. Because Mrs. Surgte has an extra wide walker, she must walk sideways in the hallway. She also has to maneuver her walker to get through the doors to the kitchen and dining room.

What suggestions should the OTA make to Mrs. Surgte for independence in her home? What home modifications might be needed? What assistive equipment will Mrs. Surgte require upon discharge home? She will be on hip precautions for 8 weeks. Should bilateral UE strength be increased? Did the OTA incorporate enough activities in the treatment sessions? What else should the OTA focus on?

There is no bathroom downstairs. The patient's husband sat sullenly in the living room throughout the entire visit. He stated that he was not going to "pick up after her. She should do things by herself now that she got that hip fixed. I'm sick and tired of preparing her meals, I'm not going to do it anymore."

Should the OTA make any referrals for Mrs. Surgte's discharge? What, if anything, should be done about the husband's attitude toward his wife? Should the OTA incorporate the patient in leisure activities? Review the progress note written by the OTA and discuss any issues or concerns.

JUVENILE RHEUMATOID ARTHRITIS

JRA usually begins at 2 to 4 years of age. JRA affects about 71,000 children in the United States (Cook, 1999, p. 175). There are 3 forms of JRA: pauciarticular, polyarticular, and systemic. Pauciarticular involves 4 joints or less and is generally asymmetrical (affecting a particular joint on one side of the body). Joints most commonly affected are the knee, hip, ankle, and elbow. The pauciarticular form may also cause eye inflammation called iridocyclitis. If iridocyclitis is not treated early, it can result in blindness. Polyarticular involves 5 joints or more.

The systemic form affects joints and internal organs and is the least common form of JRA (Cook, 1999). JRA can present as a mild condition or can be severe, leading to serious complications. Symptoms may change on a daily basis, with the child experiencing severe pain one day and mild discomfort the next. It is also significant to note that a child may experience discomfort in the morning but feel fine in the afternoon (Cook, 1999). As noted previously, there is no known cause for JRA; however, it is known that it involves abnormalities of the immune system (Cook, 1999).

Symptoms and Management

The arthritis must be present for 6 or more consecutive weeks for a diagnosis. There is no single test for the diagnosis of JRA. JRA can result in joint damage, joint contracture, and altered growth. JRA is a chronic disease that may last for many years and might have periods when the child experiences no symptoms, which is referred to as remission. Remissions may last for months, years, or forever. JRA may lead to joint deformity, altered growth, or, for children with pauciarticular JRA, there is a higher risk for chronic eye infection (Cook, 1999).

Signs and symptoms vary with each child, however, symptoms of pauciarticular and polyarticular include joint inflammation, pain, heat, altered growth, and decreased ROM. Symptoms of the systemic form include high fever that can last weeks or months, a rash on the chest and thighs, and joint inflammation that may be present with the fever or may not develop until much later. Inflammation of the heart lining, heart, or lungs may also occur. Anemia and enlarged lymph nodes, liver, or spleen are also symptoms that may be present (Cook, 1999).

ROM exercises, eye and dental care, and nutritional counseling are indicated for the child with JRA. NSAIDs are used to decrease swelling and pain. Slow-acting anti-inflammatory drugs (SAAIDs) might also be prescribed. These drugs do not immediately reduce pain or swelling. They are used to modify the natural progress of joint disease and might not be effective for weeks or months after therapy has begun (Cook, 1999).

Evaluation

OT evaluation for the child with JRA will include ROM, strength, endurance, performance of ADL and play, and gross and fine motor skills.

Case Study 2

Johnny is a 5-year-old male with a diagnosis of JRA involving his left and right knees, left and right elbows, and both hands. Johnny was an active child with normal development. He engaged in gross and fine motor activities without difficulty. Shortly after his fifth birthday, Johnny began complaining of pain in his knees. His mother noted a little swelling in one knee and assumed Johnny had fallen or bumped his knee. She also attributed Johnny's complaints to "growing pains." Johnny's complaints diminished for a week or so and then he began complaining again. At this point, Johnny's mother did notice swelling in both knees. Johnny also reported that it hurt his hands when he had to draw in kindergarten, and he did not like to play ball because it hurt his elbows. Johnny's mother scheduled an appointment with Johnny's primary care physician. The doctor diagnosed JRA. The doctor prescribed anti-inflammatory medication, provided Johnny's mother with information on JRA, and made a referral for outpatient OT.

Assessment and Evaluation Process

The OT met with Johnny and his mother. Johnny's mother removed his coat for him and had him sit on her lap. The OT suggested that Johnny play with some of the toys in the clinic while she spoke with his mother. Johnny expressed an interest in doing this and asked his mother if it was all right. After slight hesitation, Johnny's mother gave permission but told Johnny to be very careful and play gently with the toys.

The OT observed Johnny's movements. He walked stiffly and sat down slowly and deliberately. He was guarded in all movements. He began building a tower out of blocks, occasionally letting go of the blocks and stretching his fingers.

Johnny's mother reported that her son's activity level had decreased. He tended to sit and watch TV more than in the past. In fact, she stated that she would permit Johnny 1 hour of TV a day prior to this diagnosis. "Now, because of my son's sickness, I think it better that he sit quietly, so watching TV for a length of time is OK with me." Johnny's mother reported that she now dresses Johnny and assists him with his bath. She does not allow him to play outside with the other children unless she is there to monitor him. Under no circumstances is he allowed to play ball or running games. She has asked that he be excused from playground activities at school.

The OT then turned her attention on Johnny. She got down on the floor and had him play with several toys that enabled her to observe Johnny's fine motor skills. She then had him imitate animal movements, for example, "How does an elephant move its trunk? How does a monkey scratch its back?" This gave the OT an opportunity to observe gross motor movements. Johnny enjoyed playing with the OT and a quick relationship of trust developed. This enabled the OT to conduct a formal evaluation of Johnny's ROM and strength. When it was time to leave, Johnny's mother began to prepare to put Johnny's coat on for him. The OT asked Johnny if he could put his coat on by himself. He seemed eager to show the OT that he could do this but asked his mother's permission first. Johnny was able to don his coat independently but with increased time and effort. He had difficulty buttoning the coat.

Evaluation results were as follows: The right UE was within normal limits for AROM throughout except the right elbow flexion, which was limited to 80 degrees. The right fingers had edema in the PIP joints of the index, middle, and ring fingers. However, Johnny was able to manipulate various sized objects such as beads, blocks, coins, tweezers, and buttons. Strength in the right UE was 3/5. The left UE was within normal limits for AROM throughout with strength grossly 3/5. Slight edema was noted in the left elbow. Gross motor performance was guarded with slow, deliberate movements. The OT realized that PT will be following Johnny for gross motor issues. However, the OT includes it in the evaluation process because of its impact on ADL and play performance. Johnny was found to be intact for cognition and perception. Sensation was also intact.

Goals

1. Increase right elbow flexion to within functional limits.
2. Prevent contracture in right elbow flexion.
3. Increase strength in bilateral upper extremities to 4+/5.
4. Educate patient and family in joint protection.
5. Educate patient and family in energy conservation.
6. Educate patient and family in JRA related to the importance of play.

Treatment Activities

The OTA will be responsible for treatment of Johnny. In this outpatient clinic, the OTs generally do the evaluations and then discuss findings with the OTA. The OT and OTA collaborate on the treatment plan. The OTA will use play as the media to treat Johnny. She will engage Johnny in fine and gross motor activities to achieve the long-term goals. The OTA will also educate Johnny and his mother on JRA. With a thorough understanding of the disease, Johnny's mother should realize that she can allow Johnny to join in many activities that she had previously believed would be harmful. The OTA will also provide Johnny's mother with information on the Arthritis Foundation and local JRA support groups for families.

Clinical Problem Solving

- Considering Johnny's areas of occupation, suggest toys/games that would address fine and gross motor. What joint protection techniques would be especially helpful for Johnny?
- Since treatment sessions alone cannot help this child reach his fullest potential, describe a home exercise program for Johnny. What concerns should the OTA have concerning Johnny's mother following through with a home exercise program?
- Johnny's mother initially wanted to be involved in the entire treatment session. She hovered around Johnny and continually asked him if his joints hurt. How should the OTA deal with this?

RHEUMATOID ARTHRITIS

RA is a chronic, systemic, autoimmune disorder. RA can affect the lungs, heart, and eyes in some people, and it affects 2.1 million (1 in 100) people in America. Onset is typically between ages 25 to 50; however, it can occur in all ages, and women are 3 times more likely to have RA than men. Presently, there is no known cause of RA; however, research has shown that genetic, environmental, and/or hormonal factors may contribute to the disease. RA is an inflammatory disease affecting joints in the body, generally in a symmetrical pattern (i.e., if one joint is affected on one side of the body such as the hand, it will be affected in the hand on the other side as well). Other parts of the body may also be affected. Accompanying joint inflammation and pain, people may experience fatigue, occasional fever, and malaise (Cook, 1999). Remissions and exacerbations may occur in the disease process (DeLisa & Gans, 1993). RA can be mild or severe, lasting variable periods of time such as a month, a few months, or years. People who have severe RA will be in the active stage of the disease for much of the time with the symptoms lasting for many years. In these cases, there may be significant joint damage and increased difficulty in performing ADL (Cook, 1999). Today's health care system allows most people with RA to lead productive lives through medication, therapy, support groups, and patient education.

Symptoms and Management

The symptoms of RA include pain, swelling, stiffness, heat at the site, and a symmetrical pattern. Stiffness and/or pain lasts greater than 30 minutes after rest. Fatigue, occasional fever, and a general feeling of not being well are commonly experienced. Because RA is a chronic condition, depression may be experienced as well (DeLisa & Gans, 1993). Management of RA includes regular medical visits to monitor the course of the RA. Medications such as aspirin and NSAIDs are prescribed to relieve pain and decrease joint inflammation. Rest and exercise must be balanced for the person with RA. Rest helps to decrease pain and inflammation and combat fatigue. Exercise maintains ROM, increases strength, increases self-esteem, and promotes a state of well-being. Patient education brings awareness of the diagnosis and its variables and teaches individuals techniques such as joint protection and energy conservation in order that they may live productive and fulfilling lives. Support groups allow for the sharing of experiences and expression of feelings. Surgery such as joint replacement or tendon reconstruction for individuals with significant joint damage might be indicated (Cook, 1999).

Case Study 3

Mr. Caroll is an 82-year-old married male with a diagnosis of right fractured humerus and RA. He has had RA for the past 25 years. Mr. Caroll was under a doctor's care when he was first diagnosed with RA. However, when he started to feel better after a course of NSAIDs, he discontinued seeing the doctor. When his medications ran out, he felt better and thought that he was free of the RA. Over the years, if he experienced pain, he would buy over-the-counter drugs to manage his condition. If he had pain, he believed that it was part of the aging process and it was something he had to live with.

Mr. Caroll was a carpenter and had his own business. He retired at age 65; however, he continues to work with wood. He enjoys making toys for his grandchildren and simple woodwork pieces for his family. He often spends 5 hours a day in his workshop. It was here that he fell tripping over an electrical cord. The fall resulted in the fractured shoulder.

Mrs. Caroll has been a homemaker throughout her 41-year marriage. She does all the housecleaning, cooking, grocery shopping, and laundry. She is in good health and is very active in her church. Mr. and Mrs. Caroll usually go out on Saturday evenings to visit friends or attend a church function. On Sundays, they spend time with their children or grandchildren, who all live in close proximity.

Mrs. Caroll states that her husband is a very proud man. He seldom complains, however, she has observed him wince and grimace when he does his carpentry. He has difficulty eating; it seems uncomfortable for him to move his arm to bring it to his mouth, and he holds his utensil in an awkward manner. His carpentry work is not nearly the quality it used to be. Mrs. Caroll contributes this to "old age and poor vision."

Referral

Referral received from the doctor is for evaluation and treatment of the fractured humerus and RA. The orders further state active/active assistive range of motion (A/AROM) exercises for right shoulder.

Assessment and Evaluation Process

The OT and OTA collaborate in the evaluation of Mr. Caroll. The OT assesses Mr. Caroll's passive/active range of motion (P/AROM) and strength. The OTA assesses Mr. Caroll's ADL through observation of him engaged in eating, dressing, grooming, brushing his teeth, functional mobility, transfers, and endurance.

A discussion between the OT and OTA determines Mr. Caroll's status as follows:

- Left UE P/AROM limited to 100 degrees shoulder flexion, 110 degrees shoulder abduction, 60 degrees external rotation, and 55 degrees internal rotation. The elbow, forearm, and wrist are within functional limits for P/AROM. The digits are limited in flexion and extension but are within functional limits (WFL) for P/AROM. Mr. Caroll is able to oppose to the middle finger. Strength at limited range is 4-/5.

- Right UE AROM is limited to 50 degrees shoulder flexion, 35 degrees shoulder abduction, and 50 degrees shoulder extension. External rotation is 30 degrees and internal rotation is 25 degrees. The elbow and forearm are within functional limits for P/AROM. Strength for elbow and forearm is 3+/5. The right hand is severely deformed. The index finger has a sublux at the MP joint, the middle finger is limited in flexion to 10 degrees at the MP, 5 degrees at the PIP, 0 degrees at the DIP. The ring finger is also subluxed at the MP joint. Movement at the PIP is 5 degrees, the DIP joint is at 0 degrees. The little finger is within functional limits for AROM. The thumb is within functional limits. Opposition is to the index finger only. Mr. Caroll stated that his hand has been like this for the past several years, "getting worse each year." He stated that he holds his tools between his thumb and index finger and sometimes he "ties the bigger tools with a string in the palm of my hand."

- Dressing the upper extremities is with minimal assist to place the shirt over the right arm. LE dressing is independent. Eating is independent after set-up, however, Mr. Caroll has to use his nondominant hand and that is awkward for him. He also had difficulty maintaining hold of the utensils. He is independent for functional mobility and transfers. Endurance is good.

EVIDENCE-BASED TREATMENT STRATEGIES

Treatment Strategies	Authors
Assistive devices	Hurren & Tomita, 1995
Life activities	Katz, 1995
Preventative intervention	Clark et al., 1997
Occupation-based and client-centered occupation	Jackson & Schkade, 2001; Laliberte, Cook, & Polatajko, 1997
Home care	Helewa et al., 1991

Goals

1. Increase AROM in right shoulder to within functional limits.
2. Increase dressing to independent.
3. Educate patient in joint protection related to roles.
4. Educate patient in energy conservation related to roles.

Clinical Problem Solving

- Review the evaluation notes. Why did the OT not test Mr. Caroll's strength in the right shoulder? Is splinting indicated for Mr. Caroll?

- Consider MOHO as a frame of reference for treatment specific to the areas of occupation of Mr. Caroll. What assistive equipment would Mr. Caroll benefit from? Should Mr. Caroll be told that he should no longer do woodwork because of the stress to his joints? Describe 2 meaningful activities the OTA could design for Mr. Caroll's treatment session.

- Mr. Caroll mentions to the OTA that it has been a long time since he "cuddled up" to Mrs. Caroll because he is always so uncomfortable in bed. How can the OTA address this sexual expression performance area?

LEARNING ACTIVITIES

1. While wearing winter gloves, attempt to dress or do other basic ADL. Chill the gloves to experience stiff joints.

2. Investigate the Internet for information about the 3 types of arthritis presented in this chapter. Judge the trustworthiness of each site. What untested quackery is available?

3. Analyze a wardrobe of clothes for items easy or difficult to wear for a person with arthritis.

REFERENCES

Clark, F., Azen, S., Zemke, R., Jackson J., Carlson, M., Mandel, D., et al. (1997). Occupational therapy for independent-living older adults: a randomized controlled trial. *Journal of the American Medical Association, 278*, 1321-1326.

Cook, A. (Ed.). (1999). *Arthritis sourcebook*. Detroit, MI: Omnigraphics, Inc.

DeLisa, J., & Gans, B. (Eds.). (1998). *Rehabilitation medicine: Principles & practice* (3rd ed.). Philadelphia, PA: Williams & Wilkins.

Helewa, A., Goldsmith, C. H., Lee, P., Bombardier, C., Hanes, B., Smythe, H. A., et al. (1991). Effects of occupational therapy home service on patients with rheumatoid arthritis. *Lancet, 337*, 1453-1456.

Hurren, D., & Tomita, M. (1995). Assistive devices used by home-based elderly persons with arthritis. *American Journal of Occupational Therapy, 19*(8), 810-820.

Jackson, J., & Schkade, J. (2001). Occupational adaptation model versus biomechanical-rehabilitation model in the treatment of patients with hip fractures. *American Journal of Occupational Therapy, 55*(5), 531-537.

Katz, P. P. (1995). Impact of rheumatoid arthritis on life activities. *Arthritis Care and Research, 8*(4), 272-278.

Laliberte, R., Cook, J., & Polatajko, H. (1997). Understanding the potential of occupation: a qualitative exploration of seniors' perspectives on activity. *American Journal of Occupational Therapy, 51*(8), 640-650.

Lohman, H., Padilla, R., & Connon, S. (1998). *OT with elders: Strategies for the COTA*. St. Louis, MO: Mosby.

Pedretti, L., & Early, M. (Eds.). (2001). *Occupational therapy practice skills for physical dysfunction* (5th ed.). St. Louis, MO: Mosby.

OT PROGRESS NOTE

[D=DATA A=ASSESSMENT G=GOALS P=PLAN]

UNIT: 5

PATIENT: _Sturgle_   PHYSICIAN: _Dr. Brown_

DATE: 9/20/04

D: _Pt seen 5x/wk, 1x/day for 45 min tx session. Pt engaged in transfer training, dressing, position & home & food management activities. Pt instructed in LB dressing & use of AE. Pt demonstrated good understanding of dressing techniques & was I following skilled instruction. Pt demonstrating 2 min standing tolerance while engaged in meal prep at kitchen counter. Pt then required 3 min rest. Standing 1 to 4 min following rest period._

A: _Pt is cooperative & pleasant. However, pt states she does not anticipate doing much around the house when she returns home. She is making slow progress. Transfers to all surface except bathe I to S. Transfers to tub seat 1 to mod A._

G: _1 tub transfer to min A. Pt will stand at counter for 5 min 5 times so B in order to prepare sandwich. Plan is to continue OT 5x/wk, 1x/day to achieve above stated goals._

S. Milton, OTA

Real record 23-1. Real record for a client with arthritis.

Key Concepts

- Arthroplasty: Creation of an artificial joint.
- Prosthesis: Replacement part, an artificial substitute.

Essential Vocabulary

acetabulum: The socket shaped area in the pelvis where the head of the femur attaches.
anterolateral: In front and to one side.
greater trochanter: The bony prominence that gives attachment to the hip abductor muscles.
NSAID: Nonsteroidal anti-inflammatory drug, such as ibuprofen or aspirin.
posterolateral: In the rear and to one side.
service competency: The ability of the OTA to obtain the same or equivalent results as the supervising OT in evaluation and treatment.
thrombosis: A clotting within a blood vessel that may cause sudden blood insufficiency to the tissues supplied by that vessel.
Trendelenburg gait: A gait pattern that can be the result of weakness of the hip abductor muscles.

Clinical Summary

Etiology

- Degenerative joint OA.
- RA.
- Hip fracture.
- Other disease process or trauma.

Prevalence

- Over 150,000 procedures performed annually.
- Prevalence increases with normal aging of joints.

Classic Signs

- Pain.
- Decreased mobility for ambulation and ADL.
- Medications, therapy interventions, and activity modifications have not managed symptoms adequately.

Precautions

- Limit hip flexion, extension, abduction, and adduction per physician orders.
- Maintain hip in alignment, avoiding external and internal rotation.
- Limit weight bearing on affected hip per physician orders.

See Figure 24-4 for specific applications to ADL.

A Plumber and Golfer With Total Hip Arthroplasty

Dairlyn Gower, BAS, COTA/L and Marcia Bowker, OTR, CHT

Total hip arthroplasty (THA) is the surgical replacement, formation, or reformation of the hip joint. It is performed to restore motion and preserve the necessary stability to a stiffened or painful joint. This procedure is becoming an increasingly common treatment for hip arthritis. The American Academy of Orthopaedic Surgeons reports more than 150,000 procedures are performed annually (American Academy of Orthopaedic Surgeons, 2001). Technological advances and advancement in surgical procedures have resulted in more successful long-term outcomes. Arthroplasty of the hip is usually necessary because of degenerative joint OA, RA, hip fracture, or other disease process or trauma. The most significant outcome is the impact THA can make in the quality of an individual's life, not only in providing the individual with pain-free function, but also in decreasing medical costs to society by decreasing nursing home use due to the disability this type of dysfunction can cause.

Surgical procedures vary depending on many factors, including severity of joint involvement, previous hip surgery, and preferences of the physician. Complications resulting from surgery can include infection, pneumonia, nerve injury, loosening or breakage of the prosthesis within the bone, pulmonary embolism, deep vein thrombosis, and blood clots (American Academy of Orthopaedic Surgeons, 2000). Treatment implementation can also vary depending on the type of surgery performed, as well as the individual's age, health, and motivation.

THA is often necessary as a result of an individual's decreasing functional mobility and/or progressive pain. THA can improve the patient's quality of life by decreasing pain and increasing ROM and mobility, therefore improving the patient's ability to perform ADL. Although time frames can differ based on various factors, the prognosis is generally good after an approximate 4 to 5 day hospitalization and a 2 to 3 month recovery period. Patients can expect continued healing to occur, including decreased pain and improved strength, for 6 to 12 months after surgery. An individual who is independent before undergoing a THA should continue to be independent after surgery. In some instances, the patient may prefer to have some assistance from a family member or a short-term nursing home stay for rehabilitation, particularly for individuals who are older or live alone, or those with complicating factors that may impact recovery (Munin, 1998).

As mentioned previously, indications for THA are varied but tend to include conditions that cause pain and limit mobility, although pain is generally the primary indicator. These include the following (DeWal, Su, & DiCesare, 2003):

- OA and RA at the hip joint.
- Certain types of hip fractures.
- Avascular necrosis.
- Hip joint tumors.
- Hip pain that has failed to respond to conservative treatment such as NSAIDs for over 6 months or that limits the ability to perform routine activities.

Preoperative planning for THA includes x-rays, assessment of type and size of component needed, and a thorough medical examination. The medical examination includes assessment of cardiac and pulmonary function, awareness of any pre-existing medical conditions that require anticoagulants, anesthesia consultation, preoperative exercises, and/or donation of patient's own blood for use in surgery if needed.

In the surgical procedure, a prosthesis replaces the worn head and neck of the femur and a socket component replaces the worn acetabulum (Figure 24-1). The components are attached to the bones of the pelvis and femoral head by means of a self-curing, acrylic resin adherent that is applied in paste form and becomes bone-like when hardened. Most procedures involve a cemented femoral stem and an uncemented acetabular component. Noncemented techniques (also called pressfit components) can also be utilized, where the prosthetic parts are intimately driven into the bone. This intimate contact allows the bone to grow into the texture of the metal component. In younger patients, generally under 50 years of age, the THA procedure is usually uncemented. The pressfit components are now being utilized in 50- to 70-year-old individuals if their bone quality is excellent.

The surgery is performed using general or spinal anesthesia. The orthopedic surgeon makes an incision along the affected side, exposing the hip joint. The head of the femur and the acetabulum are cut out and removed. The prosthetic ball and stem are inserted in the femur and the prosthetic socket component is placed in the enlarged pelvis cup. The components are placed, using either the cemented or uncemented technique, and the muscles and tendons are repaired. Surgical procedures vary for hip arthroplasty and are largely due to physician preference. The 2 most common procedures are the anterolateral and posterolateral approaches (Kelmanovich, Parks, Sinha, & Macaulay, 2003).

The anterolateral approach involves splitting the hip abductor muscles off the greater trochanter, and the patient will experience some abductor weakness. Therefore, abduction strengthening is the most important aspect of postoperative PT to lessen the incidence of Trendelenburg gait. Specific instabilities resulting from the anterolateral approach and positions that patients need to avoid include hip external rotation, excessive hyperextension, and adduction.

The posterolateral approach does not interfere with the abductor mechanism of the hip, so there is less abductor weakness but it is slightly unstable. Specific instabilities resulting from the posterolateral approach and positions patients need to avoid include movement over 90 degrees of hip flexion, adduction, and internal rotation (van Stralen, Struben, & van Loon, 2003).

With both approaches, patients are strongly advised not to cross their legs until they have physician authorization; a simple concept to teach patients is to keep their knees about shoulder width apart. If patients do not adhere closely to precautions, they are at risk for interruption of good soft tissue and muscle healing, thus increasing the risk for hip dislocation. Hip dislocation is a possibility because the new joint capsule, sometimes referred to as a pseudocapsule because it is mainly formed by scar tissue, forms over a period of 6 to 8 weeks. This is the most critical time to reinforce the importance of adhering to precautions. Regardless of the approach, the success of recovery relies on the compliance of the patient for approximately the first 3 months after surgery.

Patients generally experience moderate to severe pain after surgery, but by the second to third day postsurgery are placed on oral analgesic medications that sufficiently control pain. Patients also return from surgery wearing antiembolism stockings, which reduce their risk of blood clots, and are generally placed on chemical anticoagulation medications by their surgeon.

The team members involved in the care of the patient with hip arthroplasty usually include the following: primary physician, orthopaedic surgeon, nursing staff, OT and PT practitioners, dietitian, pharmacist, and social worker. The role of the team is to facilitate the healing of the surgical site and development of a capsule around the joint for future stability, as well as to teach proper body mechanics, mobility, positioning, and techniques related to carrying out daily activities during the recovery period.

Carl, a self-employed plumber, is married and has adult children. At the age of 57, Carl had a rapid onset of OA. Because of right hip pain and stiffness, he began experiencing difficulty in fulfilling his job requirements, which included getting in and out of his truck, along with lifting, twisting, and pulling at odd angles. At age 65, Carl became semiretired, doing only minor plumbing jobs with the assistance of one of his sons.

The next year, the family physician referred Carl to an orthopaedic surgeon who discussed the option of a THA with him.

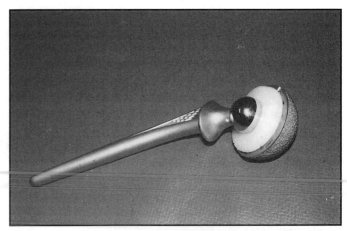

Figure 24-1. Prosthesis components.

Carl chose not to have surgery at the time because he did not want to have it until it was "necessary." He was also concerned about the expense and lost time from work during recovery.

At the age of 72, Carl was experiencing extreme hip pain, decreased joint mobility, stiffness, and a painful gait. Carl, his wife, and the orthopaedic surgeon decided it was time to have THA surgery. Being able to play "a good game of golf" was Carl's primary source of motivation. Surgery was scheduled during the winter to ensure that Carl would have adequate recovery time before the golf season.

THEORY THAT FRAMES PRACTICE

The biomechanical and rehabilitation frameworks primarily address practice following THA. The biomechanical framework focuses on the physical aspects of the body, including strength, ROM, endurance, and structural integrity. Rehabilitation addresses the patient's abilities and potential for regaining independence in ADL. Intervention addresses the use of assistive devices and modification of activities to accomplish functional goals. The 2 frameworks are intertwined throughout treatment (Sames, 2005).

ASSESSMENT

The orthopedic surgeon made a referral for OT services according to the standard THA protocol of the facility. The protocol used for OT evaluation, planning, and treatment was originally developed by the OT and OTA in cooperation with their facility orthopaedic surgeons. This protocol identifies general precautions and procedures for performance of ADL but is flexible enough to be easily adapted to the patient's individual needs, lifestyle, and home situation, as well as the specific surgical procedure.

The OTA met with Carl and his wife 1 week before his surgery in the OT clinic. Using a structured home assessment questionnaire and checklist, the OTA, who has demonstrated service competency in administering this assessment, reviewed all aspects of Carl's daily living activities, including personal care, home environment, household responsibilities, meal preparation, transportation, employment, and recreation. An example of this type of assessment is provided in Figure 24-2. The OTA then reviewed postsurgical precautions and oriented Carl and his wife to the assistive devices he would most likely find helpful and that would be issued to him in the hospital as needed. Carl was provided with a comprehensive packet of written information regarding postsurgical precautions and a list of local vendors who sell and rent equipment such as over the toilet commodes and bath benches. Carl practiced using assistive devices for LE dressing and, after discussing their home environment, decided with his wife that the installation of grab bars in his shower prior to surgery would be helpful.

Postsurgery, the OT performed a chart review and initial evaluation. The chart review allowed the OT to screen for possible complicating factors that may impair the patient's progress such as pre-existing conditions of RA, cancer, cardiac or pulmonary disorders, dementia, and any new complicating factors that may have occurred following the presurgical assessment. The initial evaluation included testing of ROM, strength, and cognitive functioning. Changes to the home environment since the preoperative assessment were briefly reviewed.

TREATMENT

At the time of the initial evaluation, the OT and the OTA established an individualized plan for OT treatment according to the standard THA protocol of the facility. The long-term goal for Carl was to return home, demonstrating independence in all ADL with all movement precautions observed. Overall functional independence is expected to be the same and, for most individuals, improved after a THA as the patient should now be demonstrating an increase in pain-free ROM. General short-term goals during the hospital stay should be, but are not limited to, the following:

- Demonstrate understanding of specific precautions and bending restrictions.
- Demonstrate independence in LE dressing through utilization of assistive devices.
- Demonstrate independence in basic homemaking skills such as meal preparation, work simplification, and energy conservation.

The action plan developed jointly by the OT and the OTA for Carl's treatment appears in Figure 24-3.

Standing orders at the hospital where Carl was a patient indicated that OT was to be initiated on the first or second day after surgery, unless otherwise indicated by the physician.

Following the initial evaluation by the OT, the OTA scheduled an initial visit with Carl. The purpose of OT intervention and the plan of care were reviewed, in addition to a brief review of the home activity inventory. Carl's wife was present and stated that she would like to attend her husband's treatment sessions to gain a better understanding of his OT program. The OTA again discussed precautions and limitations Carl must follow and highlighted precautions specific to his type of surgical procedure. All items were discussed and procedures were demonstrated whenever possible. Questions were answered and Carl and his wife indicated that they understood the impor-

tance of observing the precautions and limitations during the performance of all daily living activities. The list of precautions is shown in Figure 24-4. The OTA brought a variety of assistive devices, including a reacher, elastic shoelaces, a long-handled shoe horn, a dressing stick, a leg lifter, a walker bag/basket, and a sock aid to Carl's room. Some of these items are shown in Figure 24-5. Using the dressing devices, she demonstrated how to do LE dressing tasks such as putting on underwear, pants, socks, antiembolism stockings, and shoes. Use of a sock aid is depicted in Figure 24-6.

Carl chose to use the reacher, dressing stick, and sock aid. His loafer style shoes were easy for him to put on without any assistive devices. After practicing, Carl was able to do LE dressing safely, without flexing his hip beyond 90 degrees and without rotating his hip. The OTA taught Carl to stand by extending his knee and bringing his surgical foot forward and using his arms to push up on the chair armrests as shown in Figures 24-7 and 24-8.

Next, Carl, his wife, and the OTA went to the OT bathroom area to learn and practice shower/tub and toilet transfers. Carl indicated that the shower in their home had a 3-inch step at the entrance. Carl was shown a number of assistive devices, including a tub chair, grab bars, and a long-handled bath sponge. Carl stated that following his presurgery visit with the OT practitioners, he had grab bars installed. As a plumber, he was aware of the importance that the grab bars be securely fastened to the wall studs in his bathroom. He stated that he had a chair at home that he could use in the shower. Carl was instructed to walk to the step of the shower and turn so that he was facing away from the shower stall. He was then told to reach for the chair, sit, and lift his legs into the shower stall. Carl thought the long-handled bath sponge would "come in handy" at minimum expense.

The OTA talked with Carl and his wife about toilet use and learned that the toilet in their home was low. Using a toilet of this type would cause hip flexion beyond 90 degrees. Carl would need to use an over-the-toilet commode chair or a sturdy raised toilet seat. His wife indicated that a commode chair could be borrowed from a relative. The OTA also provided Carl and his wife with a list of local vendors who provide rental and sales of raised toilet seats, over-the-toilet commodes, and grab bars for the home. The OTA taught Carl to "back up" to the commode until he could feel the back of his knees touch. He was then instructed to reach for the arm rests, bring his surgical leg forward, and lower himself to the commode. This activity concluded the morning session, and the time of the afternoon session was confirmed.

That afternoon, Carl and his wife met the OTA in the OT kitchen. Instruction was provided in basic home management, work simplification, and energy conservation techniques. Although Carl's wife normally assumed most of these tasks, she was employed by their plumbing business 4 hours a day, 4 days per week between 10:00 a.m. and 2:00 p.m. Thus, Carl would have to prepare his own lunch, clean up, and perform other ADL independently. During this treatment session, the OTA also demonstrated specific tasks such as using a reacher, sliding items on a countertop, transporting items on a utility cart, and using a bag or basket in conjunction with a walker or crutches.

Occupational Therapy Department
Cloquet Community Memorial Hospital
512 Skyline Boulevard
Cloquet, MN 55720

ADL Inventory/Assessment Form

NAME: _____ DATE: _____ SURGERY TYPE: _____

Personal Care

Can you dress yourself? _____ Areas of difficulty _____

Can you feed yourself? _____ Areas of difficulty _____

Can you perform bathing/grooming tasks independently? _____

Were you independent in the above areas prior to your hospitalization? _____

Areas of difficulty _____

Is there someone available to help at home? _____ If yes, who? _____

Physical Layout

Do you reside in an: Apartment, House, Other _____

Is there an elevator? _____

Number of floors _____ Steps inside house _____ Steps into the house _____

Location of: Bedroom _____ Bathroom _____ Tub _____

Shower _____ Combination _____

Any areas of particular concern regarding physical layout? _____

Household Responsibilities

Which of the following activities are you currently able to perform?

Cooking _____ Grocery shopping _____ Cleaning _____

Laundry _____ Dishwashing _____ Pet care _____

Trash carryout _____ Snow shoveling _____ Care of lawn _____

Gardening _____ Maintenance _____ Other _____

Meal Preparation

Are you able to prepare meals? _____ Areas of difficulty _____

How many meals do you prepare daily? _____ For how many people? _____

Is there someone available to help? _____

Are the following available for your use? High kitchen stool _____ Microwave _____

Kitchen cart _____ Other _____

Transportation

Do you drive? _____ Is there someone available to drive, if necessary? _____

If so, who? _____

Employment

Are you employed? _____ Retired _____

Type of occupation _____

Present work status _____

Work duties (include use of stairs, lifting, bending) _____

Recreation

List hobbies/recreational activities _____

Activities discontinued because of medical condition _____

Figure 24-2. Assessment home activity inventory. (Reprinted with permission of Marcia Bowker, Director, Occupational Therapy Department of Community Memorial Hospital, Cloquet, MN.)

Postsurgery Day	Action Plan
2	Chart review by OTA; review findings with the OT and establish plan.
3 and 4 (depending on ambulation status)	**A.M. Treatment Session:**
	Initial OT contact; explain OT and treatment protocol; assessment using activity inventory.
	Provide patient with written list of postsurgical precautions; review precautions with patient and family members.
	Instruct patient in LE dressing. Assistive devices may include sock aid, elastic shoe laces, reacher, dressing stick, and long-handled shoe horn.
	Instruct patient in tub/shower and toilet transfer. Assistive devices may include a raised toilet seat or commode chair, tub chair, long-handled bath sponge/brush, and grab bars.
	P.M. Treatment Session:
	Instruct patient in basic home management, work simplification, and energy conservation techniques. Assistive devices may include a utility cart, high stool, crutch or walker bag or pail, and a firm, sturdy arm chair.
4 and 5 (depending on which postsurgical day treatment was started)	Patient demonstrates dressing techniques; patient repeats back precautions and limitations; discuss and clarify any questions or concerns patient or family may have. Provide patient with a list of area vendors for rental or purchase of commode, raised toilet seats, or grab bars.

Figure 24-3. Action plan.

Effective methods for removing and storing items in the refrigerator were also stressed, as well as using a high stool to sit on during meal preparation and dish washing. Carl was then asked to make a sandwich and a bowl of soup and to clean up, incorporating the techniques he had been taught. He completed these tasks successfully, requiring only infrequent reminders. Carl also indicated that he already had an ice cream pail and a utility cart at home that he would use for transporting items.

More general work simplification and energy conservation techniques were discussed with Carl, and important safety factors were stressed. Emphasis was placed on the following principles, which must be adhered to at home:

- Rearrange commonly used items to avoid excessive bending and reaching.
- Remove clutter, cords, and scatter rugs to prevent tripping and falls.
- Rest periodically and whenever needed to avoid fatigue.
- Sit on a firm, sturdy armchair.
- Use assistive devices as required.
- Observe all precautions and limitations when engaging in daily living activities.

At the conclusion of the afternoon treatment session, Carl, his wife, and the OTA agreed to meet the next day to review the treatment activities and procedures and to answer questions. The OTA summarized and reported Carl's progress to the supervising OT who determined that his program would be discontinued on the next day if dressing goals were met and the patient demonstrated a thorough understanding of the precautions and limitations.

The next day, the OTA saw Carl in his room. He was able to demonstrate LE dressing techniques and the effective use of assistive devices. He was able to verbally list the precautions and limitations that he must observe and related them to specific tasks and activities. Carl had several questions that the OTA answered and several that she helped Carl to answer for himself. Upon completion of this session, the OTA verified treatment and documentation with the OT, who cosigned the note and placed it in Carl's medical chart.

Treatment was discontinued after Carl met the established treatment goals. The OT and OTA met with Carl and his wife and again stressed the importance of following THA precautions and limitations discussed in OT, as well as those addressed by PT, nursing personnel, and his physician. The OTA suggested that they refer to the precautions handout when in doubt of performance techniques for activity. She also indicated that both she and the OT were available by phone if they needed assistance with unanticipated problems. The occupational therapy orthopaedic rehabilitation treatment flow sheet shown in Figure 24-9 was completed and entered in the medical chart.

Six months after his surgery, Carl was able to complete minor plumbing jobs independently for friends and family members. He had also achieved his main objective of playing golf without pain, something that he had not been able to do for years. His only regret was that he had not had the surgery several years earlier when it had been first discussed.

CONCLUSION

This case study discussed the treatment given to a patient after a THA. There are a variety of factors to consider in the treatment of THA, including the type of surgical procedure performed and the individual situation of the patient. Although treatment precautions and protocols are similar, it is imperative to follow the physician's orders for each individual's unique sit-

Precautions and Limitations Following Your Total Hip Arthroplasty

After your surgery, there are positions and activities that can cause dislocation of your hip. Special precautions must be followed for the next 6 to 8 weeks or until your doctor lifts restrictions.

Sitting

1. Sit on a firm, straight-back armchair. Avoid recliners or stools. Do not sit on soft or armless chairs. Use additional pillows or cushions or add a board under chair cushions to provide a firm surface on which to sit.
2. Keep your knees apart; avoid extreme spreading of the legs. Hip width is adequate.
3. Do not cross your legs at the knee, ankle, or in any other way.
4. Do not lean forward when sitting.
5. Do not sit for long periods of time. Try to walk around or lie down every 30 minutes.
6. Do not lift knee of surgical leg higher than hip level.

Standing

1. Do not stand with toes pointed inward or outward.
2. Do not bend forward at the trunk more than 90 degrees.
3. Do not kneel.
4. When doing a task while standing, always face what you are doing and do not overreach or twist with your upper trunk.
5. When standing up from a chair, first move to the edge of the seat, keeping your surgical leg far in front of the nonsurgical leg.

Dressing

1. Do not bend over 90 degrees at the hip to put on socks, underwear, or trousers. You will be taught to use adaptive equipment (elastic shoelaces, long-handled shoe horn, and reacher).
2. The surgical leg is dressed first and undressed last.
3. Do not wear a girdle or panty hose.

Toileting

1. Do not sit on low toilets. Use a raised toilet seat or an over-the-toilet commode to ease getting up and down.

Bathing

1. You may take a shower. You will be shown an appropriate method to do this.
2. You will need to do a sponge bath if you do not have a shower or bath chair of some type. It is important to sponge bathe from a seated position to avoid falls.
3. A long-handled bath sponge or brush is useful for washing the lower extremities.

Homemaking

1. Avoid bending and stooping to low cabinets, ovens, and dryers. Avoid making low beds.
2. Use long-handled mops, dustpans, and brooms to wash floors and sweep and dust low areas.

Car

1. The car should not have bucket seats.
2. Make sure that there is adequate leg space.
3. Transfer: The car should be away from the curb; back up to the passenger seat, sit down, slide straight back on the seat, and have someone assist you to move both legs as a unit into the car. Reverse procedure to get out of the car.

Precautions Specific to You

_____

_____

Figure 24-4. Precautions list. (Reprinted with permission of Marcia Bowker, Director, Occupational Therapy Department of Community Memorial Hospital, Cloquet, MN.)

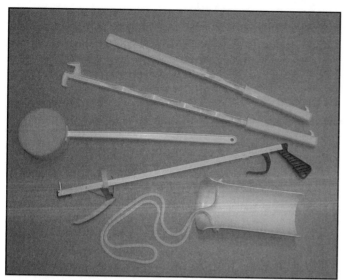

Figure 24-5. Equipment.

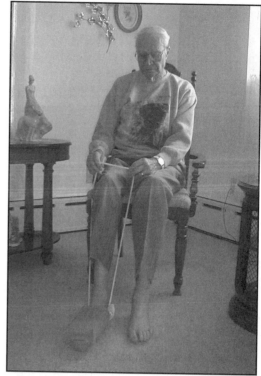

Figure 24-6. Carl using sock aid.

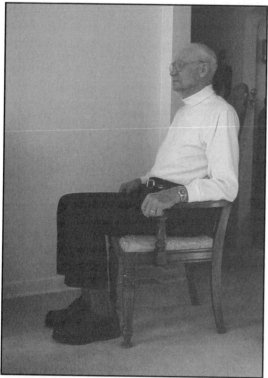

Figure 24-7. Carl in the beginning position of standing by pushing on armrests.

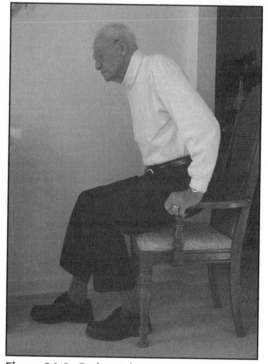

Figure 24-8. Carl standing.

Occupational Therapy Department

Dx: _____ Surgery Date: _____

PMH: _____

Living Status: Alone   w/Spouse   w/Family Member   w/Nurse-Group Home

Function Prior to Admit: _____

Support System: _____

Home Environment: House   Apartment   Mobile Home   Other

Levels_____   # Steps to enter _____ (Front/Back)   # Steps inside _____ (Handrail Yes/No)

Location of: Bedroom _____ Kitchen _____ Laundry _____ (Chute: Yes/No) Bathroom _____

          Tub _____   Walk-in-Shower _____   Tub/Shower Combo _____   Curtains/Door _____

Assistive Devices: _____

Comments: _____
_____
_____

Goals:
_____ Achieve independence with lower extremity dressing techniques.
_____ Instruct in use of adaptive equipment.
_____ Instruct in work simplification, energy conservation.
_____ Achieve independence in home management skills.

Date:		Date _____ P.O. Day: _____	Date _____ P.O. Day: _____	Date _____ P.O. Day: _____
Written Precautions	_____			
LE Dressing	_____			
Adapt. Equip.	_____			
Tub Transfer:	_____			
Home Manage	_____			
Work Smp/Energy Co	_____			
Kitchen Mobility:	_____			
Signatures:				

Patient Name: _____
Physician: _____

Figure 24-9. Occupational therapy orthopaedic rehabilitation treatment flow sheet. (Reprinted with permission of Marcia Bowker, Director, Occupational Therapy Department of Community Memorial Hospital, Cloquet, MN.)

EVIDENCE-BASED TREATMENT STRATEGIES

Treatment Strategies	Authors
Bending restrictions and precautions	Kelmanovich et al., 2003; Pedretti and Early, 2001; Trombly & Radomski, 2002
Organization and modification of the environment	Munin, 1998; Pedretti & Early, 2001
Functional performance within the environment	Munin, 1998; Pedretti & Early, 2001; Trombly & Radomski, 2002
Meaningful occupation	Pedretti & Early, 2001
Patient and caregiver education and involvement in the care plan	Pedretti & Early, 2001; Trombly & Radomski, 2002

uation regarding weight bearing, hip mobility, and positioning. Precautions apply to participation in all daily activities.

Once the OTA has demonstrated service competency working with this type of patient and treatment protocol, the OTA can usually implement the treatment program with minimum general supervision. The entry-level OTA requires closer supervision from the OT. In all cases, consultation should take place with the supervising OT after reviewing the medical chart and in preparation for discharge.

CLINICAL PROBLEM SOLVING

Frequently, a secondary diagnosis or other factors will affect the patient's ability to perform or follow routine THA treatment. Clinical reasoning is required to problem solve and adapt treatment to meet the unique needs and abilities of each individual. The following cases require such adaptations.

Read each scenario, identify "other" factors and resulting limitations, and use problem-solving strategies to identify ways to adapt or grade treatment. Remember to consider all areas of daily activities.

- Maria is 73 years old and will return to the nursing home where she has lived for the past year. Following surgery, Maria is exhibiting increased confusion.
- Bill is an 80-year-old man who lives alone in his own home. Following surgery, Bill will go to a long-term care facility for a period of 1 to 3 months, with the expectation of returning home as soon as he is able to safely function independently.
- Gary is 56 years old, is employed full time, and lives at home with his wife. Due to extreme bilateral hip pain and decreasing mobility, Gary is having both hips replaced at the same time. Gary will be returning home following surgery and is concerned about his sexual relationship with his wife.
- Elsie is 75 years old and has severe arthritic deformities in her hands that limit her functional upper extremity mobility and strength. She will return to her own home

and is having difficulty in using the assistive devices presented to her.

ACKNOWLEDGMENTS

The authors would like to acknowledge the following individuals for their contributions and assistance: Mr. and Mrs. Carl Eisenach; Joel A. Zamzow, MD; Jessica Ochis, COTA/L; Jenny Davis, COTA/L; and the staff at Community Memorial Hospital, Cloquet, Minnesota. We dedicate this chapter to Carl, who died just prior to the printing of this edition.

LEARNING ASSIGNMENTS

1. Study the list of precautions and limitations that must be adhered to following a THA. Practice demonstrating these techniques to a peer.

2. Using the same precautions and limitations, draw stick figures or take photographs to illustrate the principles. As a second activity, incorporate the figures into small posters that would be useful for teaching patients.

3. Make a list of as many work simplification and energy conservation techniques as you can think of. Compare this with those recommended for Carl. What additional ideas did you arrive at that might be useful to a person recovering from hip arthroplasty?

4. Locate assistive devices that may be useful to a patient with THA and practice using them for your own daily living tasks.

5. Identify some makeshift items commonly found in the home that can be used as an assistive device if commercially manufactured devices cannot be obtained by the patient.

6. Identify vendors and medical supply companies in your geographical area that sell or rent the type of equipment referenced in this chapter.

REFERENCES

American Academy of Orthopaedic Surgeons. (2000). Public information: Total joint replacement [on-line service]. Retrieved December 8, 2004, from http://www.aaos.org.

American Academy of Orthopaedic Surgeons. (2001). Public information: Total joint replacement [on-line service]. Retrieved December 8, 2004, from http:// www.aaos.org.

DeWal, H., Su, E., & DiCesare, P. E. (2003). Instability following total hip arthroplasty. *American Journal of Orthopedics, 32*(8), 377-382.

Kelmanovich, D., Parks, M. L., Sinha, R., & Macaulay, W. (2003). Surgical approaches to total hip arthroplasty. *Journal of the Southern Orthopaedic Association, 12*(2), 90-94.

Munin, M. C., Rudy, T. E., Glynn, N. W., Crossett, L. S., & Rubash, H. E. (1998). Early inpatient rehabilitation after elective hip and knee arthroplasty. *Journal of the American Medical Association, 279*(11), 847-852.

Pedretti, L. W., & Early, M. B. (2001). *Occupational therapy: Practice skills for physical dysfunction* (5th ed.). St. Louis, MO: CV Mosby.

Sames, K. M. (2005). *Documenting occupational therapy practice*. Upper Saddle River, NJ: Pearson/Prentice Hall.

Trombly, C. A., & Radomski, M. V. (2002). *Occupational therapy for physical dysfunction* (5th ed.). Philadelphia: Lippincott, Williams & Wilkins.

van Stralen, G. M. J., Struben, P. J., & van Loon, C. J. M. (2003). The incidence of dislocation after primary total hip arthroplasty using posterior approach with posterior soft-tissue repair. *Archives of Orthopedic Trauma Surgery, 123*(5), 219-222.

OCCUPATIONAL THERAPY DEPARTMENT

Dx: (R) THA _____ Surgery Date: 6/22/04

PMH: Osteoarthritis ; Ø other PMH _____

Living Status: ☐ Alone / (w/Spouse) ☐ w/Family Member ☐ w/ Nurse-Group Home

Function Prior to Admit: Independent ; semi-retired plumber

Support System: Wife (Florence) ; adult children (2) in town.

Home Environment: ☒ House ☐ Apartment ☐ Mobile Home ☐ Other

Levels 2 (+) Basement # Steps to enter 6/4 (☒ Front / ☒ Back) # Steps inside 12 (Handrail ☒ Yes / ☐ No)

Location of Bedroom 1st **Kitchen** 1st **Laundry** Basement (Chute ☒ Yes ☐ No) **Bathroom** 1st

☐ Tub ☐ Walk-in-Shower ☒ Tub/Shower Combo ☐ Curtains/Door

Assistive Devices: Issued walker post-op ; had grab bars installed prior to surgery

Comments: Has over-the-toilet commode @ home.
⚹ WANTS TO GOLF AS SOON AS POSSIBLE

Goals:

✓ Achieve independence with lower extremity dressing techniques.
✓ Instruct in use of adaptive equipment
✓ Instruct in work simplification, energy conservation
✓ Achieve independence in home management skills.

Date: 6/23	Date 6/24 AM P.O. Day: 3	Date 6/24 PM P.O. Day: 3	Date 6/25 P.O. Day: 4
Written Precautions 6/23 MB L/E Dressing 6/24 JD Adapt. Equip. 6/24 JD Tub Transfer: 6/24 JD Home Manage 6/24 JD Work Smp/Enrgy Co 6/23/mB Kitchen Mobility: 6/24 JD Initial - Pt c/o minimal nausea Gross eval of ROM/strength appears WNL for UE's. Alert oriented x3. Reviewed precautions/work simplification energy conservation techniques wife in attendance. Reviewed plans/goals. Reviewed home inventory	Less nauseated today states "ready to work" reviewed assistive devices. LE dress demonstration and accurate return demo performed. Issued reacher, dressing stick and sock aid. Instructed pt and wife in toilet and tub transfers, accurate return demo. by pt	Reviewed kitchen mgmt and work simplification strategies. Demonstrated functional mobility during meal prep c̄ walker use. Pt has ice cream pail and utility cart to use for transporting items.	Reviewed all precautions and instructions. Pt performed accurate return demo. of LE dressing, tub transfer and functional mobility c̄ walker for ADLs. OT department phone number issued for questions. Treatment goals met, D/C OT Thank you for your referral.
Signatures: M. Bowler, OTR/L, CHT	Jinny Davis COTA/L	Jinny Davis COTA/L	Jinny Davis COTA/L

Patient Name: Carl E. _____

Physician: Jones _____

Real record 24-1. Real record for a client with total hip arthroplasty. (Reprinted with permission of Marcia Bowker, Director, Occupational Therapy Department of Community Memorial Hospital, Cloquet, MN.)

Key Concepts

- Substance abuse treatment: An interdisciplinary program that helps individuals establish a personal plan for sobriety.
- Lifestyle management: Process of choosing and engaging in daily activities that support alcohol-free living.
- Twelve-step programs: Base recovery on total abstinence from substances, following steps that have been outlined, a sharing of personal stories, and participating in the fellowship of the program.

Essential Vocabulary

abstinence: A period of alcohol- and drug-free living.

detoxification: Process of removing the substance from the person's system; frequently done under the management of a physician.

polysubstance dependence: Characterized by using at least 3 groups of substances (in the same 12-month period) but a single substance does not predominate.

recovery: The process of regaining important life roles, developing healthy relationships with others, and establishing healthy daily routines that support abstinence and sobriety.

sobriety: Used to describe a new way of living without alcohol and drugs.

substance abuse: Includes a maladaptive pattern of use occurring within a 12-month period that is characterized by recurrent and significant adverse consequences.

substance dependence: An essential feature is a cluster of cognitive, behavioral, and physiologic symptoms within the same 12-month period.

Clinical Summary

Etiology

The etiology of substance abuse comes from a variety of factors, including but not limited to genetic predisposition; familial influences, including pathology and substance abuse; premorbid or comorbid mental disorders; availability of substances; peer influences; and role modeling.

Prevalence

It is estimated that 22 million Americans over the age of 12 (9.4%) were dependent on or abused a combination of substances (alcohol and illicit drugs). This reflects 1 in 13 American adults (nearly 14 million) abuse alcohol or are alcoholic and over 19 million Americans use illicit drugs. In general, males tend to try, use, and abuse substances more than females. According to the Substance Abuse and Mental Health Services Administration (2005), approximately 1.6 million persons were admitted for treatment in 1999 and 3% of those admissions were for prescription and over-the-counter drug abuse.

Classic Signs

Substance Dependence

- Tolerance: The need for increased amounts of the drug to obtain the same effect or diminished effect with continued use of the same amount.
- Withdrawal: A characteristic withdrawal syndrome or the use of the substance to relieve or avoid the withdrawal syndrome.
- Taking the substance in larger amounts or over a longer time period than was intended.
- A persistent desire or unsuccessful efforts to cut down or control the substance use.
- Time spent in obtaining or using the substance or recovering from the effects of substance use.
- The giving up or the reduction of important social, occupational, and recreational activities.
- The continuation of substance use despite knowledge of having recurrent physical or psychological problems caused or exacerbated by the substance (APA, 2000).

(continued)

Frank E. Gainer, MHS, OTR, FAOTA and Denise Rotert, MA, OTR

Substance Abuse

- Repeated failure to fulfill major role obligations at work, school, or home.
- Use of the substance despite obvious physical hazards.
- Use of the substance despite obvious social or interpersonal problems.
- Recurrent substance-related legal problems (APA, 2000).

Polysubstance Dependence

- Use of at least 3 groups of substances (in the same 12-month period) but a single substance does not predominate.

Precautions

Most treatment programs use total abstinence as the basis of their practice. Activities, situations, and people closely associated with use of substances probably need to be changed if the treatment is to be successful. Risky behaviors associated with substance use/abuse can lead to additional problems (e.g., injury, sexually transmitted disease, suicide, children born with Fetal Alcohol Syndrome, legal issues, marital issues, health issues).

Resources

Call the National Drug and Alcohol Information Treatment and Referral Line at 1-800-662-HELP.
Sample Internet Resources:
Substance Abuse & Mental Health Services Administration at *www.samhsa.gov*
National Institute on Alcohol Abuse and Alcoholism at *www.niaaa.nih.gov*
American Council for Drug Education at *www.acde.org*
National Institute on Drug Abuse at *www.drugabuse.gov*

INTRODUCTION

Abuse of and dependence on substances is an issue seen in virtually all areas of OT practice. Traditionally, it has been thought of as a mental health issue and OT personnel working in mental health settings may have patients with psychiatric as well as substance use diagnoses. The use/abuse of substances may also emerge as a treatment issue in acute physical disabilities treatment, rehabilitation, long-term care, or home health, for example (Stoffel & Moyers, 1997).

Substance use disorders have been identified in the *Diagnostic and Statistical Manual of Mental Disorders* (4th ed.),

also referred to as DSM-IV-TR (APA, 2000). They are viewed as diseases that are chronic, progressive, and fatal, but can be halted through abstinence from abused substances. DSM-IV-TR also distinguishes between substance dependence and abuse.

For a diagnosis of substance dependence, an essential feature is a cluster of cognitive, behavioral, and physiologic symptoms of which an individual must present with a minimum of 3 (of 7) symptoms within the same 12-month period. The symptoms as stated in the DSM-IV-TR are as follows:

- Tolerance: The need for increased amounts of the drug to obtain the same effect or diminished effect with continued use of the same amount.

- Withdrawal: A characteristic withdrawal syndrome or the use of the substance to relieve or avoid the withdrawal syndrome.
- Taking the substance in larger amounts or over a longer time period than was intended.
- A persistent desire or unsuccessful efforts to cut down or control the substance use.
- Time spent in obtaining or using the substance or recovering from the effects of substance use.
- The giving up or the reduction of important social, occupational, and recreational activities.
- The continuation of substance use despite knowledge of having recurrent physical or psychological problems caused or exacerbated by the substance (APA, 2000).

Substance abuse includes the essential feature of a maladaptive pattern of use occurring within a 12-month period that is characterized by recurrent and significant adverse consequences, including the following:

- Repeated failure to fulfill major role obligations at work, school, or home.
- Use of the substance despite obvious physical hazards.
- Use of the substance despite obvious social or interpersonal problems.
- Recurrent substance-related legal problems (APA, 2000).

Polysubstance dependence is characterized by using at least 3 groups of substances (in the same 12-month period) but a single substance does not predominate. Dependence criteria needs to be met for substances as a group but not for any specific substance. Using substances (including illicit drugs, alcohol, and/or prescription drugs) in combination or as alternates if the drug of choice is not available is a pattern of use that is frequently seen. "Generally, once a problem with alcohol or another drug arises, there is an increased vulnerability to substance dependence problems of all kinds" (Rotert & Gainer, 1993, p. 72).

The process of regaining important life roles, developing healthy relationships with others, and establishing healthy daily routines—all of which support abstinence and sobriety—is termed *recovery*. Detoxification is the process of removing the substance from the person's system and is frequently done under the management of a physician. Abstinence is a period of alcohol- and drug-free living. Sobriety is used to describe a new way of living without alcohol and drugs (Stoffel & Moyers, 1997).

Twelve-step programs have been developed to meet the needs of individuals with a desire to recover from the negative effects of substance use. Alcoholics Anonymous (AA) was the first 12-step program. Twelve-step programs base recovery on total abstinence from substances, following the steps that have been outlined, a sharing of personal stories including use of substances and sobriety, and participating in the fellowship of the program, which is based on recovering individuals assisting individuals who are new to the program (Alcoholics Anonymous, 1998). Examples of other 12-step programs that address specific needs include Narcotics Anonymous (NA) for persons abusing narcotics and Alanon for anyone in a significant relationship with a substance abuser. AA describes the progression

of the disease from spiritual to emotional to physical. Recovery is from physical to emotional to spiritual.

Individuals with substance use disorders have some common characteristics. As the disease progresses, the various areas of an individual's lifestyle performance will deteriorate. Leisure time is the prime time for individuals to use/abuse substances and work time gets protected. It is speculated that one of the reasons that work time is protected is because it is a source of revenue. The healthy activities and behaviors associated with leisure and work performance also show signs of decreasing as the use of substances increases. Role performance problems develop as the disease progresses. Relationships frequently take on attributes that enable the user to continue using. ADL tend to show a decline in skill, the amount of time, and the energy that are dedicated to related tasks. The spectrum of interests, ideas, and activities in the lifestyle of the substance user/abuser becomes constricted (Rotert, 1993).

FRAMES OF REFERENCE

Sobriety is more than abstinence and includes development of coping skills to prevent future alcohol/drug use (Stoffel & Moyers, 1997). OT's purpose can be described as guiding patients in the development of a lifestyle that is supportive of sobriety. The sober lifestyle is organized around temporal adaptation, role performance, and competency behaviors that are the components of occupational behavior.

> The function of occupational therapy is to view the individual needs of the alcoholic patients, to establish a treatment plan based on those individual needs, and to provide intervention opportunities. The overall goal is to assist the patient in development of an alcohol-free lifestyle. Short-term goals will support the overall goal and will be directed at specific deficit areas of occupational behavior. Occupational therapy teaches patients a functional, practical approach to living sober. (Rotert, 1993)

The OT process begins with an evaluation that includes development of an occupational profile and an analysis of the patient/client's occupational performance. An occupational profile will allow the OT practitioners to become familiar with the activities and patterns of the individual. Performance skills, performance patterns, contexts, activity demands, and client factors are all considered. The focus of the evaluation is on areas of occupational performance such as ADL, IADL, education, work, leisure, and social performance. The OT and OTA can join client priorities together with their expertise to develop a plan with intervention strategies that are the most effective (AOTA, 2002).

Evaluation of the occupations of individuals will provide OT personnel with the basis for an OT treatment plan. In order to complete a thorough evaluation, the full spectrum of skills, abilities, and needs must be included. In order for the evaluation to be individually determined, the clinical reasoning skills of the OT and OTA will be utilized to choose the specific assessment tools needed for each individual patient/client.

Some examples of areas of concern in the evaluation and treatment of individuals with substance use/abuse issues include self-care and personal hygiene, support system, interpersonal relationships, time management, money management, work activities, nutrition and meal preparation, safety, and engagement in leisure activities of interest. Underlying difficulties in competent role performance can be difficulties with body scheme, perceptual processing, endurance, coordination, attention span, problem solving, self-concept, interpersonal skills, and coping skills.

A key element in establishing a plan for treatment is the point of view of the client. Therefore, the client needs to be encouraged to share what occupations are important to him or her. Finally, outcomes that reflect the nature of engagement and participation in desired occupations are determined for each client. Collaboration between the client and the OT practitioners throughout the process is needed to increase the potential for successful treatment.

CASE STORY

Mrs. Nancy Jarvis, a 65-year-old white female, was referred to OT for rehabilitation of her right dominant hand after she had sustained a distal radial/ulnar fracture. She was admitted to the hospital and surgery was performed that consisted of an open reduction internal fixation (ORIF) of the distal radius/ulna. She was placed in an external fixator for 12 weeks. Mrs. Jarvis was instructed on proper care of the pin sites and on ROM exercises for the fingers and thumb. She was given follow-up appointments with the surgeon for every 2 weeks.

Mrs. Jarvis has been a widow for the past 2 years. Her husband passed away after a 5-year bout with cancer. She has 2 children, both of whom live out of the area. She has infrequent contact with them. Mrs. Jarvis lives alone in a large 3-story home. Since her husband passed away, she has limited contact with their mutual friends. She used to enjoy playing cards, going out to lunch with friends, and being active with a local community organization. She used to attend church on a regular basis but now attends only on special occasions. She has one good friend whose health has been failing. She talks to her friend daily by phone and sees her about once every other week.

Mrs. Jarvis has had difficulty making her orthopedic surgeon appointments. Her excuses have been that she has forgotten them or she has not been feeling well enough. She has had difficulty getting out of bed, getting herself cleaned and dressed, and taking a taxi to the doctor's office. The only time she would consistently make her follow-up appointments was when she needed a pain medication refill. The surgeon initially referred her to OT for ROM exercises after 4 weeks in the external fixator. However, Mrs. Jarvis never followed through with scheduling the OT evaluation.

After 12 weeks, the surgeon removed the external fixator. Mrs. Jarvis presented with very stiff and swollen fingers. The surgeon inquired about her OT treatment, and she admitted that she never followed through with making the evaluation appointment. She stated that she thought stiff and swollen fingers were normal when you had an external fixator and that it would become automatically better once you removed the fixator. The surgeon's secretary scheduled Mrs. Jarvis for her OT evaluation for that afternoon.

Mrs. Jarvis presented to the OT holding her right hand close to her chest in a very protective position. The initial evaluation consisted of the following:

- Medical background data
- ROM measurements
- Fine-motor coordination test
- Edema measurements
- Sensation testing
- Discussion of home set-up

The OT was concerned about Mrs. Jarvis' personal hygiene. She appeared unkempt and did not seem to have bathed for several days. In addition, there seemed to be an odor of alcohol on her breath. She also seemed to have an unusual dependence on her pain medication for someone who was over 12 weeks from her original date of injury. Finally, she appeared lethargic and did not seem to be overly concerned about the status of her dominant hand and the significant loss of function that was evident. The OT suspected that Mrs. Jarvis might be depressed and was using alcohol and her pain medication as a way of self-medicating. Due to the questionable pattern of substance use of both alcohol and pain medications, it was decided to include as part of the initial evaluation the following:

- ADL evaluation.
- A complete social history to include support systems.
- Leisure interests inventory.
- Time management assessment to include the structure of a typical day.

In order to begin to address the psychosocial issues that were occurring with Mrs. Jarvis, the OT had a very frank conversation with her to discuss her personal hygiene, the consistent odor of alcohol, and her seeming overdependence on her pain medication. She was counseled that all of this would have a negative impact on her realizing the best improvement she possibly could for her hand. Mrs. Jarvis related that since her injury, she was withdrawing even further from her previous interests. She was encouraged to complete a leisure interest and social history questionnaire (Figure 25-1). In addition, she was given a time clock (Figure 25-2). This allowed the OT and OTA to see how Mrs. Jarvis was structuring a typical day. They could then assess whether a certain time of the day was more problematic than another.

The OTA was responsible for completing the ADL evaluation and assessment of leisure interests and time management. The OT completed the neuromusculoskeletal evaluation as well as the social history and the assessment of substance use. Goals for Mrs. Jarvis' OT treatment program were collaborated.

General Goals

Goals included the following:
- Independence in ADL, which is supported by:
  - ROM, strength, and fine motor coordination of right dominant hand within functional limits (WFL).

Occupational Therapy Questionnaire

NAME: _____

AGE: _____ SEX: MALE / FEMALE

HOME ADDRESS: _____

WORK BACKGROUND

Current Paid Job(s):_____

Have you ever been fired from a job?   Yes / No   If yes, why? _____

_____

Other job(s): _____

Volunteer job(s): _____

What do/did you like about your job(s)? _____

What do/did you dislike about your job(s)? _____

How did you get along with others at work? _____

What are your responsibilities at home? _____

_____

EDUCATIONAL BACKGROUND

What is the highest grade that you completed in school? _____

Do you have diplomas, certificates, or degrees? (Describe) _____

_____

What do you like to study? _____

LEISURE INTERESTS

What do you do to have fun? _____

List those activities that you usually do by yourself: _____

_____

List those activities that you usually do with others: _____

_____

What clubs/organizations do you participate in? _____

_____

How would you describe your skills or talents? _____

_____

List those activities you used to participate in but no longer do: _____

_____

SOCIAL HISTORY

Do you find it easy to do the following:

Socialize with others?   Yes / No   Why or why not? _____

Start conversations?   Yes / No   Why or why not? _____

Share feelings and emotions?   Yes / No   Why or why not? _____

Describe your strongest points:_____

_____

Describe your weakest points: _____

_____

What are your goals for the future? _____

_____

What effects has substance abuse had on your life? _____

_____

Do you want to get and stay sober? _____

What would you like to change about yourself or your life to help you be sober? _____

_____

_____

Figure 25-1. Occupational therapy questionnaire.

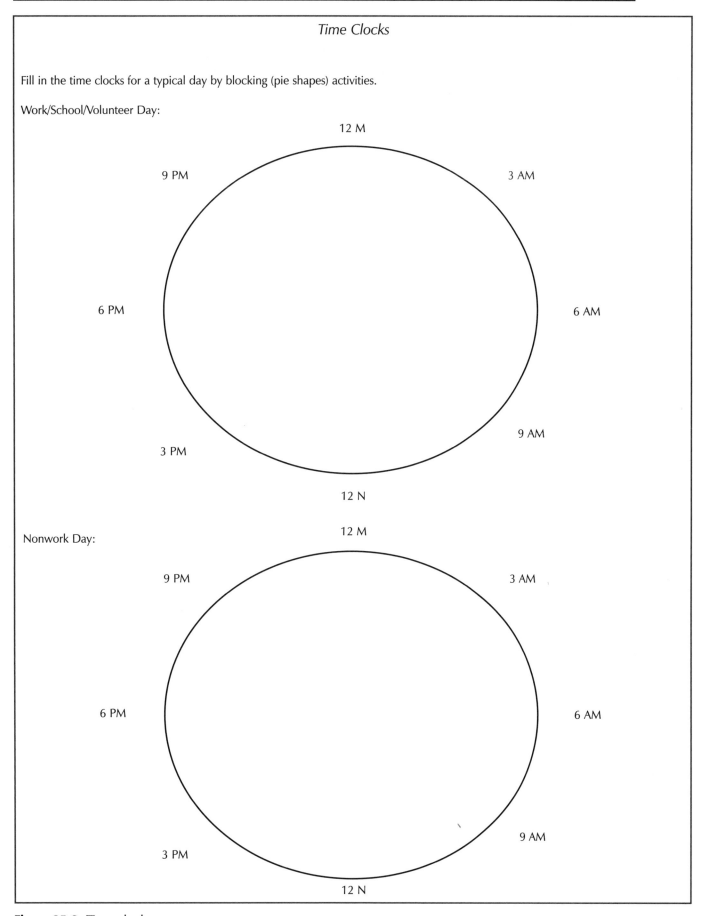

Figure 25-2. Time clocks.

○ Edema of right upper extremity WFL.
- Pursuit of identified leisure or other interests, which is supported by:
  ○ Ability to structure her day so she is up and active during the majority of the day.
- Identification of an appropriate support system.

Initially, treatment sessions were scheduled for 3 days a week, and each session was 1 hour in length. The OT and OTA worked together in treating Mrs. Jarvis. The first 20 minutes of each session consisted of using a heat modality, in this case fluidotherapy, which provides a dry heat maximizing functional activities. This was followed by a combination of exercises (AROM and PROM) and functional activities that required her to use her right hand for sustained periods of time. In addition, the patient was provided with an edema glove to wear throughout the day and at night to assist in reducing the swelling. She was also given a home program that consisted of retrograde massage, ROM exercises, and education about using routine, daily home activities to increase her competence in performance of her chosen occupations.

Mrs. Jarvis was receptive to the inquiries about her psychosocial issues as she felt that she was losing control of her life and no longer found a lot of meaning and satisfaction in the few activities she still participated in. She was concerned about her friend's failing health and how unbearable her life would be if something were to happen to her friend. The OT and OTA developed a plan of action with Mrs. Jarvis. It was decided that she would do the following:
- Abstain from using alcohol and after consulting with her physician, would take 1 pain pill 1 hour before every OT treatment session.
- Make a commitment to attend an AA meeting once a week for the next 6 weeks. She was directed to a group that consisted primarily of people in her age group so that she would be able to better relate to their issues.
- Resume attending mass once every week to try and regain the spirituality that she felt was missing.
- Make a commitment to visit her friend at least once a week and try to go to an outside activity with her.
- Commit to attending her monthly civic organization meeting.
- Contact her son and daughter a minimum of every 2 weeks for the next 6 weeks to try and reconcile her relationship with them.
- Finally, that for the next 4 weeks she would call an old friend each week and make an effort to get together and participate in some type of community activity.

Summary

The use and abuse of substances is a factor that complicates OT treatment. It can be found as an issue in the clients that receive OT services or can be seen in their caregivers. When a patient/client or caregiver uses or abuses substances, it can have an adverse effect on their ability to engage in meaningful and purposeful activities. Substance use/abuse problems may be the identified reason for attending OT or they may be issues that complicate the treatment for other issues.

The physical and/or psychosocial factors associated with substance use that emerge during the OT process can be either contributing factors or the result of heavy, chronic use/abuse of substances. From either perspective, they need to be addressed.

Clinical Problem Solving

The following are some mini cases that demonstrate some of those complicating factors. How many possibilities can you identify? How would you evaluate those factors presented? What treatment techniques might you use to reach your treatment goals?
- Nate is a retired veteran diagnosed with alcohol dependence and diabetes. He has had bilateral lower extremity amputations and uses a wheelchair full time. His friends brought alcohol when they picked him up after his discharge and they all sat outside the hospital and got drunk. Nate comes to an outpatient OT appointment for assistance with retirement planning but comes at the wrong time and on the wrong day and does not seem to recognize you. How would Nate's diabetes show up in his OT evaluation? What could you expect to find in analyzing his occupational performance?
- Susan is a 18-year-old methamphetamine abuser who has sustained a gun shot wound (GSW) to her right elbow in a domestic fight after she told her boyfriend that she is pregnant. What questions might you ask as part of Susan's occupational profile regarding occupational history, values, activity patterns, and needs? What intervention strategies might she participate in to prepare her for future changes?
- Joe is a Native American male who is returning to the reservation and has tried numerous times to get clean and sober with traditional AA. Joe's wife is also alcohol dependent and drank alcohol and smoked cigarettes throughout her pregnancy with their son who is now 5 years old and showing signs of Fetal Alcohol Syndrome (FAS). What outcomes might you identify with Joe? In looking at his role performance, what actions might you suggest?
- Evie is a 29-year-old intravenous (IV) drug user diagnosed with AIDS. Evie requests evening appointments so that she can keep everything a secret from her employer who thinks she was hospitalized for acute pneumonia and has fully recovered. What would you look for in Evie's records to determine how AIDS is having an impact on her occupational history? In setting outcomes with Evie, what are some assessments that you might use to determine her progress?

Learning Activities

1. Design a worksheet that can be used to address issues of substance abuse with a teenager.

EVIDENCE-BASED TREATMENT STRATEGIES

Treatment Strategies	Authors
Body image	Van Deusen, 2000
Cognitive-behavioral therapy	Johnson, 1987
Identity	Christiansen, 1999
Leisure participation	Hodgson, Lloyd, & Schmid, 2001; Lloyd, King, Lampe, & McDougall, 2001; Mann & Talty, 1990
Life satisfaction	Ackerson, 2000; Larsson & Branholm, 1996
Mastery, life skills, and life activities	Ackerson, 2000; Burleigh, Farber, & Gillard, 1998; Christiansen, 1999; Johnson, 1987; Kniepmann & Flanagan, 1995; Larsson & Branholm, 1996; Waid, 1993; Yerxa, 1998, 2000
Physical activity	Ussher, McCusker, Morrow, & Donaghy, 2000
Self-esteem	Kniepmann & Flanagan, 1995; Stoffel, Cusatis, Seitz, & Jones, 1992; Stoffel, 1993
Spirituality	Moyers, 1997

2. Collect data on drinking on college campuses. Have each student target a specific campus group and then add data together.

3. Investigate on-line support groups for people with substance abuse issues.

REFERENCES

Ackerson, B. J. (2000). Factors influencing life satisfaction in psychiatric rehabilitation. *Psychiatric Rehabilitation Journal, 23*(3), 253-261.

Alcoholics Anonymous. (1998). A.A. fact file. Retrieved November 23, 2003, from http://www.alcoholics-anonymous.org/default/en_about_aa.cfm.?pageid=21.

American Occupational Therapy Association. (2002). Occupational therapy practice framework: Domain and process. *American Journal of Occupational Therapy, 56*(6), 609-639.

American Psychiatric Association. (2000). *Diagnostic and statistical manual for mental disorders-IV-TR*. Washington, DC: Author.

Burleigh, S. A., Farber, R. S., & Gillard, M. (1998). Community integration and life satisfaction after traumatic brain injury: Long-term findings. *American Journal of Occupational Therapy, 52*(1), 45-52.

Christiansen, C. H. (1999). Defining lives: Occupation as identity: An essay on competence, coherence, and the creation of meaning. The 1999 Eleanor Clarke Slagle Lecture. *American Journal of Occupational Therapy, 53*(6), 547-558.

Hodgson, S., Lloyd, C., & Schmid, T. (2001). The leisure participation of clients with a dual diagnosis. *British Journal of Occupational Therapy, 64*, 487-492.

Johnson, M. T. (1987). Occupational therapists and teaching of cognitive behavioral skills. *Occupational Therapy in Mental Health, 7*(3), 69-81.

Kniepmann, K., & Flanagan, J. (1995). Violence prevention for children and families. In *Conference abstracts and resources*. Bethesda, MD: American Occupational Therapy Association.

Larsson, M., & Branholm, I. B. (1996). An approach to goal-planning in occupational therapy and rehabilitation. *Scandinavian Journal of Occupational Therapy, 3*(1), 14-19.

Lloyd, C., King, R., Lampe, J., & McDougall, S. (2001). The leisure satisfaction of people with psychiatric disabilities. *Psychiatric Rehabilitation Journal, 25*(2), 107-113.

Mann, W., & Talty, P. (1990) Leisure activity profile measuring use of leisure time by persons with alcoholism. *Occupational Therapy in Mental Health, 10*, 31-41.

Moyers, P. (1997). Occupational meanings and spirituality: The quest for sobriety. *American Journal of Occupational Therapy, 51*, 207-214.

Rotert, D. A. (1993). Occupational therapy in alcoholism. *Occupational Therapy Practice, 4*, 1-11.

Rotert, D. A., & Gainer, F. E. (1993). The adolescent with chemical dependency. In S. E. Ryan (Ed.), *Practice issues in occupational therapy: Intraprofessional team building*. Thorofare, NJ: SLACK Incorporated.

Stoffel, V. (1993). Women's self-esteem issues in substance abuse and eating disorders. *Occupational Therapy Practice, 4*, 12-18.

Stoffel, V., & Moyers, P. (1997). *Occupational therapy practice guidelines for substance use disorders*. Bethesda, MD: American Occupational Therapy Association.

Stoffel, V., Cusatis, M., Seitz, L., & Jones, N. (1992). Self-esteem and leisure patterns of persons in a residential chemical dependency treatment program. *Occupational Therapy in Health Care, 8*, 69-85.

Substance Abuse and Mental Health Services Administration. (2005). Drug and alcohol treatment. Retrieved July 14, 2005, from http://oas.samhsa.gov/tx.htm.

Ussher, M., McCusker, M., Morrow, V., & Donaghy, M. (2000). A physical activity intervention in a community alcohol service. *British Journal of Occupational Therapy, 63*, 598-604.

Van Deusen, J. (2000). The body image of four women recovered from alcohol abuse. *Occupational Therapy in Mental Health, 16*, 27-44.

Waid, K. M. (1993). An occupational therapy perspective in the treatment of multiple personality disorder. *American Journal of Occupational Therapy, 47*(10), 872-876.

Yerxa, E. J. (1998). Health and the human spirit for occupation. *American Journal of Occupational Therapy, 52*(6), 412-418.

Yerxa, E. J. (2000). Occupational science: A renaissance of service to humankind through knowledge. *Occupational Therapy International, 7*(2), 87-98.

OCCUPATIONAL THERAPY QUESTIONNAIRE

NAME: _Nancy_

AGE: _65_   SEX: MALE / ~~FEMALE~~

HOME ADDRESS:

WORK BACKGROUND

Current Paid Job(s): _Retired homemaker_

Have you ever been fired from a job?   Yes / (No)   If yes, why? _____

_____

Other job(s): _____

Volunteer Job(s): _Use to volunteer with Church_

What do/did you like about your job(s)? _____

What do/did you dislike about your job(s)? _____

How did you get along with others at work? _____

What are your responsibilities at home? _Live alone; husband_
deceased

EDUCATIONAL BACKGROUND

What is the highest grade that you completed in school? _12_

Do you have diplomas, certificates or degrees? (Describe) _No_

_____

What do you like to study? _too long ago_

Real record 25-1A. Real record for a client with substance abuse.

LEISURE INTERESTS

What do you do to have fun? _Nothing_

List those activities that you usually do by yourself: _Everything_

List those activities that you usually do with others: _Nothing_

What clubs/organizations do you participate in? _None anymore_

How would you describe your skills or talents? _Don't have any_

List those activities you used to participate in but no longer do: _cards; going out to lunch with friends_

SOCIAL HISTORY

Do you find it easy to do the following:

Socialize with others? _No_   Why or why not? _?_

Start conversations? _No_   Why or why not? _?_

Share feelings and emotions? _No_   Why or why not? _?_

Describe your strongest points: _None_

Describe your weakest points: _Many_

What are your goals for the future? _none_

Real record 25-1B. Real record for a client with substance abuse.

What effects has substance abuse had on your life? _Made me very_
lonely

Do you want to get and stay sober? _Yas_

What would you like to change about yourself or your life to help you be sober? _____
don't know where to start.

Real record 25-1C. Real record for a client with substance abuse.

Nancy

Outpatient Rehabilitation Services
__PT X OT __SLP

23 Aug 04 Pt completed the Occupational
Therapy Questionnaire this date.
She has been treated x3/weeks
for last week for s/p R distal
radius fracture. Out of fixator
x1 week now. Remains very
protective of her R dominant hand.
Assisted in completing questionnaire
w her L hand. Demonstrated some
insight into how her substance
abuse has caused significant
changes in her life style. Pt
is agreeable to implementing
some changes in her daily
routines. She reports being very
unhappy and wants to feel
better about herself.
In addition to completing the
Questionnaire this session, pt
received fluidotherapy of R wrist/hand
x 20 mins, put the AAROM exercises
of R digits/wrist and was instructed
in therapputty exercises for strengthening
R hand. Followed by completion
of simple kitchen activities. Pt
does remain protective but does
seem willing to try more tasks.
A - s/p R distal radius fx
  ↑ insight into how substance
  abuse is affecting behavior
P - ① con't outpt OT Tx x3/week
  ② con't on present home tx
  program consisting of ROM

Real record 25-2A. Real record for a client with substance abuse.

Nancy

Outpatient Rehabilitation Services
___PT   ___OT   ___SLP

23 Aug 04 (con't)
exercises + theraputty for strengthening
③ Complete the Time Clock by next
session to see how she spends
a typical day
④ will call both of her children
in order to inform them of her tx
program and progress
Next visit scheduled for 25 Aug 04

Frank E. Gainer, MHS, OTR/L

23 Aug 04
Called pt's surgeon — Dr. Michael Smith
and informed him of pt's slow,
but improving progress. He is in
agreement c̄ treatment plan.

Frank E. Gainer, MHS, OTR/L

23 Aug 04
Fax current tx plan to pt's insurance
carrier — Capital Blue Cross/Blue Shield.
They have authorized a total of 12
treatment visits over the next month.

Frank E. Gainer, MHS, OTR/L

Real record 25-2B. Real record for a client with substance abuse.

Key Concepts

- Stroke rehabilitation: A program to restore functional independence of a person after a cerebral vascular insufficiency led to the infarction of brain tissue.
- Subacute rehabilitation: An organized setting for stroke rehabilitation. Multiple disciplines provide intensive treatment for clients.
- Adaptive equipment: Devices designed to make tasks easier and safer.
- One-handed techniques: Methods of performing activities using one hand/arm to accomplish the task.

Essential Vocabulary

aphasia: A disorder of communication that affects the use and understanding of spoken and written language.
cognitive deficits: These include difficulty with problem solving, sequencing, and attention to task.
dysarthria: A disorder of articulation due to muscle weakness that is often manifested as slurred speech.
dysphagia: An impairment of the ability to eat and drink by mouth.
facilitation techniques: Manual methods used to encourage movement and sensory awareness.
flaccidity: The inability to move an extremity due to the loss of motor control.
hemiparesis: Weakness on one side of the body.
hemiplegia: The paralysis of one side of the body opposite to the site of the stroke.
infarction: Tissue death that occurs when the blood supply has been disrupted to the area.
memory loss: The inability to store new experiences or perceptions for later recall.
shoulder subluxation: The downward dislocation of the humerus.
unilateral neglect: A failure to respond to stimuli in the environment opposite to the site of the brain damage.
visual field deficit or hemianopia: Blindness in one-half of the field of vision in one or both eyes.
visual perception deficits: Often observed when the lesion is in the right hemisphere, these include difficulty with spatial relationships and form recognition.

Clinical Summary

Etiology

Stroke is the result of embolism, thrombosis, intercerebral hemorrhage, or vascular insufficiency, leading to brain tissue death or infarction. Risk factors for stroke include hypertension, atherosclerosis, diabetes, and smoking.

Prevalence

Five hundred thousand adults have a stroke each year and the incidence increases with age.

Classic Signs

The signs of stroke include sudden onset of neurological deficits of hemiparesis or hemiplegia. This weakness or paralysis of the leg and/or arm occurs on the side of the body opposite the site of the stroke. Other signs of stroke include the language deficit of aphasia, cognitive deficits, and visual difficulties. The location and extent of the stroke determines the symptoms and prognosis.

Precautions

Treatment of hypertension, cessation of smoking, weight loss, and exercise have been found to help prevent strokes from occurring.

A BUSINESSMAN WITH A STROKE

Martha Logigian, MS, OTR

INTRODUCTION

Stroke is the third leading cause of death and disability in the United States. Approximately 500,000 adults have a stroke each year. It is a rapid onset of neurological deficits that persists for at least 24 hours as a result of intracerebral hemorrhage, thrombosis, embolism, or vascular insufficiency leading to the infarction of brain tissue. Eighty-five percent of strokes are due to brain infarctions, while intracerebral and subarachnoid hemorrhages account for about 15%. Strokes occur at any age, but the incidence dramatically increases with age (Acquaviva, 1996). A stroke, which is a lesion in a hemisphere of the brain, produces motor impairment or hemiparesis of the contralateral side of the body. For example, a stroke (brain attack or CVA) in the left cerebral hemisphere is referred to as a left CVA with resulting hemiparesis on the right side of the body. Due to this weakness or lack of motion on one side of the body, the patient will experience difficulty with most ADL including self-care tasks, ambulation, and homemaking. In addition, depending on the location in the brain of the stroke, the patient may have sensory, cognitive, language, and visual deficits as well as confusion.

Many stroke survivors with impairments such as these will benefit from rehabilitation. In one study, patients who received rehabilitation achieved greater and more rapid gains in physical function than those who did not receive rehabilitation (Kelly-Hayes & Paige, 1995). Most recovery takes place within the first 3 months, and in this era of cost containment, shorter lengths of stay in the hospital and rehab setting are the norm. Thus, short-term functional gains are the focus of the OT program (Van Dyck, 1999).

THEORY THAT FRAMES PRACTICE

OT in stroke rehabilitation focuses on the functional independence of the individual following the infarction. This in turn enables the individual to resume a quality life style. Thus, the therapist provides treatment to improve performance of important occupational tasks such as dressing, grooming, and mobility.

Compensatory strategies are utilized by many therapists in the acute setting due to time and cost limitations. These include one-handed techniques for dressing and grooming beginning with simple tasks and gradually increasing in difficulty as the patient gains competency.

Alternatively, training in ADL can be approached using neurodevelopmental treatment as a remedial treatment strategy. Utilizing this approach can assist the patient in gaining independence in functional tasks and can encourage movement of the involved extremity. Moreover, as the patient progresses, more complex tasks are addressed, including meaningful life roles and avocational interests. In the case study, both strategies are utilized to provide opportunities for success utilizing the Occupational Functioning Model (Trombly, Radomski, Tresel, & Burnet-Smith, 2002).

ASSESSMENT

Areas to be evaluated in OT include functional performance, UE function, visual function, and cognition. This is done through direct observation rather than patient/family report, as there can be a significant difference between the two. In addition, to prepare for discharge planning, the assessment is completed as early as possible. The reason for this is that the patient's level of occupational performance will influence the amount of assistance needed, where the individual will live, and occupational roles in which the patient can participate.

To assess functional performance, the Barthel Index (Mahoney & Barthel, 1965) and the Functional Independence Measure (FIM) (Keith, Granger, Hamilton, & Sherwin, 1987) are standardized tools that are widely used. These are interdisciplinary assessments of self-care, bowel and bladder control, mobility, and social interaction (Gresham & Duncan, 1995). Additionally, the Philadelphia Geriatric Center Instrumental Activities of Daily Living Scale (Lawton, 1988) is utilized to determine a patient's ability to perform IADL such as using a telephone and handling finances. Some rehabilitation programs use the standardized measures at admission, several weeks later, and at discharge to help determine a patient's progress and level of function for discharge. Therapists may use a functional performance tool of their own design to document daily/weekly progress.

The assessment of UE function includes sensation testing, PROM, voluntary motion, muscle tone, motor planning, shoulder subluxation, and pain. It is useful to compare the function of the involved extremity to the uninvolved extremity of the stroke patient. This assessment typically looks at the skills and abilities of the patient in each of the above mentioned areas. Standardized measures are available, although clinical observations are most commonly utilized.

Visual function assessment includes examination of visual skills such as visual acuity and those referred to as visual perception (e.g., spatial relations, figure ground, and topographical orientation). Visual field deficits and unilateral neglect are also identified through various tasks and drawings asked of the patient.

Cognitive abilities include attention, memory, reasoning, and problem solving. These are critical to the performance of the homemaker, businessperson, or retiree interested in avocational pursuits. Formal and informal assessments are utilized to evaluate cognitive skills. An example of a formal assessment is the FIM, which contains information on cognitive performance. Informal functional assessments such as a homemaking task that includes observation of attention to task can be used. Although this type of assessment is subjective, it is useful for the patient who cannot follow verbal or written instructions.

FUNCTIONAL IMPACT

The person who has experienced a stroke has deficits determined by the location and extent of the lesion. Weakness in the extremities on one side of the body, or hemiparesis, is the most common problem. This weakness occurs on the side opposite the location of the stroke. For example, if a person has a stroke in the right hemisphere of the brain, or right CVA, weakness will be seen in the left leg and/or arm. This weakness, or in some cases total lack of movement or hemiplegia, affects the patient's ability to move in bed, bathe, groom, dress, and walk.

Shoulder subluxation due to weakness or spasticity can present a significant problem due to pain associated with this deficit. In addition, lack of proper positioning can lead to hand edema in the involved UE. This can be painful and interfere with function.

Other functional deficits may occur depending on the location of the stroke. A person with a left CVA may experience difficulty with communication or aphasia, whereas a person with a right CVA may neglect the left side of the body as well as exhibit impulsive behavior.

An important issue relative to the functional impact of stroke is the amount of assistance needed to complete self-care activities once the patient returns home. Moreover, consideration must be given to the design of the patient's home so as to enable full participation in meaningful activities.

IADL need to be addressed as well so that the person with a stroke can resume vocational and avocational interests.

TREATMENT

The acute phase of rehabilitation care for the stroke patient begins as soon as the neurological condition is stabilized and life-threatening problems are under control. In most cases, this phase is short, with patients being discharged to a subacute level of care or home within 3 days of admission. During this stay, treatment is focused on early mobilization through ADL such as bed mobility and grooming, positioning, and ROM to maintain the integrity of the skin and prevent contractures. Patient and family education is provided in terms of emotional support and explanation about what has happened to the individual and the acute phase of care. Discharge planning begins at the time of admission to the acute care facility.

The rehabilitation phase begins with an assessment followed by the identification of a problem list, short-term goals, long-term goals, treatment plan, and discharge recommendations. The primary goal of OT is to improve the performance of daily living tasks. Additionally, based on the impairments of the patient, occupational performance goals are set. These may include bilateral use of the upper extremities, visual and/or cognitive retraining, and the use of compensatory strategies for dressing and grooming such as one-handed techniques (Poole, 1997). Adaptive equipment may be utilized (e.g., a sling for the involved UE may help to reduce pain in the shoulder and hand edema).

Among the general strategies found helpful for the patient with a stroke are the following:

- Provide verbal, visual, and/or tactile cues to aid in the completion of a task.
- Divide a complex activity such as dressing into manageable parts.
- Practice the task in a consistent and systematic routine.
- Use real objects in a natural setting.
- Gradually reduce the amount of assistance and cues given as the patient progresses.
- Adapt the environment to facilitate performance.

Discharge planning occurs early as the team of rehabilitation specialists needs to be aware of the patient's physical and cognitive deficits relative to the discharge location. For example, if a patient with a left hemiparesis lives in a house with a series of stairs to enter the home, alterations must be made to enable entry, such as a ramp. However, a ramp takes time to construct, thus the team needs to plan for the return to home early on to enable an efficient discharge.

CASE STUDY

Mr. Callahan is a 65-year-old businessman who experienced a sudden onset of weakness on the left side of his body with slurred speech. He lives in a large, single-story home with his wife, and he has 3 married sons who live in the area. He was brought from home by ambulance to the hospital emergency room where the neurologist diagnosed a right middle cerebral artery infarct. He began treatment in the emergency room and was transferred to a patient care unit in the hospital. In the

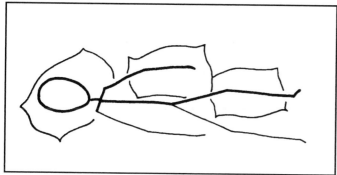

Figure 26-1. Supine position. When the patient is totally dependent, position with pillows under head and under shoulder for protraction; under extended arm and hand, with hand elevated if edematous; under calf with some knee flexion and no pressure on heel. Trunk should be aligned. (Reprinted with permission from Logigian, M. K. [1982]. *Adult rehabilitation: A team approach for therapists.* Boston, MA: Little, Brown and Co.)

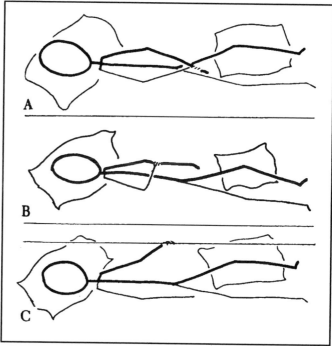

Figure 26-2. When the patient is more independent, use fewer pillows with: A. Arms extended, hands clasped together, resting on abdomen; B. Involved arm extended by side, in supination if possible, with sound hand keeping involved elbow extended; C. Involved hand on side rail, legs extended, pillow under the calf with some knee flexion, and no pressure on heel. (Reprinted with permission from Logigian, M. K. [1982]. *Adult rehabilitation: A team approach for therapists.* Boston, MA: Little, Brown and Co.)

acute phase of illness, the patient's medical condition is evolving with stabilization of accompanying neurological symptoms and the beginning stages of recovery. During these critical days in the acute care hospital, UE ROM, bed mobility, and positioning are the primary concerns of the OT program. On day 2 of hospitalization, the OT was asked by the PT to see Mr. Callahan at bedside, as his left hand and arm were flaccid and swollen. In addition, his arm had impaired sensation. He was unable to complete any self-care activities, and he had difficulty articulating his responses to the OT screening as he was dysarthric.

Mr. Callahan could move in bed from side to side, although he was uncomfortable doing so, as his arm became tangled in the sheets. He was usually found slipped down in bed and unable to regain a comfortable position. Mr. Callahan transferred bed to chair with the maximum assistance of the OT. He used a wheelchair to get to the bathroom, although he was unable to independently move the wheelchair. With maximum assistance of the OT, he was able to transfer onto the toilet. Mr. Callahan could feed himself if all of the food on the tray was set up, cut up, and opened. He could wash his face during a bed bath but was unable to bathe the rest of his body, dress, or shave.

It was anticipated that Mr. Callahan would remain in the acute care hospital for 2 more days. Due to the limited time, the OT program focused on UE ROM, positioning while in bed, bed mobility, and bed-to-chair transfers. ROM exercises for the left UE were demonstrated to Mr. Callahan, although he had difficulty doing them. His son, who was in attendance during the treatment session, learned to do the ROM exercises, and the therapist suggested that he do them daily for his father. The OT demonstrated positioning (Figures 26-1 through 26-3) and bed mobility (Figures 26-4 through 26-7) to the nurses caring for Mr. Callahan, to ensure he was comfortable in bed. Mr. Callahan's son was instructed in bed-to-chair transfers (Figures 26-8 and 26-9). The OT checked back with Mr. Callahan on day 3 and found that he was comfortable and his son was carrying out the ROM program.

It was decided that Mr. Callahan had excellent rehabilitation potential, and the plan was that as soon as his neurological symptoms stabilized he would be transferred to a subacute care rehabilitation unit with the long-term goal of return to home. On day 4, the OT wrote a discharge summary that included a statement on the program he participated in while in the acute care hospital. He was transferred to the subacute program later in the day.

The following morning, the OT at the subacute program began a complete assessment of Mr. Callahan following a review of his medical record. During the record review, medical issues are identified, including age, general health, vital signs, medications, and precautions. The assessment included sensation and motor status of the involved UE such as muscle tone, edema, and hand use; hand dominance; perception; vision status (e.g., are glasses worn?); visual field; praxis; cognition; and ADL. In addition, through discussion with Mr. Callahan and his family, information was gained concerning his level of function, work, and leisure activity (Chang & Hasselkus, 1998) prior to the stroke. Their goals, expectations, and plan for discharge from the subacute program were discussed. The family provided information on Mr. Callahan's home environment, as return to home was part of the plan. The OT reviewed the findings with the OTA and a plan of care was developed.

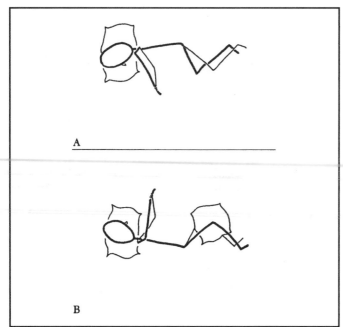

Figure 26-3. Side-lying. When the patient lies on either side (A and B), position with scapula protracted, arms extended with hands clasped together, or sound hand holding involved wrist; or knees and hips flexed, pillow between legs if necessary to keep bony prominences apart. Elevate hand on pillow if it is edematous (not shown). (Reprinted with permission from Logigian, M. K. [1982]. *Adult rehabilitation: A team approach for therapists.* Boston, MA: Little, Brown and Co.)

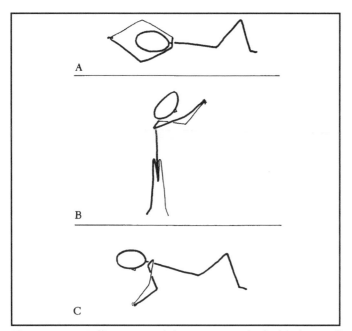

Figure 26-5. Rolling. A. With legs to one side, hold, then roll to other side, upper body relaxed. B. Arms and head to one side, hold, then to other side, lower body relaxed. C. Combine first 2 motions in opposite directions. Resist or assist patient as needed. Practice separately and together. Combine motions in same direction (one segment at a time) for rolling sequence. (Reprinted with permission from Logigian, M. K. [1982]. *Adult rehabilitation: A team approach for therapists.* Boston, MA: Little, Brown and Co.)

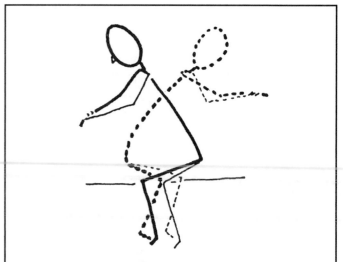

Figure 26-4. Shifting and sitting. The patient transfers all weight to feet, and lifts and moves hips to one side and sits gently on that side. The patient continues moving down one side of the mat or bed by lifting and shifting weight, repositioning feet each time, with assistance as needed. Reverse directions; keeping involved foot behind sound foot, maintain sitting balance and move slowly with control. (Reprinted with permission from Logigian, M. K. [1982]. *Adult rehabilitation: A team approach for therapists.* Boston, MA: Little, Brown and Co.)

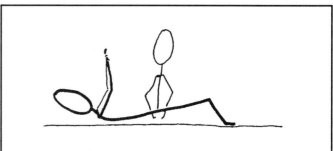

Figure 26-6. Bridging. Raise hips up, hold, lower. Keep knees together and weight evenly distributed. Repeat with knees in more flexion. Use resistance and joint compression. Hold up position and shift weight to left and right, keeping knees upright. Hold up position and abduct and adduct knees evenly. (Reprinted with permission from Logigian, M. K. [1982]. *Adult rehabilitation: A team approach for therapists.* Boston, MA: Little, Brown and Co.)

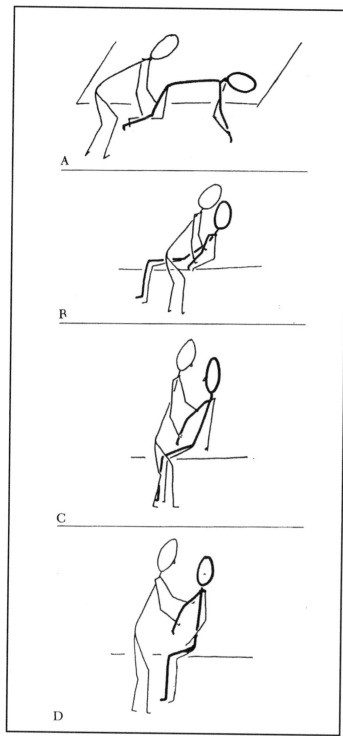

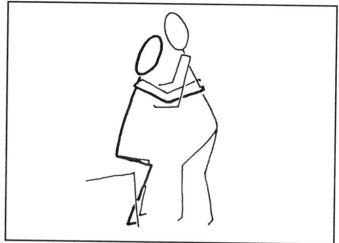

Figure 26-8. Sitting to standing. The therapist's hands are under the patient's elbow, patient's hands are around therapist's waist or elbows extended, hands are clasped together. The patient leans forward so some weight is shifted forward onto the legs, increasing the amount of leaning and weight-shifting as tolerated. Involved foot is positioned slightly behind sound foot. Lean forward so weight is transferred more on involved leg as the patient leans forward. (Reprinted with permission from Logigian, M. K. [1982]. *Adult rehabilitation: A team approach for therapists.* Boston, MA: Little, Brown and Co.)

Figure 26-7. To sitting position from sound side. A. Feet over edge, sound foot involved as necessary. Hands clasped together, arms extended. B. Prop up onto sound elbow with head turned toward involved side. Hands are still clasped, if possible, or therapist holds arm extended and scapula protracted. C. Push up onto sound hand, elbow extended. Hands are still clasped, if possible, or therapist holds extended. D. Come to full sitting position, hands in lap, feet flat on the floor. Therapist assists balance as needed. (Reprinted with permission from Logigian, M. K. [1982]. *Adult rehabilitation: A team approach for therapists.* Boston, MA: Little, Brown and Co.)

The results of the assessment indicated that Mr. Callahan was in good health prior to his stroke. He worked 4 days a week in the construction business he had established, which his sons now managed. He lived with his wife in a large, ranch-style home in the suburbs. He has a ranch-style vacation home on the ocean, which is where he spends every weekend year round. At the vacation home, he had been doing all the cooking, his specialty being Italian cuisine. Although his wife enjoyed this home, she preferred to remain in the suburban home, and Mr. Callahan frequently went to the vacation home alone or with friends.

Mr. Callahan had a flaccid left UE with shoulder subluxation, although slight movement and sensation was noted in the fingers. The shoulder was painful when passively moved and his hand was swollen. Shoulder subluxation is the downward dislocation of the humerus and a common problem for a patient with a flaccid or weak UE. In the flaccid extremity, the supraspinatus, part of the rotator cuff muscles, along with all the other scapular and humeral muscles, can no longer hold the humerus in place, as they are weak or paralyzed. The upward motion of the glenoid fossa is no longer maintained as gravity, the weight of the arm, spasticity, or a tendency to lean toward the weak side bring the scapula into a downward position. Prolonged subluxation can be extremely painful.

Mr. Callahan had good trunk mobility and was able to move in bed with minimal assistance (Table 26-1). He could transfer bed to chair and chair to toilet with moderate assistance of one. At present, he was using a wheelchair for mobility, although he needed assistance to move it any distance. The PT planned to have him ambulating with a quad cane. The speech pathologist was consulted and provided the team with suggestions for dealing with Mr. Callahan's dysarthria.

On the ADL index, he was found to have difficulty in bathing, dressing, and personnel hygiene due to left side weakness and neglect. He required moderate assistance to sponge bathe in bed and don/doff his shirt. He needed maximum assistance of one to don/doff his underwear and pants. He was able to shave himself although he had frequent cuts, as he insisted on using his single blade razor. He was able to feed himself if the food had been set up on the tray (e.g., cartons and packages opened, meat cut, and rolls buttered). He exhibited neglect of his left visual field, yet in all areas of perception, praxis, and cognition he was within the norm.

The plan of care included the following long-term goals:
- Mr. Callahan will return home with his family.
- Mr. Callahan will be independent in ADL, including bathing, dressing, toileting, shaving, brushing teeth, and feeding.
- Mr. Callahan will be independent and safe in kitchen activities with the use of adaptive equipment for food preparation.

Short-term goals (within 2 weeks) are:
- Mr. Callahan will be independent in UE dressing and require minimal assistance in LE dressing.
- Mr. Callahan will be independent in feeding, brushing teeth, and shaving with the use of compensatory techniques.
- Mr. Callahan will maintain appropriate positioning of his UE while in bed, chair, and standing.
- Mr. Callahan will prepare a simple snack in the kitchen using adaptive equipment and one-handed techniques.

Although daily notes are written by the OT and OTA following each treatment session, a progress note is written every 2 weeks. At this time, short-term goals are reviewed and updated or, if needed, new goals established. The OT discussed the assessment and plan with Mr. Callahan and his wife, and they were in agreement with it.

All records are kept in the patient's medical record so that team members have access to the information. In addition, the results of the assessment and treatment plan were presented at the weekly patient care team meeting to ensure consistency.

The OT and OTA worked as a team to initiate the program to improve Mr. Callahan's left UE function, ADL ability, and kitchen skills. Initially, the OT sought to eliminate Mr. Callahan's subluxation with manual support and mobilization of the humerus in the glenoid fossa. With support, the force of gravity is reduced, articular surfaces are in place, and pain diminished. An arm sling is one means of support, and it was decided that it would be tried due to his arm pain. Whatever type of sling is utilized, it must be evaluated routinely with special attention given to its effectiveness in eliminating subluxation, ease of use, and ability to control pain. It is not intended for 24-hour use. It is most useful when worn during standing, ambulation, and transfer activities. The hand must be positioned within the sling, maintaining wrist and finger extension.

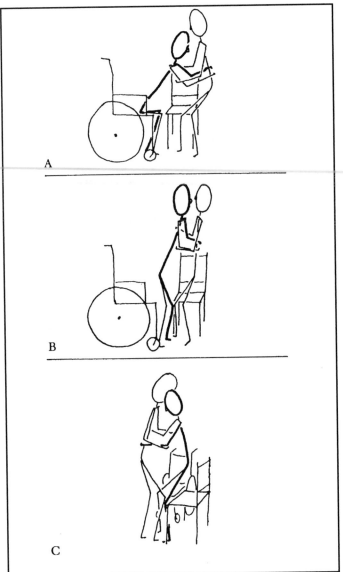

Figure 26-9. Moderate to maximum assistance toward involved side. A. Patient transfers all weight to feet, B. pivots toward involved side, and C. sits by leaning forward. Therapist assists to maintain knee extension and to keep trunk forward, as needed. (Reprinted with permission from Logigian, M. K. [1982]. *Adult rehabilitation: A team approach for therapists.* Boston, MA: Little, Brown and Co.)

The elbow should be at 80 degrees of flexion and the strap should fit comfortably on the back and neck.

A lap tray was found to be useful when Mr. Callahan was in his wheelchair, and pillows continued to be helpful while he was in bed. The lap tray and pillows are used for scapula support and normal alignment (Figure 26-10). A therapy program of scapular mobilization was initiated by the OT. It focused on the scapular upward rotators and supraspinatus portions of the rotator cuff muscles (Figures 26-11 through 26-15). Although the therapist anticipated that Mr. Callahan would need to learn one-handed techniques to accomplish self-care and daily living tasks, mobility techniques were a part of Mr. Callahan's program to enable maximum mobility of his left side. Mr. Callahan

---

Table 26-1

Scales to Measure Functional Performance

- Total assistance: The need for 100% assistance by one or more persons to perform all physical activities and/or cognitive assistance to elicit a functional response to an external stimulation.
- Maximum assistance: The need for 75% assistance by one person to physically perform any part of a functional activity and/or cognitive assistance to perform gross motor actions in response to direction.
- Moderate assistance: The need for 50% assistance by one person to perform physical activities or provide cognitive assistance to sustain/complete simple, repetitive activities safely.
- Minimum assistance: The need for 25% assistance by one person for physical activities and/or periodic, cognitive assistance to perform functional activities safely.
- Standby assistance: The need for supervision by one person for the patient to perform new activity procedures that were adapted by the therapist for safe and effective performance. A patient requires standby assistance when errors and the need for safety precautions are not always anticipated by the patient.
- Independent status: No physical or cognitive assistance is required to perform functional activities. Patients at this level are able to implement the selected courses of action, consider potential errors, and anticipate safety hazards in familiar and new situations.

Adapted from Health Care Financing Administration. (1996). *Medicare intermediary manual, Publication 13, Section 3906.4*. Washington, DC: U.S. Government Printing Office, 21-21.

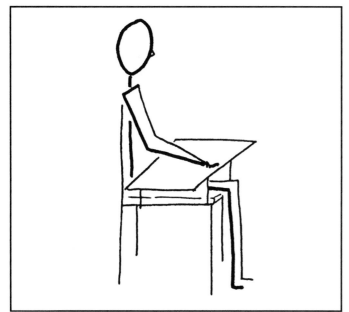

Figure 26-10. When sitting in a wheelchair or standard chair, the patient is positioned with head in midline (may need head support), trunk aligned with pillows or side supports, buttocks with special cushion to protect skin and provide comfort, thighs parallel to floor, weight evenly distributed along thighs, knees with 90 degree flexion, if possible. Feet are flat, with weight evenly distributed on both feet, foot rests, or floor; seat belt is used as indicated. Arms are extended in front and supported on a pillow, rolled-up blanket, lapboard, arm board, or table. If legs are elevated, put cushion under calves, heels free and ankles dorsiflexed. (Reprinted with permission from Logigian, M. K. [1982]. *Adult rehabilitation: A team approach for therapists*. Boston, MA: Little, Brown and Co.)

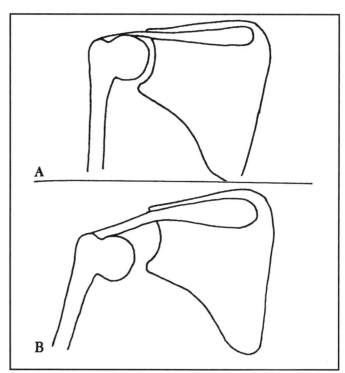

Figure 26-11. Subluxation. A. Position of the humerus in the glenoid fossa and the supraspinatus muscle in the locking mechanism. B. Position of the humerus and scapula during subluxation. Note downward rotation of the scapula and horizontal motion of the humerus. (Reprinted with permission from Logigian, M. K. [1982]. *Adult rehabilitation: A team approach for therapists*. Boston, MA: Little, Brown and Co.)

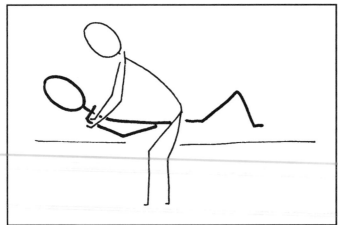

Figure 26-12. Scapular mobilization. The therapist moves the scapula through ROM by placing a hand over it, fingers on the medial border. The humerus is kept approximated in fossa so it works with the scapula as one unit. Supine. With a hand on the scapula and one under the axilla, the patient's arm relaxed by side, hand on abdomen, and keeping humerus and scapula together, passively 1. elevate and rotate upward, then depress and rotate scapula downward. 2. Protract and retract scapula by pulling and pushing on the medial border. (Reprinted with permission from Logigian, M. K. [1982]. *Adult rehabilitation: A team approach for therapists.* Boston, MA: Little, Brown and Co.)

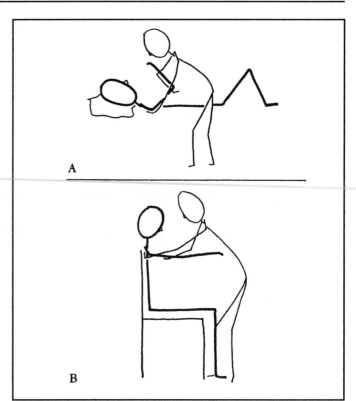

Figure 26-13. A. Supine. B. Sitting. Passively flex the humerus, staying in the pain-free range. Elbow may remain flexed or be extended. Mobilize the scapula through the following ranges: 1. Protraction and retraction using hand on the medial border while passively pulling the humerus and scapula together, forward, and back. 2. Rotate upward using a hand on the medial border and inferior angle of the scapula and increasing flexion of the humerus (it is important for humerus and scapula to work together). 3. With the humerus in abduction, rotate upward, retract and protract the scapula. Increase humeral range as tolerated. (Reprinted with permission from Logigian, M. K. [1982]. *Adult rehabilitation: A team approach for therapists.* Boston, MA: Little, Brown and Co.)

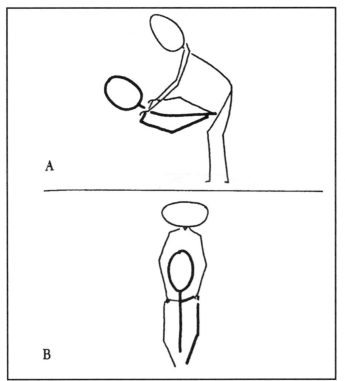

Figure 26-14. Scapula elevation (shrugging). A. Supine. B. Sitting. Active assistance to elevation; tapping on the upper trapezius; resistance to active elevation; quick stretch of the upper trapezius; associated reactions by resisting the sound side; combinations of above. (Reprinted with permission from Logigian, M. K. [1982]. *Adult rehabilitation: A team approach for therapists.* Boston, MA: Little, Brown and Co.)

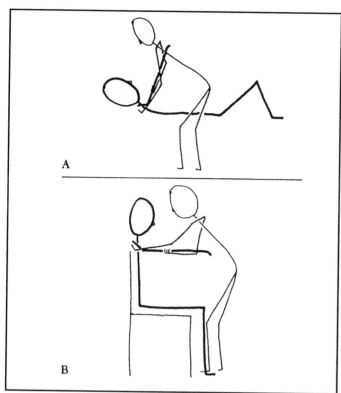

Figure 26-15. Scapula protraction and upward rotation. A. Supine. B. Sitting. With scapula placed in protracted position, the patient is asked to "hold," "reach arm forward," or "make arm longer"; quick stretch to scapula protractors then actively assisted through protraction (feel for catching reaction), giving resistance to protraction. (Reprinted with permission from Logigian, M. K. [1982]. *Adult rehabilitation: A team approach for therapists.* Boston, MA: Little, Brown and Co.)

hoped that he would regain normal movement of his left arm and hand.

In addition, PROM to the shoulder, elbow, and wrist as well as active motion of the fingers were continued daily by Mr. Callahan's son. The OTA taught Mr. Callahan how to put on the sling and position his arm and monitored the use of the sling. The assistant also provided joint mobilization through PROM, ultimately teaching Mr. Callahan how to do the exercises.

The OT program also addressed Mr. Callahan's ability with self-care activities. The OTA saw Mr. Callahan each morning for 30 minutes for bathing, grooming, and dressing/undressing. She suggested that Mr. Callahan use an electric razor for shaving and an electric toothbrush for cleaning his teeth. He completed these tasks while seated at the sink. The OTA reinforced that Mr. Callahan look to the right and left of his face while shaving, cleaning teeth, and brushing hair. Balancing safety and Mr. Callahan's wishes, it was agreed that he would use a straight razor when his son was able to help him shave.

He preferred a shower to a bed bath, so the OTA arranged for him to shower each morning while seated on a shower chair. He was instructed in one-handed methods for bathing and dressing.

A long-handled bath sponge and shoe horn were provided by the OTA to enable independence in bathing and LE dressing. Within 2 weeks, he was independent in bathing and UE dressing but required minimal assistance with LE dressing. A new short-term goal was established to address the issue with LE dressing. One week later, Mr. Callahan was independent in dressing and undressing, and the morning session with the OTA was discontinued.

During the first few days of treatment, the OTA stopped by at lunch time to demonstrate one-handed techniques for self-feeding. She also reinforced compensatory techniques for his left side visual neglect during feeding. By reminding him to turn his head to look at and feel the entire edge of the tray, Mr. Callahan quickly learned not to neglect items in his left visual field.

The OT made arrangements for Mr. Callahan to be loaned a wheelchair with hand controls on the right side, thus making it easier for him to manipulate it independently. Each afternoon, the OTA accompanied Mr. Callahan to the therapeutic kitchen. During the trip to the kitchen, Mr. Callahan was able to wheel the wheelchair independently. Initially, Mr. Callahan had to do all kitchen activities seated, but after 2 weeks he was able to stand using a quad cane for support. During this half-hour session, Mr. Callahan practiced simple kitchen activities incorporating one-handed techniques and adaptive equipment. He began with preparing a cup of tea, and by the end of 2 weeks he was able to complete a snack of cheese and crackers. He used a cutting board to secure the cheese and Fiskar scissors to cut open packaged goods. By the third week he was able to prepare pasta, yet needed to use a bottled sauce, opening it with the help of a jar opener. He was disappointed about this, as his specialty was marinara sauce. The OTA used counseling techniques to address his initial disappointments.

The OT saw Mr. Callahan daily for 30 minutes to provide a UE mobilization program that included facilitation techniques to encourage movement and sensory awareness of the left side. Mr. Callahan demonstrated a reduction of shoulder subluxation and improvement in scapular and humeral motion. As a result, it was decided that Mr. Callahan would discontinue using a sling when ambulating.

Although Mr. Callahan was making progress in his OT program and he and his wife were anxious for him to return home, he was extremely concerned about his ability to return to his weekends at his oceanside home. These concerns were shared with the OTA while working in the kitchen with Mr. Callahan. The OTA discussed this with the OT, and it was decided that a family team conference be held to develop a plan. At the conference, which was attended by Mr. Callahan and his family, as well as all team members, it was decided that the OTA would make a home visit to the vacation home with Mr. Callahan to determine accessibility. The social worker would investigate the option of having an aide go with Mr. Callahan to the vacation home each weekend. As Mr. Callahan was not able to drive a car due to his visual deficits, the aide would need to drive them to the ocean home.

The home visit was useful, as an exact layout of the kitchen and living area was determined that enabled suggestions to be made for several environmental changes to enable maximum mobility. The house had only one step into it and one step up from the kitchen to the living room. A railing was recommended for the entrance to the house and living room. The master bedroom and bath were near the living room and kitchen. Toilet rails and a shower chair were recommended for the bathroom. The kitchen was spacious and had adequate counters to allow Mr. Callahan to slide objects from the refrigerator to the stove. All of the adaptive equipment Mr. Callahan had been using was suggested for installation in the kitchen.

Following the home visit, the team and family decided that Mr. Callahan would be discharged by the end of his fourth week in the subacute program. Thus, during this final week, Mr. Callahan spent 1 hour each day in the kitchen practicing his one-handed techniques in final preparation for making his famous sauce. Two days prior to discharge, he invited the OTA, OT, and his wife to the OT kitchen for a pasta feast with his homemade sauce. He took great pride in preparing it independently.

Mr. Callahan was discharged home with his wife at the time anticipated by the team. He was able to arrange for an aide to accompany him to his vacation home on weekends and resumed his cooking activities on a regular basis. The OT note at discharge included a statement on the progress he made, as well as indicators for follow-up care. It was suggested that Mr. Callahan continue his UE mobilization program twice a week for 6 weeks as he was continuing to make gains in this area. A follow-up phone call 1 week after discharge found that Mr. Callahan was receiving a mobilization program at an outpatient ambulatory clinic near his suburban home.

CLINICAL PROBLEM SOLVING

- If Mr. Callahan had been younger, he would need to return to work to support his family. If this had been the case, what would you have done to assist him with this situation?
- A work site visit would be useful to make suggestions for modifications. One-handed techniques for office activities, such as a telephone holder and use of a computer for written communication, can make return to work easier. In addition, the OTA could suggest office modifications to enhance accessibility, such as removal of carpets and positioning of a desk and chair to allow ease of movement.
- Mr. Callahan had a great deal of difficulty accepting that his left arm was non-functional. What would have happened if he had refused to accomplish his ADL utilizing one-handed techniques and adaptive equipment? A family team conference could be useful to discuss the situation with all involved, making compromises about what activities Mr. Callahan would accomplish independently with devices and those for which the family agreed to provide assistance. For example, a clean, neat shave was important to Mr. Callahan and no matter how hard he tried he could not accomplish it to his satisfaction. Perhaps his son could shave him with the understanding that Mr. Callahan would bathe and dress himself.

LEARNING ACTIVITIES

1. Make a chart of functional problems that compares deficits of a left stroke and those of a right stroke.
2. Develop a pamphlet that describes energy conservation techniques.
3. Develop a list of activities that a retiree with a stroke might have interest. Consider cognitive problems by looking at Allen's Diagnosis Module.

REFERENCES

Abreu, B. C. (1995). The effect of environmental regulations on postural control after stroke, *American Journal of Occupational Therapy, 49*(6), 517-525.

Acquaviva, J. (1996). *OT practice guidelines for adults with stroke.* Bethesda, MD: American Occupational Therapy Association.

Angeleri, F., Angeleri, V. A., Foschi, N., Giaquinto, S., & Nolfe, G. (1993). The influence of depression, social activity and family stress on functional outcome after stroke. *Stroke, 24*(10), 1478-1483.

Bernspang, B., & Fissher, A. G. (1995). Differences between persons with right or left CVA on the assessment of motor and process skills. *Archives of Physical Medicine and Rehabilitation, 76*(12), 1144-1147.

Bohannon, R. W., & Andrews, A. W. (1990). Shoulder subluxation and pain in stroke patients. *American Journal of Occupational Therapy, 44*(6), 507-510.

Bourbonnais, D., & Vanden Noven, S. (1989). Weakness in patients with hemiparesis. *American Journal of Occupational Therapy, 43,* 313-319.

Brodie, J., Holm, M. B., & Tomlin, G. S. (1994). Cerebrovascular accident: Relationship of demographic, diagnostic and occupational therapy antecedents to rehabilitation outcomes. *American Journal of Occupational Therapy, 48,* 906-913.

Chang, L. H., & Hasselkus, B. R. (1998). Ots' expectations in rehabilitation following stroke: Sources of satisfaction and dissatisfaction. *American Journal of Occupational Therapy, 52*(8), 629-637.

Duncan, P. W. (1997). Synthesis of intervention trials to improve motor recovery following stroke. *Topics in Stroke Rehabilitation, 3*(4), 1-20.

Duncan, P., Studenski, S., Richards, L., Gollub, S., Lai, S. M., Reke, S., et al. (2003). Randomized clinical trial of therapeutic exercise in subacute stroke. *Stroke, 34,* 2173-2180.

Flinn, N. (1995). A task-oriented approach to the treatment of a client with hemiplegia. *American Journal of Occupational Therapy, 49,* 560-569.

Griffin, J. W. (1986). Hemiplegic shoulder pain. *Physical Therapy, 66,* 1884-1893.

Gresham, G. E., & Duncan, P. W. (Eds.). (1995). *Post-stroke rehabilitation. Clinical practice guideline 16.* Rockville, MD: U.S. Agency for Health Care Policy and Research.

Hajek, V. E., Gagnon, S., & Rudeman, J. E. (1997). Cognitive and functional assessments of stroke patients: an analysis of their relation. *Archives of Physical Medicine and Rehabilitation, 78*(12), 1331-1337.

EVIDENCE-BASED TREATMENT STRATEGIES

Treatment Strategies	Authors
Motor control	Bourbonnais & Vanden Noven, 1989; Duncan et al, 2003; Flinn, 1995; Logigian, Samuels, Falconer, & Zagar, 1983; Nakayama, Jorgenson, Raaschou, & Olsen, 1994; Taub et al., 1992
Functional performance	Abreu, 1995; Nakayama et al., 1994; Tooth et al., 2003; Trombley, 1995; Trombley & Wu, 1999
Hemiplegic shoulder	Bohannon & Andrews, 1990; Griffin, 1986; Van Dyck, 1999
Return to valued roles	Duncan, 1997; Vestling, Tufvesson, & Ivasson, 2003
Neurologic deficits	Bernspang & Fissher, 1995; Brodie et al., 1994; Hajek, Gagnon, & Rudeman, 1993; Osmon, Smet, Winegarden, & Gandhavadi, , 1992; Warren, 1993
Patient and family education	Angeleri, Angeleri, Foschi, Giaquinto, & Nolfe, 1993; Law, Baptiste, & Mills, 1995; Maeshima et al., 2003; Sabari, 1998

Keith, R. A., Granger, C. V., Hamilton, B. B., & Sherwin, F. S. (1987). The functional independence measure: a new tool for rehabilitation. *Advances in Clinical Rehabilitation, 1,* 6-18.

Kelly-Hayes, M., & Paige, C. (1995). Assessment and psychologic factors in stroke rehabilitation. *Neurology, 45*(Suppl. 1), S29-S32.

Law, M., Baptiste, S., & Mills, J. (1995). Client-centered practice: What does it mean and does it make a difference? *Canadian Journal of Occupational Therapy, 62*(5), 250-252.

Lawton, M. P. (1988). Scales to measure competence in everyday activities. *Psychopharmacology Bulletin, 24*(4), 609-614.

Logigian, M. K., Samuels, M. A., Falconer, J., & Zagar, R. (1983). Clinical exercise trial for stroke patients. *Archives of Physical Medicine and Rehabilitation, 64*(8), 364-367.

Maeshima, S., Ueyoshi, A., Osawa, A., Ishida, K., Kunimoto, K., Shimamoto, Y., et al. (2003). Mobility and muscle strength contralateral to hemiplegia from stroke: Benefit of self-training with family support. *American Journal of Physical Medicine and Rehabilitation, 82,* 456-462.

Mahoney, F. C., & Barthel, D. W. (1965). Functional evaluation: the Barthel index. *Maryland State Medical Journal, 14,* 61-65.

Nakayama, H., Jorgenson, H. S., Raaschou, H. O., & Olsen, T. (1994). Compensation in recovery of upper extremity function after stroke: The Copenhagen study. *Archives of Physical Medicine and Rehabilitation, 75,* 852-857.

Osmon, D. C., Smet, I. C., Winegarden, B., & Gandhavadi, B. (1992). Neurobehavioral cognitive status examination: Its use with unilateral stroke patients in a rehabilitation setting. *Archives of Physical Medicine and Rehabilitation, 73,* 414-418.

Poole, J. L. (1997). Rehabilitation: Occupational therapy for stroke. In K. M. A. Welch, L. R. Caplan, D. J. Reis, B. K. Seisjo, & B. Weir (Eds.), *Primer on cerebrovascular diseases* (pp. 744-747). San Diego: Academic Press.

Sabari, J. S. (1998). Occupational therapy after stroke: Are we providing the right services at the right time? *American Journal of Occupational Therapy, 52,* 299-302.

Taub, E., Miller, N. E., Cook, A., Flemming, E. W., Nepomuceno, W. C., Connell, C. S., et al. (1992). Technique to improve chronic motor deficit after stroke. *Archives of Physical Medicine and Rehabilitation, 74,* 347-354.

Tooth, L. R., Ottenbacher, K. J., Smith, P. M., Illig, S. B., Linn, R. T., Gonzales, V. A., et al. (2003). Effect of functional gain on satisfaction with medical rehabilitation after stroke. *American Journal of Physical Medicine and Rehabilitation, 82,* 692-699.

Trombley, C. A. (1995). Occupation: Purposefulness and meaningfulness as therapeutic mechanisms. *American Journal of Occupational Therapy, 49,* 960-972.

Trombly, C. A., Radomski, M. V., Tresel, C., & Burnet-Smith, S. E. (2002). Occupational therapy and achievement of self-identified goals by adults with acquired brain injury: Phase II. *American Journal of Occupational Therapy, 56*(5), 489-498.

Trombley, C. A., & Wu, C. Y. (1999). Effect of rehabilitation tasks on organization of movement after stroke. *American Journal of Occupational Therapy, 53,* 333-344.

Van Dyck, W. R. (1999). Integrating treatment of the hemiplegic shoulder with self-care. *OT Practice, 4*(1), 32-37.

Vestling, M., Tufvesson, B., & Ivasson, S (2003). Indicators for return to work after stroke and the importance of work for subjective well-being and life satisfaction. *Journal of Rehabilitation Medicine, 35*(3), 127-131.

Warren, M. (1993). A hierarchical model of evaluation and treatment of visual perceptual dysfunction in adult acquired brain injury: Part 2. *American Journal of Occupational Therapy, 47,* 55-66.

Rehabilitation Services
Occupational Therapy Evaluation

Evaluation type: Initial

Diagnosis
R MCA infarct

Orders/Precautions
OT Consult: Pt. W/ large R MCA stroke. Needs assist to mobilize.

SBP goal 150-180

PMH: HTN, PVD.

HPI: Pt. In USOH until 10/2/03 found by son w/ dysarthria, L
hemiparesis. Pt. To ED where CTA showed R ICA clot extending to M1
of ACA. Pt. w/ worsening gaze preference. Interventional radiology
w/ Merci retrieval after 6 passes for revascularization. (-) bubble study,
EF of 60%. 10/7/03 awaiting LENI's. Per MD on 10/8/03, less concern
for DVT as no clinical evidence at this time. Appropriate for OOB
activity. 10/9/03.

Social/Environmental:
Following information obtained from care coordination notes- Pt lives
Rochester NY (+) stairs to enter. Bedroom/bathroom on first floor.

Prior Functional Level
Per chart, pt was indep with ambulation, self care and driving.

Current Functional Level
Bed Mobility
Roll side to side: Maximum
Comments: Max assist to roll to L side
Supine to sit: Maximum
Comments: Max assist rolling to L side to come to
sitting. Pt participating in task. Once sitting, required mod assist to
maintain balance (prevent fall posteriorly and to L).
Sit to supine: max assist
Transfers
Sit to stand: Max assist of 1
Stand to sit: Max assist of 1

Real record 26-1A. Real record for a client with stroke.

Bed to chair: Max assist of 1, mod/max assist of 2 with transfer to L.
Self Care
Total
Comments: Max assist for dressing, grooming. Able to was face, max assist with bed bath. Able to feed self if tray prepared.

Physical Status
On Initial Eval 10/14/03

Observation: Pt sitting in bed with head rotated to L side.
R peripheral IV in place.

MS: Pt follows 3 step commands, mildly slurred speech.

Perception: Pt able to track w/ eyes beyond midline to L/R. Able to locate Objects and reach for them on L side of body.

Pain: +3 pain in L shoulder.

ROM: Grossly WFL's throughout extremities; however, developing Significant edema in L hand that limits motion.

Tone: Hypotonic LUE.

Sensation: Impaired light touch, pin prick LUE.

Strength: RUE moving spontaneously/ purposefully.
LUE 0/5, no movement spontaneously or on command.

Balance: Seated: fair (pt is unable to sit upright w/o assist of another person.

Activity Tolerance: Tol 5 min sitting edge of bed with c/o fatigue.

Patient/Family Education
Pt informed of purpose of OT evaluation; importance of increasing time OOB. Pt agreed to try and sit OOB for 30 min this AM.

Problem List
Impairments:
Potential loss of ROM
Decreased sitting and standing balance
Hypotonic LUE
No movement LUE

Real record 26-1B. Real record for a client with stroke.

Edema L hand
Pain L shoulder
Dependent for functional mobility, ADL's

Short Term Goals
    To be met by 10/28/03:
    1. Rolling with mod assist
    2. Supine to sit with mod assist
    3. Tol 30 + minutes OOB
    4. Transfer bed to chair mod assist
    5. Demonstrate ROM- LUE

Long Term Goals
    To be met over next 4 weeks:
    1. Indep bed mobility
    2. Indep sit to stand transfers
    3. Indep bed to chair
    4. Pt to achieve 2/5 strength LUE
    5. Indep ADL's

Treatment Plan
    In-house OT services 3-5x/wk, with re-evaluation in 1-2 weeks, to
    include: neurofacilitation techniques, bed mobility and transfer training,
    functional activity progression, pt instruction re: max safety with ADL's.

Discharge Plan/Recommendations
    Pt p/w multiple deficits detailed above; currently dependent for most
    ADL's, large decline from baseline. Plan is for inpatient rehab
    placement when medically ready. Will continue to follow as per above
    Plan while awaiting placement.

Modality/Equipment
    Issued arm sling; to be worn when standing.

Real record 26-1C. Real record for a client with stroke.

Key Concepts

- Etiology of Parkinson's disease (PD): All factors that may be involved in PD, including the nature and course of the disease.
- Signs and symptoms of PD: Common problems and deficits associated with PD.
- ADL: Skills identified as self-care, mobility, communication, and environmental hardware.
- IADL: Skills identified as home management, community living, health management, safety management, and environmental hardware.
- Proprioceptive neuromuscular facilitation (PNF): Therapeutic technique that helps initiate a proprioceptive response.
- Considerations for exercise and activity: Use of exercises and activities unique to the symptoms of persons who have PD.
- Home program: Exercises and activities to be completed at home, usually after discharge from OT treatment.

Essential Vocabulary

akinesia: An abnormal state of motor hypoactivity or muscular paralysis.
bradykinesia: General loss of spontaneous movement.
dopamine: A chemical messenger, deficient in the brains of patients who have PD.
dysarthria: Difficult and poorly articulated speech due to poor muscle control.
festination: A symptom characterized by small, quick forward steps.
micrographia: Abnormally small writing.
postural instability: Impaired balance and coordination, often causing patients to lean forward or backward and to fall easily.
progressive resistive exercises (PRE): A method of increasing the strength of a weak muscle by gradually increasing the resistance against which the muscle works.
proprioceptive neuromuscular facilitation (PNF): Therapeutic technique that helps initiate a proprioceptive response.
rigidity: A symptom of the disease in which muscles feel stiff and display resistance to movement even when another person tries to move the affected part of the body.
substantia nigra: Movement-control center in the brain where loss of dopamine-producing nerve cells triggers the symptoms of PD. Substantia nigra means "black substance," so called because the cells in the area are dark.
tremors: Shakiness or trembling, often in a hand, which in PD is usually most apparent when the affected part is at rest.

Clinical Summary

Etiology

- PD occurs when certain nerve cells, or neurons, in an area of the brain known as the substantia nigra die or become impaired. The cause of this cell death or impairment is not known. This disease is both chronic (i.e., it persists over time) and progressive (i.e., its symptoms grow worse over time). There are many theories about the cause of PD. Researchers have reported families with apparently inherited PD. Until recently, however, the prevailing theory held that one or more environmental factors caused the disease.

Prevalence

- PD affects 1 million Americans. PD affects about 50,000 Americans each year, with more than half a million Americans affected at one time. PD strikes men and women in almost equal numbers and it knows no social, economic, or geographic boundaries. PD does not affect everyone in the same way. The disease can progress quickly in some patients and is more insidious in others. The majority of individuals with PD are older than 60 years of age. However, PD occurring before the age of 40 years accounts for 4% to 12% of all individuals who have PD.

(continued)

A HOMEMAKER AND VOLUNTEER WITH PARKINSON'S DISEASE

Kathryn Melin Eberhardt, MAEd, COTA/L, ROH

Classic Signs

- Early symptoms of PD are subtle and occur gradually. Individuals may be tired or notice a general malaise. Some may feel a little shaky or have difficulty getting up from sitting. They may notice that they speak too softly or that their handwriting looks cramped or small. The individual may feel irritable or depressed for no apparent reason. Often family members are the first to notice changes. As the disease progresses, the shaking or tremors may begin to interfere with daily activities.

- Major symptoms of PD:
  - Tremors (generally nonintention tremors)
  - Rigidity
  - Bradykinesia
  - Postural Instability

- Other symptoms commonly seen with PD:
  - Depression
  - Emotional changes
  - Difficulty in swallowing or chewing
  - Speech changes
  - Urinary problems
  - Skin problems (most common in oily skin)
  - Sleep problems

Precautions

- One of the more dangerous symptoms of PD is the lack of postural stability. Ten to fifteen percent of individuals who have PD also exhibit hypotension, usually caused by the medication levodopa. The combination of poor postural stability and hypotension leads to a significant risk of falls.

- Approximately 30% of individuals who have PD will develop some degree of dementia. Often this may be caused by the PD medication. However, the dose at which the mind is clear often means that the level of mobility had been reduced to an unsatisfactory level.

- Vision is also affected in many individuals who have PD. Being able to rapidly move the eyes to a target, track a moving object, and perceive information of limited contrast may be affected.

INTRODUCTION

James Parkinson, a British physician, first described the disease in 1817 when he published a paper on what he called "the shaky palsy." In the early 1960s, researchers identified a fundamental brain defect that is a hallmark of the disease: the loss of brain cells that produce a chemical called dopamine, which helps direct muscle activity. The 4 primary symptoms are as follows:

1. Tremors of the arms, legs, jaw, and face.
2. Rigidity or stiffness of the limbs and trunk.
3. Bradykinesia or slowness of movement.
4. Postural instability or impaired balance and coordination.

PD occurs when dopaminergic neurons in the substantia nigra die or become impaired. Normally, these neurons produce a brain chemical known as dopamine. Dopamine is a chemical messenger responsible for transmitting signals between the substantia nigra and the next "relay station" of the brain, the corpus striatum, to produce smooth, purposeful muscle activity. Loss of dopamine causes the nerve cells of the striatum to fire out of control, leaving individuals unable to direct or control their movements in a normal manner. There are 400,000 nerve cells in the nigra. Symptoms of PD become apparent after approximately 240,000 nerve cells (60% of the total) die. In normal, unaffected individuals approximately 2,400 nigral cells die each year. Thus, if an unaffected individual lives 100 years, he or she will most likely develop PD (Lieberman, 2003). The cause of this cell death or impairment is not known. This disease is both chronic (i.e., it persists over time) and progressive (i.e., its symptoms grow worse over time). PD is a disease of late middle age, usually affecting people over the age of 50. The average age of onset is 60 years. However, PD occurring before the age of 40 years accounts for 4% to 12% of all individuals who have PD. Individuals who develop PD between the ages of 21 to 40 years are called young onset PD (YOPD). Individuals who develop PD before the age of 21 years are called juvenile parkinsonism (JP). JP is a mix of diseases, which is designated as Parkinsonism (or Parkinson syndrome) not PD (Sanchez-Ramos, 2003). There are many theories about the cause of PD. Researchers have reported families with apparently inherited PD. Until recently, however, the prevailing theory held that one or more environmental factors caused the disease. Severe Parkinson's-like symptoms have been described in people who took an illegal drug contaminated with the chemical MPTP (1-methyl-4-phenyl-1,2,3,6-tetrahydropyridine) and in people who suffered a particularly severe form of influenza during an epidemic in the early 1990s. Fifteen percent of individuals who have PD have a family history of one or more members of 1 or 2 generations who have PD. It is unknown if this results from a genetic factor, a shared environmental toxin, or both. In several of these families, a PD gene has been found (Lieberman, 1999; National Institute of Health, 1998).

In 2001, a study reported strong evidence that several genes may influence the development of PD. The researchers detected evidence for genetic linkage to 5 distinct regions on chromosomes 5, 6, 8, and 17. Chromosome 6 contains the Parkinson gene, which was previously thought to be involved in the rare early-onset form of Parkinson's. The new study suggests that the Parkin gene is important in early-onset Parkinson's, and the multiple genetic factors may be important in the development of late-onset Parkinson's. The cause of PD is unknown; however, it is thought to have both genetic and environmental factors. Past research has shown that environmental factors, such as exposure to pesticides, may contribute to development of Parkinson's in genetically susceptible individuals (National Institute of Neurological Disorders and Stroke, 2001; Pericak-Vance, 2001).

There is no way to predict or prevent PD at this point. However, researchers are now looking for biomarkers (a biochemical abnormality that all individuals with PD might share) that could be picked up by screening techniques. Positron emission tomography (PET) scanning may also lead to important information regarding PD. PET scans of the brain produce pictures of chemical changes as they occur in the living brain. Research scientists can study the brain's dopamine receptors to determine if the loss of dopamine activity follows or precedes degeneration of the neurons that make the chemical. This information could help scientists better understand the disease process and may potentially lead to improved treatment (National Institute of Neurological Disorders and Stroke, 2001).

SIGNS AND SYMPTOMS OF PARKINSON'S DISEASE

PD affects about 50,000 Americans each year, with more than half a million Americans affected at one time. PD strikes men and women in almost equal numbers and it knows no social, economic, or geographic boundaries. PD does not affect everyone in the same way. The disease can progress quickly in some individuals and is more insidious in others (National Institute of Neurological Disorders and Stroke, 2001).

PD has been characterized as having 3 common stages. In Stage 1, the disease is mild with signs of slowing and tremor. The duration of this stage is from onset to 4 years. In Stage 2, the disease is moderately severe. The duration of this stage is 5 to 10 years from onset. By Stage 3, the disease has exceeded 10 years from its onset and has become severely involved (Lazaruk, 1994). Tremors are one of the major symptoms of PD; however, many other symptoms are just as troublesome.

Major Symptoms of Parkinson's Disease

Tremor

The tremor typically takes the form of a rhythmic back-and-forth motion of the thumb and forefinger at 3 beats per second. This is sometimes called "pill-rolling." Tremors usually begin in the hands and are most obvious at rest, especially during the first stage; this may also be described as nonintention tremors. The tremors often disappear during sleep and improve with intentional movement (Miller & Keane, 1997).

Rigidity

In PD, rigidity is apparent in response to signals from the brain, and the delicate balance of opposing muscles is disturbed. The muscles remain constantly tensed and contracted so that the person aches and feels stiff and/or weak. The rigidity can be classified as ratchet-like, jerky movements called "cogwheel" rigidity, or no movement, called "lead-pipe" rigidity (Miller & Keane, 1997).

Bradykinesia

Bradykinesia is the slowing down of movements, which causes a slowness of initiating and executing movements. Fine motor deficits and difficulty in performing repetitive movements are common problems with this symptom (Miller & Keane, 1997).

Postural Instability

Impaired balance and coordination causes the individual with PD to develop a forward or backward lean and to fall easily. When balance is disturbed from the front or when starting to walk, the patient with a backward lean has a tendency to step backward, which is known as retropulsion. This deficit can cause stooped posture in which the head is bowed and the shoulders droop (Miller & Keane, 1997).

Festination

Festination is walking in rapid, short, shuffling steps. This symptom is also a leading cause of falls with persons who have PD (Miller & Keane, 1997).

Akinesia

Akinesia is the term given to impaired ability to initiate voluntary and spontaneous motor responses. It is characterized by the interruption of performance of an ongoing movement or "freezing" when attention is distracted (Miller & Keane, 1997).

Other Common Symptoms of Parkinson's Disease

Depression

This is a common problem and may appear early in the course of the disease, even before other symptoms are noticed. Depression may not be severe but may be intensified by the drugs used to treat other symptoms of PD (Borcherdt, 2003; Burn, 2002; Leentjens, 2003; Noh & Posthuma, 1990).

Dementia

Dementia refers to slow loss of memory and other intellectual abilities that interfere with an individual's ability to function. Thirty percent of individuals who have PD develop dementia. Most vulnerable are individuals over 70 years of age. The symptoms of PD are similar to the process responsible for the symptoms of dementia. Both sets of symptoms arise from the loss of nerve cells (Richard, 2002).

Difficulty Swallowing and Chewing

Muscles used in swallowing may work less efficiently in later stages of the disease. Food and saliva may collect in the mouth and back of the throat, which can result in choking or drooling (National Institute of Neurological Disorders and Stroke, 2001).

Speech Changes

Individuals who have PD may speak softly or in a monotone, hesitate before speaking, slur or repeat their words, or speak too fast (National Institute of Neurological Disorders and Stroke, 2001).

Urinary Problems and Constipation

Bladder and bowel problems can occur due to the improper functioning of the autonomic nervous system, which is responsible for regulating smooth muscle activity. The prevalence ranges from 38% to 71%. Some individuals may become incontinent while others have trouble urinating. Constipation may occur because the intestinal tract operates more slowly, because of inactivity, eating a poor diet and/or drinking too little fluids (Singer, 1998).

Skin Problems

It is common for the skin on the face to become very oily, particularly on the forehead and at the sides of the nose. The scalp may become oily also, resulting in dandruff. In other cases, the skin may become very dry. These problems are also the result of an improperly functioning autonomic nervous system. Excessive sweating, another common symptom, is usually controllable with medication used to treat PD (National Parkinson Foundation, 1999).

Anxiety

This is a prominent feature in 40% of individuals who have PD. Whether it is part of the disease or a reaction to the disease in unknown. The anxiety may or may not be associated with depression. In addition, many individuals have panic attacks (i.e., episodic outbursts of anxiety). The attacks are characterized by a variety of symptoms, including fear of dying, fear of going insane, breathlessness, sweating, chest pain, choking, and dizziness. Panic attack may simulate a heart attack, and occasionally, a panic attack must be distinguished from a heart attack. In many individuals, the panic attacks are situationally cued and are linked to sudden immobility (National Parkinson Foundation, 1999).

Sleep Disturbance

This may present as inability to sleep at night and daytime drowsiness. The sleep disturbance may be related to anxiety, depression, the anti-Parkinson drugs, the inability to turn in bed, or it may be unrelated to any of the above. The sleep centers are in the brainstem near the substantia nigra and may be altered in PD. It must be remembered that von Economo's encephalitis, which between 1918 and 1926 resulted in 6 million cases of parkinsonism, was called "sleeping sickness" because sleep disturbances were so prevalent (National Parkinson Foundation, 1999).

Other Secondary Symptoms

- Micrographia (i.e., small, cramped handwriting).
- Reduced arm swing.
- Slight foot drag.
- Freezing (i.e., the phenomenon of being "stuck in place" when attempting to initiate movement).
- Hypomimia (i.e., decreased facial expression due to rigidity of facial muscles).
- Decrease in automatic reflexes such as blinking and swallowing.

MEDICAL MANAGEMENT

PD is diagnosed if an individual has 2 or more major symptoms, one of which is bradykinesia or resting tremors. Resting tremors alone, or a combination of it and bradykinesia, is sufficient to diagnose PD. Generally, within 2 to 5 years, other PD symptoms appear and the diagnosis is confirmed.

At present, there is no cure for PD. However, a variety of medications and treatments are available to provide dramatic relief from the symptoms. Levodopa is the most commonly prescribed medication for relief of the symptoms of PD. Levodopa helps to replace the missing dopamine levels in the brain (National Institute of Neurological Disorders and Stroke, 2001; National Parkinson Foundation, 1999).

Rehabilitation management by a treatment team consisting of the physician as well as the occupational, physical, and speech therapy practitioners can do much to assist the individual who has PD to achieve his or her maximum occupational performance.

Individuals who are well maintained on medication (levodopa/carbidopa) may continue to be very functional for usually about 2 to 5 years. After that "Levodopa honeymoon," the individuals' level of motor function begins to fluctuate and is identified as the wearing off phenomenon. Individuals who have PD compare their "on-off" periods to a light switch. Therefore, it is critical to the individual and the practitioner to determine the on-off periods to maximize the individuals' abilities. Physicians may also ask the individual and his or her practitioner to keep a record of the on-off periods, often identified as a motor diary. This will enable the physician to optimize medication levels to stabilize motor fluctuations (Hutton, 2003).

SURGICAL MANAGEMENT

None of the surgical procedures offers a definitive cure for PD; most patients continue to require medications to manage symptoms postoperatively. Many of the operations are relatively new, and the indications and long-term results are not yet well defined. The surgical procedures currently used are as follows (National Institute of Neurological Disorders and Stroke, 2001):

- Pallidotomy: Surgical destruction of the globus pallidus, internal segment.
- Thalamotomy: Surgical destruction of a subdivision of the thalamus called "vim."
- Xenograft: Transplant cells taken from a different species (such as using a pig fetus for human brain cell transplantation).
- Allograft: Transplant cells taken from a different member of the same species (such as using a human fetus for a human brain cell transplantation).

FRAME OF REFERENCE

Rigidity and akinesia produce a stiff individual who is limited in active movement. PNF techniques such as chopping, lifting, and unilateral diagonal patterns may assist in improving trunk mobility, which will assist in overall functional movement. Since PNF techniques lend themselves to functional tasks, it allows the individual with PD to complete the performance skills necessary to be independent and at the same time assist with the difficult mobility problems that affect persons with PD. Rapid, rhythmical movements are most appropriate for remediation of the mobility deficits seen in this diagnosis. PNF patterns could be set to music to assist in fluency of movement and create more automatic and purposeful smooth movements. Rhythmic initiation is used to improve the ability to initiate movement. This technique involves passive rhythmic motion, followed by active motion. Once again, this technique is used during functional activities to assist in fluid movement and to allow for independence in various performance components (Newman, Echevarria, & Digman, 1995; Platz, Brown, & Marsden, 1998).

CASE STUDY

Elizabeth is a 65-year-old woman who has been admitted to a skilled nursing facility from the local hospital after being admitted for medication adjustment for the treatment of PD. Elizabeth is married with 2 grown children and 2 grandchildren. She is a full-time homemaker who volunteered at the local hospital gift shop 2 days a week. She was diagnosed with PD 5 years ago and was well managed up until the last 2 months, when her symptoms became much more intense and she was unable to function independently at home. She was admitted to the hospital to re-evaluate her medication and is now responding well to the new regimen but has suffered setbacks due to her immobility for the last several months. Elizabeth demonstrates a moderate resting tremor with consistent cogwheel rigidity. She requires moderate assistance for all self-care activities and mobility due to her fair standing balance with symptoms of akinesia. Elizabeth's active movement is limited due to her rigidity, and her coordination skills are fair due to her resting tremors. She expresses great concern regarding her personal self-care and has verbalized how depressed she feels now that her husband must assist her in her personal self-care skills. Her goal is to return home with her husband and to be able to take care of her own needs. Elizabeth lives in a raised ranch home with a 2-step entrance to the home. Her husband and children are very supportive and are willing to assist her as necessary. Her attending neurologist who prescribed evaluation and treatment as needed referred Elizabeth to OT.

Occupational Therapy Evaluation and Assessment

Evaluation

The evaluation process must focus on the performance deficits seen in the individual who has PD. The OT determines the performance deficits that the person exhibits and then chooses the evaluative procedure for each deficit. Commonly used evaluations include ROM, muscle tone, righting reactions and other automatic postural movements, speed and accuracy of voluntary movements, coordination, cognitive skills, and functional performance in daily living tasks. Other areas of concern may be addressed based on the individual and possible multiple diagnoses. The OT performs the evaluation/s and after demonstrating service competency, the OTA may assist in the assessment process. Various standardized assessments are available to determine performance deficits and the OT/OTA team together will decide which assessments are necessary and who will be performing them. State regulations may dictate the role of the OTA in the evaluation process. The OTA must be aware of the legislation that pertains to his or her practice and adhere to those standards (AOTA, 1995).

In Elizabeth's case, the evaluation began with an initial interview. During the initial interview, the OTA explained the role of OT to Elizabeth and began obtaining some information that was identified on the standard evaluation form for the facility. The OTA asked about the architecture of her home, emphasizing the stairs and kitchen and bathroom layout, as well as the characteristics of other rooms. The OTA inquired about what type of assistance she has at home for the performance areas of shopping, laundry, and heavy cleaning.

Other questions focused on her goals, knowledge of her disability, and awareness of her prognosis. After the initial screening, the OTA organized all of the data and reported it to the supervising OT. The OT then analyzed the screening data to determine the appropriate assessment to be completed and conferred with the OTA as to the delineation of the assessments. In this case, the OT identified the following areas of evaluation: ADL and IADL, sensorimotor components, and psychosocial components. Before conducting the evaluations, the OT discussed her concerns with the OTA and explained the other areas that she wanted the OTA to focus on, such as using her observational skills during the evaluation to further assess Elizabeth's functional motor skills. Because the OTA had demonstrated service competency, the OT felt comfortable delegating the following assessments: ADL and IADL skills, upper and lower extremity status, fine and gross motor coordination, and strength and endurance during the ADL/IADL assessment.

Occupational Therapy Assistant Assessment

The OTA began by having Elizabeth fill out a structured interview form that gathered additional data about her family history, self-care abilities, school and work history, and her leisure interests and experiences. The OTA performed the assessments in the following area:

- ADL
  - Grooming
  - Head/neck and oral hygiene
  - Dressing: upper and lower extremity
  - Functional mobility: transfer skills (bed, toilet, tub)
  - Functional communication skills: telephone and writing skills
  - Balance and endurance while sitting and standing related to ADL skills
- UE and LE Status
  - Observation of AROM/PROM in functional ADL activities
  - Testing of gross and fine motor coordination with standardized assessments
  - Observation of strength and endurance during functional activities

After completing her evaluation, the OTA summarized the data and reported the findings to the OT. Together they discussed the OTA findings and determined what additional assessment would be needed.

Occupational Therapist Assessment

The OT assessed Elizabeth's neuromuscular status, concentrating on AROM and PROM and the quality of movement to include tremors and rigidity (refer to initial evaluation report). The OT performed a manual muscle test and noted that Elizabeth was not experiencing any pain or discomfort. When all the assessments were completed, the OT analyzed the data collected, documented the findings, and made recommendations regarding the course of treatment. It was determined that Elizabeth was experiencing decreased AROM in the upper extremities, problems with gait, balance, and tremors, which led to her lack of independence in ADL skills. Both the OT and OTA found Elizabeth to be motivated toward OT treatment and willing to work on her deficits. These findings were shared with Elizabeth, priorities were set, and a treatment plan was developed based on the overall OT findings and Elizabeth's needs.

General Goals

Upon completion of the formal evaluation, the OT and the OTA will confer and develop a problem list. This list must include the goals of the patient and/or significant others and the identified occupational role to which the individual will be returning or adapting. In general, the goals for individuals who have PD are as follows (Ber, 1998; Newman et al., 1995):

- To increase mobility and prevent deformity.
- To improve initiation of movement and to increase the fluency of movement.
- To improve psychosocial status.
- To improve or maintain independent performance of daily life tasks.
- Improve ability to participate in leisure activities.
- Provide education and support to the patient and family.

In the case of Elizabeth, the OT and OTA began to develop long-term and short-term goals for a program of treatment to be carried out by the OTA. The main areas of concentration in treatment included the improvement of ADL skills, motor proficiency, improvement in general mobility and balance skills, investigate leisure opportunities, and education and adjustment to her disability. During this process, a discussion regarding Elizabeth's IADL skills should take place. These areas may not be applicable until Elizabeth has developed improved postural stability, increased mobility, and improved motor proficiency. However, Elizabeth's priority was to return to her former occupational role as a homemaker, so treatment activities should focus on these areas. In addition, goals regarding an ongoing home program should be addressed during the treatment planning process.

Treatment Precautions

One of the more dangerous symptoms of PD is the lack of postural stability. Ten to fifteen percent of individuals who have PD also exhibit hypotension, usually caused by the medication Levodopa. The combination of poor postural stability and hypotension leads to a significant risk of falls. This must be taken into account during all mobility activities (Ber, 1998; Clemson, Manor, & Fitzgerald, 2003; Cram, 2003; Kinn & Galloway, 2000).

Treatment Activities/Techniques

The OT treatment for the individual who has PD is often developed on a trial and error basis. Since PD is unique to each individual and the response to medications varies for each individual, the course of treatment is dependent on the deficits of each individual and a combination of techniques to remediate the performance deficits. The maintenance of normal muscle tone and function is an important aspect of the treatment of PD. In part, the medication for this disease achieves this goal. However, to realize the full benefit of the medication, daily exercises and activity are essential. The following are suggestions based on the frame of reference noted earlier and common techniques that have worked with many individuals who suffer from PD. Each individual may react differently to these suggestions (Ber, 1998; National Parkinson Foundation, 1999; Newman et al., 1995).

Increase Mobility and Prevent Deformities

Rigidity and akinesia put an individual with PD at great risk of developing contractures and becoming deconditioned. A daily self-ROM program that includes rhythmical exercises is recommended. This program should be continued upon discharge from OT services. Family and/or significant others should be instructed in the home program as well as in the techniques of passive stretch if the individual has difficulty with completing the ROM exercises independently. Verbal cues and written instructions may be necessary for improved follow through. PNF techniques, such as chopping, lifting, and unilateral diagonal patterns, may be beneficial for improving trunk mobility. These activities lend themselves to functional activi-

ties and should be incorporated in ADL and IADL tasks. Auditory commands, counting out loud, and music may be beneficial in improving the fluency of movement and assist with difficult mobility tasks, such as transfer training. Anticipatory activities such as balloon volleyball or catch are excellent activities that can improve strength as well as postural stability and general mobility (Ber, 1998; National Parkinson Foundation 1999, Newman et al., 1995). The Schenkman model suggests a progression of treatment within the treatment session and over time. The model is as follows: 1) relaxation, 2) breathing exercises, 3) passive muscle stretching and positioning,(4) AROM and postural alignment, 5) weight shifting, 6) balance response, 7) gait activities, and 8) home exercises (Christiansen & Baum, 1991; Harburn & Miller, 1990).

Activities of Daily Living

Akinesia presents great challenges for the individual who has PD to complete occupational performance tasks. Issues of postural instability greatly interfere with ADL and IADL success. The use of adaptive equipment such as long-handled shoehorns, reachers, sock aids, and a dressing stick are helpful to eliminate bending for individuals who have poor balance. Feeding devices such as built-up handles, weighted utensils and cups, scoop dishes, or plate guards may assist in independent feeding for individuals with tremors and decreased hand function. Zipper pulls, buttonhooks, and Velcro closures can assist in dressing tasks for individuals with poor coordination and/or tremors. Safety issues must be addressed when dealing with bathroom considerations. Due to the high incidence of falls among individuals with PD, bathroom safety equipment will be most essential. The use of a tub bench or seat, nonskid mats rather than throw rugs, toilet frames, and possibly a raised toilet seat are most helpful.

Individuals should be cautioned not to use towel bars, soap dishes, or sinks as mobility aids and should have grab bars professionally installed to assure the grab bars are anchored in the wall studs. The use of toilet frames and tub grab bars can be commercially obtained without having to install grab bars on the wall. Family and/or significant others should also be instructed in the use of adaptive devices and equipment to ensure safety with all ADL skills at home (Ber, 1998; National Parkinson Foundation, 1999; Newman et al., 1995).

Communication

Individuals who have PD often have problems with dysarthria. The symptoms are usually described as a monotone voice and low volume speech. This is often due to poor vital capacity and postural difficulties. The OT intervention used most often is to teach deep breathing and postural control exercises. Also, counting out loud during all exercises or reading out loud has been successful in increasing communication skills. Singing is another activity that incorporates the rhythmical component of treatment as well as improving overall volume of speech. Because of the indication of micrographia, handwriting exercises encouraging large letter formation are helpful; if the individual becomes fatigued or the letter formation becomes significantly smaller, the activity should be discontinued. Use of built-up pens, markers, or felt tip pens can assist with this deficit. Telephones with automatic dialing and large buttons may also assist communication for the individual with poor hand skills (Ber, 1998; National Parkinson Foundation, 1999; Newman et al., 1995).

Psychosocial Status

The individual who has PD faces several difficult issues regarding psychosocial skills. The absence of facial expressions, incidents of depression, impaired communication skills, and mobility deficits all contribute to social isolation. Lack of facial expressions and slowness of movement is often misunderstood for the individual not being interested in a conversation or being lazy. These misunderstandings can lead to continued social isolation, especially if the individual has severely impaired communication and mobility. Education of family and/or significant others is key to avoiding these misunderstandings. Support groups for both the individual who has PD and for his or her family are paramount in battling stereotypes and misinformation. The National Parkinson Foundation offers support groups, literature, a Web site, advice, and education regarding issues related to PD. The individual who has PD may also benefit from adult day treatment programs and group counseling. Providing an emotional outlet will assist the individual who has PD in successfully adjusting to his or her disability (Ber, 1998; National Parkinson Foundation, 1999; Newman et al., 1995).

Leisure Skills

The disease process of PD often makes it difficult for individuals to participate in leisure skills. Adaptive devices such as a cardholder, craft frames, and adaptive board games are available to assist individuals with limited mobility and hand function. Exercise groups offered by local Parkinson's Foundation support groups can become a new leisure opportunity. Local exercise activities such as swimming and walking clubs may also be helpful (Ber, 1998; National Parkinson Foundation, 1999).

Home Evaluation

A home evaluation is an extremely important component of the overall treatment program for an individual who has PD. The home evaluation is critical for safety because of the incidence of increased falls among individuals who have PD. Individuals who demonstrate impaired mobility often have a shuffling gait, which prevents them from picking up their feet upon ambulation. This impairment can lead to significant safety concerns if the individual has carpeting and/or rugs in his or her home. It is imperative that scatter or throw rugs be removed and any carpeting that is loose should be removed or tacked down. Doorway thresholds may also be a problem and should be removed or altered to be flush with the floor surface on each side of the threshold. As mentioned earlier in this chapter, the use of adaptive bathroom equipment is recommended for safety in the bathroom. A firm mattress, chair, and sofa are necessary to assist with transfers. This furniture may be adapted by using a solid surface under the cushions. Also, the height of the furniture may need to be increased by putting blocks under the legs of the furniture. This will also assist in safe and efficient transfer skills. In the kitchen the individual should consider the items used most often and place those items in easy to reach areas. Incorporating a pushcart or purchasing a walker basket will assist in homemaking activities (Ber, 1998; National Parkinson Foundation, 1999).

Home Program

PD is known to be a progressive disorder and as stated earlier every individual responds to treatment differently. For these reasons a home program is essential to the maintenance of function. The home program should be initiated while the individual is receiving therapy services. The individual and the family and/or significant others must understand the importance of remaining active. These activities should be practiced during the treatment session with the family and/or significant others present. Written materials and possibly audio or video tapes should be given to reinforce the home program. The home program should include exercises to maintain ROM, mobility, and postural stability. It may also contain suggestions for leisure skills, outside exercise activities, video list of appropriate exercise tapes, support group names and numbers, and any other information that would assist the individual to maintain his or her present status. The National Parkinson Foundation offers pamphlets regarding exercises and suggestions for several problems seen in PD (Ber, 1998; National Parkinson Foundation, 1999).

Treatment Implementation for Elizabeth

The following is a brief overview of Elizabeth's treatment program utilizing the theories and treatment techniques discussed in this chapter. The treatment plan was implemented by the OTA. Elizabeth was scheduled for the OT AM Dressing Program as well as 2 additional treatment times during the day. During the AM Dressing Program, the OTA focused on the use of a reacher, sock aid, and built-up handles for hygiene activities. Elizabeth was successful with the use of the equipment, and was also able to successfully manage her personal hygiene by utilizing a wash mitt and soap-on-a-rope. The OTA also had Elizabeth complete a shower in the OT mock apartment. She was able to utilize a tub bench, extended shower hose, soap on a rope, and a long-handled bath brush. Elizabeth's husband was also trained in the supervision of Elizabeth and the appropriate equipment to install in their home prior to Elizabeth's return home. During the morning and afternoon treatment sessions, Elizabeth participated in ROM exercises, coordination activities, mobility/balance activities, and group discussions with other residents. Elizabeth was taught to complete self-ROM exercises and was given directions to begin her home exercise program. PNF patterns of chopping and lifting were incorporated into homemaking activities, such as filling and emptying the dishwasher, putting away groceries, and light meal preparation. Work simplification and energy conservation techniques were also incorporated into the homemaking activities. Elizabeth was given several worksheets to practice handwriting skills starting with shapes, progressing to printing, and then to cursive skills. This activity was also added to Elizabeth's home program. Elizabeth participated in group exercise programs, which included several anticipatory activities, such as balloon volleyball, football fling, and catch. During these activities, Elizabeth was encouraged to count out loud and each treatment session began and ended with deep breathing exercises. Elizabeth was exhibiting difficulty in using a standard cup for drinking due to her tremors. The OTA suggested a weighted cup and practiced with Elizabeth, who found it very beneficial. Elizabeth also participated in a leisure skills discussion group in which she identified her leisure interests. During a treatment session, the OTA assisted Elizabeth in finding solutions to assist her in returning to her desired leisure skills. Elizabeth also discussed with the OTA her concerns regarding other individuals' reactions to her disability. The OTA suggested that a community outing might be helpful in practicing and anticipating how others would react to her. Elizabeth agreed and participated in a group outing. A follow-up discussion was helpful to Elizabeth and the other group members to discuss their feelings about issues related to architectural barriers, stereotypes of persons with disabilities, and other issues related to social interaction. A home visit was completed 2 weeks prior to Elizabeth's anticipated discharge date. The OT, OTA, PT, social worker, Elizabeth, Elizabeth's husband, and son were all participants in this visit. Elizabeth demonstrated her mobility skills by getting into and out of bed, a kitchen chair, the living room sofa, and the bathtub. Elizabeth's husband and son were directed in the type of supervision that was needed for Elizabeth, and the home program was discussed. Elizabeth also demonstrated her ability to prepare a light meal utilizing her utility cart and the skills learned in OT treatment. During this evaluation, it was noted that Elizabeth's sofa and bed were too soft, which made it difficult to be independent in mobility skills. Elizabeth's husband and son were given suggestions on how to remediate this problem. Architectural barriers were also discussed with Elizabeth and her family regarding the entranceway, discarding of the throw rugs, and removing the carpet runners. Upon returning to the skilled nursing facility, Elizabeth continued to refine her mobility skills, coordination activities, ADL training, and homemaking activities. Elizabeth also continued to work on her home program daily.

Discharge Planning

Because of the progressive nature of this diagnosis, it is imperative that individuals with PD continue a regimen of exercise and movement. Referrals to the Parkinson Foundation support groups, respite care, service agencies that provide attendant care and home management assistance, and local adult day care facilities are essential. In the case of Elizabeth, she began to attend support group meetings while in the skilled nursing facility and intends to continue going with her husband. Elizabeth's husband was given information regarding respite care and homemaker services. Both Elizabeth and her husband were instructed in the home exercise program and appear motivated to follow through with the activities. A written home program with diagrams and pictures was given to Elizabeth upon discharge as well as several pamphlets from the National Parkinson Foundation.

Clinical Problem Solving

Taking the case of Elizabeth, what accommodations or additions to her treatment plan would you include in the following situations:

- Elizabeth will be returning home alone, with minimal supervision from an elderly neighbor. What services could you recommend to assist Elizabeth? Where would you find these services? Who might you talk to first regarding these issues?
- Elizabeth's husband is working full time and is not available during the day to assist her. What community assistance is available during the day to assist Elizabeth and her husband?
- Elizabeth is a 40-year-old female who is working full time when she becomes unable to function without assistance. She has 2 teenagers and a husband who works full time. What services may be helpful to Elizabeth? What would be your focus of treatment? What is Elizabeth's occupational role and how would you assist her in returning to that role?
- What recommendations/suggestions would you give to Elizabeth and her family regarding the process of aging and how it affected this disease? What should they expect? What is normal?

Utilizing the OT evaluation of Elizabeth, complete the following:

- Write a problem list for Elizabeth.
- Write long- and short-term goals based on the problem list.
- Describe the treatment activities you would use with Elizabeth.
- List and prioritize all safety concerns.
- What would you identify as Elizabeth's major obstacle(s) for independence in ADL?
- How could you document psychosocial issues on the initial evaluation? What issues might be important considering the clinical problem-solving cases presented above?

Utilizing the OT daily progress reports regarding Elizabeth, complete the following:

- List all abbreviations and symbols and the correct term for each.
- Write a weekly summary of the patient's skills based on the daily progress notes.
- Convert these narrative notes into the SOAP format.

EVIDENCE-BASED TREATMENT STRATEGIES

Treatment Strategies	Authors
Active exercise to improve mobility	Bridgewater & Sharpe, 1996; Hurwitz, 1989; Majsak, Kaminski, Gentile, & Flanagan, 1998; Tse & Spaulding, 1998
Initiating movement	Gauthier, Dalziel, & Gauthier, 1987; Platz et al., 1998; Quintyn & Cross, 1986
Awareness of depression	Borcherdt, 2003; Burn, 2002; Leentjens, 2003; Noh & Posthuma, 1990
Environmental adaptations	Clemson, Roland, & Cumming, 1997; Sanford, Pynoos, Tejral, & Browne, 2002; Sevigny, 2000
ADL	Gaudet, 2002; Montgomery, Singh, & Fries, 1994; Murphy & Tickle-Degnen, 2001
Fall prevention	Clemson et al., 2003; Cram, 2003; Kinn & Galloway, 2000

LEARNING ACTIVITIES

1. Access the following Internet resources:

National Parkinson Foundation, Inc.
Education, announcements, links to related sites.
www.parkinson.org

National Family Caregivers Association
Extensive education and support services for family caregivers.
www.nfcacares.org

National Alliance for Caregiving
Advocacy and support organization. Parent site for the highly recommended Karen Henderson care giving seminars.
www.caregiving.org

The American Parkinson Disease Association, Inc.
Headquartered in New York, the organization focuses its energies on research, patient support, education and raising public awareness of the disease.
www.apdaparkinson.org

American Parkinson Disease Association
Young Parkinson's Information & Referral Center
2100 Pfingsten Road
Glenview , IL 60026
Toll-free: 800-223-9776

Web site for caregivers of people with Parkinson's disease
www.myparkinsons.org

2. Attend a meeting of a PD support group in your community. Identify local resources available to individuals who have PD.
3. Depending on the individual interest, what are additional functional activities that can be used to increase and/or maintain strength, endurance, and coordination skills?
4. Assess your own home for architectural barriers and make recommendations based on an individual who has PD.
5. Visit an adult day care center in your community. Assess the current program in regards to an individual who may have PD. What are the motor activities for this center? How are the clients stimulated cognitively? What leisure opportunities do they provide?
6. Investigate community programs that might benefit an individual who has PD. Look for exercise groups, walking clubs, swimming activities, and older adult programs.
7. Review video exercise programs for the elderly and choose several to recommend to individuals who have PD.

ACKNOWLEDGMENT

I would like to thank my OTA students for their never-ending source of inspiration to me; my grandfather, Ernest Melin, who lived with PD for more than 20 years and taught me the meaning of patience; and to my daughter Elizabeth, who inspires me daily!

REFERENCES

American Occupational Therapy Association. (1995). Guide for supervision of occupational therapy personnel. *American Journal of Occupational Therapy, 49*, 1027-1028.

Ber, P. (1998). Degenerative diseases of the central nervous system. In M. B. Early (Ed.), *Physical dysfunction skills for the occupational therapy assistant* (pp. 481-484). St. Louis, MO: Mosby.

Borcherdt, B. (2003). Shaking without being shaken: A rational emotive behavioral therapy (REBT) approach to managing and coping with Parkinson's disease. *Parkinson Report, Spring*, 16-17.

Bridgewater, K., & Sharpe, M. (1996). Aerobic exercise and early Parkinson's disease. *Journal of Neurological Rehabilitation, 10,* 223-241.

Burn, D. (2002). Beyond the iron mask: Towards better recognition and treatment of depression associated with Parkinson's disease. *Journal of Movement Disorders, 17,* 445.

Christiansen, C., & Baum, C. (1991). *Occupational therapy: Overcoming human performance deficits.* Thorofare, NJ: SLACK Incorporated.

Clemson, L., Manor, D., & Fitzgerald, M. H. (2003). Behavioral factors contributing to older adults falling in public places. *The Occupational Therapy Journal of Research, 23,* 107-117.

Clemson, L., Roland, M., & Cumming, R. G. (1997). Types of hazards in the homes of elderly people. *Occupational Therapy Journal of Research, 17,* 200-213.

Cram, D. (2003). Orthostatic hypotension in Parkinson's disease. *Parkinson Report, Spring,* 22-23.

Gaudet, P. (2002). Measuring the impact of Parkinson's disease: An occupational therapy perspective. *Canadian Journal of Occupational Therapy, 69,* 104-113.

Gauthier, L., Dalziel, S., & Gauthier, S. (1987). The benefits of group occupational therapy for patients with Parkinson's disease. *American Journal of Occupational Therapy, 41,* 360-365.

Harburn, K. L., & Miller, J. A. (1990). Parkinsonian mechanisms of rigidity and occupational therapy approaches. *Occupational Therapy Practice, 1,* 34-43.

Hutton, J. (2003). *Motor fluctuation: On, off and dyskinesias.* Miami, FL: National Parkinson Foundation.

Hurwitz, A. (1989). The benefit of a home exercise regimen for ambulatory Parkinson's disease patients. *Journal of Neuroscience Nursing, 21,* 180-184.

Kinn, S., & Galloway, L. (2000). Do occupational therapists and physiotherapists teach elderly people how to rise after a fall? *British Journal of Occupational Therapy, 63,* 254-259.

Lazaruk, L. (1994). Visuospatial impairment in persons with idiopathic Parkinson's disease: A literature review. *Physical and Occupational Therapy in Geriatrics, 12*(2), 37-38.

Leentjens, A. (2003). Higher incidence of depression preceding the onset of Parkinson's disease. *Journal of Movement Disorders, 18,* 414.

Lieberman, A. (1999). Curing Parkinson's disease in our lifetime: Part I. *The Parkinson Report, XX*(3), 3-4.

Lieberman, A. (2003). *Understanding proteins, understanding Parkinson disease.* Miami, FL: National Parkinson Foundation.

Majsak, M., Kaminski, T., Gentile, A., & Flanagan, J. (1998). The reaching movements of patient with Parkinson's disease under self-determined maximal speed and visually cued conditions. *Brain, 121,* 755-766.

Miller, B. F., & Keane, C. B. (1997). *Encyclopedia and dictionary of medicine, nursing, and allied health* (5th ed.). Philadelphia, PA: WB Saunders.

Montgomery, E., Singh, G., & Fries, J. (1994). Patient education and health promotion can be effective in Parkinson's disease: A randomized controlled trial. *American Journal of Medicine, 97,* 429-435.

Murphy, S., & Tickle-Degnen, L. (2001). The effectiveness of occupational therapy-related treatments for persons with Parkinson's disease: A meta-analytic review. *American Journal of Occupational Therapy, 55,* 385-392.

National Institute of Health. (1998). *NIH researchers find Parkinson's disease gene.* Bethesda, MD: Polymeropoulos.

National Institute of Neurological Disorders and Stroke. (2001). *Parkinson's disease: Hope through research.* Bethesda, MD: National Institute of Neurological Disorders and Stroke.

National Parkinson Foundation. (1999). *The Parkinson handbook.* Miami, FL: National Parkinson Foundation.

Newman, E. M., Echevarria, M. E., & Digman, G. (1995). Degenerative diseases. In L. W. Pedretti (Ed.), *Occupational therapy for physical dysfunction* (4th ed., pp. 745-747). Baltimore, MD: Williams and Wilkins.

Noh, S., & Posthuma, B. (1990). Physical disability and depression: A methodological consideration. *Canadian Journal of Occupational Therapy, 57,* 9-15.

Pericak-Vance, M. (2001). Complete genomic screen in Parkinson disease: Evidence for multiple genes. *Journal of the American Medical Association, 286,* 2239-2244.

Platz, T., Brown, R., & Marsden, C. (1998). Training improves the speed of aimed movement in Parkinson's disease. *Brain, 121,* 505-514.

Quintyn, M., & Cross, E. (1986). Factors affecting the ability to initiate movement in Parkinson's disease. *Physical & Occupational Therapy in Geriatrics, 4,* 51-60.

Richard, I. (2002). Parkinson's disease and dementia with lewy bodies: One disease or two? *Journal of Movement Disorders, 17,* 1161.

Sanchez-Ramos, J. (2003). *Parkinson disease at an early age.* Miami, FL: National Parkinson Foundation.

Sanford, J. A., Pynoos, J., Tejral, A., & Browne, A. (2002). Development of a comprehensive assessment for delivery of home modifications. *Journal of Physical and Occupational Therapy in Geriatrics, 20,* 43-55.

Sevigny, J. (2000). The value of OT in home safety: More than just an assessment. *Occupational Therapy Practice, 5,* 10-13.

Singer, C. (1998). Urinary dysfunction in Parkinson's disease. *Journal of Neuroscience, 5,* 78-86.

Tse, D. W., & Spaulding, S. J. (1998). Review of motor control and motor learning: Implications for occupational therapy with individuals with Parkinson's disease. *Physical & Occupational Therapy in Geriatrics, 15,* 19-38.

Eberhardt Rehabilitation
Occupational Therapy Department
Initial Evaluation

Name: *Elizabeth*	Room#:		Age: *65y/o*	Payment: *BC/BS, Medicare A*

Initial Evaluation/Status Report

Diagnosis: *Parkinson's disease*

Special Precautions: *Postural instability*

S: *(Social information, goals, complaints)*

Elizabeth is married with 2 grown children and 2 grandchildren. Elizabeth volunteers' 2x a week at the local hospital in the gift shop. She was dx with PD 5 years ago. Elizabeth is concerned regarding her personal self-care skills. She lives in a raised ranch home with a 2-step entrance to the home. Her family is very supportive.

Goals: *Elizabeth's goals are to return home and be able to take care of her personal needs. She would also like to resume her volunteer work.*

O: **EVALUATION RESULTS:**

I. Behavior/Cognitive Function	II. Perceptual Function	Formal Evaluation	Functional Carryover
Alert/Variable: *Alert*	Hemianopsia R L	*NA*	*NA*
Oriented: *X3*	Neglect R L	*NA*	*NA*
Attention Span: *Good*	Figure Ground	*Intact*	*Intact*
Carryover of Instructions: *Good*	Form Constancy	*Intact*	*Intact*
Emotional: *Exhibits lability in stressful situations.*	Position in Space	*Intact*	*Intact*
Exhibits symptoms of depression, especially with	Depth Perception	*Intact*	*Intact*
Issues regarding her self-care skills	Visual Body Scheme	*Intact*	*Intact*
	Spatial Relations	*Intact*	*Intact*

III.   **COMMUNICATION/COMPREHENSION:**

Verbal: *Impaired, exhibits mild dysarthria*   **Auditory**: *Intact*   **Writing Skills**: *Poor-exhibits micrographia*

Vision: Functional ☒ Impaired ☐   **Glasses**: *Yes* **Hearing:** Functional ☒ Impaired ☐   **Hearing Aid**: NA

IV.   **UE FUNCTION:**

Hand Dominance: Right ☒   Left ☐   **Grasp**: Right - *60#* Left – *45#*

Tone/Joint Changes: *Moderate Rigidity, worsens during medication "off" periods*

Other: *Moderate resting tremors in both UE's, Exhibits ↓AROM, especially in the shoulder movements.*

ROM/STRENGTH

Movement	PROM (R) UE	PROM (L) UE	Strength (R) UE	Strength (L) UE
Shoulder Flexion	*WFL*	*WFL*	*4/5*	*4/5*
Shoulder Abduction	*WFL*	*WFL*	*4/5*	*4/5*
Shoulder Extension	*WFL*	*WFL*	*4/5*	*4/5*
Internal Rotation	*WFL*	*WFL*	*4/5*	*4/5*
External Rotation	*WFL*	*WFL*	*4/5*	*4/5*
Elbow Flexion	*WFL*	*WFL*	*4/5*	*4/5*
Elbow Extension	*WFL*	*WFL*	*4/5*	*4/5*
Pronation	*WFL*	*WFL*	*4/5*	*4/5*
Supination	*WFL*	*WFL*	*4/5*	*4/5*
Wrist Flexion	*WFL*	*WFL*	*4/5*	*4/5*
Wrist Extension	*WFL*	*WFL*	*4/5*	*4/5*
Hand Flexion	*WFL*	*WFL*	*4/5*	*4/5*
Hand Extension	*WFL*	*WFL*	*4/5*	*4/5*

SENSATION/ COORDINATION

Skill	(R) UE	(L) UE
Sharp/dull	*Intact*	*Intact*
Proprioception	*Intact*	*Intact*
Steriognosis	*Intact*	*Intact*
GMC	*Fair*	*Fair*
FMC	*Poor*	*Poor*

V.   **MOBILITY SKILLS**

Mobility Skills	Level of Function	Comments (Cues, equipment, etc.)
Rolling Right	*Moderate Assist (3)*	*Verbal cues*
Rolling Left	*Moderate Assist (3)*	*Verbal cues*
Supine to Sit	*Moderate Assist (3)*	*Verbal and Physical cues 2° LE rigidity & postural instability*
Sit to Supine	*Moderate Assist (3)*	*Verbal and Physical cues 2° LE rigidity & postural instability*
Sit to Stand	*Moderate Assist (3)*	*Verbal and Physical cues 2° LE rigidity & postural instability*
Stand to Sit	*Moderate Assist (3)*	*Verbal and Physical cues 2° LE rigidity & postural instability*

Real record 27-1A. Real record for a client with Parkinson's disease.

VI.   TRANSFER SKILLS

Transfers Skills	Level of Function	Comments (Cues, equipment, etc.)
Bed	Moderate Assist (3)	LE rigidity & balance
Toilet/commode	Moderate Assist (3)	LE rigidity & balance
Tub	Total Assist (1)	LE rigidity & balance

VII.   WHEELCHAIR SKILLS

Mobility Skills	Level of Function	Comments (Cues, equipment, etc.)
Wheelchair	N/A	Ambulates with a rolling walker, but
Ambulation	Minimal Assist (4)	he does not like to use it and tries to ambulate by holding onto the furniture.

VIII.   BALANCE SKILLS

Balance Skills	Level of Function	Endurance Skills	Comments on Function
Sitting	Fair	Fair	↓trunk control, especially unsupported
Standing	Poor	Poor	Rigidity in the LE which ↑with activity

IX.   SELF-CARE SKILLS

Self-Care Skills	Level of Function	Comments (Cues, equipment, etc.)
Feeding	Modified Independent (6)	2°tremors
Oral hygiene	Moderate Assist (3)	Set-up & coordination
Facial/make-up	Moderate Assist (3)	Set-up & coordination
Shave- Electric/Straight	Moderate Assist (3)	Set-up, coordination & ↓postural stability
Hair–comb/style	Moderate Assist (3)	Set-up & coordination
UE Bathing	Moderate Assist (3)	Must sit at sink, ↓postural stability
UE Dressing	Moderate Assist (3)	↓postural stability & coordination
LE Bathing	Moderate Assist (3)	↓postural stability & coordination
LE Dressing	Moderate Assist (3)	↓postural stability & coordination
Sock/Stocking/TED Hose	Total Assist (1)	2°hypotension & ↓postural stability
Shoe/Slipper	Independent (7) - Total Assist (1)	Independent with slip-ons, Dependent with tie

A: Overall Skills
- **Overall Endurance**: Fair
- **Participation**:   Very motivated towards treatment

X. PROBLEM AREAS

P: Goals

Real record 27-1B. Real record for a client with Parkinson's disease.

OCCUPATIONAL THERAPY TREATMENT NOTES

DATE	NOTES	SIGNATURE
1/23 (AM)	Pt. seen bedside for AM ADLs. Pt. required moderate assist to complete UE dressing and bathing 2° ↓ postural security. Pt. also required moderate assist to don pants in a sitting position. Pt. exhibited poor standing balance when attempting to pull pants up over her hips. Pt. exhibited ↑ rigidity in both upper & lower extremities. Conferred with nursing re: the possibility of taking medication earlier to ↑ fluency of movement during AM activities. Pt. also exhibited ↓ FMC skills when performing facial & oral hygiene activities. Pt. appeared disappointed with overall skill level at this RX session--------	KME, COTA/L
1/24 (PM)	Pt. seen in clinic. Pt. demonstrated the ability to come to standing with moderate assist for ↓ postural security. Pt. was instructed in rhythmical/rocking techniques to ↑ her ability to come to standing. Pt. was able to return demonstrate the technique with a noticeable ↑ in her balance skills & ↓ in LE rigidity. Pt. was able to maintain a dynamic standing posture while performing an UE activity for ~3 minutes. Pt. also c/o feeling fatigued during PM RX session.-----------	KME, COTA/L
1/25 (PM)	Pt. seen in clinic for ↑ fluency of movement in (B) UEs. Pt. was able to complete a set of PNF/diagonal activities, utilizing both chopping & lifting patterning. Pt. exhibited ↑ rigidity initially, however improved upon repetition. Pt. also exhibited ↑ FMC skills following the patterning & was able to manipulate small items in the kitchen with ↑ ease. Pt. demonstrated an ↑ in dynamic balance as well, during home management activities, utilizing PNF patterning. Pt's affect during these activities appeared to be bright & responsive to her ↑ skill level. --	KME, COTA/L
1/26 (AM)	Pt. seen for AM ADLs following her medication by ~1 hour. Pt. exhibited a ↑ in her balance skills & ↓ in LE rigidity throughout all UE & LE ADLs. Pt. required Min. assist for UE dressing, primarily for fastening. Pt. continues to require Mod. Assist for LE dressing, 2° ↓ postural security. Pt. demonstrated an ↑ in dynamic balance over previous RX session, however, continues to require assistance when attempting multiple tasks in standing. Pt. required Min. assist for facial hygiene, 2° manipulation of small items, however, this has ↑ from last AM session. Pt. also appears more motivated towards her goals of independence in ADLs, stating "The medication really does make a difference". Will confer with OTR re: pt. status.-----------	KME, COTA/L

Real record 27-2. Real record for a client with Parkinson's disease.

Key Concepts

- Blindness: Refers to the eye's total inability to perceive light.
- Legal blindness: Legal, not functional, definition of vision problems developed to determine qualification for services.
- Low vision: A variety of conditions in which vision loss affects the ability to carry out daily activities.
- Vision rehabilitation: Refers to programs of training and adaptation to vision loss.
- Visual impairments: Any type of reduction in the ability to see.

Essential Vocabulary

accommodation: The eye's ability to shift focus between objects at close range and those at a distance.
cataracts: Refers to clouding of the lens of the eye and occurs naturally with aging.
center vision: The central part of what one sees when looking straight at an object.
continuous reading: Reading long, connected passages, such as a book or magazine.
diabetic retinopathy: A vision disorder associated with diabetes that can cause total loss of vision if not controlled.
eccentric viewing techniques: Using side vision or turning head to maximize remaining vision.
glaucoma: A disease causing loss of vision when fluid pressure within the eye damages the optic nerve.
macular degeneration: An incurable disorder of the eye affecting the ability to see objects in the center of the visual field.
ophthalmologist: A medical doctor specializing in the eye.
optometrist: A medical professional specializing in the correction of vision.
peripheral vision: Side vision, or seeing out of the corner of the eye.
presbyopia: Loss of ability to see details at close range due to aging.
scotoma: "Blind spots" that often occur as a result of disease or injury.
spot reading: Reading of a few words at a time, such as a sign or label.
visual acuity: The eye's ability to focus on details, at any range.
visual fields: Areas or angles of vision that can be seen without moving the head or eyes.

Clinical Summary

Etiology

- Aging: Declines in hearing and vision begin in midlife but become more pronounced with age and include decreased flexibility of the lens of the eye and clouding of the lens.
- Disease: Cataracts (most common, but treatable), macular degeneration, diabetic retinopathy, glaucoma, stroke may result in visual field deficits.
- Trauma: Includes hearing loss due to exposure to high noise levels; accidents that affect organs of vision or hearing, closed head injuries.

Signs and Symptoms

- Common types of vision deficits:
  - Decreased visual acuity
  - Central field impairments
  - Peripheral field impairments
  - Inability to see contrasting colors or tones, which has a greater impact on function than visual acuity
  - Sensitivity to glare
  - Light sensitivity, or photophobia
- Common types of hearing deficits:
  - Presbycusis, with loss of ability to hear higher pitched sounds first
  - Tinnitus, a high-pitched ringing or "whistling" sound in the ears
  - Decreased ability to hear speech sounds

(continued)

A Retired Librarian With Sensory Deficits

Paula W. Jamison, PhD, OTR

Prevalence

Ages 70 to 74:   12% of males with visual impairments, 15% of females
35% of males with hearing impairments, 22% of females

Ages 75 to 79:   17% of males with visual impairments, 18% of females
41% of males with hearing impairments, 27% of females

Ages 80 to 84:   25% of males with visual impairments, 23% of females
47% of males with hearing impairments, 36% of females

Age 85+   26% of males with visual impairments, 34% of females
58% of males with hearing impairments, 49% of females

Precautions:

- Social isolation.
- Depression.
- Diminished self-esteem.
- Decreased mobility and independence.
- Decreased participation in occupation (ADL, IADL, leisure and social activities).
- Potential for untreated disease due to "silent" onset of these conditions.

Adapted from Hoyer, W. L., & Roodin, P. A. (2003). *Adult development and aging* (5th ed., pp. 65-66). New York: McGraw Hill.

INTRODUCTION

Sensory Loss and Normal Aging

Vision loss related to aging is one of the most common disabling conditions affecting the elderly, ranking third after arthritis and heart disease (Warren, 1999). The National Eye Institute has predicted that by 2020, the number of Americans who are blind or visually impaired will double, as the Baby Boomer generation ages (2002). Vision loss often goes unmanaged, in part because it is often difficult to distinguish it from the gradual sensory loss that accompanies the normal aging process. Natural changes most noticeably affect what have been called the distance senses—vision and hearing. The ability to see and hear makes it possible to explore and survey the world from afar, to scan a crowd for a friend's face, or hear an oncoming car on a dark street. Even partial loss of these abilities can have a profound effect on a person's sense of independence, restricting mobility both at home and in the community. Gradual disturbances in sight and hearing can also affect interpersonal relationships; it may become impossible to recognize a familiar face or hear a conversation. These impairments can have a significant impact on the quality of function in the older adult, who may additionally be suffering from other chronic or acute conditions. The OT and OTA working with older people need to be particularly alert to problems posed by vision and hearing loss.

Beginning in midlife, many individuals begin to experience visual impairments and deficits in hearing. During natural aging, the eye's ability to receive and process visual input is affected as the lens becomes less clear and the photoreceptor cells in the retina—the actual visual sensory receptors—decline in number. The eye also loses its ability to accommodate, or adjust its focus, as it moves from objects at a distance to those close at hand, such as reading material. This age-related deterioration of close-up vision is called presbyopia and occurs in most people (Hoyer & Roodin, 2003). By the ages of 50 to 60, most individuals require corrective lenses, at least for reading, and people who have worn glasses or contact lenses for years may now require bifocals.

Night-time vision also becomes less reliable, as the eye no longer accommodates as well to dim light or glare. Even for otherwise healthy individuals, activities such as driving and reading may require special adjustment; older adults may prefer not to drive in low-lighted conditions, such as on rural roads at night, or they may find that there is too much glare to read a magazine with glossy pages. Moreover, because their reaction times have slowed, joints are stiffer, and balance has become impaired, many older adults find themselves at increased risk of falling. As a result, they may also experience increased fear and anxiety about venturing out into the community, leading to a sense of isolation. Formerly pleasurable leisure activities such as reading or television may no longer be as satisfying.

Vision Loss

Older adults undergoing normal changes in vision and hearing are usually able to adapt to these losses, and in many cases corrective lenses or hearing aids may drastically improve their quality of life. However, more severe vision loss is also common among older people. It has been estimated that 15% of people aged 65 and older, and at least 23% of those aged 75 and older, are visually impaired (Meyers, 2002; Stuen & Offner, 1999; Warren, 1999). While OT practitioners have not traditionally reported serving large numbers of individuals with vision problems, vision loss touches the lives of many middle-aged and older adults, either directly or through a friend or family member. Vision loss is a major contributor to decreased independence among older adults and increases the likelihood of falls or injury (Alliance for Aging Research, 1999; Burmedi, Becker, Heyl, Wahl, & Himmelsbach, 2002a). Additionally, vision loss has been correlated to depression and other mental health concerns (Burmedi et al., 2002b; Horowitz & Reinhardt, 2000).

Despite these large numbers, older persons with vision loss have been an underserved population. Many reasons contribute to this. First of all, for many people, vision deteriorates slowly, and changes in the ability to see are often difficult to pinpoint. One may have the perception that ability is still present. Because the eyes function together, and changes in one eye can often be compensated for by the other eye, people may become habituated to dimmer and fuzzier images on the television, for

example. In addition, since most individuals began to experience changes in vision as a result of normal aging, many people—including health care professionals—fail to distinguish between normal, age-related visual impairments and disease-related vision loss.

It has been estimated that older adults wait 5 to 7 years between the onset of vision problems and seeking rehabilitation (Warren, 1995). Delayed intervention means increasing possibilities for social isolation and such mental health issues as anxiety and depression as well as needless loss of dependence (Horowitz & Reinhardt, 2000). When vision loss is complicated by additional chronic medical problems, it is often overlooked or considered to be a factor that interferes with recovery or adaptation to new circumstances. Finally, while a variety of techniques and assistive technology devices are available to assist older adults in maintaining as independent a life as possible, the general public is largely unaware of available options.

How Vision Problems are Defined

Specialists describe and measure vision in a number of different ways. Standardized terms have come into use to help everyone understand the varying degrees of vision loss. This type of uniform terminology is useful in helping professionals and lay people alike to understand levels of function and dysfunction as well as to understand the standards applied that determine eligibility for services. For example, visual impairment refers to decreased visual ability as it impacts on daily activities and applies to a range of impairments, from total blindness at one extreme to partial vision at the other (Freeman, 2002). Table 28-1 lists the common classifications of degrees of vision loss, along with accompanying problems with activities.

Low vision is a term used when an individual retains some amount of usable vision but is unable to carry out desired tasks because of impaired visual functioning. It is a broad term that refers to a wide range of disability. Older adults with low vision may be experiencing loss of function related to aging or chronic conditions as well. However, even with the additional limitations in function resulting from low vision, older adults with visual deficits continue to reside in their own homes and to live alone.

One measurable quality of vision is acuity, or the eye's ability to see details with clarity. Acuity is measured with a Snellen chart, the familiar eye chart that contains rows of letters or figures of decreasing size. Results are given in the form of a fraction. For example, an individual with 20/40 vision is able to see at a distance of 20 feet what a normal individual could see at 40 feet (Scheiman, 2002). Low vision is defined as visual acuity of 20/70 in the better eye with the best possible correction. In addition, specialists also refer to the visual field, a term that refers to the area that the eye is able to see while remaining focused. People with low vision may also have a reduced visual field. Low vision may occur throughout the lifespan and does not necessary lead to total vision loss, or blindness (Scheiman, 2002).

The individual with low vision still has some usable sight; however, he or she may require training in compensatory strategies or the use of adaptive equipment to function independent-

Table 28-1

Visual Impairment in Terms of Visual Acuity

	(Snellen Chart)
Normal Vision	
Range of normal vision	20/12
- normal reading distance	20/20
- normal reading performance	20/25
Near normal vision	20/30 to 20/60
- normal reading using shorter reading distance	
Low Vision	
Moderate low vision	20/80 to 20/160
- near normal performance using magnifiers, other aids	
Severe low vision	20/200 to 20/400
- slower than normal, with aids; "legal blindness" in the United States	
Profound low vision	20/500 to 20/1000
- limited reading with aids	
- problems with orientation and mobility	
Near Blindness	
Near blindness	20/1250 to 20/2500
- vision unreliable	
Total blindness	No light perception (NLP)
- no vision	

Adapted from Colenbrander, A., & Fletcher, D. C. (1995). Basic concepts and terms for low vision rehabilitation. *American Journal of Occupational Therapy, 49*, 865-869.

ly. Some forms of low vision, such as macular degeneration, may affect the individual's central or center vision (i.e., the ability to see objects straight on) (Mogk & Mogk, 1999). Other forms may affect peripheral or side vision. In addition to reduced visual acuity, low vision may cause problems with discerning contrasting images, impaired depth perception, difficulties with color vision, or the development of blind spots (i.e., scotomas) and field cuts that limit the angle of vision (Hellerstein, 2002). Other forms of low vision may be the result of cataracts or scarring of the cornea or retina, and cause overall blurred or distorted vision. However, the individual still has some ability to perceive light and may, depending on the services available, other contributing illnesses, and family and social support, be able to successfully adapt to this major loss (Kleinschmidt, 1999). While low vision can affect people of any age, the older adult faces special challenges and conditions.

It is important not to confuse low vision with legal blindness, another phrase often used to describe persons with visual impairments. "Legal blindness" is used by the federal government to determine eligibility for government and agency services and benefits. A person who is legally blind has at best a corrected vision of 20/200 in the better eye or a visual field of 20 degrees or less (Mogk & Mogk, 1999). Often, individuals who experience low vision are not classified as legally blind. Until 1999, when Medicare guidelines were changed to include low vision as a physical impairment appropriate for rehabilitation, many individuals with vision loss did not meet the criteria of

legal blindness and found it difficult to receive services (Warren, 1999).

THE FUNCTIONAL IMPACT OF LOW VISION

If normal vision loss requires management and adaptation on the part of the individual, low vision poses additional problems that require skilled intervention. At any age, vision loss can occur because of congenital, hereditary, or acquired medical conditions. Disabling conditions associated with aging, such as diabetes or stroke, contribute greatly to the incidence of low vision among the aging population. For example, each year thousands of adults become visually impaired as the result of strokes. It has been estimated that approximately 90% of persons who have suffered some type of neurological damage, either through stroke or injury, experience visual impairments (Hellerstein, 2002). Visual impairments often persist long after motor and cognitive function have been recovered and can continue to have a major impact on function (Meyers, 2002).

Since older adults have enjoyed normal or correctable vision throughout their lives, the changes they now experience may be a source of anxiety and frustration. Applying makeup or picking out matching socks becomes difficult, and finding lost objects, such as a dropped coin or bottle cap, no longer seems worth the bother. Previously enjoyable activities such as playing cards, visiting with friends, reading, or sewing become next to impossible. Friends and loved ones may respond with anger or concern because the person with low vision appears to ignore them by failing to greet them. It may become difficult to walk safely in low-lighted areas, such as restaurants, or to see the edge of a chair when the carpet beneath it is of similar color. It becomes increasingly challenging to see low-lying tables and scatter rugs, and while it is still possible to move through familiar surroundings, venturing into the street or a shopping mall becomes difficult and anxiety provoking.

With some conditions, the individual's ability to see may vary widely from day to day. On a good day, he or she may be able to read without difficulty or recognize a friend's face. The following day, these activities may be difficult or impossible, leading to acute feelings of frustration and problematic social interactions. Family and friends may find the older person's behaviors puzzling, and their reactions may further aggravate feelings of isolation or anger.

COMMON CAUSES OF LOW VISION IN THE ELDERLY

The most common causes of low vision in the elderly are cataracts, age-related macular degeneration (ARMD), diabetic retinopathy, and glaucoma. Strokes and injuries to the brain may also result in damage to vision.

Cataracts are the result of a continued clouding of the lens that may eventually make it impossible to see at all. Cataracts grow slowly and in most cases may be surgically removed and the lens replaced. Surgical techniques using lasers have made cataract removal a relatively simple and common procedure. Once the most common cause of blindness in the elderly, cataracts are now medically manageable for most people.

ARMD is an extremely widespread but as yet little understood degenerative condition causing scarring in the area in the center of the retina of the eye known as the macula. The result is the progressive loss of central vision. There is no cure, and vision losses of this type cannot be corrected. Individuals with ARMD experience problems with reading small print or seeing details, such as facial features, and find that their center vision becomes increasingly blurred. They may have trouble distinguishing between similar colors. Glare may pose a problem, due to the eye's inability to adjust to higher light levels, and night vision deteriorates. In addition, about 10% to 40% of individuals diagnosed with ARMD complain of what has been called "phantom vision" in which they see objects such as patterns of flowers that they know are not actually there (Mogk & Mogk, 1999). In cases of ARMD, however, the individual retains use of peripheral vision and thus is able to detect objects on the edge of the visual field.

Although ARMD is extremely distressing to the people who suffer from it, it does not lead to total loss of vision. Indeed, many times people with ARMD can learn to use eccentric viewing techniques, in which they use their peripheral vision to compensate for lost center vision. However, if the individual does not learn how to adapt, the results are limitations in the ability to perform ADL and work and leisure activities, which in turn have an impact on the individual's sense of independence and relationships with others.

Despite the fact that ARMD is the most widespread cause of low vision in the elderly, it is relatively little known. The reason for this lies in part with the gradual and painless onset of the condition. ARMD usually begins in one eye, and most people do not notice any troubling symptoms for a long time. Not only does the unaffected eye compensate for the loss, it is easy to make simple adaptations without noticing them (e.g., by turning on an extra lamp because light levels no longer seem sufficient). Thus, an individual who has not had regular eye checkups may not notice any changes in vision until the condition has progressed significantly. Sadly, one of the contributing factors to recognizing ARMD, as with other types of low vision, is hearing loss. People who have spontaneously used auditory cues, such as listening for a friend's voice, and lose this aid as their hearing deteriorates, may suddenly be confronted with the realization that they may have to learn to rely on other ways of interacting with friends and loved ones.

Diabetic retinopathy is a condition caused by diabetes, a disease that if left untreated has a profound effect on the body's circulatory system. The tissues of the retina become swollen and abnormal blood vessels develop, which can bleed, constrict, or lead to a detached retina. If detected in its early stages and the underlying diabetes is controlled, laser surgery may be successful in repairing the damaged tissue.

Unlike ARMD, which affects only the center, or macula, of the retina, diabetic retinopathy can affect the entire retinal surface. Vision losses associated with diabetic retinopathy may disrupt both center and peripheral vision. If the underlying diabetes is not managed, diabetic retinopathy can lead to blindness. Vision may also fluctuate according to blood sugar levels, if medication and diet have not been properly adjusted. In addition to blurred center vision, individuals with diabetic retinopathy may have difficulty in shifting focus from near to distance vision and may experience a decrease in their color vision.

Glaucoma has been termed the most feared disease of vision. At the same time it is the most preventable. Glaucoma is characterized by an increase in the pressure of the internal fluid of the eye, which can then damage the optic nerve, resulting in blindness. In the acute stage it may be painful as a result of the increased intraocular pressure; however, the chronic state is usually painless. Regular eye examinations using a pressure test can provide early detection, and medication in the form of eye drops is successful in keeping the intraocular pressure under control. Individuals who have required frequent prescription changes to correct their vision, who complain of seeing halos around lights or mild headaches, or who find that their eyes have problems adapting to darkness may be experiencing symptoms of glaucoma and should be seen by an eye care professional immediately.

Vision loss due to neurological damage from strokes and head trauma can cause a wide range of impairments. Most common among these are diplopia, or double vision, and visual field cuts, such as homonymous hemianopsia, in which the temporal and nasal aspect of each visual field no longer appears to the individual. In addition, other visual impairments may be the result of brain lesions affecting the oculomotor nerves; as a result, for example, it may become difficult or impossible for a person to read because the ability to visually track, or follow a written line with the eyes without moving the head, has been lost.

OCCUPATIONAL THERAPY INTERVENTIONS

Service-Delivery Models

Older adults with vision problems can benefit from the skills provided by an OT and OTA. Traditionally, services for individuals with visual impairments are provided through the blind rehabilitation model. This includes government and community agencies established to help the blind or those with severe visual impairments. It was for this purpose that the term *legally blind* was adopted. Individuals whose impairments meet the specifications are eligible to receive training in such areas as orientation and mobility, which focuses on techniques and the use of equipment such as the familiar white cane or aids such as guide animals to determine position and move in familiar and unfamiliar environments. Training is also offered in communication skills, including but not limited to teaching the use of Braille, a tactile system based on a grouping of 6 raised dots arranged in various ways to represent letters, numbers, and abbreviations. The overall goal of such programs has traditionally centered on providing the severely visually impaired with vocational skills and enough education to be self-supporting, independently functioning members of the community.

Programs devoted specifically to blind rehabilitation are found throughout the world. They include specialists who provide comprehensive rehabilitation and training and play a key role in helping countless numbers of individuals with severe visual impairments to live independently in a sighted world. In addition, service clubs and special organizations, such as the Lions Club and Lighthouse for the Blind, have dedicated their efforts toward fundraising and community-based activities to provide services for those who qualify.

The traditional blind rehabilitation model for service delivery has been of less immediate help to many of the elderly suffering from low vision (Orr & Huebner, 2001). There are a number of reasons for this. First of all, in order to qualify for services, one has to be identified as legally blind. Many elderly people who are experiencing gradual deterioration of their sight have severe functional limitations even though they do not qualify. Second, since the focus of blind rehabilitation services has been to prepare people for vocational and educational performance, older individuals who may be retired, already disabled due to other conditions, or who are preparing to leave the workforce are at a lower priority for services. Third, specialized blind rehabilitation programs are centralized. At present, there are only 7 visual rehabilitation training centers and 19 orientation and mobility programs in the United States (Orr & Huebner, 2001). Many people living in small towns or rural areas find it impossible to travel the distances needed to participate in these programs.

Vision specialists in the health care field include ophthalmologists, who are physicians who treat diseases of the eye, and optometrists, who usually specialize in correcting vision with glasses and lenses. Until recently, these professionals primarily focused on treating correctable vision problems. Lately, increasing numbers of optometrists, in particular, have begun to turn their attention to providing assistance to individuals with low vision (Mogk & Mogk, 1999). They provide an important resource in communities without specifically defined vision rehabilitation programs. Increased help for elderly adults with low vision became available in 1999, when the Medicare guidelines changed to include visual impairment as a category eligible for rehabilitation services.

Services specially targeted at helping people with low vision are available from OTs and OTAs working in the medical model and now, increasingly, in community-based practice. As a result, OTs and OTA have the opportunity to become more active in servicing clients with low vision. Their contributions are particularly valuable in teaching techniques for increasing functional performance of ADL, such as grooming, dressing, feeding, home and money management, leisure activities, and community mobility.

OTs and OTA who wish to devise and deliver a full spectrum of services to the person with low vision, particularly to teach reading and orientation skills, require specific training (Riddering, 1999). However, the skills that OTs and OTAs have in clinical observation, combined with their abilities to grade and adapt activities, make them uniquely suited to helping individuals adapt to vision and other sensory losses. As a general rule, OTs and OTAs working with older people should be especially aware of the potential for sensory problems in the aging population, even if these problems have not been formally diagnosed.

Frames of Reference

Professionals in the field of low vision specialize in vision rehabilitation. Like any other type of rehabilitation, vision rehabilitation focuses on developing an individualized strategy to teach the individual ways to compensate for his or her impairment (Freeman, 2002). Vision rehabilitation can be a key component of the services provided to a person suffering from other chronic conditions, such as arthritis, heart or pulmonary disease, or diabetes. As in other forms of rehabilitation, the individual's needs and personal desires must be evaluated prior to treatment by means of a thorough assessment of his or her current abilities along with problems with functional skills. Particularly when low vision is suspected, a home-site evaluation, ideally followed by training in the home, is crucial to understand and then make it possible for the patient to learn key strategies for adapting to the specific characteristics of the home environment.

Once the assessment has been completed, vision rehabilitation focuses on training individuals with low vision to use their remaining vision. The emphasis may be on ADL, mobility, leisure, or vocational interests. Vision rehabilitation can also include adapting the patient's home environment, either through the use of lighting, the removal of clutter, or providing

---

Table 28-2

Principles of Low Vision Management of Older Adults

- Distinguish the effects of normal aging from the effects of disease.
- View the older individual as a whole person.
- Use teamwork; employ a multidisciplinary team approach.
- Develop interventions that focus on the person's goals.
- Improve quality of life by facilitating independence and meaningful activity.

Adapted from Watson, G. R. (1996). Older adults with low vision. In A. L. Corn & A. J. Koenig (Eds.), *Foundations of low vision: Clinical and functional perspectives* (pp. 363-394). New York: American Foundation for the Blind.

---

high color contrast between furniture and carpeting to permit higher visibility. Vision rehabilitation may also include helping the client select appropriate household appliances, such as talking thermometers, or special adaptive equipment such as professionally fitted magnifiers or high powered lenses for reading, and then offering training in their use (Freeman, 2002).

The illnesses and dysfunctions associated with aging are often accompanied by other losses. People who are struggling with changes in their accustomed mobility, familiar leisure activities, work roles that may have to be abandoned, or the companionship of friends due to an inability to drive are responding to both physical and psychological stressors. Depression in particular is a risk (Burmedi et al., 2002b). When an ongoing rehabilitation program focuses on the needs of the whole person, the regular one-on-one contact provided during OT allows OTs and OTAs opportunities to monitor crucial shifts in the patient's emotional state as well as changing physical abilities. In some communities, counseling and support groups especially designed to meet the needs of people with low vision are available. In addition to providing important local resources and encouragement to help people cope with the frustrations of learning new ways of carrying out familiar tasks, these groups offer emotional support and may help counteract the feeling of isolation so often experienced.

Other frames of reference that are particularly useful to the OTA who is treating an individual with low vision focus on the importance of occupation and its role in helping individuals adjust to the major life changes brought about by any physical, cognitive, or emotional dysfunction. The Model of Human Occupation stresses the creation of an environment in which it possible for the client to regain feelings of competence and mastery. This model offers OTs and OTAs alike a way of organizing and grading meaningful activities, all the while keeping the patient's goals in mind. The professional also serves as a problem-solver and offers counseling, as client and professional cooperate to find the most workable solutions to problems in carrying out accustomed roles and activities. Likewise, although it has a slightly different emphasis, the Occupational Adaptation frame of reference looks at the client's interactions with his or her environment. Here the focus is on the client's adaptive responses. Occupational therapy evaluation and treat-

ment are aimed at fostering the achievement of a sense of mastery over these environmental challenges. In short, all of these frames of reference provide a way in which the client's unique personality, life history, strengths, and weaknesses can be taken into account in order to create a personalized plan of client-centered treatment. Overall goals focus on ensuring the safe performance of daily activities, including mobility, and either increasing or maintaining the ability to perform ADL, leisure, and vocational tasks (Table 28-2).

TREATMENT PRINCIPLES

Wide ranges of adaptations have been devised to assist persons with low vision (for the following and other examples, see especially Duffy, 2002; Duffy, Huebner, & Wormsley, 2002; Freeman, 2002; Mogk & Mogk, 1999; Riddering, 1999; Warren, 1999). Some of the general principles that are useful for individuals with little or no vision can be useful to people with low vision. For example, since people with low vision rely more on memory than fully sighted individuals, it is important to make the environment as predictable and uncluttered as possible. Organizing shelves with toiletries or medications in a logical way and always returning items to the same place makes self-care activities manageable. Keeping pathways clear inside the house decreases the risk of falling. For people with severely impaired vision, such mobility techniques as memorizing the number of steps into the house or the bus stops between home and one's destination can be useful. In addition, being able to locate landmarks using other senses, such as the smell of a bakery, may make it possible to move independently in the community.

Other principles of adapting to low vision focus on utilizing the patient's remaining vision to the maximum possible. Light levels must either be raised or adjusted to provide sufficient brightness but avoid glare. High contrasting colors can be used to make it possible to distinguish between the edge of a table, for example, and the floor beneath it. Printed materials can be magnified into a larger format, or optical magnifiers can be used. Adaptations that permit the user to employ tactile cues, such as folding money into different sizes according to denomination, are also useful (Table 28-3).

Table 28-3

Resources for the Person With Low Vision

National Organizations

The following is a partial list of organizations serving individuals with low vision. Many national organizations also have local chapters.

American Foundation for the Blind
1-800-232-5463
www.afb.org

The Lighthouse International Information and Resource Caller Service
1-800-829-0500
www.lighthouse.org

Foundation Fighting Blindness
1-888-394-3937
www.blindness.org

Macular Degeneration International
1-800-683-5555
www.maculardegeneration.org

National Association for the Visually Handicapped
1-800-677-9965

U.S. Department of Veteran Affairs, Blind Rehab Services
1-800-827-1000 (also, contact the local VA hospital and ask for a Blind Liaison)

Association for Macular Diseases
1-212-605-3719
www.macula.org

Glaucoma Foundation
www.glaucoma-foundation.org

Prevent Blindness America/National Society to Prevent Blindness
1-800-331-2020

United States Association of Blind Athletes
1-719-630-0422
www.usaba.org

Reading Materials, Audiotapes, etc.

Library of Congress Talking Book Program. Free audiotapes of books, magazines, descriptive videos, and large print books. Contact local library or 1-800-424-8567

Choice Magazine Listening. Selected readings, free if person is registered with the Library of Congress.
1-516-883-8280

The Bibles Alliance. Free Bible on audiocassette. Several languages are available.
1-941-748-3031

In addition, the American Printing House for the Blind offers free cassette tapes of *Reader's Digest* and *Newsweek* articles on tape. 1-800-223-1839. Many publishers have large type formats, and both books and newspapers, such as *The New York Times*, can be found on tape.

Adapted from Riddering, A. T. (1999). Low vision rehabilitation: An introduction. Paper presented at the meeting of the Michigan Occupational Therapy Association, Mackinaw Island, MI; and the American Foundation for the Blind Information Center. (2003). Retrieved December 9, 2004, from http://www.afb.org.

Specific Problems and Adaptations

A variety of techniques and equipment are available to permit individuals with low vision to maintain or increase their level of independence in the performance of self-care, home management, and money management tasks, to name a few. These can often be further adapted for individuals with special needs, which can vary according to the nature and degree of visual impairment. In addition, individual preferences and the presence of other chronic or acute conditions affect the selection of suitable, usable equipment. Older adults may be less receptive to high technology alternatives or be unable to afford extensive outlays for new equipment, for example.

Self-Care

Many individuals with vision loss experience difficulties with once-simple tasks, such as seeing in the mirror to comb their hair, apply makeup, or shave. For people with moderate vision loss, changing the lighting may be sufficient. It is important to consider the possibility that glare is a factor; both brightness and the position of the lighting may need to be adjusted. It may also be necessary to position the patient's face closer to the mirror. Magnifying mirrors, sometimes with lighted frames, may also be useful. Tasks such as shaving, combing hair, or applying toothpaste to a toothbrush can be performed using tactile cues rather than relying on vision. Bathing can be made easier by using a wash mitt instead of a washcloth, and using soap on a rope may make it easier for the person to keep track of that slippery item. For safety in tub transfers, tub or shower areas should have nonskid surfaces and bath mats should be nonskid or be eliminated.

In keeping with the general principle of predictability, self-care products and medicines should be organized. Items should also be clearly marked, either with high-contrast, easy-to-read labels or with tactile cues, such as rubber bands, tape, or Velcro strips. For individuals who have learned simple Braille, labels can be produced either using a special stylus designed for that purpose or made on a computer using a special Braille printer. Avoiding clutter and using trays with built in compartments can do much to make important items easier to find and use.

Eating and Food Preparation

Kitchen and eating areas should be assessed for sufficient lighting and be free of glare. It is helpful to have simple, unbreakable dishware in both white and dark colors to make it easier to see foods of different colors. Using the principles of high contrast is helpful. Plates and kitchenware should contrast with the surface underneath them, and this principle applies to serving food as well. It can be very difficult to see mashed pOTAtoes served on a white plate, for example. Pouring milk into a dark mug may help avoid spills. When pouring cool or cold liquids, a finger can be placed inside the container to determine liquid levels; liquid level indicators are also available that beep when the cup or bowl is full. Liquids should always be poured over the sink or kitchen counter, to avoid spills on the floor. Persons with extremely low vision may find it helpful to organize their plate using a clock face as a guide: peas are at 2 o'clock, meat loaf at 6:00, etc.

Cutting should be done with care. Cutting boards should be available in white and dark surfaces to contrast with food. Many items are now available prechopped. Stoves and appliance settings can be marked with large print or tactile labels, using Velcro dots, for example, on commonly used settings. Oven mitts should be used instead of potholders, as they provide better protection against burns. So-called spatter screens made of mesh that can be placed over cooking pots are available at most stores selling household goods. Again, it is important to organize and label shelves. Salt shakers can be distinguished from pepper shakers by wrapping a rubber band around the salt shaker. Tactile cues are helpful when spreading margarine or mayonnaise on bread.

Clothing and Laundry

Many people with low vision experience difficulties seeing subtle variations in color and find selecting clothes difficult. Whenever possible, increase the lighting in closets, which again should be free of clutter and organized in an understandable and easy to use fashion. For example, clothes can be arranged so that like colors are hung together, or "outfits" can be hung together on a hanger to prevent confusion. Safety pins placed on tags to color code clothing is another helpful idea. Using tactile cues can also be helpful in identifying items; socks of like colors can be marked with thread made into one or two knots near the top. Limiting one's wardrobe to two or three basic colors can also eliminate the need for much marking, guessing, and rearranging.

If laundering is done at home, efforts should be made to spot treat clothing immediately after a spill; stain remover sticks are useful for this purpose and are readily available at the grocery store. One way to check for stains is to use a scanning technique. This task should be carried out in a well-lighted area. To do this, the person mentally divides up the area of clothing being examined, and then, just as one would mow a lawn, strip by strip, makes a tactile or visual search (perhaps using a magnifying device) until the entire area has been covered. This is also a useful technique to use when looking for an item that has been dropped. The laundry area should be lighted and kept clean. Commonly used settings on the washer and dryer can also be marked with high contrast labels or tactile markings. Small hand-held magnifiers can also be used for reading dials and placed in a pocket when not in use.

Appliances and Safety Devices

Today, many simple and useful adaptations of common household items are available, often at local stores. Telephones may be purchased with large buttons and can be programmed to make dialing frequently used numbers simple and accurate. Thermostats embossed or printed with large, bold, and easy-to-read numbers can be found in large home supply stores. Clocks are available with faces printed in many sizes; digital displays may be difficult to read, however, as there often is insufficient contrast. Alarm clocks with alarms that can be adjusted to variable pitches or that have a vibration setting may be helpful for people who also have hearing loss. Alarms can also be connected to a lamp to turn on the lights.

Reading and Writing

People who are adjusting to low vision may experience significant problems when reading. Professionals distinguish between spot reading, in which small amounts of information need to be visually processed, and continuous reading, in which more lengthy amounts of text are read. Spot reading is necessary for reading labels, addresses, dials, pill bottles, or restaurant menus. For these short bursts of reading, hand-held magnifiers can be useful, as they can be easily adjusted for distance and do not need to be held for long periods of time. For continuous reading, which takes more time, stand magnifiers that rest on the page and can cover a whole line may be more practical. For people whose vision is less than 20/400, video magnifiers or closed circuit televisions (CCTVs) may be most useful for both spot and continuous reading.

As mentioned above, individuals with severe visual impairment may also be trained to read simple Braille, which is useful for labeling medicines or storage bins. High contrast labels made with felt markers can also be used by people with more moderate impairments.

A number of adaptations and pieces of equipment can be used to make handwriting easier and more legible. Contrast between ink and paper should be maximized, which can most easily be done by writing with a black felt-tip pen on white paper. Dark lined paper or a dark guide sheet can be used to as a guide for handwriting. In addition, big-print check registers, checks, calendars, and date books are all available. For those who use computers, some adjustment to the monitor may be all that is necessary to make items on the screen more visible. Purchasing a larger monitor will increase the text size by up to 40%. Otherwise, software programs are available that can enlarge the text on the screen up to 16 times the normal size. Before suggesting the purchase of any new hardware or software, however, make sure that the software is compatible with the computer in use and that there is enough space on the hard drive and enough memory to store the program. Often the state's commission for the blind or department of rehabilitation offers advice to consumers and even opportunities for computer demonstrations and training.

OTHER SENSORY LOSS

In the United States, approximately 25% to 40% of the population over age 65 is estimated to have a hearing impairment (Brennan, 2003; Hoyer & Roodin, 2003). While the joint occurrence of severe visual and hearing loss is relatively rare, older people with visual impairments are also susceptible to hearing losses brought about by the normal aging process. Sensitivity to high frequencies normally begins to diminish in midlife, affecting the ability to detect higher pitched sounds. As a result, it may become difficult for individuals to hear women's voices yet still be able to hear the ranges of a male voice. Individuals who may benefit from using "talking" books and products should order them with male voices, as these may be easier to hear and understand.

Hearing aids do not provide a sure remedy. While many people with hearing loss related to nerve damage have been unable to be satisfactorily fitted with a hearing aid, recent technology has made them more comfortable and effective, if fitted by a trained professional (Hoyer & Roodin, 2003). However, the newer devices are often expensive and, like all hearing aids, are typically not covered by Medicare or other insurers. Additionally, while these devices are extremely useful to some individuals, they do not restore "normal" hearing. It is usually necessary to learn how to screen out normal background or ambient noise, as all sounds are amplified to the same degree. Without proper fitting and training, many older adults abandon their hearing aids or turn them off, finding the noise level confusing and unhelpful. Furthermore, in situations with large amounts or high levels of background noise, many hearing aids are not practical. Newer, more expensive models now may contain gain controls, which automatically dampen the amplification level when noise reaches a certain volume or can even selectively amplify the frequency levels (pitches) where losses have occurred. However, even users of such devices may have to go through an adjustment period to learn how to use the device properly.

When hearing loss is an issue, compensatory strategies can be useful in preventing social isolation and other loss of function. When communicating with individuals with residual hearing, the following strategies can be useful:

- Eliminating competing background noise makes it possible to focus on what is being said.
- Pitch may be as important as volume: lower pitches are generally more easily heard than higher frequencies.
- If more than one speaker is present, speak in turn.
- Speak slowly and clearly, and avoid unfamiliar words.

Devices to ensure safety in the home for individuals who are experiencing the loss of both vision and hearing are particularly important. Alarm systems, such as smoke detectors, may have to be modified to set off a flashing light, such as a lamp, for example. Telephones for the hearing impaired are also available; telephone devices for the deaf (TDD) are systems requiring a special device that holds the receiver and transmits and receives typed messages. If an individual is able to read using a magnification system, these adaptations can be useful. Appliances and equipment that provide auditory cues can sometimes be adapted by varying the pitch and volume. Additionally, people who experience loss of both vision and hearing must rely increasingly on the so-called near senses (i.e., touch, movement, taste, and smell).

When older people are away from home, explicit identification is an important safety precaution. Persons with visual impairments may require a white cane, typically associated with low vision, as an aid to navigation as well as a means of identifying them to others. Carrying a laminated card with important information, including blood type, known allergies, and emergency contact information, can be vital in providing needed attention in case of an accident or illness. Elderly persons with specific impairments or physical conditions (e.g., diabetes, heart conditions, or allergies) may wish to wear Med-Alert bracelets or pendants containing this information. Furthermore, monitoring systems are available for use in the home. These range from devices that permit the monitoring of health conditions, such as respiratory failure, sleep disorders, cardiovascular function, or falling, to simple push-button pendants that can be used to notify designated friends or neighbors in case of an emergency.

CASE STUDY

Louise is a 76-year-old former librarian who has a history of falling, cardiac disease, and hypertension. She is taking several medications and uses at least 2 inhalers for asthma and bronchial problems. She was born in Hungary and came to the United States as a refugee shortly after the end of World War II. While her English is fluent, she speaks with a pronounced accent, especially when upset. Her husband died a year ago, and she is currently living alone in the house that they shared for over 40 years. Her oldest daughter lives in the area and has been concerned because she believes that her mother is losing her ability to take care of herself; her personal hygiene appears to have deteriorated and the house is increasingly untidy and dark. The daughter also states that her mother has been withdrawn, frightened, and unwilling to communicate. "She doesn't seem her old self. She's not getting Alzheimer's, is she?"

Two weeks ago, Louise fell again and fractured her right hip. She has made a good physical recovery, but the medical team has expressed concern about Louise being able to manage on her own. However, since her daughter has offered to stay with Louise, she is being discharged to her home from inpatient rehab. She will receive home health visits from PT and OT, and the OTA will be providing most of the OT treatments.

The OT evaluation included assessments of ADL and cognitive abilities as well as clinical observations and functional testing. The OT evaluation revealed that Louise was able to follow hip precautions that were task specific, such as during bathing or dressing. However, the OT observed her starting to cross her legs while the 2 were talking, and she had to remind Louise of her hip precautions.

Louise was able to perform UE dressing with set-up but was unable to appropriately identify and match clothing, which bothered her a great deal. She was unable to identify the foods placed before her by sight and demonstrated difficulty pouring milk from a small carton into a glass without spilling. She continually turned her head to one side when speaking to another person. She was unable to identify money independently or differentiate between medications. She became frustrated when she was unable to open small containers.

These results confirmed the health care team's suspicion that Louise was having difficulties with center vision, even with her glasses, and that she demonstrated some hearing loss as well. Based on this information, the physician recommended a vision check, which revealed ARMD in her right eye. This condition, which had been undetected (it had been 6 years since Louise had been to the eye doctor), had progressed to the point that Louise was unable to read, watch television, or go outside the house safely alone. A hearing exam revealed that Louise had

moderate loss in the higher frequency ranges. Louise's cognition was within normal limits for her age. As her score on the Short Form of the Geriatric Depression Scale was a 10, Louise was prescribed an antidepressant to reduce symptoms of anxiety and social withdrawal.

With input from Louise and her daughter, the following goals were established:

- Louise will be able to dress independently while maintaining hip precautions, including identifying, sorting, and selecting clothing.
- Louise will be able to bathe and groom herself independently while maintaining hip precautions.
- Louise will be able to manage her medications independently.
- Louise will adopt 3 new or adapted leisure/social activities.

In addition, an appointment was set for a home evaluation to permit adoption of environmental adaptations that would facilitate independence in mobility and overall function.

The OTA working with Louise began by reviewing techniques for LE dressing and reinforcing hip precautions during tub transfers. She also stressed to Louise's daughter and other children that their mother needed to be reminded of the precautions when socializing. The family kept a log of when their mother needed reminders, and after a week the reminders had dropped to none. The OTA included the family in discussions about adaptive techniques and home modifications.

The OTA assisted Louise in developing a system to sort her clothing by color and attach identifying markers that Louise could use. All of her blue outfits were coded by putting 2 small safety pins on the labels; green had 1. Using a simple eccentric viewing technique Louise was able to read very large print; her medications were labeled and stored where she could see them more easily. Because she used the inhalers so often, the one used most was marked by winding several layers of tape around it, so she could easily determine it by touch. With the assistance of Louise's daughter, brighter lighting was brought into the house, in most cases by choosing safe light bulbs with higher wattage. Simple white and black plastic dishware replaced the pastel floral pattern Louise had used before to make it possible for her to see what she was eating. Louise qualified for Meals on Wheels, which meant that her need to prepare her own meals was kept to a minimum, and her daughter took care of the laundry.

In addition to removing all scatter rugs, Louise's daughter put bright yellow tape on the edges of all the chairs she used, which provided a contrast with her dark green carpeting. Although Louise began to demonstrate increasing ability to dress herself and move through the house safely, she continued to voice concerns about her loneliness and her fears of falling. She began to complain to the OTA that she was fearful at night, though she did not tell her daughter.

OT sessions began to focus on improving Louise's leisure skills and encouraging her to be in touch with friends. Card games with large format playing cards were attempted, but Louise, who had been receptive at first to the idea, was clearly bored. Although Louise had loved to read, she was frustrated trying to use a magnifier, and on more than one occasion threw the book across the room. The OTA had suggested that Louise's daughter check out talking books from the library, but Louise resisted the idea, saying she could not concentrate. She insisted on keeping the television on but did not seem to be paying any attention to it. Neither Louise nor her daughter followed up on any recommendations for local support groups or to take part in activities at the local senior center.

After 2 weeks, Louise seemed to become impatient with the OTA and began to talk about "firing" her. She told the OTA that the OTA could do nothing for her loneliness and that the OTA could not bring back Louise's old life. Louise added that she was an old lady who had to learn to "get on" with what she had left.

At the end the month, Louise was able to meet her goals for independence in upper and LE dressing, bathing, and grooming. However, she was unable to adapt her old leisure skills to her reduced level of vision and hearing. Despite her expressed concerns about loneliness, she resisted participating in activities that took her outside of the house or placed her in contact with other people of her age group, whom she said did not understand her.

SUMMARY

People who suffer from low vision find that their lives are affected in multiple ways. OTAs play a crucial role by providing skilled interventions that make it possible to regain a lost sense of independence and dignity or maintain current levels of functioning. For the older adult, the adaptation process may be particularly difficult. Cognitive changes, such as the onset of mild dementia, may interfere with the learning of new habits or the ability to use memory and other mental organization techniques. Even in cases where independent function cannot be achieved, however, the use of adaptations for low vision such as tactile cues or large print formats can enable the older client to take part in self-care activities and make communication easier. These interventions can help diminish the sense of isolation and helplessness that often intensifies the pain of coping with the chronic and progressive conditions that may accompany aging. It is important to remember, however, that like any other rehabilitation process, adapting to low vision and hearing loss requires a great deal of energy and concentration on the part of the elderly client. Successful adaptations are most likely to occur when the client is able to focus on his or her personal goals and not those of family members, peers, or even clinicians.

CLINICAL PROBLEM SOLVING

- Review Louise's medical history and treatment records. What are some other ideas you could use to address her problems with leisure activities? How would you respond to Louise's discouragement with treatment?
- Do you think that Louise's life history and cultural background have a role in her response to treatment? Why or why not?

- Looking at her records, why do you think that Louise was able to adapt to her hip precautions successfully in some cases but not in others? Based on this observation, how confident are you that Louise can maintain her precautions while alone?
- As you work with Louise, it becomes clear to you that she is having difficulties hearing you. What are some techniques that you could use to communicate with Louise? How would you change her treatment activities? How do you document what you have observed?
- Other than the magnifier, which Louise has difficulty using, are there any kinds of adaptive or specialized equipment that she might use?
- Based on her response to treatment, as indicated in her records, do you think Louise is still depressed? Why or why not? What is your role as an OTA in addressing this problem?
- After spending part of a treatment session with Louise in the kitchen, you have concerns because she leaves the gas burner on after removing the teakettle. How do you respond? How can you explain her behavior, when her cognitive performance was within normal limits on her assessment?
- You notice the smell of alcohol on Louise's breath one day when you are working together and are concerned that she may be drinking too much. What would you do?
- Look at Louise's treatment records. Do you understand all the terminology?

LEARNING ACTIVITIES

1. Bring in a remote control from home. Using sunglasses with a bit of petroleum jelly on them, evaluate your remote and classmates' remotes. Determine which is best for someone with low vision.
2. Stock the ADL kitchen with canned goods of approximately the same size. Include cans of household cleaners as well. Grab cans to make a fictitious meal while your eyes are closed.
3. The teacher will bring in a bag full of tubes (e.g., toothpaste, body lotion, hair gel). Pick the tube of toothpaste from the bag without looking in the bag.

REFERENCES

Alliance for Aging Research. (1999). Independence for older Americans: An investment for our nation's future. Retrieved December 9, 2004, from http://www.agingresearch.org.

Brennan, M. (2003). Impairment of both vision and hearing among older adults: Prevalence and quality of life. *Generations, 27,* 52-56.

Burmedi, D., Becker, S., Heyl, V., Wahl, H. V., & Himmelsbach, I. (2002a). Behavioral consequences of age-related low vision: A narrative review. *Visual Impairment Research, 4,* 15-45.

EVIDENCE-BASED TREATMENT STRATEGIES

Treatment Strategies	Authors
Maintain existing perceptual skills	Freeman, 2002; Warren, 1999
Incorporate health education and wellness awareness into treatment	Dahlin Ivanoff, Sonn, & Svensson, 2002; Jackson, Carlson, Mandel, Zemke, & Clark, 1998
Teach adaptive techniques for ADL and IADL	Duffy, 2002; Duffy et al., 2002; Freeman, 2002; Lindo & Nordholm, 1999
Teach adaptive viewing techniques and introduce acceptable low vision aids	Freeman, 2002; Riddering, 1999; Warren, 1999
Introduce environmental adaptations to maximize safety and independence	Freeman, 2002; Meyers, 2002; Riddering, 1999
Provide education to family and friends about condition and communication strategies	Horowitz & Reinhardt, 2000; Riddering, 1999
Incorporate family members and friends in treatment activities	Duffy et al., 2002; Warren, 1999
Monitor emotional responses to condition and assist in development of healthy coping strategies	Freeman, 2002; Lindo & Nordholm, 1999

Burmedi, D., Becker, S., Heyl, V., Wahl, H. V., & Himmelsbach, I. (2002b). Emotional and social consequences of age-related low vision: A narrative review. *Visual Impairment Research 4*, 47-71.

Dahlin Ivanoff, S., Sonn, U., & Svensson, E. (2002). A health education program for elderly persons with visual impairments and perceived security in the performance of daily occupations: A randomized study. *American Journal of Occupational Therapy, 56*, 322-330.

Duffy, M. A. (2002). *Making life more livable: Simple adaptations for living at home after vision loss.* New York: American Foundation for the Blind Press.

Duffy, M. A., Huebner, K. M., & Wormsley, D. P. (2002). Activities of daily living and individuals with low vision. In M. Scheiman (Ed.), *Understanding and managing vision deficits: A guide for occupational therapists* (2nd ed., pp. 289-306). Thorofare, NJ: SLACK Incorporated.

Freeman, P. B. (2002). Low vision: Overview and review of low vision evaluation and treatment. In M. Scheiman (Ed.), *Understanding and managing vision deficits: A guide for occupational therapists* (2nd ed., pp. 265-288). Thorofare, NJ: SLACK Incorporated.

Hellerstein, L. F. (2002). Visual problems associated with brain injury. In M. Scheiman (Ed.), *Understanding and managing vision deficits: A guide for occupational therapists* (2nd ed., pp. 177-186). Thorofare, NJ: SLACK Incorporated.

Horowitz, A., & Reinhardt, J. P. (2000). Mental health issues in vision impairment: Research in depression, disability, and rehabilitation. In B. Silverstone, M. Lang, B. Rosenthal, & E. E. Faye (Eds.), The *Lighthouse handbook on vision impairment and vision rehabilitation* (pp. 1089-1109). New York: Oxford University Press.

Hoyer, W. L., & Roodin, P. A. (2003). *Adult development and aging* (5th ed.). New York: McGraw Hill.

Jackson, J., Carlson, M., Mandel, D., Zemke, R., & Clark, F. (1998). Occupation in lifestyle redesign: The well elderly study occupational therapy program. *American Journal of Occupational Therapy, 52*, 326-336.

Kleinschmidt, J. (1999). Older adults' perspectives on their successful adjustment to vision loss. *Journal of Visual Impairment & Blindness, 93*, 69-81.

Lindo, G., & Nordholm, L. (1999). Adaptation strategies, well-being, and activities of daily living among people with low vision. *Journal of Visual Impairment & Blindness, 93*, 434-446.

Meyers, J. R. (2002). Low vision and occupational therapy: Developing an occupational therapy specialty in low vision. In M. Scheiman (Ed.), *Understanding and managing vision deficits: A guide for occupational therapists* (2nd ed., pp. 307-323). Thorofare, NJ: SLACK Incorporated.

Mogk, L. G., & Mogk, M. (1999). *Macular degeneration: The complete guide to saving and maximizing your sight.* New York: Ballantine Books.

National Eye Institute. (2004). Vision loss from eye diseases will increase as Americans age. Available at: http://www.nei.nih.gov/news/pressreleases/041204.asp. Accessed February 25, 2005.

Orr, A. L., & Huebner, K. M. (2001). Toward a collaborative working relationship among vision rehabilitation and allied health professionals. *Journal of Visual Impairment & Blindness, 95*, 468-82.

Riddering, A. T. (1999). Low vision rehabilitation: An introduction. Paper presented at the meeting of the Michigan Occupational Therapy Association, Mackinaw Island, MI.

Scheiman, M. (2002). Optometric model of vision, part one: Acuity, refractive, and eye health disorders. In M. Scheiman (Ed.), *Understanding and managing vision deficits: A guide for occupational therapists* (2nd ed., pp. 17-44). Thorofare, NJ: SLACK Incorporated.

Stuen, C., & Offner, R. (1999). A key to aging in place: Vision rehabilitation for older adults. *Physical and Occupational Therapy in Geriatrics, 16*, 59-77.

Warren, M. (1995). Providing low vision rehabilitation services with occupational therapy and ophthalmology: A program description. *American Journal of Occupational Therapy, 49,* 877-884.

Warren, M. (1999). *Occupational therapy practice guidelines for adults with low vision.* Bethesda, MD: American Occupational Therapy Association.

PLAN OF TREATMENT   CARR'S INLET HEALTH CARE

(X) Initial ( ) Update		Type: ( ) PT (X) OT ( ) SLP	
Patient Last Name	First Name MI		DOB
	Louise D		
Primary Diagnosis	Treatment Diagnosis		Onset Date
(R) hip fx	low vision		12-28-02

PROVIDER #   CERTIFICATION/RECERTIFICATION DATES

ullu   FROM: 1·21-03   TO: 2·21·03

I HAVE REVIEWED THIS TREATMENT PLAN AND CERTIFY CONTINUING NEED FOR SERVICES. PHYSICIAN
SIGNATURE (APPROVAL)   DATE
Meeng, MD   1-21-03

PATIENT SIGNATURE   DATE
Louise   1-21-03

THERAPIST NAME   PHYSICIAN NAME
X YF Jones, OTR   Muuu

PRECAUTIONS: falls, depression

PROBLEM
LIST: ↓'d LE dressing
    ↓'d mgmt of clothing, ↓'d UE dressing
    ↓'d feeding
    ↓'d leisure & socialization

PLAN: Pt & family education re THP, home safety
    Instruct in eccentric viewing techniques
    Home eval & modifications
    A.E. as tolerated
    monitor depression, socialization

REHABILITATION
POTENTIAL:

GOALS: SERVICE PERIOD SUMMARY MUST ADDRESS FUNCTIONAL PROGRESS FOR EACH GOAL
    (1) LE dressing to (I)
    (2) UE dressing to (I)
    (3) ↑ medication mgmt to (I)
    (4) ↑ leisure participation

Real record 28-1. Real record for a client with sensory deficits.

GERIATRIC DEPRESSION SCALE: SHORT FORM*

DIRECTIONS: Ask all questions, then total the score. One (1) point for each response found in the bracket. Zero (0) points if no response differs from bracket.

1. Are you basically satisfied with your life? (No)	NO
2. Have you stopped many of your activities and interests lately? (Yes)	Yes
3. Do you feel that life is empty? (Yes)	Yes
4. Do you often feel bored? (Yes)	Yes
5. Are you in good spirits most of the time? (No)	NO
6. Are you afraid that something bad is going to happen to you? (Yes)	NO
7. Do you feel happy most of the time? (No)	Yes
8. Do you often feel helpless? (Yes)	Yes
9. Do you prefer to stay in your room rather than go out to do new things? (Yes)	Yes
10. Do you feel that you have more problems with memory than most people? (Yes)	NO
11. Do you think it is wonderful to be alive now? (No)	NO
12. Do you feel pretty worthless the way you are now? (Yes)	Yes
13. Do you feel full of energy? (No)	NO
14. Do you feel that your situation is hopeless? (Yes)	NO
15. Do you think most people are better off than you are? (Yes)	NO
Score	10

SCORING
0–3	No Depression
4–7	Mild Depression
8–11	Moderate Depression
12–15	Severe Depression

Comments:

KP Smith, MSW
Evaluator, title

Louise D
Name

_1-20-03_
Date

(signature) MD
Physician

Real record 28-2. Real record for a client with sensory deficits.

Carr's Inlet Health Care
Occupational Therapy
Weekly Treatment Summary

Client: Louise D —

Date: 2-15-03

Problem: ↓ ADLs & ↓ IADLs

Goal: See initial eval

Objective: Pt will utilize tactile & memory cues to identify & correctly organize meds; Pt will perform LE dressing safely (THP)

S: "This is so confusing, but I understand what you want."

O: Pt identifies Albuterol inhaler 3/5 x with tactile cues
Pt requires verbal cues x 25% to use eccentric viewing to ID medicine bottles
Pt selects pants & matching shirt using tactile cues (safety pins)
Dons pants seated & given verbal instructions to daughter on THP, Ø errors

A: Continued progress toward goals, although ↑'d tactile contrast required to differentiate inhalers
Pt confusion appears to ↓ with daughter's participation
Appears to understand techniques for adapted vision

P: Continue as planned

A.E. Jones, OTR
(Therapist signature)

Real record 28-3. Real record for a client with sensory deficits.

Key Concepts

- Brain functions: In Alzheimer's disease, the brain atrophies and loses functional connections, which impairs the nervous system's ability to process the sensory information it receives from the environment.
- Brain dysfunction: An individual with Alzheimer's disease becomes unable to process information, access memory, utilize language, and perform motor acts.
- Function and behavior: Baum (1993) found that individuals who remained engaged in activities displayed less difficulty with dressing, feeding, bathing, and grooming and had fewer occurrences of disruptive behaviors.
- Caregiver roles: For individuals to remain engaged in activities as the disease progresses, it is necessary for the caregiver to compensate for the planning and organizational deficit and memory loss. Family members derive satisfaction from providing care when the caregiving activities are predictable and controllable (Kinney & Stephens, 1989).

Essential Vocabulary

agnosia: The inability to recognize objects and/or people.
aphasia: Absence/impairment of the ability to communicate through speech, writing, or signs.
apraxia: Form of brain damage that results in a motor planning deficit.
clinical dementia rating: Staging instrument that categorizes the level of the disease experienced by the patient.
declarative memory: Memory for general knowledge.
episodic memory: Memory for personal episodes or events that have contextual reference.
occupation: Meets the individual's needs for self-maintenance, expression, and fulfillment (see Figure 29-1).
procedural memory: Knowing how to perform an activity.
prospective memory: Difficulty remembering what to do.
semantic memory: Memory of facts.
short-term memory: Working memory, holds recent events.

Clinical Summary

Etiology

Two types of Alzheimer's disease, one familial caused by genetics and one sporadic with causes unknown.

Prevalence

Genetically caused Alzheimer's disease is rare and typically before age 60. Most common is the type associated with aging that begins after age 60 but more likely later in the 70s and 80s. By age 85 the risk of the disease is near 50%. Four and a half million people are affected with the disease in the United States with a cost of 100 billion dollars in services (Alzheimer's Association, 2004).

Clinical Signs

Early signs include functional decline in IADLs, Leisure, and Work. Moderate signs include required assistance in BADLs such as dressing and meals. Late stage signs include loss of speech, incontinence, and dependence in all ADLs.

Precautions

Safety is a major issue for people with Alzheimer's disease. At home, the family must be educated in making the home safe such as appropriate places for locks. Driving is of grave concern and may require not only ending the license to drive but locking away the keys. Extra household keys should be safely stored outside the home in case the family member is locked out by the person with Alzheimer's disease. Filling out missing person's reports with photos before the person wanders will speed the process of finding a person who leaves home.

A MARRIED COUPLE DEALING WITH ALZHEIMER'S DISEASE

Carolyn M. Baum, PhD, OTR/C, FAOTA

INTRODUCTION

Alzheimer's disease robs the mind of its capacity to make decisions and carry out activities that define the individual. OT offers a client-centered, occupational performance-oriented approach to the person and family as they build the strategies to live their lives. This chapter will provide information for the OTA to employ with persons with cognitive loss, and although it will focus on Alzheimer's disease, the strategies presented will be helpful in interacting with clients or patients who are experiencing cognitive problems or cognitive decline (e.g., multiple sclerosis, PD, stroke, head injury, schizophrenia, and learning disabilities).

Dementia of the Alzheimer's type (DAT) is a progressive, degenerative, and devastating disease for which there is no cure. The DSM-IV-TR (APA, 1994) characterizes DAT by memory loss, impaired abstract thought and judgment, and abnormalities in higher cortical function with resulting personality changes. As it progresses, the disease increases impairment in cognitive function, reflected in deterioration of the ability of the individual to perform tasks and interact socially with family and others.

For centuries, senility was viewed as an inevitable consequence of old age. Only within the past 20 years have doctors applied the medical diagnosis of DAT (Ramsdell, Rothrock, Ward, & Volk, 1990). The search for a cure has spurred families overwhelmed by the consequences of the disease to demand action from Congress, which responded by allocating monies for research and services (Fox, 1989). Currently, 7.5% of the population over 65 have DAT (Gurland, 1985). The prevalence rises to over 20% in individuals over the age of 80 (Magaziner, 1989). Twenty percent of our seniors suffer from some disability that affects function (Alzheimer's Association, 2004; American Association of Retired Persons, 2002) and establishes DAT as a major societal problem.

The family, as the primary caregiver, is faced with the functional, behavioral, and neurological problems of the person with DAT, often without having access to treatment because DAT is not a diagnosis that requires acute medical intervention, therefore, they and their families are not given access to many insti-tutional-based rehabilitative services. Community programs must emerge to help families learn to manage the problems associated with neurological deficits.

Cognitively impaired persons experience anxiety and display disrupting behaviors that may be related to their diminished ability to process information to perform instrumental, self-care, and social activities. Such behaviors may be indications that the person with cognitive loss is bored or not able to do what he or she wants or needs to do. It can be posited that if the caregiver can set up and support the environment to keep the impaired person engaged in a routine of activities, the effort could potentially minimize the disruptive behaviors of his or her loved one and reduce his or her stress.

OTs and OTAs play a critical role in helping families acquire the knowledge and skills to support their loved one's behavior as they strive to maintain dignity and engage in activities. There is consensus that activity is important to maintain cognitive and physical health (Almli, 1993; Christiansen, 1991; Fidler & Fidler, 1963; Kielhofner, 1992; Lawton, 1990).

ALZHEIMER'S DISEASE AND ITS FUNCTIONAL PROGRESSION

The brain processes information and organizes behavior. In DAT, the brain atrophies and loses functional connections, which impairs the nervous system's ability to process the sensory information it receives from the environment. Persons with DAT often have primary sensory impairments (visual, olfactory, gustatory, auditory) because the key centers of the brain that interpret information do not allow the person to create appropriate responses. This means that his or her vision, taste, smell, and hearing may be impaired, complicating his or her ability to participate with others.

Cognition is the process by which sensory input is transformed, reduced, elaborated, stored, recovered, and used (Duchek, 1991). Since behavior is dependent on sensory input, DAT interferes with the individual's performance. As the disease progresses, the individual with DAT becomes unable to process information. People experience losses in their ability to

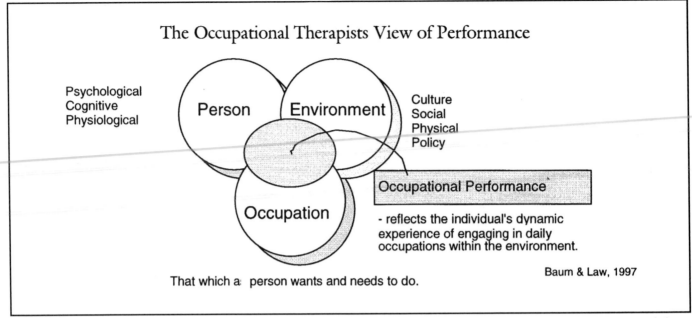

The Occupational Therapists View of Performance

Psychological
Cognitive
Physiological

Person   Environment

Culture
Social
Physical
Policy

Occupation

Occupational Performance

- reflects the individual's dynamic experience of engaging in daily occupations within the environment.

Baum & Law, 1997

That which a person wants and needs to do.

Figure 29-1. Conceptual framework. (Modified from Christiansen, C., & Baum, C. M. [Eds.]. [1991]. *Occupational therapy: Overcoming human performance deficits.* Thorofare, NJ: SLACK Incorporated; Christiansen, C., & Baum, C. M. [Eds.]. [1997]. *Occupational therapy: Enabling function and well-being.* Thorofare, NJ: SLACK Incorporated; and Law, M., Cooper, B., Strong, S., Rigby, P., & Letts, L. [1996]. The person-environment-occupation model: A transactive approach to occupational performance. *Canadian Journal of Occupational Therapy, 63*, 9-23.)

access memory, use language, and perform motor acts (Baum, Edwards, Leavitt, Grant, & Deuel, 1988). The loss is demonstrated when the person has trouble carrying out tasks of daily living and interacting socially. He or she also has difficulty in solving problems (Baum, Edwards, & Morrow-Howell, 1993; Edwards & Baum, 1990).

DAT has been thought to be a deficit of memory. Memory is a problem, however, and individuals can exhibit many different neurological deficits. These deficits are not always present, and if they are present, they may be displayed differently in different stages of the disease. This means that a person with DAT requires accurate assessment to determine the extent of the deficit and how it contributes to the person's occupational performance.

People with Alzheimer's disease may display the following:

- They may not be able to discriminate facial expression or voice tone qualities (Allender & Kaszniak, 1989; Eslinger & Damasio, 1986). This can explain why people have difficulty recognizing staff and family. If someone were to change his or her glasses or hair color or style, the person with DAT would not be able to recognize him or her.

- Aphasia may limit or obscure the person's ability to comprehend or express language (Faber-Langendoen et al., 1988). Just because someone cannot speak, it does not mean he or she cannot communicate. A speech pathologist can help identify successful strategies, such as having the person read. Some people have difficulty initiating speech, and sometimes just starting a story will help them speak.

- Agnosia is an even greater difficulty for families because a person's inability to recognize objects and/or people is impaired (Mendez, Mendez, Martin, Smyth, & Whitehouse, 1990). People who cannot recognize objects need labels on the items and need a helper to be sure they have the right tool for the task they are trying to accomplish.

- Organized or purposeful movements are often difficult due to apraxia (Edwards, Baum, & Deuel, 1991). Families have great difficulty with apraxia, not understanding how the person can do some things and not others. Families sometimes think persons with apraxia are willful and difficult until they understand that the inability to move is a brain deficit.

- Impairment also exists in problem solving, judgment, organization, and sequencing due to frontal and temporal lobe damage (Baum & Edwards, 1993; Sullivan, Sagar, Gabrieli, Corkin, & Growdon, 1989). These functions are basic to people who are able to engage in activities. When these deficits exist, the person needs a caregiver who can get them started on tasks.

- Memory is affected in persons with DAT. Short-term memory is the memory that holds recent events prior to the event being stored. Persons with DAT cannot retain items in short-term memory. This is why you never want to ask a person with DAT "What did you have for breakfast?", "Was your daughter here this morning?", or "What did the announcer say about the weather?"

- Long-term memory is more complex; it can also be used if you can figure out strategies to tap it. Episodic memory is memory for personal episodes or events that have contex-

The Occupational Performance Assessment	
Person factors	The Kitchen Task Assessment (Baum & Edwards, 1993)
	The Functional Behavior Profile (Baum & Edwards, 2000; Baum et al., 1993)
Occupation factors	The Activity Card Sort (Baum, 1993; Baum & Edwards, 2001)
Environment factors	The Memory and Behavior Problems Checklist (Zarit & Anthony, 1986)
	The Zarit Burden Interview (Zarit & Anthony, 1986)

Figure 29-2. Model to guide the assessment process.

tual reference. You can often trigger episodic memory with stories, pictures, and smells. Semantic memory is the memory for facts. It is difficult to tap semantic memory unless the person has extensively used information in their daily life. Some persons retain information about birds, flowers, or other categories of knowledge. Declarative memory is memory for general knowledge and is not often preserved. Prospective memory is the memory that we use to remember what to do. This is impaired in DAT, yet it is amenable to adaptive strategies and cues. The final type of long-term memory is procedural memory. This type of memory is knowing how to do something. We most often think of procedural memory when we think about how we know how to ride a bike, even though we have not done it since childhood. If we know what the person has done in the past, we can tap his or her procedural memory to perform tasks and activities that he or she could not do if it required new learning.

A FRAMEWORK FOR ASSESSMENT

Occupational Therapy Evaluation

Information to frame treatment must be collected from both the person with the impairment and the caregiver. Because treatment involves training of the caregiver to construct opportunities for the person to stay engaged in occupational tasks, it is important to have a clear picture of the pattern of the person's deficits, a history of interests and activities, and the expectations and skills of the caregiver. Figure 29-2 presents a model to guide the assessment process. Each of the instruments included in the model is described below.

The Kitchen Task Assessment (KTA) (Baum & Edwards, 1993) requires the person with DAT to make a cooked pudding from a mix. It allows the clinician to administer a standardized measure without employing an artificial task. The KTA is a valid and reliable measure that can be used as a clinical as well as a research tool because it discriminates the performance of individuals across all stages of the disease. It records changes in the person's performance in initiation, organization, sequencing, incorporation of all steps, safety and judgment, and task completion. The information gained from the administration of the KTA can be used by the clinician to train the caregiver to

assist the impaired individual in daily living tasks. The person must be directly observed in the performance of the task. The test takes approximately 15 minutes.

The Functional Behavior Profile (FBP) (Baum & Edwards, 2000; Baum et al., 1993) is a reliable and valid assessment that documents the caregiver's observation of the task, social, and problem-solving behaviors of a person with DAT. The FBP can help the caregiver focus on the presence of productive behaviors useful in managing the impaired person. When used with the KTA, it helps the clinician understand how the caregiver sees the capabilities of the person with the impairment and how that might differ from the responses that the therapist can elicit from the impaired person with the appropriate level of cueing. It can be completed in checklist or interview format.

The Activity Card Sort (ACS) (Baum, 1993; Baum & Edwards, 2001) is a card sort of 61 activities including 13 instrumental, 36 leisure, and 12 social activities identified by older adults as activities they typically do. Using this assessment, it is possible to calculate the person's previous and current level of engagement in activities from the information provided by the caregiver. The ACS gives the clinician information about the interests, activities, and hobbies of persons to use in planning care. It can be completed in card sort or checklist format.

The Memory and Behavior Problem Checklist (MBPC) (Zarit & Anthony, 1986) reports the problems identified by the caregiver in managing the person with cognitive impairment. The instrument has 2 sections: one documenting the presence of the behavior and the second documenting the caregiver's tolerance for the behavior, if it is observed. In addition to recording the presence of disturbing behaviors, such as wandering, rudeness, losing things, and not recognizing others, it also reports the help needed to perform basic and instrumental tasks of daily living. The instrument can be completed in interview or checklist format by the caregiver and provides information that can help the clinician help the caregiver.

The Zarit Burden Interview (Zarit & Anthony, 1986) reports the burden experienced by the caregiver in managing the person with cognitive impairment. It includes questions that address both demand and emotion-focused stress. Demand stress involves issues such as time for self, dependency, access to resources, and social life. Emotion-focused stress addresses issues such as guilt, anger, fear, and embarrassment. The instrument is completed in interview or checklist format by the caregiver.

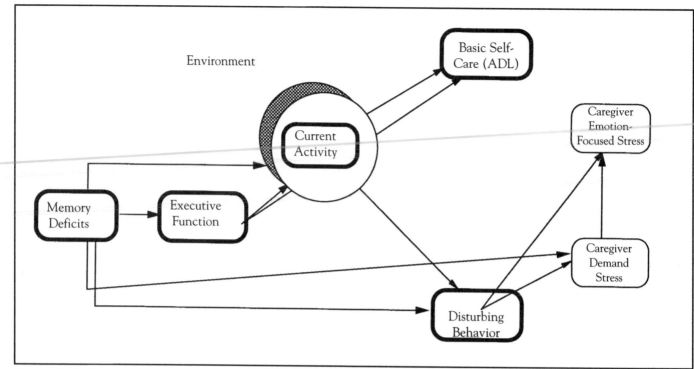

Figure 29-3. Determining management strategies for persons with Alzheimer's disease.

A FRAMEWORK FOR INTERVENTION

Baum (1993) found that individuals with DAT who remained engaged in activities displayed less difficulty with dressing, feeding, bathing, and grooming and had fewer occurrences of disruptive behaviors. Some have suggested that caregivers should be given formal or informal support with tasks such as bathing and dressing (Miller, McFall, & Montgomery, 1991; Vitaliano, Russo, Breen, Vitello, & Prinz, 1986). Help with the self-care tasks alone would not alleviate the caregiver's stress, as the stress is related to the disturbing behaviors, not the frequency with which help is required in self-care. Some disturbing behaviors may surface during dressing and bathing tasks, particularly if the tasks are presented at a level beyond the impaired person's capability. Figure 29-3 describes relationships that can guide OT intervention.

For individuals to remain engaged in activities as the disease progresses, it is necessary for the caregiver to compensate for the planning and organizational deficit and memory loss. The caregiver must be taught how to provide the organizational strategies and memory supports that the person with the impairment can no longer provide for him- or herself. Productive behaviors in the form of instrumental, leisure, and social tasks become the mechanism to minimize the disturbing behaviors. To minimize disturbing behaviors, activities important and meaningful to the person must be organized into routines that are consistent from day to day.

Family members derive satisfaction from providing care when the caregiving activities are predictable and controllable (Kinney & Stephens, 1989). Using this explanation, the caregiver would not be stressed by the actual tasks of caring, but by the unpredictability of the occurrence of disturbing behaviors.

The following is a description of the changes that occur in the individual's performance as the disease progresses. The following is also a summary of the performance reported by the caregiver on the FBP (Baum et al., 1993) and staged using the Clinical Dementia Rating (Berg, 1988).

During the earliest stage of the disease, the individuals usually are appropriate in activities and can do what they are asked to do if the instructions are simple. They usually perform activities without frustration and in a reasonable time frame. They may need encouragement to begin a task. It is impossible for persons to learn a new complex activity, but they can perform complex tasks that are overlearned without assistance. The caregivers begin to face problems at this level. One problem concerns the person's ability to drive. Additional problems involve the ability to manage money and maintain relationships.

In the mild stage of the disease, individuals remain appropriate in activities and independent in grooming and hygiene. They can independently do a simple task; however, they often need encouragement to begin the activity and will do better if the tools and supplies they need are placed at the point of use. They need assistance in doing more complex tasks (those with multiple steps).

The next stage of the disease (moderate) is very problematic for the caregiver, as the impaired person can no longer perform any activity without either verbal or physical assistance, meaning that the person cannot be left alone. Impaired persons can still identify familiar persons, and their behaviors are usually appropriate.

In the severe stage, persons cannot do anything for themselves. Often individuals are in nursing homes but for many reasons (costs ranging from $24,000 to $40,000 per year being just one), a substantial number remain at home. Individuals in this stage can still carry out a response to a one-step command. However, the request must take into consideration their physical capabilities. Specific verbal guidance must be provided to elicit every movement. If you were feeding a person with DAT, you would have to say, "Here, hold this bread. Put it to your mouth. Open your mouth. Take a bite. Chew." The important thing to remember is even though the person appears quite disabled, he or she still has a social need to be part of his or her family social unit and enjoys being a part of interactions (Baum et al., 1993).

Cognitively impaired persons experience anxiety and display disrupting behaviors that may be related to their diminished ability to process information to perform instrumental, self-care, and social activities. Disruptive behaviors include aggressiveness, outbursts, combativeness, wandering, disturbed sleep, incontinence, agitation, insecurity, decreased responsiveness, decreased cheerfulness, irritability, selfishness, crudeness, sexually inappropriate behavior, suspiciousness, the hiding of objects, and repetitive actions (Buckwalter, 1990; Rabins, Mace, & Lucas, 1982; Sinha et al., 1992; Swearer, Drachman, O'Donnell, & Mitchell, 1988). Such behaviors may be indications that the person with cognitive loss is bored or not able to do what he or she wants or needs to do. It can be posited that if the caregiver can set up and support the environment to keep the impaired person engaged in a routine of activities, the effort could potentially minimize the disruptive behaviors of his or her loved one and reduce his or her stress.

OTs and OTAs play a critical role in helping families acquire the knowledge and skills to support their loved one's behavior as they strive to maintain dignity and engage them in activities. There is consensus that activity is important to maintain cognitive and physical health (Almli, 1993; Christiansen, 1991; Fidler & Fidler, 1963; Kielhofner, 1992; Lawton, 1990).

OCCUPATIONAL THERAPY PRINCIPLES GUIDING TREATMENT

OT offers guiding principles that are basic to developing and implementing a client-centered program for people with cognitive loss.

- An individual's performance results from the relationship between that individual and the specific environment in which the activity occurs (Bronfenbrenner, 1979; Christiansen, 1991).
- Engagement in activity makes it possible for individuals to influence their own physical and cognitive well-being (Csikszentmihalyi, 1988; Fidler & Fidler, 1963).
- There is a dynamic interaction among the biological, social, and environmental factors that underlies the individual's capacity for performance in instrumental, leisure, and social activities (Almli, 1993; Kielhofner, 1992; Lawton, 1990).
- Individuals whose activity is within their capabilities do not demonstrate anxiety or boredom related to the task (Csikszentmihalyi, 1988).

Problems Experienced by Individuals With Cognitive Deficits

Most individuals with cognitive impairment have predictable behaviors associated with their deficits. The following are common; however, nothing should substitute for assessments that focus on the client's and the caregiver's needs as a treatment plan is developed:

- Difficulty with awareness—They have difficulty making insightful statements, and it is particularly difficult to modify behavior.
- Poor impulse control—They have difficulty thinking before acting.
- Poor short-term memory, although long-term memory is well-preserved.
- Perseveration—They often display inappropriate and repetitious behaviors.
- Difficulty initiating and organizing tasks.
- Difficulty recognizing objects, people, and sounds.
- They present safety problems for family and themselves.
- Changes in their sensory systems limit vision, they do not smell as well, and they do not have the same level of taste, making food not as appetizing.

TREATMENT STRATEGIES

The social science and occupational science literature provides guidance to practitioners with general strategies to teach the family members of the person with the cognitive loss. The strategies in Table 29-1 have been determined to be effective.

General Strategies to Support Occupation

The following specific strategies can be used by the OTA to help the family member acquire the understanding and skills to help his or her loved one maintain independence.

- Build a consistent schedule; build routines around activities he or she has previously enjoyed.
- Do not expect new learning; perform activities that have been previously overlearned.
- Speak with the person about issues that he or she will hold in long-term memory, as he or she will not be able to store more recent events (e.g., Did you have a nice visit with your daughter yesterday? What did you have for breakfast?).
- Play music from the person's era, not current music.
- Use strong lighting.
- Create contrast on surfaces.
- Avoid distractions, and work in a quiet environment.
- Alter recipes to give them more spice or herb flavor.
- Engage the family in care so they can learn cueing skills and see their loved one perform successfully.
- Find activities that couples can do together.

Table 29-1

Evidence-Based Treatment Strategies

Strengthen remaining capacity of person with impairment	Averbuch & Katz, 1992; Baum & Edwards, 1993
Keep them active and involved	Burns & Buell, 1990; Corcoran, 1994; Dougherty & Radomski, 1993; Oakley, 1993; Zarit & Anthony, 1986
Practical advice to caregiver	Baum & Edwards, 1993, 1993; Cohen, Kennedy, & Eisforder, 1984; Corcoran, 1994; Dooley & Hinojosa, 2004; Dougherty & Radomski, 1993; Haley, Levine, Brown, Berry, & Hughes, 1987; Josphsson, Backman, Nygard, & Borell, 2000; Oakley, 1993; Quayhagen & Quayhagen, 1988; Vitaliano et al., 1986
Organization of a schedule	Baum, 1993; Cohen et al., 1984; Corcoran, 1994; Dougherty & Radomski, 1993; Oakley, 1993
Organization of the environment	Dooley & Hinojosa, 2004; Dougherty & Radomski, 1993; Gitlin, Corcoran, Winter, Boyce, & Hauck, 2001; Oakley, 1993; Toglia, 1992; Zarit & Anthony, 1986
Exercise	Quayhagen & Quayhagen, 1988
Maintenance of interpersonal relationships	Cohen et al, 1984; Corcoran, 1994; MacDonald, 1978; Motenko, 1989
Family included in care plan	Clipp & George, 1990; Cohen et al, 1984; Corcoran, 1994; Dougherty & Radomski, 1993; Quayhagen & Quayhagen, 1988
Training in communication skills	Bourgeois, 1993; Dooley & Hinojosa, 2004; Quayhagen & Quayhagen, 1988; Rabins et al., 1982

- Do not expect caregivers to do things for which they need skills.
- Talk openly about the issues of driving and refer the family member to resources.

Environmental Strategies

- Organize daily activities (occupations) into a consistent pattern.
- Build a message center in the home. Post a weekly schedule and specific daily schedule at the center.
- Provide choices in menu items, activities, and clothing.
- Construct memory books, and ask for the help of the children and grandchildren.
- Pets are great companions and offer a temporal aspect to the day.
- Keep patterns of church attendance or visiting with friends.
- Go to the same restaurant to maintain familiarity with surroundings and menu.
- Continue walking or exercise programs.

- Build a work station. Create a stable environment with tools and items needed to do a task.
- Lay out clothes or items that will be used in a task.
- Continue activities that offer socialization.
- Enroll in a support group (for both the client and caregiver).
- Attend a work-oriented day program.
- Teach the family to engage the person in activities even if he or she is not capable of interacting.
- Help the family choose activities to do together so that socialization is maintained.

Some individuals in the early stage of the disease are able to use self-instruction strategies. These are suggested by Sholberg and Mateer (1989).

- Verbalize out loud each move and the reason for the move before and during execution of the task.
- Whisper rather than verbalize out loud.
- Talk to yourself during the task.
- Switch tasks and repeat the preceding steps.

Note: Generalizations occur only after direct extended training using real-life situations. With an individual with DAT, only activities that have been previously performed can be used, as the potential for new learning is very limited.

Self-Instruction Interventions

- Make lists (gauge improvement on the completeness of the list).
- Proceed with verbalization sequence (above).
- Time management training (Sholberg & Mateer, 1989).
- Time estimation—estimate time it will take as part of planning.
- Creating time schedules, generate a plan for the activities to be accomplished.
- Execute a plan within scheduled time constraints.
- Calendar, day planner.
- Schedule, have a schedule center in home.
- Sticky notes.

Most persons with DAT require compensatory interventions. Usually, the compensatory strategy is provided by the caregiver, aides, and attendants who often fulfill that role and require training. Interventions that are compensatory include the following:

- Person directed by another person (Luria, 1963).
- Organize the setting.
- Build a daily schedule to foster daily routines.
- Help families learn why their loved ones have difficulty initiating and organizing tasks and activities, and teach them how to cue and organize environments for successful interactions.

Individuals with DAT have lives to live (some live 15 years from the time of diagnosis), as do those who are providing care. The OTA is a key professional to help families learn how to manage their loved one, and how to manage without disrupting the lives of the family.

The ideas presented in this chapter seem intuitive and simple. They are not. Families who are experiencing the behavioral changes of their loved one have a hard time recognizing the behaviors as a neurological problem. Deficits such as agnosia, apraxia, and memory are complex neurological problems, and families have no context to understand them. They know their loved ones are acting differently and making demands on them. The OTA can have a major role in helping them understand that their loved one's behavior is not willful but a plea for help to make sense out of experiences that are too complex or too fast for them to process.

The following case is presented to highlight how effective strategies can help family members manage their loved one with mild stage DAT. A person in the mild stage of the disease was chosen because OT intervention can make a difference in helping the family manage these individuals at home.

Case Study

Mr. and Mrs. Johnson

For several years, Mr. Johnson, age 63, had been having difficulties that his family found out of character. He misplaced things, would miss appointments with his plumbing clients, became lost when driving and got frustrated, and frequently lost his keys. He had always been responsible for keeping his company books. Mrs. Johnson took him to the geriatric clinic after the bank talked to her son-in-law about problems with the business account.

On medical examination, there appeared to be no other medical explanation for the symptoms. There was no evidence of hypothyroidism, vitamin B-12 deficiency, or other potentially reversible causes of dementia, such as severe hypertension, stroke, kidney, or heart disease. Additionally, there was no evidence of drug abuse or psychiatric illness. The physician gave the Johnsons the diagnosis of probable Alzheimer's disease and referred them to the social worker and OT. Additionally, she gave them a packet of information about services available through the Alzheimer's Disease and Related Disorders Association.

Social History

The Johnsons have a strong marriage. Each had their own interests and together they shared their family, church, bowling, and camping interests. They raised 3 children, 2 of whom lived within 6 blocks of their parents. Mr. Johnson finished high school and completed an apprenticeship as a plumber. He worked for a company for 35 years before it closed. For the past 10 years, he managed a small plumbing company with his son-in-law. His wife is a secretary in the chemistry department at a small private college. She is 61 years old and in relatively good health. Since she began a low fat, sugar-free diet and a daily walking program, she had brought her blood sugar under control and lost 25 pounds.

Occupational Therapy Assessment Results

Mr. Johnson displayed no evidence of apraxia, and previous neuropsychological testing had not revealed aphasia nor agnosia. He did have some facial masking that made it difficult for family to read his emotional status. The physician team had identified his level of impairment as CDR (Clinical Dementia Rating) 1 (mild Alzheimer's disease). Characteristics of mild DAT include moderate memory loss, especially for recent events; deficits that interfere with everyday activities; and moderate difficulty with time relationships. These characteristics were descriptive of Mr. Johnson.

From the KTA, Mr. Johnson's executive skills were impaired. He required verbal cues to initiate, organize, perform all steps, and sequence the kitchen task. He also needed verbal assistance in managing the stove and pouring the hot liquid. He did recognize that the task was finished. He was capable of performing all aspects of the task but needed the presence of a person to verbally cue him throughout the task.

From the FBP, Mrs. Johnson reported that her husband was able to concentrate for long periods of time as evidenced by his daily activity of continuing with plumbing tasks around the house. (She had encouraged him to continue with his plumbing at home after he no longer went to work.) He usually finished tasks that he started (when he had done them in the past), performed his work neatly, and had no trouble using tools or manipulating small items like buttons on clothing. He did need help with his razor, so Mrs. Johnson got him an electric razor, which he could manage. His activities were usually appropriate to the time of day, however, lately he had been waking at night and going to the kitchen to get something to eat. He continued to make decisions concerning what to wear and what to eat, but Mrs. Johnson found that he was better at this when he was given choices. He continued to bathe and groom with only a little encouragement. He really enjoyed getting out to church activities and being with the children and grandchildren. However, Mrs. Johnson reported that he did not want to stay at events as long as she did. He continued to recognize family and most friends, however, friends helped by saying their name when they greeted him. He rarely initiated conversation but conversed when others started the conversation. Family and friends prompted him when he got lost in a story. Rarely did he know what day it was and he could no longer make independent decisions or problem solve.

From the ACS, Mr. Johnson gave up the tasks of managing personal finances, investments, and general car maintenance. He continued to do home repairs and frequently drove on familiar routes in the neighborhood. He managed the telephone, as his wife had programmed and labeled the frequently called numbers. He read the newspaper and watched sports on TV.

He had given up his church committee activities, however, he still enjoyed going to church. He and Mrs. Johnson went bowling each week in a couples' league and went dancing with friends at least twice a month. They did less family visiting and went out to eat less frequently than 1 year ago. He had given up fishing and hunting, but still did woodworking, camping, and gardening, although less frequently than before because he needed to find time when his son or son-in-law could help him. He had always taken a Sunday afternoon ride in the country.

He watched birds in the backyard but could no longer name them all, and he tended his flowers, but not carefully. He needed help to get started and move from task to task. He had given up reading the Bible and reading in general.

Mrs. Johnson still worked full-time and worried how she would finish the year so she could collect her early retirement from Social Security. She had help from the daughter and son and their families, but all of them worked so she had limited assistance during the day. Mr. Johnson had worked alongside his son-in-law until 6 weeks ago. Mrs. Johnson reported that the future was frightening to her.

From the Zarit Behavior Problem Checklist, Mrs. Johnson reported that Mr. Johnson occasionally had gotten lost, and she thought it was time to take away the car. She reported that he asks repetitive questions and that it was beginning to get on her nerves. She also indicated that he was misplacing things. She reported that he did not destroy things or do things that could be dangerous to himself or others. However, she said he was frustrated frequently, as evidenced by his yelling at her and the dog; and recently she had found him wandering about the neighborhood. She did not recall that he had reported hearing voices or having hallucinations. If she laid out his clothing, he could dress himself. She indicated that he did not have difficulty with self-care tasks, however, she did have to help him with money. She had programmed the telephone so he could get in touch with her during the day. She admitted that he called her frequently and her office seemed to understand, but she felt that it would be a problem soon. She reported being very committed to providing care for him. She reported that they have had a good marriage and that she continued to feel very close to him.

Intervention

Strategies suggested by the OT based upon information obtained from the assessment interview and preferences stated by the Johnsons included:

General Strategies

- Mrs. Johnson was helped to build a consistent schedule. She filled out daily schedules for several weeks until she realized that a consistent schedule had been constructed. She noticed an improvement in Mr. Johnson's behavior when he functioned in a routine.

- Mrs. Johnson was taught to deliver cognitive support. Mr. Johnson mostly required verbal cues and functioned fairly independently when the environment was organized to cue him. It was important to help Mrs. Johnson understand that Mr. Johnson needed help in getting started (initiation) with an activity and also required assistance in getting the task organized. She learned that his difficulty with initiation was not due to stubbornness, but due to the related neurological deficit.

- The family was introduced to cueing strategies, and they chose activities that each of them would be able to do with their father/grandfather, including taking walks, growing flowers, playing with the dog, watching birds, managing house plants, and bowling. Mrs. Johnson integrated these activities into the weekly schedule.

- The family was taught about the related neurological deficits. Because Mr. Johnson displayed some facial masking, it was important for the family to learn to look beyond his facial expression when he was expressing feelings and emotions.

Strategies to Support Behavior in the Absence of Ability to Solve Problems

- The family built a message center in the home so that Mr. Johnson would have a place to go to find out where Mrs. Johnson was, even if she was in the yard. The weekly schedule and specific daily schedule was posted at the center. The children learned to use the center when they were in the home.

- Mrs. Johnson found that when she gave Mr. Johnson choices in menu items that he eats better. He loves French fries and rather than let him choose them daily, she includes them as a menu choice twice a week. He had never been one to help with dinner preparation, but Mrs. Johnson found that he preferred to be with her and that he would do simple tasks like tearing lettuce or stirring a pot of soup or stew. He can do most any task when she chooses to guide him verbally through the task.

Strategies to Support Socialization

- A memory book was constructed with the help of the children and grandchildren. This book was to be used to engage Mr. Johnson in conversation and help him remember familiar people and important past events. A special section on birds was included so that he could keep up with his bird watching.
- Bowling and dancing have been an important part of their routine, so Mrs. Johnson is trying to keep them going. His attention span is decreased but he enjoys the socialization that they offer.
- Mr. Johnson is very fond of his dog. The dog actually cues him to let him out and feed him. They are great companions. The dog is always by his side when he is working in the garage. The problem is the dog is old, so the therapist suggested that a younger dog might be a good investment to maintain the companionship in the future.
- Mr. Johnson no longer can manage Sunday School, but he does sit patiently through church. Mrs. Johnson noted that he does better when they go consistently.
- Mrs. Johnson wanted Mr. Johnson to have a process to express his frustrations and concerns, so she enrolled him in the group for persons with mild DAT sponsored by the local Alzheimer's Disease and Related Disorders Association. He goes to the group weekly. While he is there, Mrs. Johnson can run errands or meet with the other spouses.
- The Johnsons had always enjoyed going out to dinner. They always go to the same restaurant so that Mr. Johnson can manage the menu and visit with the staff and friends that frequent the restaurant.

Strategies to Support the Performance of Tasks

- Mr. Johnson began a work-oriented day program where he could use his handyman skills to make toys for underprivileged children.
- A plumbing work station was built in the garage where Mr. Johnson could safely work with his tools and keep busy while at home. His time in this task gave Mrs. Johnson time to do her activities at home.
- He continues to dress himself when she places the clothes in the same order each day.

- Mr. Johnson's driving skills were evaluated by an OT in an on-the-road assessment. It was determined that it was no longer safe for him to drive. Mrs. Johnson takes him to day care on her way to work and picks him up after work. Because Mr. Johnson always liked to see the hills in the country, either his son or son-in-law takes him for a weekly drive to keep him in touch with nature.
- Mrs. Johnson continued with her walking program but included Mr. Johnson. In good weather they used the college track; in inclement weather they walked in the mall.
- The entire family came to understand how important a stable environment was to support Mr. Johnson's function. The grandchildren have learned why his paper should be in the same place, why his tools should not be moved. The family marked their father's bathroom door with a picture of him shaving. A card labeling the TV stations with news (Channel) 4, sports (Channel) 2, etc., was pasted on the back of the remote control so that he could watch his shows. The power button was painted white. The remote is always in a basket on the table by his chair.

When Mr. Johnson stays involved in activities that are important to him, he does not exhibit as many disturbing behaviors as when he is bored or anxious. He particularly enjoys working in his garage workshop. Mr. Johnson's memory has not improved, but the modifications that the family has made is providing an environment that maximizes his function and keeps him active and engaged. Mrs. Johnson reports that she is able to continue working, which is an important goal for both of their long-term security.

Discussion

Mrs. Johnson was a caregiver with a mission: to maintain a purposeful relationship with her husband, to be a successful caregiver, and to remain at work. She was meeting and continues to meet those goals. Of course there were difficult days, but she had a sense of humor, a very supportive family, and a friendship network at home and at work to help her. She was particularly happy when the Family Leave Bill passed, knowing that she had the resources to manage problems as they arrive and can take some time off if it is necessary.

An adaptive approach was the treatment of choice, not only because it makes good clinical sense, but it was what the family wanted and needed. They were willing to take on their role of caring, they just needed the skills to be successful.

CLINICAL PROBLEM SOLVING

Mr. and Mrs. Johnson had excellent diagnosis and treatment options as they addressed the problems of Alzheimer's Disease. Consider the following case typical of uncertainty in the early stages of proper diagnosis:

- Frances is a 72-year-old woman who lived with her family in a major East Coast city. She was admitted to a subacute rehabilitation facility following an acute care hospitalization of 10 days after a fall in the bathtub. Although being treated initially as a person with a head injury, information about her preaccident functioning hinted at other problems. The family was guarded about sharing information and there seemed to be conflicts within the family about "protecting family assets." The client was cooperative but clearly confused. As time went on, information came forward that Frances had been taking a shower, fully clothed including sneakers, when she fell and experienced the head injury. The social worker was concerned about the safety of the home and for Frances' well-being, and asked the treatment team to assess and treat the client keeping in mind that litigation or protective services may become involved.

The OT then completed the Bay Area Functional Performance Evaluation (BaFPE) along with other formal assessments to get a better handle for the client's behavioral functioning. Serious cognitive deficits were documented. The client was first handed a packet of money ($5.00) and asked to complete a budget sheet using a grocery list. Second, the client was asked to draw a house floor plan (5 by 7 inches rectangle) using a list of required rooms. Lastly, the client was asked to draw a person "doing something." Copies of Frances' work are in the record section.

Considering the evidence from the BaFPE, what discharge plans seem appropriate? How can the family become involved in the treatment process? What signs of cognitive disabilities are present in the 3 sub-tasks of the BaFPE?

LEARNING ACTIVITIES

1. Design a family education tool that addresses how to deal with the frustration that comes with the patient "slowing down."

2. Investigate Internet sites that provide services or supports for people with Alzheimer's. Evaluate the trustworthiness of each site.

3. Design a leisure check sheet for a person with Alzheimer's. Keep in mind the motor and cognitive issues that can interfere with movement.

This chapter was updated by the editor. Dr. Baum was president of the American Occupational Therapy Association at the time of this writing.

REFERENCES

Allender, J., & Kaszniak, A. W. (1989). Processing of emotional cues in patients with dementia of the Alzheimer's type. *International Journal of Neurosciences, 146*, 3-4, 147-155.

Almli, C. R. (1993). Abstract: Motor system, development, and neuroplasticity: Implications of theory and practice in OT. AOTF Research Colloquium, Seattle, WA, June, 1993.

Alzheimer's Association. (2004). Fact sheets. Retrieved October 5, 2004, from http://www.alz.org/Resources.

American Association of Retired Persons. (2002). *America in 2011: A new vision.* Long Beach, CA: Author.

American Psychiatric Association. (1994). *Diagnostic and statistical manual of mental disorders* (4th ed.). Washington, DC: Author.

Averbuch, S., & Katz, N. (1992). Cognitive rehabilitation: A retraining approach for brain-injured adults. In N. Katz (Ed.), *Cognitive rehabilitation: Models for intervention in OT* (pp. 219-239). Boston, MA: Andover Medical Publishers.

Baum, C. M. (1993). The effects of occupation on behaviors of persons with senile dementia of the Alzheimer's type and their caregivers. Dissertation. George Warren Brown School of Social Work, Washington University, St. Louis, MO.

Baum, C. M. (1995). The contribution of occupation to function in persons with Alzheimer's disease. *Journal of Occupational Science, 2,* 59-67.

Baum, C. M., & Edwards, D. F. (1993). Cognitive performance in senile dementia of the Alzheimer's type: The Kitchen Task Assessment. *American Journal of Occupational Therapy, 47*(5), 431-436.

Baum, C. M., & Edwards, D. (2000). Documenting productive behaviors: Using the functional behavior profile to plan discharge following stroke. *Journal of Gerontological Nursing.*

Baum, C. M., & Edwards, D. F. (2001). *The Washington University Activity Card Sort.* St. Louis, MO: Penultimate Publications.

Baum, C. M., Edwards, D. F., Leavitt, C., Grant, B., & Deuel, R. M. (1988). Performance components in senile dementia of the Alzheimer's type. *OT Journal of Research, 8,* 356-364.

Baum, C. M., Edwards, D. F., & Morrow-Howell, N. (1993). Identification and measurement of productive behaviors in senile dementia of the Alzheimer type. *The Gerontologist, 33*(3), 403-408.

Berg, L. (1988). Clinical dementia rating (CDR). *Psychopharmacology Bulletin, 24*(4), 637-638.

Bourgeois, M. S. (1993). Using memory aids to stimulate conversation and reinforce accurate memories. In *Gerontology Special Interest Section Newsletter* (pp. 1-3). Rockville, MD: AOTA.

Bronfenbrenner, U. (1979). Purpose and perspective. In U. Bronfenbrenner (Ed.), *The ecology of human development* (pp. 1-15). Cambridge, MA: Harvard University Press.

Buckwalter, K. C. (1990). Alzheimer's disease: Supportive interventions at home and in the institution. Recent Advances in Alzheimer's Disease: Conference Proceedings. University of Kentucky.

Burns, T., & Buell, J. (1990). The effectiveness of work programming with an Alzheimer population. *OT Practice, 1*(2), 64-73.

Christiansen, C. (1991). OT: Intervention for life performance. In C. Christiansen & C. M. Baum (Eds.), *Occupational therapy;: Overcoming human performance deficits* (pp. 4-43). Thorofare, NJ: SLACK Incorporated.

Clipp, E. C., & George, L. K. (1990). Caregiver needs and patterns of social support. *Journal of Gerontology, 45*(3), S102-S111.

Cohen, D., Kennedy, G., & Eisforder, C. (1984). Phase of change in the patient with Alzheimer's dementia: A conceptual dimension for defining health care management. *Journal of the American Geriatrics Society, 32*(1), 11-15.

Corcoran, M. A. (1994). Management decision made by caregiver spouses of persons with Alzheimer's disease. *American Journal of Occupational Therapy, 48*(1), 38-45.

Csikszentmihalyi, M. (1988). A theoretical model for enjoyment. In M. Csikszentmihalyi (Ed.), *Beyond boredom and anxiety* (pp. 35-54). San Francisco, CA: Jossey-Bass.

Dooley, N. R., & Hinojosa, J. (2004). Improving quality of life for persons with Alzheimer's disease and their family caregivers: Brief occupational therapy intervention. *American Journal of Occupational Therapy, 58*(5), 561-569.

Dougherty, P. M., & Radomski, M. V. (1993). *The dynamic assessment approach for adults with brain injury: The cognitive rehabilitation workbook.* Gaithersburg, MD: Aspen Publications.

Duchek, J. (1991). Cognitive dimensions of performance. In C. Christiansen & C. M. Baum (Eds.), *Occupational therapy: Overcoming human performance deficits* (pp. 284-303). Thorofare, NJ: SLACK Incorporated.

Edwards, D. F., & Baum, C. M. (1990). Caregiver burden across stage of dementia. *OT Practice, 2*(1), 17-31.

Edwards, D. F., Baum, C. M., & Deuel, R. M. (1991). Constructional apraxia in senile dementia: Contributions to functional loss. *Physical and Occupational Therapy in Geriatrics, 9*(3), 53-68.

Eslinger, P. J., & Damasio, A. R. (1986). Preserved motor learning in Alzheimer's disease: Implications for anatomy and behavior. *Journal of Neuroscience, 6*(10), 3006-3009.

Faber-Langendoen, K., Morris, J. C., Knesevich, J. W., LaBarge, E., Miller, J. P., & Berg, L. (1988). Aphasia in senile dementia of the Alzheimer type. *Annuals of Neurology, 23*(4), 365-370.

Fidler, G., & Fidler, J. (1963). *OT: A communication process in psychiatry.* New York, NY: Macmillan.

Fox, P. (1989). From senility to Alzheimer's disease: The risk of the Alzheimer's disease movement. *Milbank Quarterly, 67*(1), 58-102.

Gitlin, L. N., Corcoran, M., Winter, L., Boyce, A., & Hauck, W. W. (2001). A randomized controlled trial of a home environmental intervention: Effect on efficacy and upset in caregivers and on daily functioning of persons with dementia. *Gerontologist, 41,* 4-14.

Gurland, B. J. (1985). Public health aspects of Alzheimer's disease and related dementias. In Kelly (Ed.), *Alzheimer's disease and related disorders: Research* (pp. 146-158). Springfield, IL: Charles C. Thomas.

Haley, W. E., Levine, E. G., Brown, S. L., Berry, J. W., & Hughes, G. H. (1987). Psychological, social, and health consequences of caring for a relative with senile dementia. *Journal American Geriatric Society, 35*(5), 405-411.

Josphsson, S., Backman, L., Nygard, L., & Borell, L. (2000). Non-professional caregivers' experience of occupational performance on the part of relatives with dementia: Implications for caregiver program in occupational therapy. *Scandinavian Journal of Occupational Therapy, 7,* 61-66.

Kielhofner, G. (1992). *Conceptual foundations of OT.* Philadelphia, PA: F. A. Davis.

Kinney, J. M., & Stephens, M. A. (1989). Hassles and uplifts of giving care to a family member with dementia. *Psychology of Aging, 4*(4), 402-408.

Lawton, M. P. (1990). Environmental approaches to research and treatment of Alzheimer's disease. In E. Light & B. D. Lebowitz (Eds.), *Alzheimer's disease treatment and family stress: Directions for research* (pp. 340-362). New York, NY: Hemisphere Publications Co.

Luria, A. R. (1963). *Restoration of function after brain injury.* New York, NY: Oxford University Press.

MacDonald, M. L. (1978). Environmental programming for the socially isolated aging. *Gerontologist, 18,* 350-354.

Magaziner, J. (1989). Demographic and epidemiologic considerations for developing preventative strategies in the elderly. *Maryland Medical Journal, 38*(2), 115-120.

Mendez, M. F., Mendez, M. A., Martin, R., Smyth, K. A., & Whitehouse, P. J. (1990). Complex visual disturbances in Alzheimer's disease. *Neurology, 40*(3), 439-443.

Miller, B., McFall, S., & Montgomery, A. (1991). The impact of elder health, caregiver involvement and global stress on two dimensions of caregiver burden. *Journal of Gerontology, Social Sciences, 46*(1), S9-S19.

Motenko, A. K. (1989). The frustrations, gratification and well-being of dementia caregivers. *Gerontologist, 29*(2), 166-172.

Oakley, F. (1993). *Understanding the ABC's of Alzheimer's disease: A guide for caregivers.* Rockville, MD: American Occupational Therapy Association.

Quayhagen, M. P., & Quayhagen, M. (1988). Alzheimer's stress: Coping with the caregiving role. *Gerontologist, 28,* 391-396.

Rabins, P., Mace, H. L., & Lucas, M. J. (1982). The impact of dementia on the family. *Journal of the American Medical Association, 248,* 333-335.

Ramsdell, J. W., Rothrock, J. F., Ward, H. W., & Volk, D. M. (1990). Evaluation of cognitive impairment in the elderly. *Journal of General Internal Medicine, 5,* 55-64.

Sholberg, M. M., & Mateer, C. A. (1989). *Introduction to cognitive rehabilitation: Theory and practice.* New York, NY: The Guilford Press.

Sinha, D., Zemian, F. P., Nelson, S., et al. (1992). A new scale for assessing behavioral agitation in dementia. *Psychiatry Research, 41,* 73-88.

Sullivan, E. V., Sagar, H. J., Gabrieli, J. D., Corkin, S., & Growdon, J. H. (1989). Different cognitive profiles on standard behavioral tests in Parkinson's disease and Alzheimer's disease. *Journal Clinical Experimental Neuropsychology, 11*(6), 799-820.

Swearer, J. M., Drachman, D. A., O'Donnell, B. F., & Mitchell, A. L. (1988). Troublesome and disruptive behaviors in dementia. Relationships to diagnosis and disease severity. *Journal of the American Geriatric Society, 36*(9), 784-790.

Toglia, J. P. (1992). A dynamic interactional approach to cognitive rehabilitation. In N. Katz (Ed.), *Cognitive rehabilitation: Models for intervention in OT* (pp. 104-143). Boston, MA: Andover Medical Publishers.

Vitaliano, P. P., Russo, J., Breen, A. R., Vitello, M. V., & Prinz, P. N. (1986). Functional decline in the early stages of Alzheimer's disease. *Psychology of Aging, 1*(1), 41-46.

Zarit, S. H., & Anthony, C. R. (1986). Interventions with demential patients and their families. In M. L. M. Gilhooly, S. H. Zarit, & J. E. Biren (Eds.), *The dementias: Policy and management.* Englewood Cliffs, NJ: Prentice Hall, 66-92.

Zarit, S., Reever, K., & Bach-Peterson, J. (1980). Relatives of the impaired elderly: Correlates of feeling of burden. *The Gerontologist, 20*(6), 649-655.

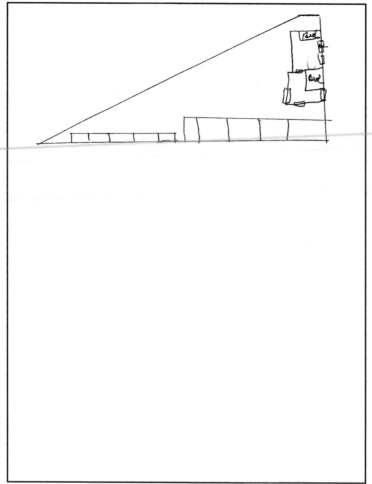

Real record 29-1. The client was asked to draw a 5 x 7 inch rectangle floor plan for 4 people, including a kitchen, bath, and 2 bedrooms. A ruler was provided by the therapist.

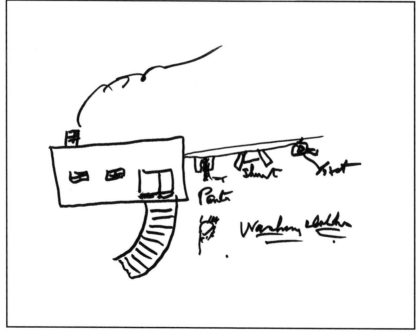

Real record 29-2. Following the floor plan task, the client was asked to draw a person doing something. The client continued with the house theme and drew a person washing clothes, although the person is unclear.

Worksheet

1. Total cash in the envelope: $ *$110.00*

2. The items you are to buy are:

   SOAP – $.65; EGGS – $.90; SHAMPOO – $1.98; APPLES – $1.10;

   PEANUT BUTTER – $2.75; BREAD – $.99; TOOTHPASTE – $.78

COST OF PURCHASE: Please copy amounts from above.

Shampoo	*1.0 0*
Toothpaste	*2.0 5*
Bread	*$1.0*
Apples	*1.00 apples*
Eggs	*Breast*
Soap	*soda*
Peanut Butter	*2.00*
TOTAL	$ _____

3. Is the money from the check needed for the purchase?

                    Yes: _____   No: _____

If "Yes," please put today's date on the front of the check and endorse it by signing your name on the back, and give it to the examiner. The examiner will give you money in exchange for the check.

4. Will you have money left after the purchase? If so, how much?

Total money available: $ _____

Cost of purchase: $ _____

Difference: $ _____

Real record 29-3. Real record for a client with Alzheimer's disease.

TREATMENT TECHNIQUES, PROCEDURES, AND CONCEPTS

Key Concepts

- Evidence-based practice: The utilization of research to qualify effective intervention strategies.
- Experiential learning: Learning by doing.
- Therapeutic use of self: A complex concept used by therapists who form a therapeutic relationship with clients and actively use their own intrapersonal and interpersonal knowledge to foster change in their clients.
- Group dynamics: Conscious and unconscious forces within a group.
- Group process: Deliberate reflection on the intersection patterns between group members following a group experience.
- Social microcosm: Enactment of one's typical interpersonal style.
- Interpersonal learning: Yalom's therapeutic factor describing a complex process that leads to therapeutic change within groups.
- Cohesiveness: Stage of group development where members feel bonded to each other, share mutual identification, and can tolerate conflict among themselves.
- Group development: Sequential and predictable stages of growth in group functioning.
- Seven step process for activity groups: Cole's format for an OT group that encourages interpersonal communication skill development but can be adapted for lower functioning needs as well.

Essential Vocabulary

consensual validation: Comparing one's personal perceptions with other members in a group and receiving feedback.
content: Actual words spoken or used within a group.
"here and now": Pertaining to what is experienced in the present only.
interpersonal: Occurring between one's self and others.
intervention: Strategies used for practice implementation.
intrapersonal: Occurring within one's self.
norms: Codes or rules for behavior.
ontogeny: Normal course of development.
projection: A defense mechanism; taking the unacceptable parts of one's self and unconsciously placing them onto a person or environment.
process: Pertaining to the relationships within a group.
roles: Expected social behavior or position.
task: An activity or process with a tangible end product.
therapeutic communication: Verbal and nonverbal interaction that occurs within a therapeutic relationship.

30

GROUP INTERVENTION

Roseanna Tufano, LMFT, OTR

INTRODUCTION

The intervention process in OT is complex. There are a vast amount of intervention choices and methods that could be used by practitioners. According to the new *Occupational Therapy Practice Framework* (AOTA, 2002), *intervention* is a term that describes the processes and methods used by OT practitioners to assist clients in the achievement of one's chosen occupational performance goals. Intervention plans should describe a strategy or method that creates/promotes, establishes/restores, maintains, modifies, and/or prevents occupational performance (AOTA, 2002).

The recent publication of the *Occupational Therapy Practice Framework* (AOTA, 2002) has reorganized our clinical view of the intervention process. Within the *Framework* document, occupational performance areas such as ADL, IADL, work, play, leisure, education, and social participation (AOTA, 2002) are defined. Interventions are organized by these categories and are meant to impact occupational performance within these performance areas. All OT interventions have inherent methods for their implementation, like requiring certain objects or following a particular sequence of steps. The demands of any activity intervention must also match the body functions and structures of a client as defined within the *Framework* document. For example, a client may have poor short-term memory, a function of one's mental state. An appropriate OT intervention to remediate short-term memory may be the recommendation that a client write daily notes to him- or herself in a portable notebook that he or she could look up as needed. This intervention will only be successful if the client has the ability to read and write, has the motivation to carry around a notebook, and agrees to write important details in it everyday. Interventions are also meant to impact a client's skills (motor, process, communication, interaction) and patterns (habits, routines, role performance). Successful occupational performance is invariably influenced by context, which includes cultural, physical, social, personal, spiritual, temporal, and virtual factors within the client's life. Interventions are typically most effective when conducted in a natural environment that is familiar to the client (AOTA, 2002).

Occupational therapists must use effective clinical reasoning to evaluate a client and integrate all of the above stated variables into the intervention process. A reliable intervention plan not only reflects the practitioner's clinical perceptions and evaluation findings but also represents a client's occupational profile and goals, values, interests, and needs (AOTA, 2002). OTAs are expected to implement the interventions in an effective, therapeutic manner that matches the desires and abilities of the client. OT practitioners specialize in the ability to impact a person's quality of life via occupational performance.

The following chapter describes a type of intervention commonly used by OT practitioners within a predominantly social context. Group interventions include varied social methods and expectations, and it is very important for the practitioner to recognize how the client's mental functions and processing, communication, and interaction skills all impact occupational performance outcomes. The client's role performance patterns also have a significant impact on participation within any type of OT group. Group interventions could be structured to enhance all areas of occupational performance—ADL, IADL, work, play, leisure, social participation, and education—as well as to address various health conditions that reflect a client's body functioning and/or structural concerns. Group interventions also require that the practitioner have a competent "therapeutic use of self." An effective practitioner/group leader will be able to apply all methods for intervention as defined by the *Framework* document—create/promote, establish/restore, maintain, modify, and prevent—within the group structure. Group interventions have been a critical intervention strategy used by OTs since the origins of the profession and continue to provide a valuable means of enhancing occupational performance.

Within the current mental health system, group forms of therapy are steadily growing in popularity. There appears to be several reasons for the prominent use of groups in today's health delivery system. Research has demonstrated that group therapy can have significant impact for people of various ages, socioeconomic backgrounds, educational status, and various health conditions (Roback, 2000). A second factor is the impact of managed care and financial and political pressure to utilize less costly intervention strategies (Roback, 2000; Scheidlinger,

2000). Groups are an effective means of minimizing costs because several clients can receive treatment with one therapist at the same time. A third consideration is the shift away from medical model and the implementation of health care practice toward community- and school-based settings. An example of a community practice intervention is a peer support group, a popular and effective resource for clients of various conditions that also requires a minimal fee-per-service.

Specifically, within the profession of OT, evidence-based practice has become an important trend. Mary Law and Carolyn Baum, 2 prolific OTs, have defined evidence-based OT practice as "...the use of research evidence together with clinical knowledge and reasoning to make decisions about interventions that are effective for a specific client" (Law & Baum, 1998, p. 131). Although OT is in the early stages of conducting and publishing research on its practice, studies have emerged regarding group effectiveness in managing various mental health issues. It is essential to our profession that we validate the effectiveness of our practice, not only to substantiate what we do as practitioners, but also to meet the current health care delivery system's focus on outcomes. Simply stated, insurance companies will seek to pay for those services that demonstrate effective results, or outcomes and will deny interventions that have no research to support their reliability and validity.

The purpose of this chapter is to discuss various components of group intervention, group models, and group dynamics typically found within OT practice. The reader will find the following:

- A brief history of the origins of group activities that have influenced the profession.
- A selection of OTs who have founded a specific model for OT group intervention and practice.
- An overview of group theory, the process of therapeutic communication, and the typical developmental stages of groups.
- Leadership styles and membership roles that influence group interaction both positively and negatively.
- A format for creating an integrative communication group as an intervention.
- An inclusion of evidence-based research concerning group effectiveness specifically in OT practice as well as related group therapy studies.

It is this author's intention that the reader will be briefly introduced to various OT group practice models and come to appreciate group therapy as a valid intervention strategy. It will be critical for the reader to understand the general concepts of group process, how these dynamics impact outcome, and how group interventions can enhance occupational performance in clients when seeking to use these group therapy interventions in the clinical setting.

OCCUPATIONAL THERAPY GROUPS AND THE EXPERIENTIAL LEARNING PROCESS

Groups, as a model of intervention, have their roots in anthropology, sociology, communication, and psychology theories. In the 1920s, OT originally included treating patients in groups for the sole purpose of working on projects or performing activities. The therapeutic value of the group experience was not fully recognized at that time, however.

During the 1940s, a social psychologist named Kurt Lewin founded the first training for human relations group, also known as T-groups (Yalom, 1995). His research was to have significant impact on the development of group theory principles. The state of Connecticut had passed a Fair Employment Practices Act and Lewin was asked to train group leaders who could effectively deal with individual tensions regarding racial issues evident in social groups at that time. The goal of these groups was to change the racial attitudes of the public. These discussion groups were held in a unique way. Observers recorded the behavioral interactions of the group members while the therapy process was occurring in a room. Although not part of the original plan, eventually group participants, group leaders, and group observers met together to analyze and discuss the interactions that took place within the group experience. These discussion meetings reflected the concept of experiential learning, a term that has come to be associated with Kurt Lewin and this research project. When used in a group setting, the concept of experiential learning describes a unique way to instruct members about their behavior. Simply stated, experiential learning is learning from your personal experiences. As an intervention, observations are made about a person's behavior and feedback is given immediately to this member during the group process, just like Lewin's T-groups. Observations can be made by the group leader and participating group members. This feedback is offered to assist a person in learning how one's behavior influences him or her as well as others.

Experiential learning is an effective way to increase one's awareness of interpersonal relationships and/or social skills and is an integral part of OT interventions. Therapeutic observations are given most effectively when the OT practitioner makes clear statements and shows respect for the person, regardless of his or her behavior. Therapeutic communication is a learned skill that is different from our everyday, personal style of interaction. It takes practice to learn how to give constructive feedback in a nonjudgmental way, especially when a client shows a different set of values and behaviors from the practitioner. Giving constructive feedback is an art that enhances group process.

An OT practitioner who uses the group model as a form of intervention should have knowledge of group theory and be skilled at effective communication. Therapeutic communication refers to the ways that practitioners and clients exchange information, thoughts, and ideas (Tufano, 1997). An essential component of group work is to establish trust and rapport with the members, which can be enhanced by both nonverbal and verbal interactions. A competent practitioner is self-aware of strengths and limitations and continuously works at developing a style that is therapeutic and conducive to the various needs of clients. This self-understanding contributes to the development of one's "therapeutic self."

THE DEVELOPMENT OF OCCUPATION-BASED GROUPS

During the early 1900s, many large hospitals, such as Sheppard-Pratt in Maryland, McLean Hospital in Massachusetts, and Bloomingdale Hospital in New York, developed occupation programs for their patients with mental illness. Significant contributors of this time included Dr. William Rush Dunton, Jr., who has also been referred to as the "father of OT." Dr. Dunton was among the first to recognize that crafts provided a positive distraction for persons with mental illness. He was highly influenced by the work of Dr. Adolph Meyer, a psychiatrist who founded the psychobiological approach to psychiatry. Dr. Meyer believed that mental illness was composed of physical and psychological causes. Dr. Dunton noted how occupations helped patients become healthier, and he proposed that research be conducted to understand why "occupation therapy" worked. So began a long-standing professional relationship between Eleanor Clark Slagle, who was a social worker, and Dr. Dunton. This relationship eventually led to the founding of the AOTA (Quiroga, 1995) (see Chapter 1).

OT continues to promote the role of occupation and its significance for healthy functioning. In its origins, activities were used for diversion, to decrease boredom, and as a productive way to keep patients active. In the 1920s, patients worked on projects that included crafts, basketry, and work-related activities. Patients worked in parallel fashion, side-by-side on their own individual projects without specific treatment goals, or a clear therapeutic focus. There was no emphasis on their socialization and interpersonal skills (Quiroga, 1995).

In the 1950s, significant contributions were made to activity groups as a form of intervention by OTs. The Azimas (1959) recognized the therapeutic value of creative activities such as art, music, poetry, drama, dance, and clay/sculpting. These activities are also referred to as projective media. The purpose of projective media groups is to increase self-awareness and promote self-understanding to encourage intrapersonal change. The Azimas were influenced by psychodynamic concepts, including Freud's psychoanalytic theory. OT practitioners who use the psychoanalytic frame of reference as a theory base for activity groups believe that unconscious conflicts and unresolved issues from one's past influence one's personality development. The goal of projective groups is to increase a person's self-awareness by uncovering conflicts buried within one's unconscious. Groups such as art therapy and music/dance therapy, activities such as journal writing and poetry, and projects such as sculpting and pottery provide an opportunity for clients to freely express feelings in a symbolic way. An OT practitioner who leads projective groups reminds the clients that there are no "rights or wrongs" and that it does not matter whether one has had art, music, or dance lessons. The activity process itself becomes significant. Once a client overtly expresses and recognizes his or her internalized conflicts that have now been triggered by the projective arts media, he or she is free to change these identified feelings into productive behaviors. The energy that was once used to repress these conflicts and bury them into one's unconscious is now freed and available to use again in the here and now. A healthy person is free to love, work, and play in ways that are satisfying to one's self and society; in other words, to engage in productive and meaningful occupations (Stein & Cutler, 2002).

While the Azimas promoted the use of projective assessments and interventions based on psychodynamic theories, Kurt Lewin (1945) took another therapeutic route. He believed that behavior is an outcome of one's personality traits plus one's interaction with the social environment. The blending of one's personality (intrapersonal) traits and one's interpersonal experiences comprise our "life space." According to Lewin, "life space" is in a state of constant change since it is influenced considerably by one's social environment. Lewin focused his research on group process and how social behaviors develop and change among persons. Along with the development of the notion of experiential learning, he also defined another significant concept pertaining to group process. Group dynamics (Edelson, 1964) are the forces within a group that encourage social interaction between members. Lewin recognized how powerful and influential these forces, or dynamics, are toward a person's change process. Examples of dynamics include group process, development, and norms, as well as leadership and membership roles. OT practitioners recognize the various group dynamics that are found in every group and use them to promote healthy functioning in members as they attempt to improve their occupational performance.

FIDLER'S TASK-ORIENTED GROUP MODEL

An OT who was influenced by both psychodynamic theory and Lewin's experiential learning is Gail Fidler (1969). Fidler founded the task-oriented group, which she developed from her research at New York State Psychiatric Institute and her work with male patients who were diagnosed with schizophrenia. According to Fidler (1969), "tasks" are any activity or process that result in an end product or demonstrable service. Examples of task groups include arts and crafts, cooking, horticulture, work/vocational activities, and volunteer or charity projects, such as participating in a soup kitchen or collecting toys for underprivileged children. Gail Fidler believed that the purpose of a task-oriented group was to create a working and sharing environment where a client's productive and nonproductive behaviors could be observed as he or she attempts to complete an end product. It is assumed that clients will naturally show their abilities and dysfunctional patterns in the OT group similar to what they do in their own social environments. She recognized how the process of completing a task allowed the group leader and fellow members an opportunity to observe the relationship between one's feelings, thoughts, and behaviors (Fidler, 1969). Activity groups served as a vehicle to analyze the patient's conflicts and to promote the ability to work through the unconscious themes that become evident in the here and now of the activity group. The group leader is expected to interpret the symbols that emerge unconsciously during the activity group. The internal drives, conflicts, and repressed emotions are expressed while completing the task and the end product comes to represent these internalized themes (Tallant, 2002).

The task-oriented group emphasizes how a person functions in such areas as decision making, problem solving, task initiation and engagement, cause and effect, sharing and cooperation with others, reality testing, and task accomplishment. Emphasis is not on the end product itself but rather on the process of completing the task project According to Fidler, the task becomes the driving force in which healthy, productive behaviors can be learned and eventually transferred into the client's everyday life. An OT practitioner constantly notices how a client's feelings, thoughts, and behaviors impact the completion of a task and influence occupational behavior. The group leader shows concern for the client's feelings about the group process, encouraging appropriate expression and self-understanding. The task group provides an excellent opportunity for experiential learning to take place because feedback about one's performance and feelings are immediately given by the group leader and members. This feedback is essential to accomplishing the needed goals of self-discovery and insight by the client. The client, in response, has an opportunity to experiment with new, more productive behaviors in the group process and to receive continued feedback about his or her new behaviors (Fidler, 1969).

The OT practitioner also identifies how the behaviors of a client, represented in the "here and now" of the group activity, influence his or her functioning ability to complete meaningful activities. Clients are encouraged to transfer their learning from the OT task group into their own natural environments. The group leader encourages and guides the therapy process without taking responsibility for the task. Learning from our mistakes can have advantages for problem solving and understanding consequences of our actions, although it is hard for practitioners to sometimes let clients experience the natural impact of their behavior. It is not the job of the OT practitioner to make the end product successful, but to encourage and teach productive occupational behaviors that the client could use in the present as well as in the future. The OT practitioner is also concerned about the client's feelings regarding group process and encourages appropriate self-expression and self-understanding during the group discussion.

Gail and Jay Fidler have had a notable impact on the field of OT since the 1950s. They authored the first textbook in mental health practice in 1954, *Introduction to Psychiatric Occupational Therapy* and followed it with a second edition,

Occupational Therapy: A Communication Process in Psychiatry (1963). They emphasized the role of activity as a therapeutic method to resolving personality conflicts based on psychoanalytic theory (Tallant, 2002).

Critics of psychoanalytic theory believe that it is an impractical method for treatment. Regarding its application to the present health care delivery system, psychoanalytic approaches are typically long-term and often suitable for persons with a good degree of ego functioning. Contrast this statement with the fact that the long-term clients of today include those with the most severe forms of pathology, such as schizophrenia. Critics also voice a concern regarding research of psychoanalytic concepts. How does one measure the unconscious if it is invisible (Corey, 1996)?

Nonetheless, there are many aspects of psychoanalytic theory that can be applied and modified by OT practitioners. A recent study was conducted by Victoria Schindler (1999) who compared the effectiveness of an activity group, structured discussion group, and control group on the social interaction skills of 25 individuals with mental health disabilities. The outcome of this study showed that the persons who participated in the activity group demonstrated significant improvement in scores. In comparison, there were no significant changes in scores of participants who participated in the structured discussion group or the control group (Schindler, 1999). These findings suggest that activity groups have a more positive impact on fostering social interaction than the discussion group format or lack of treatment. Schindler's recent study on activity effectiveness is validating to the practice of group intervention. This study supports Fidler's original idea of the task group model. Schindler further comments in her article *Group Effectiveness in Improving Social Interaction Skills* (1999) that:

> The results of the study support the premise that involvement in typical life activities can promote the learning of necessary skills, including social skills, in a natural manner. Because normal social interactions are part of everyday activities, an individual simply has "to do" or participate in these activities. The therapist facilitates this process through the careful selection and introduction of the activity in addition to the therapeutic use of self (Fidler, 1969; Mosey, 1970). The presence of a task can provide a nonthreatening focus for individuals who have difficulty interacting in social situations (McDermott, 1988).

The reader is encouraged to consult Gail Fidler's (1969) article *The Task-Oriented Group as a Context For Treatment* for the original study and further appreciation about this OT group model.

MOSEY'S DEVELOPMENTAL GROUP MODEL

Another significant contributor to OT group intervention is Anne Cronin Mosey (1970). Mosey was influenced by Fidler's task-oriented group. However, her frame of reference was different from the psychodynamic origins of Fidler. Mosey attempted to apply a developmental approach to OT group treatment. She believed that treatment should be a "recapitulation of ontogeny." In other words, OT should repeat the normal course of development (Jacobs, 1999).

According to Mosey (1970), developmental groups are nonfamilial, task-oriented groups that imitate common experiences in normal development. They were specifically designed to address group interaction skills described by Mosey as "...the ability to engage in a variety of primary groups." A person's ability to successfully participate and live in one's community is dependent on group interaction skill formation. OT practitioners give positive reinforcement in a step-by-step and graded fashion, encouraging success and a feeling of social accomplishment.

Mosey (1970) identified 5 stages of developmental groups that occur in sequential order. They are called parallel, project, egocentric-cooperative, cooperative, and mature. Here is a brief description of each level.

1. Parallel group: This is the most basic level of group interaction, typically occurring in children ages 18 months to 2 years of age. Clients are involved in their own individual tasks with little required interaction between members. The group leader helps with task accomplishment and takes major responsibility for meeting the social-emotional needs of each client.

2. Project group: This level of group participation is typically shown in children ages 2 to 4 years of age. Clients are involved in short-term tasks with the main emphasis on task accomplishment. There is some group interaction required, such as sharing of tools. Cooperation between members is encouraged, as it is related to the completion of the task. The group leader once again responds to the social-emotional needs of group members.

3. Egocentric-cooperative group: Participation at this level is typical of children ages 5 to 7 years of age. Members select, implement, and execute their tasks, which may be moderately long-term and require some social-emotional satisfaction from each other. The group leader provides any needed support and guidance for group members to achieve task accomplishment and continues to supply emotional need satisfaction.

4. Cooperative group: This level of social interaction is typically accomplished between 9 to 12 years of age. This group experience includes a very supportive atmosphere where both task accomplishment and social-emotional needs are met by fellow members. The group leader is often an advisor and may not be present at all group meetings.

5. Mature group: This is the highest level of group interaction skill typically seen in adolescents between the ages of 15 to 18 years old. All task accomplishment needs and social-emotional needs are met by members. The group leader acts as a co-equal.

Mosey's developmental group model has been selected as a source for evidence-based practice research among two OTs. Sisko Salo-Chydenius designed a "Group Interaction Skills Survey" (1996) based on Mosey's Developmental Group Model. This survey was used in a study that investigated the development of coping and social skills for persons with long-term mental illness. Outcomes were measured for those clients who participated in a weekly structured OT group that met for 1.5 hours each session. Changes in social skills were monitored over a period of 12 weeks. An interesting aspect and adaptation within this study is that the theoretical base for this program was the cognitive-behavioral theory rather than the developmental theory as originally used by Mosey. The OT facilitated social skills training through various psychoeducational media and used client self-assessment and therapist observations to document conclusions based on the developmental sequence of acquiring social skills as identified by Mosey. The results of the study showed that social skills can be learned effectively in structured groups based on the strategies of cognitive-behavioral theory. Implications of this study are important for several reasons. First, it supports the role of OT in providing an effective group intervention for persons with long-term illness who require social skills training. Second, it also highlights the continued need for further research.

In her 1999 study, Schindler identified several remaining questions for further research regarding social skills training. They include:

- How can the effectiveness of social skills training be most usefully measured?

- What are the factors inherent and distinctive in OT that promote desired change?

- What is the meaning to the patient of the process of activity in this change? Are therapeutic factors in OT groups as effective (or more effective) in promoting change as in those groups using discussion only?

A second research study has been initiated and conducted by Mary Donohue (2003). Dr. Donahue examined the validity of Mosey's "Group Profile" and concluded that the profile is a unifactorial measure of group level functioning. Dr. Donahue (2003) summarizes:

> It has validated the importance of the concepts of both Parten and Mosey for examining and assisting the social development of children's participation/interaction. Now the "Group Profile" can be used to measure the levels and changes in levels of group functioning skills in OT activity groups because it has adequate preliminary validity.

Dr. Donahue plans to conduct further research and continue this study. The reader is encouraged to consult Anne Cronin Mosey's (1970) article *The Concept and Use of Developmental Groups* for further clarification and understanding of this group model.

KAPLAN'S DIRECTIVE GROUP

Kathy Kaplan (1988) is also an OT who designed a group intervention specifically for acutely ill and minimally functioning clients. Similar to Fidler and Mosey, Kaplan's directive group is a structured experience. It is suited for persons in an inpatient unit who are often not appropriate for verbal psychotherapy groups. Clients who are referred to this group often show chronic functional impairments such as decreased verbal communication, limited self-initiative, and poor judgment. Kaplan used group dynamic principles and the Model of Human Occupation frame of reference as foundation theories for this intervention model.

The directive group is designed to provide a consistent and structured experience as a way to increase the adaptive functioning level of clients. In other words, this group is meant to assist clients with disorganized thinking and behaviors to structure their expressions and social interactions into productive actions within the OT activity. Kaplan described that the purpose of the group is to "… assist patients in reorganizing their behavior to a beginning level of competence" (Kaplan, 1986). The group is meant to be offered daily, at the same time and place, for a duration of 45 minutes. There is a predictable sequence of events that should take place in every group. The group sequence includes 1) reality orientation, 2) introduction of the group members, 3) a warm-up activity, 4) an activity experience, and 5) a wrap-up/summary. The OT practitioner acts as a role model who readily supports and guides clients to meet their cognitive, social, and emotional needs (Kaplan, 1988).

There are 4 main short-term goals to the directive group. These goals include 1) to participate in the activities of each session, 2) to interact verbally with others around the common tasks, 3) to attend the group on time and for the full 45 minutes, and 4) to initiate relevant ideas for group activities (Kaplan, 1986). The group leader documents daily on each client, using a "Directive Group Progress Sheet." This progress sheet is a type of grid with a numbered rating scale beginning at level #1 (lack of skill) and progressing to a level #5 (skill adequately demonstrated for 45 minutes). The OT practitioner notes a client's daily progress and/or regression by using this progress sheet and comparing the scores. Clients are discharged from the directive group when they demonstrate readiness to engage in other OT experiences such as a task-oriented group or communication group.

Kaplan intended that this group intervention model could be adapted for different populations, including clients with head injuries, stroke, mental retardation, dementia and disorientation, and chronic psychiatric histories. An example of a recent application and research study related to this model was conducted by Trace and Howell (1991) who applied this directive model to a geriatric population. Group topics included the benefits of purposeful activity, life roles, memory enhancement, environmental adaptation, and medication education. Group goals such as "preserving autonomy, enhancing integrity, and increasing personal and community safety" were enhanced in the group participants. Trace and Howell (1991) noted that an effective group outcome for this particular elderly population was maintaining abilities rather than creating new skills (Tallant, 2002).

The reader is encouraged to consult Kaplan's (1988) book, *Directive Group Therapy: Innovative Mental Health Treatment*, for further group description and explanation as well as examples of suitable activities designed for clients with low level functioning. At the present time, there is no available information about a future outcome study regarding this group model.

ROSS' INTEGRATIVE GROUP

Mildred Ross (1991) created a unique OT group experience that is composed of 5 steps or stages. Similar to Kaplan, Ross designed a group model that is highly structured, predictable, and consistent in its format. It is best suited for persons who show limitations in sensorimotor development and who require stimulation and cueing to engage with their environment in meaningful ways. While it can be used with all age groups, the integrative group is primarily designed for persons with developmental disabilities, mental retardation, chronic mental illness, and cognitive disorders due to dementia, stroke, head trauma, and severe physical dysfunction (Ross, 1997).

Ross (1991) based her integrative group on concepts from neurophysiology and sensory integration principles. The OT practitioner selects various activities that provide sensory stimulation in meaningful ways to each client. The goal of this group is to facilitate organized sensory, motor, affective, and/or cognitive responses while the client demonstrates the following occupational behaviors: good social interaction, competency, and choice (Ross & Bachner, 2004). Ross & Bachner (2004) define the Five-Stage Group as follows:

> …a systematic and sequential method for organizing the presentation of activities in a group format. It is developmental… and hierarchal, in that each stage is dependent on the stage before it to enhance its acceptance. Tasks chosen for each stage must be able to be graded up or down.

While most OT activities may be suitable intervention methods for this group approach, the practitioner must adapt the activities to fit within the 5 stages as defined by Ross. A summary of the purpose for each of the 5 specific and sequential steps are listed below (Ross, 1997). It is expected that the group leader will maintain the same group format for every session, as a way of fostering familiarity with repetition for persons who are typically disoriented and confused.

- Stage 1: Acknowledge each member, use activities to alert and arouse attention, and discuss the purpose of the group in simple and clear terms.
- Stage 2: Use simple and repetitive movement activities to foster physical and cognitive readiness and to foster a sense of well-being.
- Stage 3: Select visual motor activities to increase self-awareness, awareness of others, encourage reality testing when appropriate, and encourage an appropriate and planned adaptive response.
- Stage 4: Promote the cognitive integration of prior behaviors and responses by incorporating various cognitive activities and encouraging shared leadership by members, offer reinforcement and support to appropriate cognitive responses while maintaining a calm and focused group tone.
- Stage 5: Use familiar activities to close the group, reinforce all accomplishments, and decide whether group needs additional alerting or calming techniques.

In general, the OT practitioner selects activities that provide sensory stimulation, movement, visual motor responses, and cognitive reasoning. These activities may be selected to provide alerting or calming responses based on the needs of the clients. The desired outcome goal of each group is to acquire calm alertness that increases one's ability to interact in an organized and adaptive fashion. A benefit of this group experience is to enhance the quality of a client's life, even if it is for a brief period of time. The reader is encouraged to consult Mildred Ross and Susan Bachner's most recent book *Adults with Developmental Disabilities: Current Approaches in Occupational Therapy* for further information and examples of sensorimotor activities.

OTHER COMMON GROUP MODELS FOUND WITHIN OCCUPATIONAL THERAPY PRACTICE

There are various other group models and methods that have been designed by OTs. The reader may want to further explore some of the following examples:

- Claudia Allen (1985), who designed cognitive disabilities theory, believes that function is an outcome of one's cognitive level. Earhart (1985) described 9 OT groups to match the 6 levels of cognitive dysfunction as defined by Allen. Each level has a specific set of activities that are suited for intervention.

- Lorna Jean King pioneered the use of sensory integration approaches, originally researched by Jean Ayres, for the treatment of persons with mental illness. King's (1978) Gross Motor Activities are designed to stimulate the sensory processing systems, particularly of persons with schizophrenia.

Since the profession's origins, OT practitioners have developed group methods and intervention strategies (e.g., self-awareness groups, reality-oriented groups, role-oriented groups, social skills training groups, prevocational groups, ADL groups, arts and crafts groups, psychoeducational groups, leisure skills groups, assertiveness training groups, stress management groups, values clarification groups, etc.). While this list may appear overwhelming to the novice practitioner, it verifies that OT practice is an ever-evolving and changing profession that embraces occupational performance for the enhancement of one's quality of life.

GROUP PROCESS

The reader has now been introduced to a brief history of the origins of OT group treatment and various group models that influence our profession. It is evident that activity groups are an inherent and significant form of intervention in OT practice. The following sections of this chapter will review group theory principles, including a discussion of various dynamics that are used in OT group intervention.

A paramount notion that acts as a basis for all group therapy is a concept called social microcosm (Yalom, 1995). Members who are allowed to freely interact in group with minimal structural restrictions will naturally show their interpersonal style. Regardless of the frame of reference used by the group leader, group members will eventually show more and more of their typical social behaviors, for better and for worse! Both adaptive and maladaptive patterns of behavior will be evident. A therapeutic value of recognizing the social microcosm dynamic is that the group leader can also observe triggers of one's behaviors and come to understand the meaningfulness of one's actions.

Consider the following example. John, a group member, becomes anxious because the OT group leader is 15 minutes late for group. He begins to fear that something catastrophic has occurred and that the leader is seriously injured. His anxiety is high and John begins to have signs of a panic attack. As the group leader arrives, she apologizes and describes how she got stuck in traffic for 1 hour. John is so nervous that he is unable to listen. The OT practitioner recognizes that John's response is an over reaction to this particular situation. In the course of discussion, John reveals that he was abandoned by his mother at an early age. To this day, he struggles with anxiety attacks when he fears that someone of significance may leave him.

Another significant dynamic evident in all groups is that each client will have a unique and different reaction to the same event. Using the above example, which described the arrival of the late therapist, an effective group leader would consult with other members of the group to seek their views of what happened. Did everyone panic? Did everyone think that a catastrophic accident occurred to the therapist? The concept of comparing one's thoughts and feelings with others, within a group context, is called consensual validation (Fidler, 1969). A benefit to using consensual validation is that a client could hear a different perspective than his or her own and use this feedback to formulate an adaptive response that he or she may have learned from others in the group. To set this dynamic in motion, the OT practitioner asks other members to comment on how they feel about a similar situation or event. This inquiry can be done very easily in groups because there are several members who are present and hearing the same information at the same time. Using the example above, John would hopefully hear that other members may have been concerned about the "missing therapist" but did not have a panic response. In this way, John may come to understand that his reaction was different and out of proportion in relation to others. The client can be encouraged to understand that "waiting for someone who arrives late" may be a trigger or reminder for feelings of abandonment, which leads to feelings of intense anxiety and panic. The skilled OT practitioner can appreciate differences among group responses and allows each member to express his or her opinions honestly and appropriately. Members will refrain from sharing their reactions if they perceive that they are about to be judged.

In order to promote interpersonal learning, a group leader must guide a group to understand its process. According to Yalom, the term *process* refers to the "nature of the relationship between interacting individuals" (Yalom, 1995, p. 130). Process is different from content in client discussions. The content refers to the actual words or topics used by the speaker. Content can be described by quotes. Refer once again to the above example. John said to the OT group leader as she arrived late to group, "Where have you been? I was beginning to panic. I thought that you were dead." These 3 statements refer to the content of John's concern. Group leaders who are process oriented are concerned with why a client says what he or she did, at a certain time, in a certain manner, and to a certain person (Yalom, 1995). Focusing on the process is a main component of experiential learning and experiential groups.

Interpersonal learning is another significant therapeutic factor inherent within group therapy. This learning can occur within experiential groups by giving and receiving feedback about the various behaviors shown during the group process (Yalom, 1995). The skill of giving feedback is challenging for all group leaders and members. It often takes practice to become a good observer and then to figure out how to verbally express these observations in a therapeutic and nonjudgmental way. An effective group leader continues to develop his or her therapeutic sense of self and communication techniques so that he or she could offer feedback in clear and nonbiased ways.

When giving feedback, there are 3 steps or levels that an OT practitioner should follow (Yalom, 1995). These steps should occur in sequence because each statement builds upon the other. You will also notice that each step gets deeper into a client's emotions and behaviors. You do not have to use all 3 levels each time you give feedback. The art of running a therapeutic group includes having a good sense of timing and knowing when a client is ready to hear and accept feedback from others.

- Step 1 involves giving information about how a client's behavior is being noticed and understood by others. It includes making observations about a client's verbal and nonverbal behaviors. These statements are often concrete and very specific. They often begin with "I see...," "I notice...," or "I hear..." An example of such a statement is, "John, I notice that you have tears in your eyes while you are talking about how worried you became when I did not arrive for group on time." Notice that the OT practitioner does not make any interpretations about the client's behavior at this step. It is now up to the client to affirm or deny what is being stated and observed.

- Step 2 involves more depth and understanding on the group leader's part. This level of feedback can be made when the OT practitioner has established a rapport with a client and has come to understand patterns of behavior. In step 2, a group leader comments on how a client's behavior reflects his or her self-image to others. This feedback is an attempt at interpreting what a person's behavior says about him or her. In keeping with the example above, the following statement could be made as part of step 2: "John, you appear frightened and panicked about the possibility of being left or abandoned." Notice how this statement is different from the first one. The OT practitioner is commenting on how the client's self is reflected by both the verbal and nonverbal behaviors observed during the group event.

- Step 3 includes statements about how a client's behaviors impact the group leader and/or fellow members of a group. The purpose of this feedback is to offer perspectives on

how one's behavior is affecting other people in the environment. It provides information about the consequences of a client's behaviors. For example, one group member may respond to John in this way, "When I saw you crying and feeling scared, I wanted to comfort you and tell you that everything is going to be all right." Another member of the group may have a different perspective to offer, "I find that it is hard to be around you because you are so anxious and high strung. I get nervous just from being around you!" These different responses allow John to understand how people may respond to him both in group as well as socially in the surrounding community. Remember, the group becomes a social microcosm of the real world. John has gained some awareness as to how his behaviors may draw some people closer to him while also pushing others away. The client should be encouraged by the group leader to respond to these feedback statements and discuss what, if any, changes he would like to make about his behavior. Remember, a benefit for using an experiential approach is to encourage immediate behavioral change by practicing within the group setting.

OT groups can provide the opportunity to use experiential learning and processing. Some examples of group interventions that are suited for experiential learning include self-awareness, communication, task, social skills, self-esteem, self-management, and projective arts. In general, clients who are suited for these group experiences have adequate motivation, verbal skills, and the ability to reflect and explore the meaning of their behaviors. The group leader is often a facilitator who probes members about their behaviors, provides feedback, and supports the group to take risks and experiment with new behaviors.

On the other hand, there are also OT groups whose therapeutic value is in the experience of an activity. Examples include developmental groups, sensory integrative groups, directive groups, and psychoeducational groups that teach basic ADL skills such as cooking, budgeting, doing laundry, etc. Clients suited for these interventions are often nonverbal, have low motivation and self-awareness, with chronic maladaptive behavioral patterns and illness. The group leader is active and provides varying degrees of structure to maintain both physical and emotional safety.

An effective OT practitioner is knowledgeable of various types of groups that are suited for a range of functioning levels. It takes both experience and knowledge of group dynamics theory and competent therapeutic communication to become a skilled leader.

GROUP NORMS

A dynamic that influences group process is group norms (Yalom, 1995). Norms may be described as the rules of behaviors or expectations within a group. They can be stated verbally or implied nonverbally. The group leader has a basic responsibility to guide the development of norms. The leader's influence is significant in setting up rules of both acceptable and nonacceptable behaviors, similar to how parents establish expectations within a family. An example of a positive group norm is confidentiality, which is usually discussed during a first session. A group leader typically initiates conversation about confidentiality and explains its purpose for increasing a feeling of emotional safety within the group. Other examples of positive norms include arriving on time for group, remaining for the entire duration of group, giving constructive feedback, supporting members in nonjudgmental ways, and disclosing one's thoughts and feelings. Sometimes, members are asked to sign a contract that states they are in agreement with the group norms and commit to following those rules.

Norms evolve within every group that we partake in within our society (Yalom, 1995). For example, a typical norm within a classroom is that students raise their hand to get their teacher's attention before speaking. These rules are often set early in the group experience and are often difficult to change. Norms are expressed in both direct and nondirect ways, otherwise called explicit or implicit norms (Yalom, 1995). An explicit norm may be the verbal decision of group members to attend every group unless there is an emergency. This example of a norm is typically discussed explicitly and directly in group, while members decide together what constitutes an emergency and an acceptable absence. On the other hand, indirect or implicit norms get unconsciously set by factors such as imitating the behaviors of others and social reinforcement. For example, a group member begins to cry and the group leader extends a tissue to her. This act of support is a nonverbal and implicit way of giving the member permission to cry and nonverbally "stating" that it is acceptable to express sad feelings in this group.

Norms have both a positive and negative influence on group process (Yalom, 1995). Examples of nonproductive norms are interrupting others when one is talking, sub-grouping, avoiding topics, criticizing and/or blaming others, talking through the group leader rather than directly to each other, and talking about members outside of group. Negative norms create dissension rather than cohesiveness and trust. An effective leader will address both the positive and negative norms of group, inviting members to discuss and take responsibility for their own actions. Sometimes, there are serious consequences for breaking group rules, and a member may be asked to leave a group. An effective way to address inappropriate behavior in a group is to give the member a choice; he could either comply with the group expectations and rules or choose to leave. This technique should be used after various attempts have been made to discuss the problem behavior. In a cohesive group, members are willing to negotiate and compromise their needs for the benefit of the whole group. The group leader should role model behaviors and values such as respect and concern for others, while also standing up for group principles and setting limits on inappropriate behaviors, especially those that violate others. Asking a member to leave a group should be used as a last resort because it creates tension between members and the leader. A natural response for other members is to wonder if they will also be asked to leave the group by this leader, and they may begin to question the level of trust and balance of control within the group.

GROUP DEVELOPMENT

There is a sequential set of stages that often occur as part of group development. Several theorists have researched the phases of group process and have titled these stages in different ways. Regardless of the theorist, there is overall agreement about the typical patterns, themes, and dynamics that occur within any therapy group.

According to Yalom (1995), a group passes through a beginning phase of orientation whereby members are looking for direction, structure, goals, and behavioral expectations (norms) from the leader. This stage is similar to early childhood development, where we are dependent on our parents for nurturance and support, eventually feeling ready to distinguish ourselves and become more independent. The catalyst of this stage is the search for individual purpose and meaning and to establish a significant role within the group.

Phase two (Yalom, 1995) includes an individual's awareness of differences and conflicts among others in the group. A common group tension is that members both desire approval and closeness from the group, yet strive to keep self-control and independence. This stage resembles adolescence and can therefore be challenging and confusing for both the leader and members as they try to balance the formation of both a personal identity as well as a group identity. The group leader will likely be confronted during this stage and must be able to discriminate between an attack on one's person versus an attack of one's role. An effective group leader will demonstrate the ability to understand differences and conflict and appreciate that a member's rebellion is a way to try and reclaim some personal control. A confident and secure leader will respond, negotiate, and compromise the various themes and issues that are presented in group without trying to control or dominate the members. A leader who implicitly or explicitly supports suppression of anger and conflict will create other group problems. Members will remain inhibited and, therefore, unable to fully express who they are or what they want from the therapy experience. Another dynamic that is evident of group suppression is the emergence of a scapegoat. Members will displace anger felt toward the leader onto a "safe" member, one who is willing to become the sacrificial lamb for the group. It is the responsibility of the group leader to point this out and redirect the anger toward him or her in order to preserve group functioning.

Yalom's (1995) third stage is called cohesiveness. During this phase, members report feeling close, trusting, and supportive of each other. Self-disclosure is heightened, with a desire for mutual acceptance and positive group spirit. True cohesiveness cannot be reached without members working through the conflict stage. This phase resembles early adulthood, when children healthily return to their families as adults, with their own separate identity, and feel proud to be part of the family unit, recognizing both its strengths and limits.

It is worth noting other theorists, besides Yalom, who have researched and labeled the stages of group development. Schutz

(1958) focused on the interpersonal needs of group members, believing that groups follow a similar sequence to normal child development. He called these phases inclusion, control, and affection. Bion (1961) focused his research on task accomplishment within corporations rather than interpersonal development. He called his stages flight, fight, and unite. Lastly, Tuckman (1965) believed that there are 4 consistent stages of group regardless of whether they are short-term or long-term based. He called his stages forming, storming, norming, and performing.

The OT practitioner must have an understanding of group development to support healthy and productive occupational functioning among members. Within this social microcosm, the practitioner becomes a role model for ways to manage both effective and noneffective communication patterns and the working through of dependent versus independent functioning.

LEADERSHIP STYLES

The OT practitioner must decide what style of leadership will compliment his or her own personality and the functioning level of group members. Your style of leadership is an example of how you incorporate your therapeutic use of self. Practitioners who are self-confident with good self-esteem will model a positive, accepting regard for clients because they accept who they are in real life. This means that the practitioner accepts both the positive and negative parts of him- or herself without self-degradation. In turn, the OT leader can provide nonjudgmental and unconditional positive regard for every person in treatment, aside from his or her diagnosis, labels, or history.

In general, clients with low functioning abilities will need more direction and structure from the leader, which requires an active, attentive leader. Examples include Mosey's parallel and project level groups (1970), Kaplan's directive group (1986, 1988), and Ross' integrative group approach (1991). When members show high cognitive functioning, evident by their ability to communicate with good insight and judgment, the group leader acts as a facilitator of group process. Sometimes, the leader can even act as a fellow member. For example, Mosey's egocentric-cooperative level group requires that an OT practitioner facilitate the process, while Mosey's mature level group allows the leader to act like a member or adviser.

According to Yalom (1995), the effective group leader guides the group through an experience and then encourages members to reflect and learn about the process. OT practitioners must decide what style of leadership is best suited to guide both the experiential and processing aspects of group. Levels of control and direction must match the needs of clients and suit the type of group model that is selected for intervention.

Kurt Lewin (Lewin & Lippitt, 1938) identified 3 main styles of leadership: autocratic, democratic, and laissez-faire. Autocratic leadership reflects complete control, similar to a dictatorship. There is no input or feedback sought from the members. It is hard to imagine that an OT practitioner would use such a leadership style. Even under extraordinary circumstances, where one may be giving PROM to a client who is comatose, the practitioner is always monitoring the potential response of the client. A more humane, acceptable approach that is suited for low functioning clients is the directive style of leadership. A group leader who is directive will recognize that clients may have impairment in communication, judgment, and reasoning; therefore, the practitioner will set goals, determine group structure, set limits on inappropriate and unsafe behaviors, and closely monitor the social-emotional needs of clients. It is common for OT practitioners to use the directive style of leadership because we provide many group interventions for clients with impaired cognitive abilities.

A democratic style of leadership allows for feedback to be exchanged between the group leader and group members. Freedom and choices, expression of wants and needs, and personal self-disclosure are all encouraged by the OT practitioner who uses this approach. Lewin (Lewin & Lippitt, 1938) believed that a group is most likely to become cohesive if the leader is democratic. Another way to define this level of leadership is facilitative. A facilitator guides the group to accomplish their goals and reach their highest level of functioning by empowering members to take risks and make good decisions. This style of leadership is suited for persons who have adequate self-awareness and the verbal ability to express personal wants, desires, and needs.

A group leader who uses a laissez-faire approach appears passive and nondirective. All goal setting, decision making, and problem solving is accomplished by group members, without any influence from the leader (Lewin & Lippitt, 1938). The group's functioning is the total responsibility of its members. This approach can be used with a mature and high functioning group in which members are capable of leading and processing their own group experience, without any direction or guidance from the leader. An OT practitioner who is laissez-faire deliberately refrains from interfering in the process, a different role from acting like a fellow member or advisor. An example of a positive group experience that is run with minimal guidance from a leader is a community meeting. Members hold office (president, vice-president, secretary, and treasurer) and independently conduct daily or weekly informational meetings with both fellow clients and staff present.

GROUP MEMBERSHIP ROLES

As discussed, the OT practitioner can have significant impact on group development and process by his or her leadership role. Another important influence that greatly impacts group functioning is the membership roles. In 1948, 2 researchers, Kenneth Benne and Paul Sheats, defined 3 categories of membership roles. In general, they defined group roles as predictable behavioral patterns that will emerge in every group experience regardless of who participates in them. Roles are interchangeable and assumed by various members who reenact their interpersonal style in the social microcosm experience. A healthy functioning individual can assume many roles and accommodate the needs of the group by relating to others in a variety of ways. A goal for every OT practitioner is to develop as many healthy, productive roles as possible. A group leader can enhance group functioning and development by supporting and role modeling an assortment of roles.

Benne and Sheats (1978) defined three categories of group roles from their research at the National Training Lab in Group Development. They are group task roles, group building and maintenance roles, and individual roles. The following is a brief summary of these descriptions.

- Group task roles describe behaviors that contribute to how work gets done and how solutions can be reached. These roles impact discussions and problem solving, evident within the content of group. There are 12 roles:

  1. Initiator contributor: Provides ideas and new perspectives.
  2. Information seeker: Seeks clarification and factual information.
  3. Opinion seeker: Wants clarification of values and attitudes.
  4. Information giver: Readily provides facts as needed.
  5. Opinion giver: Offers values and attitudes to others.
  6. Elaborator: Expands on suggestions.
  7. Coordinator: Assembles/organizes ideas.
  8. Orientor: Reminds the group of its intent and purpose.
  9. Evaluator critic: Offers standards used to measure accomplishments.
  10. Energizer: Motivates the group to decide and/or take action.
  11. Procedural technician: Takes on various duties and jobs.
  12. Recorder: Keeps notes on group and recalls information.

- Group building and maintenance roles are those that promote a relationship between members and sustain functioning within the group. These roles are identified by exploring the group process. There are 7 supportive roles:

  1. Encourager: Supports others in positive ways.
  2. Harmonizer: Attempts to mediate differences of opinions.
  3. Compromiser: Will accommodate and trade off own position for good of whole.
  4. Gatekeeper and expediter: Keeps lines of communication open and flowing.
  5. Standard setter: Sets expectations and ideals for group.
  6. Group observer and commentator: Shares views and interpretations.
  7. Follower: Passively goes along with members.

- Individual roles describe behaviors that serve personal needs rather than group needs. They distract a group from becoming cohesive because they have a negative impact on group development and interfere with group functioning rather than encourage it. There are 8 individual roles:

  1. Aggressor: Demeans and attacks the status of others by expressing negativity.
  2. Blocker: Resists group progress.
  3. Recognition seeker: Attracts attention to self.
  4. Self-confessor: Attracts attention by inappropriate disclosures.
  5. Playboy: Uses joking and provocative behavior to distract attention onto self.
  6. Dominator: Shows inappropriate authority by monopolizing others.
  7. Help seeker: Appears needy; seeks pity.
  8. Special interest pleader: Disguises own prejudices through social positions.

A productive and healthy functioning group exhibits a balance of task and group building/maintenance roles and shows a scarcity of individual roles. The reader is encouraged to complete the role analysis worksheet found in Cole (2005) as an experiential exercise to increase understanding and application of these concepts.

CREATION AND DESIGN OF AN ACTIVITY GROUP

Now that the reader has come to understand basic components of group dynamics, this next section will focus on a group format, designed by Marli Cole (2005), that will encourage group process and the integration of experiential learning. Cole adapted her "seven step process for activity groups" from Pfeiffer and Jones' *Reference Guide to Handbooks and Annuals* (1977). While this group format is easily suited for high functioning groups with good cognitive ability, it can be adapted to meet the goals of any group. Here is a summary of the 7 sequential steps (Cole, 2005).

1. Introduction: In this step, both the leader and members introduce themselves to each other. The purpose of this step is to acknowledge every person in group and to begin the process of building trust and rapport among members. Within this step, the OT practitioner must include the following components:

   a. Warm-up
   b. Expectations/norms of the group
   c. Explanation of purpose and goals reflecting OT domains of practice
   d. Brief outline of the group structure, including the time frame

2. Activity: This step includes the experience portion of the group. The OT practitioner explains the directions of the activity in ways that can be optimally understood by members. For example, the group leader may give directions verbally, in writing, and/or through demonstration. Depending on the cognitive level, directions may be provided in a step-by-step fashion or in a series of steps. Inherent in this step, the OT practitioner must have adequately considered the therapeutic goals and desired outcome of the activity, physical and mental capacities of the members, knowledge and skill of the leader, and grading needs and adaptation of the activity to the clinical setting.

3. Sharing: Each member is asked to share his or her experience with others. The group leader models effective verbal and nonverbal communication such as listening,

attending, asking open questions, and conveying empathy. Members should once again be acknowledged for their participation and self-expression. It is important not to exclude anyone in the group; therefore, every member should be invited to participate in the experience.

4. Processing: This is the most challenging aspect of group. It is where interpersonal learning (Yalom's therapeutic factor) can occur between members. In this step, the members are guided by the leader to reflect on what they have learned from the experience or activity. An OT practitioner who is knowledgeable about group dynamics will incorporate this understanding, asking members to discuss norms, developmental stages, leadership and membership role functioning, as they all reflect the interaction patterns of members. A group leader will encourage expression of feelings and the development of self-awareness about both intrapersonal and interpersonal aspects.

5. Generalizing: The group leader in this step addresses the cognitive learning aspects of the group. Principles are highlighted and discussed in preparation for the next phase of group.

6. Application: Here, members are asked to consider how they will transfer what they learned during this group into their own lives. The meaning and/or significance of the group activity is discussed and members are encouraged to think about how this group reflects issues and concerns that are part of their everyday relationships outside of groups. In other words, this is where members explore the social microcosm experience and apply it to their own individual lives.

7. Summary: This is the final step of group. The most important learning principles of the experience are reviewed and summarized. It is also highly effective for the group leader to remind the group of its original purpose and goals and discuss what goals have and have not been reached. Members are asked to define goals for their future and summarize what other learning they would like to accomplish outside of this group. Each member is thanked for his or her contribution.

The reader is encouraged to consult Cole (2005) for further explanation of this group format, including other factors that contribute to a successful group experience.

Summary

The profession of OT began in the 1920s as a group-oriented approach for the treatment of persons with mental illness. "Occupation therapists" observed how purposeful occupations increased the adaptive functioning of their patients, although they did not understand the reasons why. With the ascent of further research from various theorists and current evidence-based practice studies showing the different benefits of clinical practice and group therapy, OT practitioners can validate the use of group models for their practice. This chapter summarizes some

of the most recent and significant group models founded by OTs from a variety of theoretical perspectives. These well-known contributors include the Azimas, Fidler, Mosey, King, Kaplan, Allen, Ross, and Cole.

To utilize group therapy as an effective intervention, OT practitioners must have comprehensive knowledge about the various group models, their foundation constructs, and the applicable domains of practice that are needed by the client. Following an assessment of a client's clinical needs, the practitioner must select an appropriate group intervention that matches his or her occupational profile. The OT practitioner also needs to understand basic group dynamic principles to appreciate how the group model can be used for experiential learning and the achievement of positive social outcomes in members. Social microcosm theory is a basic assumption that underlies all group work. Other significant components of group intervention include the formation of norms, stages of development, interpersonal learning, the development of cohesiveness, group process, leadership style, and membership roles.

Even though the OT practitioner may understand group dynamics, he or she must develop a communication style that fosters a therapeutic relationship with the members. Therapeutic communication is different from the typical ways of interacting and socializing with people in our natural environments. Practitioners who exemplify a proficient "therapeutic use of self" demonstrate core qualities such as respect for others, genuine and unselfish concern for others, authentic expression of attitudes and behaviors, and dignity in valuing the uniqueness of every individual. Practitioners who are self-aware and self-accepting will naturally model ways to encourage the formation of intrapersonal and interpersonal aspects of the self.

OT practitioners who are knowledgeable about group theory, possess a repertoire of group models for practice, and manifest proficient therapeutic communication are likely to become competent group leaders. They can create, design, and adapt any therapy group to suit a variety of performance areas and components as defined by the *Occupational Therapy Practice Framework*.

Learning Activities

1. Lead a group on a developmental level:
   - Craft group with peers
   - Communication worksheet with peers
   - Self expressive activity with peers
   - Task group with peers assigned to be patients
   - Task group with well elderly
   - Task group with people with a disability

2. In a lab group, plan and perform an activity without feedback from the educator. After it is completed, write a paper using the role list in the chapter. Who was the blocker or help seeker, etc? What behavior or statement documents the role?

EVIDENCE-BASED TREATMENT STRATEGIES

Treatment Strategies	Authors
Developmental groups (Mosey) and group profiles	Donohue, 2003
Geriatric group intervention	Gregory, 1996; Menks, Sittler, Weaver, & Yanow, 1997; Trace & Howell, 1991
Group therapy and abuse	Talbot et al., 1999
Individual vs. group therapy	Marques & Formigoni, 2001; Renjilian et al., 2002
Psychoeducational skills groups—anger and depression management	Coon, Thompson, Steffen, Sorocco, & Gallagher-Thompson, 2003; Yakobina, Yakobina, & Tallant, 1997
Short-term group therapy	Littlefield, 2001; Prior, 1998; Snyder, Kimissis, & Kessler, 1999
Social skills training groups	Dobson, McDougall, Busheikin, & Aldous, 1995; Kopelowicz, Liberman, Mintz, & Zarate, 1997; Marder et al., 1996; Salo-Chydenius, 1996; Schindler, 1999

REFERENCES

American Occupational Therapy Association. (2002). *Occupational therapy practice framework*. Bethesda, MD: Author.

Azima, H., & Azima, F. (1959). The therapeutic use of self. *American Journal of Occupational Therapy, 12*, 215-225.

Allen, C. K. (1985). *Occupational therapy for psychiatric diseases: Measurement and management of cognitive disabilities*. Boston, MA: Little, Brown, & Co.

Benne, K., & Sheats, P. (1978). Functional roles of group members. In L. Bradford (Ed.), *Group development* (2nd ed.). La Jolla, CA: University Associates.

Bion, W. (1961). *Experiences in groups and other papers*. New York, NY: Basic Books.

Cole, M. B. (2005). *Group dynamics in occupational therapy. The theoretical basis and practice application of group intervention* (3rd ed.). Thorofare, NJ: SLACK Incorporated.

Coon, D. W., Thompson, L., Steffen, A. Sorocco, K., & Gallagher-Thompson, D. (2003). Anger and depression management: Psychoeducational skill training interventions for women caregivers of a relative with dementia. *Gerontologist, 43*(5), 678-689.

Corey, G. (1996) *The theory and practice of counseling and psychotherapy* (5th ed.). Monterey, CA: Brooks/Cole.

Dobson, D. J., McDougall, G., Busheikin, J., & Aldous, J. (1995). Effects of social skills training and social milieu treatment on symptoms of schizophrenia. *Psychiatric Services, 46*, 376-380.

Donohue, M. V. (2003). Group profile studies with children: Validity measures and item analysis. *Occupational Therapy in Mental Health, 19*(1), 1-23.

Earhart, C. (1985). Occupational therapy groups. In C. Allen (Ed.), *Occupational therapy for psychiatric diseases :Measurement and management of cognitive disabilities* (pp 235-264). Boston: Little & Brown.

Edelson, M. (1964). *Ego psychology, group dynamics, and the therapeutic community*. New York, NY: Grune & Stratton.

Fidler, G. (1969). The task-oriented group as a context for treatment. *American Journal of Occupational Therapy, XXIII*(1), 43-48.

Gregory, S. (1996). Memory maintenance groups in the community. *British Journal of Occupational Therapy, 59*, 25-26.

Jacobs, K. (1999). *Quick reference dictionary for occupational therapy*. Thorofare, NJ: SLACK Incorporated.

Kaplan, K. (1986). The directive group: Short-term treatment for psychiatric patients with a minimal level of functioning. *American Journal of Occupational Therapy, 40*, 474-481.

Kaplan, K. (1988). *Directive group therapy: Innovative mental health treatment*. Thorofare, NJ: SLACK Incorporated.

King, L. J. (1978). A sensory-integrative approach to schizophrenia. *American Journal of Occupational Therapy, 28*(9), 529-536.

Law, M., & Baum, C. (1998). Evidence-based occupational therapy. *Canadian Journal of Occupational Therapy, 65*(3), 131-135.

Lewin, K., & Lippitt. (1938). *An experimental approach to the study of autocracy and democracy: A preliminary note. Sociometry, I*, 292-300.

Lewin, K. (1945). *Dynamic theory of personality*. New York: McGraw Hill.

Marder, S. R., Wirshing, W. C., Mintz, J., McKenzie, J., Johnston, K., Eckman, T. A., et al. (1996). Two-year outcome of social skills training and group psychotherapy for outpatients with schizophrenia. *American Journal of Psychiatry, 153*, 1585-1592.

Marques, A. C., & Formigoni, M. L. (2001). Comparison of individual and group cognitive-behavioral therapy for alcohol and/or drug-dependent patients. *Addiction, 96*(6), 835-846.

Menks, F., Sittler, S., Weaver, D., & Yanow, B. (1997). A psychogeriatric activity group in a rural community. *American Journal of Occupational Therapy, 6*, 376, 381-384.

Mosey, A. (1970). The concept and use of developmental groups. *American Journal of Occupational Therapy, XXIV*(4), 272-275.

Pfeiffer, J., & Jones, J. (1977). *Reference guide to handbooks and annuals* (2nd ed.). LaJolla, CA: University Associates.

Prior, S. (1998). Determining the effectiveness of a short-term anxiety management course. *British Journal of Occupational Therapy, 61*, 207-213.

Quiroga, V. A. M. (1995). *Occupational therapy: The first 30 years: 1900 to 1930*. Bethesda, MD: American Occupational Therapy Association.

Renjilian, A., Nezu, R., Shermer, M., Perri, W., McKelvey, W., & Anton, S. (2002). Individual versus group therapy for obesity: Effects of matching participants to their treatment preferences. *Journal of Consulting and Clinical Psychology, 69*(4), 717-721.

Roback, H. (2000). Adverse outcomes in group psychotherapy. *Journal of Psychotherapy Practice and Research, 9*, 113-122.

Ross, M. (1991). *Integrative group therapy: The structured five-stage approach* (2nd ed.). Thorofare, NJ: SLACK Incorporated.

Ross, M. (1997). *Integrative group therapy: Mobilizing coping abilities with the five stage group.* Bethesda, MD: American Occupational Therapy Association.

Ross, M., & Bachner, S. (2004). *Adults with developmental disabilities: Current approaches in occupational therapy.* Bethesda, MD: American Occupational Therapy Association.

Salo-Chydenius, S. (1996). Changing helplessness to coping: An exploratory study of social skills training with individuals with long-term mental illness. In R. Cottrell (Ed.), *Proactive approaches in psychosocial occupational therapy.* Thorofare, NJ: SLACK Incorporated.

Scheidlinger, S. (2000). The group psychotherapy movement at the millennium: Some historical perspectives. *International Journal Group Psychotherapy, 50*, 315- 339.

Schindler, V. (1999). Group effectiveness in improving social interaction skills. *Psychiatric Rehabilitation Journal, 22*, 349-355.

Schutz, W. (1958). The interpersonal underworld. *Harvard Business Review, 36*(4), 123-135.

Snyder, K. V., Kimissis, P., & Kessler, K. (1999). Anger management for adolescents: Efficacy of brief group therapy. *Journal of the American Academy of Child & Adolescent Psychiatry, 38*, 1409-1416.

Stein, F., & Cutler, S. K. (2002). *Psychosocial occupational therapy. A holistic approach.* San Diego, CA: Singular Publishing Group.

Talbot, N. L., Houghtalen, R. P., Duberstein, P. R., Cox, C., Giles, D. E., & Wynne, L. C. (1999). Effects of group treatment for women with a history of childhood sexual abuse. *Psychiatric Service, 50*(5), 686-692.

Tallant, B. (2002). Applying the group process to psychosocial occupational therapy. In F. Stein & S. K. Cutler (ed), *Psychosocial occupational therapy. A holistic approach.* San Diego, CA: Singular Publishing Group.

Trace, S., & Howell, T. (1991). Occupational therapy in geriatric mental health. *American Journal of Occupational Therapy, 45*(9), 833-838.

Tuckman, B. (1965). Developmental sequence in small groups. *Psychological Bulletin, 63*(6), 384-399.

Tufano, R. (1997). Therapeutic communication. In K. Sladyk (Ed.), *OT student primer. A guide to college success.* Thorofare, NJ: SLACK Incorporated.

Yakobina, S., Yakobina, S., & Tallant, B. (1997). I came, I thought, I conquered: Cognitive behavior approach applied in occupational therapy for the treatment of depressed (dysthymic) females. *Occupational Therapy in Mental Health, 13*, 59-73.

Yalom, I. D. (1995). *The theory and practice of group psychotherapy.* New York, NY: Basic Books.

Key Concepts

- Crafts and OT: A historical legacy in OT.
- Crafts and frames of reference: Different theories emphasize different uses for crafts, and there is a vast variety of crafts available for use with clients and patients.
- Crafts and occupation: How someone does a craft is an example of how he or she lives his or her life.

Essential Vocabulary

art: A skilled way of decorating or illustrating.
craft: An object usually made by hand using tools and skill.
kits: Preprepared materials for a craft project.
theory: An explanation of why the world is the way it is and why things work the way they do.

31

ARTS AND CRAFTS AS MEANINGFUL OCCUPATION

Margaret Drake, PhD, OTR, FAOTA

INTRODUCTION

Crafts are occupations using special skills such as manual arts. They are part of our OT legacy from founders and professional elders. Despite the fact that the world has changed so that computer technology and information management occupy a good part of many people's work lives, crafts continue to engage our creative impulses. The proliferation of craft supply stores and craft departments in super stores attests to this. In the early part of the 20th century, industrialization removed workers from direct contact with the materials they were shaping into objects. Assembly lines removed the opportunity for workers to put their individual mark on their work or to see the manufacture from raw materials to finished product. The parallel development of the craft movement provided this connection that had previously been an integral part of many workers' lives. As crafts came to be thought of as leisure activities, they were no longer as worthwhile in our culture, a culture in which work is a central value. Crafts were no longer considered work (Drake, 1999).

Though crafts are no longer the main treatment modality in OT, more than half of OT clinics still use some crafts. This is not reflected in our textbooks and journals (Dickerson & Kaplan, 1991; Drake, 1999; Taylor & Manguno, 1991). It may be likened to the way that cleanliness was an early and integral value for nurses, and while nurses are still taught techniques of cleanliness even as they learn the newer technologies, they have not abandoned this central practice of their profession. The nursing journals and books have little about cleanliness, just as our literature has little about crafts and art.

DO THEORIES INFLUENCE HOW CRAFTS ARE USED?

Theories are ideas about why things work the way they do. In OT, theories and ideas continue to change. OT practitioners call their theories models. Each model listed has some central concepts. Each has an example of how a paper weaving craft might be used.

- The neuromotor behavior model concept is that dysfunction comes from chemical or structural problems in the nervous system. Problems can be remedied by restructuring the nervous system or compensating for chemical imbalance with medication. A craft would be used to overcome a brain dysfunction by stimulating activity that would cause chemical changes or would enhance neuron restructuring in the brain. An OTA might choose paper weaving because it has repetitive features that cause a person's neurological system to produce more or less of a chemical or reroute information in the brain around the damaged pathways.

- The learning/cognitive disabilities model believes task performance shows the level of cognitive function or ability to learn. Levels of conscious awareness are given numerical values. The type of craft used would be on the level the patient can do without too much challenge and stress. The OTA might choose paper weaving because it is the right amount of challenge for a person functioning at a lower level.

- The developmental/spatiotemporal model views human life as a series of stages. Dysfunction is the failure to pass through the appropriate life stages and to achieve certain milestones. A craft would be expected to assist the person to grow toward the next stage of development. The OTA might choose paper weaving to help the person to learn a lesson that will help him or her to grow mentally so that he or she can do the things expected at the next life stage.

- The lifestyle/adaptive performance model is based on the idea that a person has 4 domains. Each domain includes needs that each human must satisfy in order to function in a healthy way. The domains are interpersonal relationships, welfare of others, self-care, and intrinsic gratification. A craft would be expected to assist the person to satisfy the needs of his or her 4 basic domains. The OTA might help the patient make a paper weaving gift to satisfy the interpersonal need or to gain intrinsic gratification from creating something attractive.

- The rehabilitation model emphasizes the team approach in which continued challenge is part of a patient's treatment. The therapist is considered a teacher. A craft would be used to challenge the individual to learn new skills. The OTA might choose paper weaving in order to challenge a patient who needs to improve fine motor control and dexterity.

- The Model of Human Occupation is based on the idea that all things are connected. The mind, brain, and body cannot be separated in therapy. There are 3 subsystems that deal with level of motivation, habitual learning, and functional performance of the combined mind-brain-body. The craft would be used to integrate skills and learned behavior with understanding of one's own values, motivations, and acceptance of personal responsibility for his or her life. The OTA might offer paper weaving as a choice with some other crafts to assist the individual in increasing responsibility in decision making and personal choice.

- The occupational adaptation model deals with how individuals adapt to changing conditions in their lives. Crafts would be used to assist individuals to experiment with adapting to changes in life by adapting to changes in projects and materials. The OTA might use paper weaving to assist the person in adapting him- or herself to the simple paper materials available.

An OTA may work in a situation in which one theory is used; however, it is more usual to combine theories in using crafts with patients. The best therapists are able to use whatever model most thoroughly explains why a patient needs the craft activity. Such a therapist is an eclectic thinker. Eclectic means to use whatever best fits the situation (Drake, 1999).

WHEN ARE CRAFTS THERAPEUTIC?

Most people feel more capable when they are able to prove to themselves that they can complete a craft. Some crafts are also associated with self-care such as mending and sewing to maintain clothing, cooking to provide adequate nutrition. While these crafts apply to almost everyone, there are specific crafts that fit a specific dysfunction better than other crafts. The best way to assess whether or not a craft will be therapeutic is to look at the OT treatment goals for that person. Will the craft help achieve either the short-term objectives or the long-term goals? Can the craft be finished in the time the patient is expected to be receiving OT treatments? Is the craft likely to make the person feel good about him- or herself, his or her work, and his or her relationship to other people? Does it fit with the patient's interests? If the answer to these questions is yes, the craft is probably therapeutic.

Not all people respond well to craft occupations. They may have had little experience working with their hands or little experience in creatively expressing themselves. For them, a craft may not be therapeutic. It may make them feel inadequate or frustrated.

FRAMEWORK, AREAS OF OCCUPATION, AND PERFORMANCE SKILLS

The profession's practice framework helps organize the knowledge garnered over the last 85 years of the profession. This framework defines for the profession what activities and processes fall within the range of our responsibilities. The areas of occupation into which most crafts can be categorized are play and leisure, though some could possibly be categorized as work (AOTA, 2002).

Performance skills are the abilities necessary to do the different activities, be they ADL or IADL. A craft such as assembling a wooden birdhouse kit involves motor skills, process skills such as paying attention, organizing objects and space, and compensating for problems. These performance skills help OTs organize how we think about the many ways our clients perform without neglecting an important skill.

Performance patterns includes habits, roles, and routines, which are ways of operating that the person has developed over time. These patterns have been developed in contexts such as where the person lives, works, relates with others, and interacts with technology. Each of these can affect how a person will react to craftwork. Knowing the client's performance contexts can guide the OTA to focus on the person's stage of life, social groups, family attitudes, home situation, and financial status. These contexts offer guidance in being appropriate in craft choices for individuals (see Chapter 5).

WHICH IS ART AND WHICH IS CRAFT?

Crafts have often been thought of as lesser than arts. The problem of distinguishing art from craft is an old one. Both craftspeople and artists have felt undervalued by Western cultures, as their pay was never equivalent with hourly pay of other workers. Some think of art, such as drawing and painting, as more skilled than craftwork, such as ceramics and woodworking. Almost every craft requires the use of some skill from art. In some art shows, work that has been judged to be a craft rather than art has been rejected. This may have to do with pricing, as the prices of art are often much higher than craft. Those who judge work by its monetary value may adhere to the idea that art is higher than craft. OT practitioners and art therapists seldom make those distinctions because therapists know that all personal expressions have value and meaning.

KITS: THE MODERN EQUIVALENT OF A CAKE MIX

OT practitioners have traditionally prepared their materials in large quantities for the sake of efficiency. Some therapists are more skilled in using raw materials than others. The modern health care environment does not encourage therapists to use their time in materials preparation, as the time we spend with patients is billable. The time we spend preparing craft materials is not billable. Even nonprofit hospitals want their therapists to pay for themselves through their work. Consequently, therapists are encouraged to use kits because they can spend most of their time with their patients and be paid for it, rather than preparing materials and not being paid for it. Nonetheless, it is still a valuable skill for an OTA to know how to prepare and use raw materials. Some kits are not readily available, but the OTA can still utilize crafts if the raw materials are available in the same way a modern cook may have to fall back on baking a cake from scratch if a cake mix is not available. Kits take up less space in the modern clinic than raw materials just as a cake mix takes up less space than a canister of flour, a canister of sugar, a can of shortening, and a can of baking powder. The eggs and milk are raw materials that must be kept separate and refrigerated for both cake and cake mix. A wooden birdhouse requires that the finishes be kept separate whether it is made from a kit or from boards.

COOKING

"…Cooking is the most commonly practiced craft in all OT clinics" (Drake, 1999, p. 157). Cooking is a craft media that appeals to childhood memories. Food fills the needs of nutrition, symbolizes love, and provides opportunities for creative expression. Food appeals to everybody. Each culture has food that has special meaning. It is important to explore these meanings with clients before actually cooking. Some cultures and religions have foods that are prohibited. For example, pork is prohibited in both Judaic and Islamic religions. Some patients have food restrictions that are part of their treatment regime. For example, people with diabetes have dietary guidelines they must follow as do people with eating disorders, high blood pressure, and cholesterolemia. These are all considerations the OTA must resolve before cooking with patients.

Cooking is an activity that lends itself to group cooperation. Each person can be responsible for one small piece of the cooking activity in the same way that potlucks offer the opportunity to be part of a larger production that gives pleasure to many.

WOODWORKING

Crafts made with wood can range from something as simple as assembling a kit to complex projects such as designing furniture. Woodworking has a special mystique because traditionally it involved skills and knowledge not easily acquired. The feel of the smooth finish on wood products has been called sensual. Wood products remind us that we, too, are a part of nature. Woodworking has the classic features of constructive/destructive materials. While creating something with it, we are also destroying its previous state. This is the constructive/destructive feature.

In the past, many clinics had big floor tools, powered either by electricity or foot pedals. Modern clinics are more apt to have one cupboard with hand tools purchased at the hardware store. Some use kits, which require only sandpaper, glue, and a hammer. Woodcarving on softwood, such as balsa, still offers the opportunity to whittle like our ancestors did.

Woodworking was traditionally identified as man's work. Currently, it is considered appropriate for women, men, children, and the elderly. Age or gender is not a qualification for woodworking. Strength, endurance, and awareness of safety measures are important qualifications in this craft. Because so many woodworking tools are capable of inflicting wounds, therapists in psychiatric settings need to be especially careful to prevent their use as weapons, for self-mutilation, or as safety hazards for the cognitively impaired.

LEATHERWORK

Few of us live our lives without leather clothes, games, or tools. While many mammals and reptiles produce leather, most therapists use cowhide, which comes in several thicknesses. Cowhide is readily available, and most leather kits are made of this.

Leatherwork offers a spectrum of crafts from very difficult to extremely simple. Examples are a complex leather briefcase to a simple keychain. Leather can easily be graded. It can be tooled in intricate designs by higher functioning patients. Stamping tools provide quick, uncomplicated patterns for lower functioning patients. Plastic templates can be used to press predrawn pictures onto the leather. Leather can be colored with stains and paint. There are a variety of laces for piecing leather together.

Few younger children are able to benefit from leatherwork. Adolescent and older children may enjoy it. Since hand strength is so important in leatherwork, it is a challenge for many elderly (Drake, 1999).

NEEDLE CRAFTS

One out of five OT clinics uses needlework at least once per week in patient treatment (Drake, 1999). Sewing and needlework are among the easiest and most controllable crafts for very sick patients. Needlework includes simple sewing of clothing and home furnishings; quilting; and surface decorations such as embroidery, needlepoint, knitting, and crocheting. These crafts traditionally have been considered women's work. For this reason, it may be difficult to motivate males to try them, although many famous male athletes have used needlework to improve fine motor skills. Small children may not know about the gender stereotyping of needlework and be eager to try sewing. For them, sewing can be just another way to make a picture.

Most movement in sewing is in the hands and arms. It is good for improving dexterity but can cause repetitive motion injuries in some patients. Sewing can be adapted for patients with vision problems by using contrasting threads, such as dark thread on light-colored cloth. Tools such as left-handed scissors make this craft accessible to almost everyone. Those with immune disorders and poor circulation, such as diabetes, need extra precautions when using needles to avoid infection in a needle-prick wound. Many sewing tools are capable of inflicting wounds. Therapists in mental health facilities need to be especially careful to prevent their use as weapons, for self-mutilation, or as safety hazards for the cognitively impaired.

METAL CRAFTS

Metalworking is a skill that few people learn before they experience it in OT. Shaping a flat piece of metal, such as in cooper tooling, is one method. Piercing metal in a pattern is another. More sophisticated metal treatments include soldering, etching, enameling, and riveting. All these methods require extra safety precautions. Grading of metalwork can start with simple plastic template copper tooling to a sophisticated metal sculpture.

All metal work requires good strength, eye-hand coordination, and sensory awareness. The simplest techniques require few supplies or tools and can be done at bedside with therapists completing in the clinic what cannot be done in the patient's room. Almost complete assurance of a pleasing outcome makes copper tooling an ideal project for patients who need immediate gratification. Children can use simple tools and materials, such as piercing copper or aluminum foil with a toothpick. For the elderly with cognitive impairment, copper tooling or piercing does not challenge their capabilities, while still providing a pleasing outcome.

MOSAICS

Mosaic is an ageless craft in which colored pieces of materials, such as tile, are assembled to make a picture or design. One-third of clinics have mosaic as a treatment occupation (Drake, 1999). This craft is part of several formal OT assessments because it is able to determine a patient's color discrimination, spatial awareness, dexterity, and motor skills. A client can complete a tile trivet in 2 sessions, which appeals to therapists whose patients only stay a few days. It can be done by bed patients, by one-handed patients, by low functioning mental health patients, and the elderly. The attention span of children is usually not long enough to do traditional mosaics; however, there are ways to hasten the process to adapt to short attention spans, such as mosaics made with paper "tiles."

FIBER CRAFTS

Fiber crafts include things made from reeds, grasses, paper, yarn, cord, and string. It is basically the same process for all fiber crafts (i.e., intermingling one strand of fiber with another strand of fiber). In weaving, the warp and weft fibers cross each other at square angles. Macramé and tatting are special forms of knotting fibers. Rug hooking involves special knots through a coarse cloth to make a nap on one side. In Turkish knotting, special knots are tied around 2 warp strands. While needlework was often the responsibility of females, in some cultures, males had the responsibility for fiber crafts.

Men learned how to make nautical knots and nets as well as weaving carpets. Currently, some clinics use these crafts for fine motor strengthening as well as to increase bilateral dexterity.

CERAMICS

While whole buildings can be built of fired ceramic clay, for the purposes of OT, small projects are best. The clay used in ceramics has special properties that make it harden in the intense heat of the ceramic oven, often called a kiln. Many newer manufactured materials have appeared that mimic ceramics. Some of these imitators are very adaptable to the clinic. They can be baked in the clinic oven (Dierks, 1994). However, traditional ceramic clay pieces are more durable and impervious to water.

One in 3 therapists uses clay or one of its imitators in therapy. In psychiatry, it is often used as part of a battery of assessment for patients. Because of its malleability, clay helps therapists understand how patients deal with structure and control. Wet clay allows a person to reshape his or her mistakes without penalty. The pottery wheel is seldom used in clinics now because it requires advanced skills not acquired in short hospital stays. It also requires upper body strength, which many sick people do not have. Most ceramics currently used in treatment are hand built or slip cast, which is liquid clay poured into a plaster mold, allowed to harden, and dried before firing.

Clay imitators, called therapy putties, are used daily in physical rehabilitation for strengthening, increasing ROM, and developing coordination. The visually impaired respond to the tactile quality of clay. Some psychiatric patients use clay as a method of expressing ideas that are difficult to verbalize. Children find clay a natural toy, which they manipulate in a way developmentally parallel to drawing (i.e., first the head, then the body, and so on). The elderly have sensory losses that can both enhance or cause endangerment through clay work. Ceramic clay is inexpensive, however, the kiln, kiln wiring, and kiln furniture to hold pieces being fired can be major expenses (Drake, 1999).

COMPUTER CRAFTS

Most new computers already come equipped with a graphics drawing program. Graphics programs come in all levels of complexity. Some are for people who like to draw freehand. Others are predrawn images assembled like a collage. Computer crafts are especially helpful for those patients whose self-image is tied to the age of information technology. Journal writing, poetry writing, and other forms of expressive language are easy on the computer. There are programs for music composition and programs for assisting children to create stories. If scanners are available, computers can be used in conjunction with photography. Many skills can be the focus of treatment while using a mouse, a trackball, or a joystick to control the pictures (Cook & Hussey, 2002). Screen magnifiers and enlargers assist the visually impaired.

FOUND MATERIALS

In many situations, therapists are called upon to improvise with available noncommercial materials that were not intended for crafts. These could include household items like empty containers, natural materials such as pinecones, scraps of cloth, paper, or small metal items. The found items can be assembled into wall decorations, sculptures, mobiles, puppets, or decorated containers. The possibilities are limited only by the creativity of the therapist and the patient and availability of glue, staples, string, and tape. Therapists have always resorted to found materials when their budget did not provide for more expensive supplies. The capability to see possibilities in the humblest materials is the skill of a superior therapist.

OTHER CRAFTS

Some departments have a category of crafts called "minor media." This usually includes decorative processes not included in the above categories. Some of these are printing, which includes silkscreen, linoleum blocks, and vegetable prints; decoupage, in which pictures are glued to wooden plaques; suncatchers, which are small transparent window decorations; and other specialty crafts. New products are developed constantly. This by no means covers all the craft possibilities. An alert therapist keeps his or her eyes open for such new treatment options for patients. Some places to look for these new ideas are in home magazines, the craft-book section of bookstores, craft catalogues, home decorating programs on television, on the Internet, and from other therapists.

MISCELLANEOUS MEDIA

Therapists have often used creative media, some of which are called crafts, to elicit from patients their own creative impulses. Some of these crafts are face-painting, clowning, pantomime, and magic. Another kind of media that encourages creativity is noncompetitive games, which get people to think in new cooperative ways about how to solve problems. Some of these games can be played on the playground and some on board games. These games help people have fun without the pressure to win. All these media help people approach their problems in new ways.

SUMMARY

Crafts continue to offer patients the opportunity to see their work behavior as a microcosm of their way of being in the world. When patients hold up a completed project and proclaim, "I did this," therapists are able to give real praise for a job well done. If the craft project is not well done, the therapist can use it as a teaching opportunity to discuss how the experience of working on the craft mirrors the patient's experiences in life. The "doing" of crafts is a sample of the "doing" in life. To learn more about these benefits, read *Crafts in Therapy and Rehabilitation, Second Edition* (Drake, 1999).

LEARNING ACTIVITIES

1. Learn and then teach one craft from a selected list to the class.
2. With an extremely small budget ($3.00 per group of 8 to 10 people), lead a task group. The scenario is as follows: You have been asked to lead a holiday group for 8 people in a community setting that not only has no OT services but has no budget for supplies for groups. If the administrator likes what she sees, she will consider giving you a budget in the future. The group room has 2 pencils, 2 pens, 1 pair of scissors, 1 mixing bowl, and 1 wooden spoon. You have $3.00 to buy everything else. If you buy glue for $1.00 but only use half, it still counts as $1.00. Paper or photocopies are 5 cents each. Recycled soda-pop cans are 5 cents. Free things such as newspaper, tin cans, pinecones, or paper bags are considered free only if everyone can get them free (i.e., fabric your mother was tossing out is not considered free). You may not bring anything from home unless it is part of your budget. *Editor's note:* I have done this task for many years and each year a few students surprise me with their creativity even with my craft experience.

REFERENCES

American Occupational Therapy Association. (2002). Occupational therapy practice framework: Domain and process. *American Journal of Occupational Therapy, 56*, 609-639.

Atwal, A., Owen, S., & Davies, R. (2003). Struggling for occupational satisfaction: Older people in care homes. *British Journal of Occupational Therapy, 66*, 118-124.

Boyer, J., Colman, W., Levy, L., & Manoly, B. (1989). Affective responses to activities: A comparative analysis. *American Journal of Occupational Therapy, 43*, 81-88.

Carter, B. A., Nelson, D. L., & Duncombe, L. W. (1983). The effects of psychological type on the mood and meaning of two collage activities. *American Journal of Occupational Therapy, 37*, 688-693.

Cook, A. M., & Hussey, S. M. (2002). *Assistive technologies: Principles and practice.* St. Louis: Mosby.

Dickerson, A., & Kaplan, S. H. (1991). A comparison of craft use and academic preparation in craft modalities. *American Journal of Occupational Therapy, 45*, 11-17.

Dickie, V. A. (2003). Establishing worker identity: A study of people in craft work. *American Journal of Occupational Therapy, 57*, 250-261.

Dierks, L. (1994) *Creative clay jewelry: Designs to make from polymer clay.* Ashville, NC: Lark Books.

Drake, M. (1999). *Crafts in therapy and rehabilitation* (2nd ed.). Thorofare, NJ: SLACK Incorporated.

Duncan, S. J. (1986). Knitting device for bilateral upper extremity amputee. *American Journal of Occupational Therapy, 40*, 637-638.

Gourley, M. (2000). Center for occupational therapy and lifestyle redesign. *OT Practice, 5*, 18-19.

Griffiths, S. (2002). Focus on research… The clinical utility of creative activities used as an occupational therapy treatment medium for people with mental health problems. *British Journal of Occupational Therapy, 65*, 226.

EVIDENCE-BASED TREATMENT STRATEGIES

Treatment Strategies	Authors
Pediatrics	Hardison & Llorens, 1988; Kleinman & Stalcup, 1991
Geriatrics	Atwal, Owen, & Davies, 2003; Lushbough, Priddy, Sewell, Lovett, & Jones, 1988; Perrin, 2001
Physically handicapped	Duncan, 1986; Matsushima, 1986
Mental health	Boyer, Colman, Levy, & Manoly, 1989; Haiman, 1989; Klyczek & Mann, 1986; Kremer & Nelson, 1984; Marer, 2002; Perrin, 2001; Rocker & Nelson, 1987; Steffan & Nelson, 1987
Gender	Dickie, 2003; Taylor, 2003
General	Boyer et al., 1989; Carter, Nelson, & Duncombe, 1983; Dickie, 2003; Gourley, 2000; Griffiths, 2002; Haiman, 1989; Holder, 2001; Katz & Cohen, 1991; Marer, 2002; Murphy, Trombly, Tickle-Degnen, & Jacobs, 1999; Rocker & Nelson, 1987; Steffan & Nelson, 1987

Haiman, S. (1989). Preface: Selecting group protocols: Recipe or reasoning. *Occupational Therapy in Mental Health, 9,* 1-14.

Hardison, J., & Llorens, L. A. (1988). Structured craft group activities for adolescent delinquent girls. *Occupational Therapy in Mental Health, 8,* 101-117.

Holder, V. (2001). The use of creative activities within occupational therapy. *British Journal of Occupational Therapy, 64,* 103-105.

Katz, N., & Cohen, E. (1991). Meaning ascribed to four craft activities before and after extensive learning. *Occupational Therapy Journal of Research, 11,* 24-39.

Kleinman, B. L., & Stalcup, A. (1991). The effect of graded craft activities on visuomotor integration in an inpatient child psychiatry population. *American Journal of Occupational Therapy, 45,* 324-330.

Klyczek, J. P., & Mann, W. C. (1986). Therapeutic modality comparisons in day treatment. *American Journal of Occupational Therapy, 40,* 606-611.

Kremer, E. R. H., & Nelson, D. L. (1984). Effects of selected activities on affective meaning in psychiatric patients. *American Journal of Occupational Therapy, 38,* 522-528.

Lushbough, R. S., Priddy, J. M., Sewell, H. H., Lovett, S. B., & Jones, T. C. (1988). The effectiveness of an occupational therapy program in an inpatient geropsychiatric setting. *Physical Occupational Therapy in Geriatrics, 6,* 63-73.

Marer, E. (2002). Knitting: The new yoga. *Health, 16,* 76-80.

Matsushima, D. S. (1986). Crotchet aide for the amputee. *American Journal of Occupational Therapy, 40,* 495-496.

Murphy, S., Trombly, C., Tickle-Degnen, L., & Jacobs, K. (1999). The effect of keeping an end-product on intrinsic motivation. *American Journal of Occupational Therapy, 53,* 153-158.

Perrin, T. (2001). Don't despise the fluffy bunny: A reflection from practice. *British Journal of Occupational Therapy, 64,* 129-134.

Rocker, J. D., & Nelson, D. L. (1987). Affective responses to keeping and not keeping an activity product. *American Journal of Occupational Therapy, 41,* 152-157.

Steffan, J. A., & Nelson, D. L. (1987). The effects of tool scarcity on group climate and affective meaning within the context of a stenciling activity. *American Journal of Occupational Therapy, 41,* 449-453.

Taylor, J. (2003). Women's leisure activities, their social stereotypes and some implications for identity. *British Journal of Occupational Therapy, 66,* 151-158.

Taylor, E., & Manguno, J. (1991). Use of treatment activities in occupational therapy. *American Journal of Occupational Therapy, 45,* 317-322.

Key Concepts

- Equipment clinical reasoning: Thinking that evaluates equipment procedurally, interactively, and conditionally.
- Precautions: Factors that consider safety first.
- Characteristics of good construction: Solid design, ease of use, comfort, acceptable to user.
- Equipment design process: Steps involved in developing new adaptive equipment.
- Presentation and follow-up: Education and review of equipment use.

Essential Vocabulary

adaptive equipment: Devices used to allow performance of a functional task.
bolsters: Soft therapeutic equipment that provides support under a child's axilla in the prone position.
clinical reasoning process: A type of thinking used in clinical work.
cost-effective: Equipment that is worthwhile to make considering the therapist's time and materials involved.
Cowan stabilizing pillow: An example of an adaptive device that assists a child's balance or stability when sitting.
half-lapboard: An example of an adaptive device that provides support to a client's hemiplegic arm.
life tasks: Daily activities.
specific needs: Activities the client requires in daily life.
trial use: An established period of time when equipment may be applied and evaluated as to its effectiveness.

Assistive Technology and Adaptive Equipment

Mary Kathryn Cowan, MA, OTR, FAOTA and Beth O'Sullivan, MPH, OTR

Introduction

A critical role that OT practitioners play is to assist clients in obtaining and maintaining individual occupational roles and interests. With advances in technology and the sciences, the OT profession has been able to utilize and merge technological knowledge and development into clinical practice.

The term *adaptive equipment* has been used throughout the course of OT and rehabilitation history to describe assistive devices, aids, or equipment that allow a person with a disability to perform an occupational activity that otherwise would have been difficult or impossible. Although a variety of equipment is available for purchase, time constraints, budget limitations, reimbursement problems, and/or the uniqueness of a specific participation problem may require the construction of special devices to suit a particular situation. Recently, the OT profession has incorporated the term *assistive technology* to describe any identified piece of equipment or system utilized to improve, maintain, or increase an individual's functional ability to perform areas of occupation (AOTA, 2002).

Assistive technology is selected or designed and constructed when an individual cannot perform a life task or area of occupation without some form of assistance. Appropriate aids are needed when problems with postural control, reaching, grasping, or accessing materials interfere with active participation in meaningful occupational activities. Many individuals whose intervention plan includes the possible use of assistive technology may also have goals to improve the very abilities that interfere with performance skills as well. Either on a temporary or long-term basis, change in performance skills that underlie the areas of occupation may not be extensive enough to allow independence in some activities. Assistive technology may then fill the need for this individual. By increasing the individual's independence in important life skills (i.e., activities that must be accomplished for successful living throughout the life span) and roles through use of assistive devices, a sense of achievement and satisfaction can be realized (AOTA, 2004).

Individually constructed equipment may be as simple as using a waxed paper container to hold playing cards ("low tech") or as complex as the design and use of computerized environmental control systems ("high tech"). Whether simple or complex, the focus of this chapter is to acquaint the reader with principles of selection, design, and construction that usually guide a therapist in solving a functional problem with the use of assistive technology.

Historical Uses

The earliest forms of adaptive equipment in OT included page turners, card holders, and nailboards, which allowed the person with a handicap to read a book without using his or her hands, to play cards with only one hand, and to peel a fruit or vegetable when the person did not have use of a stabilizing hand, respectively. Although adaptive equipment was originally developed to provide improved ability to perform ADL and participate in leisure pursuits, it also became commonly used as a term to apply to therapy equipment that is used to develop a person's abilities or skills in therapy. Eventually balance boards, bolsters, standing tables, prone boards, and related equipment were designed and used by one or several therapists before they became standard pieces of therapy equipment.

Therapist-made equipment was a necessity for many years and only in recent OT history have many of these innovations been mass produced, marketed through catalogs, and readily available to OT personnel. When suitable equipment is available commercially, the device must still be carefully selected. This availability of equipment from catalogs does not rule out the need for individually constructed equipment. The unique needs of the individual may require the design and construction of a device that is not commercially available or is too costly to purchase. These situations require the OT or OTA to use problem-solving skills to determine the relationship between the individual's motor skill problem and the life task that needs to be accomplished, then design and construct a helpful tool to make participation possible. These skills include studying the situation that presents uncertainty or doubt and arriving at the most appropriate solution. The process involves definition, selection of a plan, organizing steps, implementing the plan, and evaluating the results.

Occupational Therapy Personnel Roles

The *OT Roles* paper (AOTA, 1999) describes the OTA's role in program planning as dependent upon establishing service competency by the OT. Designing and constructing a positioning device for a child with CP based on the theoretical principles of neurodevelopmental treatment is an example in which OT supervision is required. A therapist with this specialized training should decide if the design and the final product do indeed fulfill the principles and intent of this therapeutic approach. A neonatal positioner that is based on such principles as well as use in a complex therapeutic environment (the neonatal intensive care unit) is another example of adaptive equipment selection or construction that requires close supervision by the OT (Monfort & Case-Smith, 1997). Frequently, the OTA who works closely with an OT in a complex treatment setting may be the individual with the most knowledge of tools and equipment and, therefore, the one who will actually construct the needed equipment once the OT/OTA team has determined the need and type of equipment required. Equipment developed in these situations requires that the OT establish the OTA's service competency, as the performance components involved need ongoing interpretation.

The OTA working in a setting where chronic conditions are prevalent is continually dealing with recurring functional problems that may not require the OT's clinical involvement in the adaptive equipment decision-making process. The selection, design, and construction of card holders, book holders, and built-up handles on recreational games for people with physical handicaps are examples of situations in which the OTA would not require close supervision. This type of equipment may be part of a generally accepted routine.

Selecting, designing, and constructing adaptive equipment at various levels can be a collaborative effort between the OTA and the OT, but it must also be emphasized that the client is the third partner in this collaboration. The individual receiving treatment will often exhibit or describe a problem that creates a need for adaptive equipment. The user gives the OT or OTA feedback on fit and comfort. Finally, the user determines the ultimate effectiveness and usefulness of the item by choosing to use it or not.

Selection of Adaptive Equipment— Clinical Reasoning Process

A study by Gitlin and Burgh (1995) involved focus groups of OTs who decided on client needs for adaptive equipment in order to determine the methods of clinical reasoning used by OTs. It was determined that the methods used were procedural (concrete steps and procedures implemented by the therapist), interactive (interacting with the client to individualize the treatment), and conditional reasoning (developing a comprehensive understanding of client's situation and potential for change). The following steps were used by therapists in this study when selecting adaptive equipment.

1. Selecting a device—Involved consideration of many factors, which were either (Figure 32-1):
   - Client-focused (client status and characteristics, role history, activity level, and performance goals)
   - External (physical and emotional environmental support factors)

2. Fitting a device to an activity—Issuing a device involved selecting an activity that had meaning to the individual or would match the client's cognitive and functional abilities in order to ensure the success of the device and its acceptance (Watson & Wilson, 2003).

3. Determining the best time to introduce a device—Often decided based on the stability of the client's condition, the client's readiness to accept the use of a device, and the future involvement of the client in rehabilitation services after leaving their facility.

4. Choice of an instructional site—Depends on the activity selected (a device used for independence in dressing might be demonstrated on the ward instead of the clinic area). Consideration for the individual's privacy in trying a new piece of equipment was often made.

5. Instruction in use—Approaches to instruction might include describing the use of the device by other individuals with similar problems, use of group training, role modeling by another client, verbal instruction, and inclusion of a family member in instruction. An exploratory study of elderly clients who were taught to use bathing and dressing devices showed that those clients "most satisfied" with the device had greater knowledge of its use (Schemm & Gitlin, 1998). Lack of knowledge about a device or inadequate instruction can be reasons clients do not continue to use a device (Finlayson & Havixbeck, 1992; Neville-Jan, Piersol, Kielhofner, & Davis, 1993).

6. Reinforcement of device use—Included providing opportunities for independent use, convincing staff in the rehabilitation setting of its location and importance, and educating the family (Gitlin & Burgh, 1995).

Whether a piece of adaptive equipment is temporary or permanent, it should meet a specific need for the individual. Unnecessary use of specialized equipment has the potential for making any person feel additionally or visibly "handicapped." Therefore, it is important for the OT/OTA team to ascertain that the individual meets the following criteria:

- Unable to complete the task without the use of an aid.
- Understands the need for additional equipment.
- Is agreeable to trial or long-term use of the needed equipment (Stark, 2004).

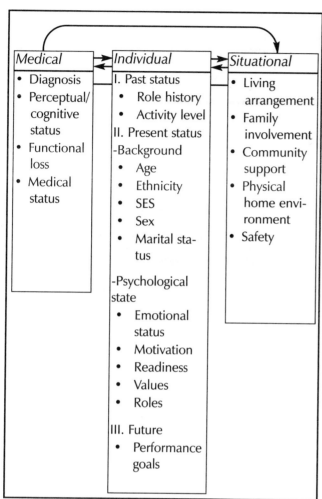

Figure 32-1. Twenty-two factors that therapists considered in selecting and training clients in adaptive equipment (SES = socioeconomic status). (Reprinted with permission from Gitlin, L. N., & Burgh, D. [1995]. Issuing assistive devices to older patients in rehabilitation: An exploratory study. *American Journal of Occupational Therapy, 49*[10], 996.)

Constructing Adaptive Equipment—Precautions

Whether a device is commercially available or constructed by the OT/OTA team, safety is a constant and essential concern. When the equipment is not available commercially and must be constructed, safety is determined during 3 stages of the process of development:

1. Design
2. Construction
3. Use

When designing equipment, safety must be considered so that time in construction is not wasted on a piece of equipment rendered useless later when it is discovered to be unsafe. In this context, safety refers specifically to the employment of measures necessary to prevent the occurrence of injury or loss of function. Some questions the OT or OTA should ask during the design phase are:

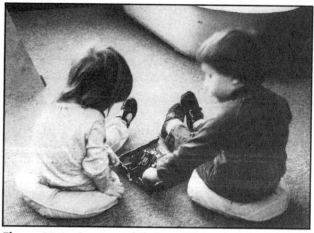

Figure 32-2. Cowan stabilizing pillow.

- Will a breakdown of materials from ordinary wear cause discomfort or injury?
- Will the shape of the equipment interfere with safe use of any other equipment regularly used, such as a wheelchair or crutches?

When constructing adaptive equipment, safety problems can be anticipated by eliminating rough finishes on wood, metal, or plastic and by sanding all surfaces, edges, and corners smoothly to prevent splinters, cuts, and bruises. It is also important to use nontoxic finishes, particularly for equipment used by children who might be likely to mouth or chew objects.

Instructing the client, family, and caretakers in safe usage of equipment is the final step in making safe equipment. Observing the individual using the equipment and discussing with him or her where, when, and how to use it properly alerts the person to any possible misuse, and therefore unsafe use, of equipment made by OT personnel.

Characteristics of Well-Constructed Adaptive Equipment

Simplicity in Design

A simple design facilitates the construction of the device and increases the likelihood of it being used more frequently. An example is provided in Figure 32-2, which shows the Cowan stabilizing pillow, an adaptive pillow for children who have balance problems when sitting on the floor (Cowan, 1988). The design's simplicity (8 sections of cloth, sewing of simple seams, filling with styrofoam pellets) makes it possible for others such as therapists, assistants, volunteers, teachers, or parents to make more pillows when recommended for other children (Figure 32-3). The chance of the next item being made improperly is also reduced by having a simple design. Because a small, soft pillow is easily transported and easily stored in a corner of the classroom, both children and teachers will be more likely to use it. If the stabilizing seat had been made from a more complicated

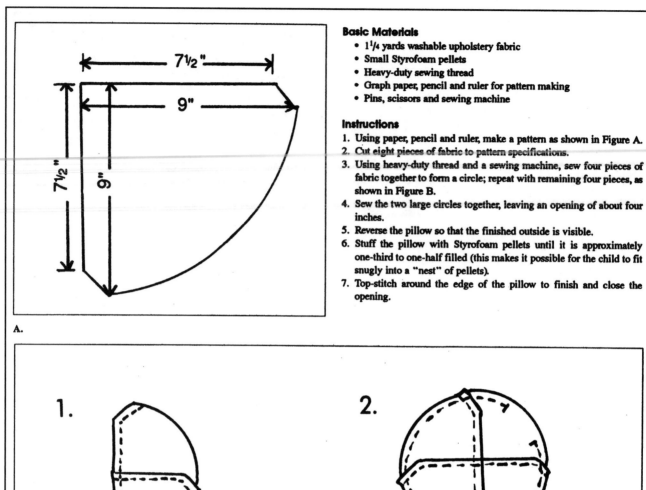

Basic Materials
- 1¼ yards washable upholstery fabric
- Small Styrofoam pellets
- Heavy-duty sewing thread
- Graph paper, pencil and ruler for pattern making
- Pins, scissors and sewing machine

Instructions

1. Using paper, pencil and ruler, make a pattern as shown in Figure A.
2. Cut eight pieces of fabric to pattern specifications.
3. Using heavy-duty thread and a sewing machine, sew four pieces of fabric together to form a circle; repeat with remaining four pieces, as shown in Figure B.
4. Sew the two large circles together, leaving an opening of about four inches.
5. Reverse the pillow so that the finished outside is visible.
6. Stuff the pillow with Styrofoam pellets until it is approximately one-third to one-half filled (this makes it possible for the child to fit snugly into a "nest" of pellets).
7. Top-stitch around the edge of the pillow to finish and close the opening.

Figure 32-3. Instructions for constructing a Cowan stabilizing pillow.

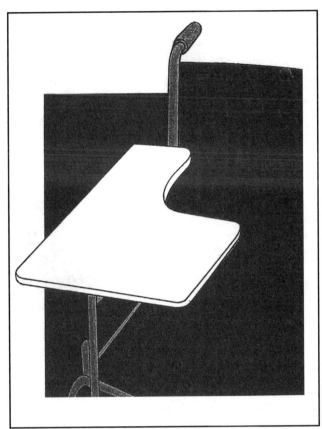

Figure 32-4. Wheelchair half-lapboard. (Adapted from Walsh, M. [1987]. Brief or new: Half-lapboard for hemiplegic patients. *American Journal of Occupational Therapy, 41*, 533-535.)

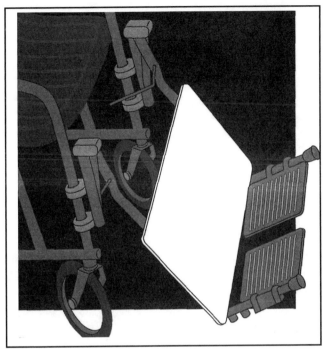

Figure 32-5. Calf board. (Adapted from Chandler, D., & Knackert, B. [1997]. Positioners for wheelchairs in long-term care facilities. *American Journal of Occupational Therapy, 51*, 921-924.)

design (e.g., a metal and leather seat with a backrest), it would be more difficult to make, move, store, and use.

Controlling the Size of Equipment

It is important that the size of equipment be limited so that it does not become awkward or cumbersome to use. An example of this might be carrying devices for wheelchairs, such as lapboards or trays, armrests, and back pockets. Although anyone in a wheelchair may want to carry large items occasionally, making the tray or pocket too large may make daily use of the wheelchair cumbersome. The half-lapboard for clients with hemiplegia, shown in Figure 32-4, demonstrates this principle by having a surface large enough to support the person's hemiplegic arm without having the surface extending out to either side (Walsh, 1987). This thoughtful consideration allows the person in the wheelchair to avoid bumping into objects and people with extra or unnecessary tray extensions, and also allows adequate space to transfer in and out of the chair. (See Walsh [1987] for specific information on how to construct this equipment.) Another example of this principle is the calf board in Figure 32-5 (Chandler & Knackert, 1997) designed to keep elderly nursing home residents' feet and legs from slipping off their wheelchair foot rests and thus causing poor position as well as skin tears on feet and ankles from rubbing against the metal edges of the foot

rests. The calf board clips on to the vertical supports of the foot rests with just enough soft surface to support and maintain the legs and feet in correct position, in this way preventing foot slippage backward. (See Chandler and Knackert [1997] for specific information on how to construct this equipment.)

Consideration of Cost of Materials and Construction Time

If a piece of adaptive technology requires expensive materials or if it takes a long time to make, the item is no longer cost-effective. The hourly wages of the OT and OTA, as well as the cost of the materials, must be considered. Many hours of therapy time spent constructing one piece of equipment may increase the cost of that equipment to such a point that purchasing a similar item may prove less expensive, as well as a better use of valuable clinic time.

The inexpensive bolsters shown in Figure 32-6 are designed for use with children under 3 years and demonstrate the use of economical materials. Mary Clark, an OTA in Portland, OR, uses vinyl or oilcloth for the covering and lightly rolled newspapers for the interior (Clark, 1990). The seam on the outside is closed with cloth tape. Larger bolsters can be made by taping empty 3-pound coffee cans together, covering them with 1-inch foam, and then adding an outside cover of vinyl (Clark, 1990). She has also used large cardboard tubes from carpet rolls to provide the inner shape of the bolster, adding a layer of foam followed by a vinyl covering to create the finished equipment (Clark, 1990). All of these bolsters involve the use of economical materials and require very reasonable construction time.

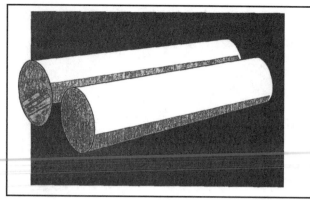

Figure 32-6. Bolsters. (Courtesy of M. Clark.)

Because the bolsters are inexpensive, they can be provided to many families. In this way, it is possible to leave assistive technology in a home, a practice that is often not possible when similar commercially made but more expensive bolsters are used.

Attractive Appearance

An unattractive piece of equipment, no matter how useful, can interfere with its potential use. People do not like to use equipment that is roughly made, battered from use, or that has unappealing surfaces. For example, a waxpaper box makes a quick and easy piece of adaptive equipment for the one-handed card player. By covering the box with attractive vinyl shelf paper or other washable, durable material, it is not only useful but pleasant to look at.

Figure 32-7 shows an example of a make-up board designed for use by women with quadriplegia (Hague, 1988). It is simple in design and attractive without being medical or therapeutic in appearance and would be a natural addition to a woman's bedroom. (See Hague [1988] for specific instructions on how to make this equipment.)

Safety in Use

Although safety as a principle has already been addressed, it is an essential characteristic of well-constructed adaptive equipment that cannot be overemphasized. For example, if a stabilizer for a bowl or a pan used on the stove is not predictably stable (i.e., it can become easily detached from the surface), it can cause spilling of hot liquids onto the homemaker. Although the equipment may serve a purpose for the individual with the use of only one hand, it can create a danger that could be avoided by more careful design and construction.

Comfort in Use

The comfort of the user is affected by the placement of the equipment when it is used, materials that touch the user's body in some way, and a comfortable fit when the item is worn by the user. A handle that requires the fit of a hand grasp or a situation in which the body or extremities are resting on the equipment are examples that illustrate the need to consider user comfort.

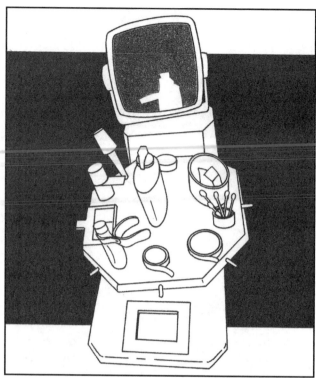

Figure 32-7. Make-up board. (Adapted from Hague, G. [1988]. Brief or new: Makeup board for women with quadriplegia. *American Journal of Occupational Therapy, 42,* 253-255.)

An example of this principle is the foam positioning device shown in Figure 32-8 (von Funk, 1989). Because it uses soft foam as a basic material, it appears to be comfortable for long periods of contact with the skin, particularly when the person is immobile. (See von Funk [1989] for specific instructions on how to make this equipment.) Possible allergy to any substance used in making equipment for a specific individual or groups of individuals should be checked. Children with spina bifida, for example, are known to have allergies to latex materials, which should not be used in any of their adaptive devices (Scoggin & Parks, 1997).

Ease in Application and Use

The ultimate test of the ease in application and usage principle is to determine if the client can apply the device to him- or herself independently. If this is not the case, the individual(s) responsible for assisting the client must be familiar with its proper positioning and use. The knitting device designed for use by a client with a bilateral UE amputation shown in Figure 32-9 is a good example (Duncan, 1986). The piece of equipment requires the use of a C-clamp and wing nuts (both of which the client can manage with the bilateral prosthesis) to attach the device to the table and tighten or loosen the tension on the yarn. (See Duncan [1986] for specific information about how to construct this equipment.)

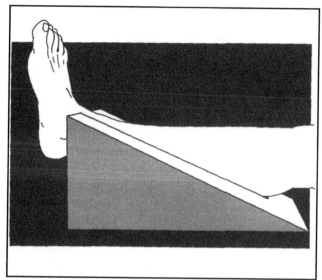

Figure 32-8. Foam positioning device. (Adapted from von Funk, M. [1989]. Positioning device has multiple benefits for patients. *Advance for Occupational Therapists, 13*, 13.)

Ease in Maintenance and Cleaning

Simplicity in the design and choice of materials for any device makes it easier to maintain and clean. A simple design eliminates corners, holes, and crevices that collect debris that is difficult to remove. If the equipment is to be used with people who have infections or are highly susceptible to infection, the construction materials must withstand the intense steam or hot water required for adequate removal of bacteria. Most clinics or schools require that all equipment be washed or cleaned period ically to promote normal infection control. Nonporous surfaces such as plastic and metal are less likely to retain dirt or agents that cause infection, and heavier, porous fabrics that can be washed easily (e.g., upholstery fabric) are recommended.

DESIGNING ADAPTIVE EQUIPMENT

A Problem-Solving Process

The design of every adaptive device begins with a therapist, assistant, and the client facing a deficit in function together in a thoughtful, problem-solving process. If the client is unable to participate in an activity or attain the position necessary for optimal work or task completion, new methods are tried and catalogs are perused for available equipment likely to alleviate the problem. In some instances, the problem will be solved only by designing a new piece of equipment.

Use of Patterns

Very early in the process of designing equipment, a pattern can be developed to guide the construction process. The Cowan stabilizing pillow (see Figure 32-2) provides a useful example.

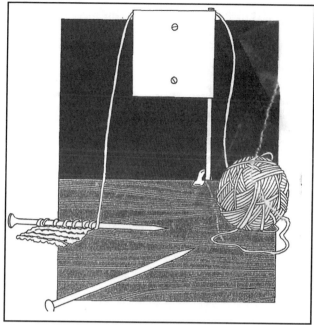

Figure 32-9. Knitting device for amputees. (Adapted from Duncan, S. [1986]. Brief or new: Knitting device for bilateral upper extremity amputee. *American Journal of Occupational Therapy, 40*, 637-638.)

One-quarter of one surface of the pillow was drawn on graph paper to establish the necessary size and shape. The paper pattern was then checked in relation to the client's body or body part, and any necessary adjustments were made. All of the other examples shown in various figures in this chapter required a basic pattern for construction. Making a pattern is an important step in the problem-solving process, as it guides the OT or OTA in estimating size and shape of the piece of adaptive equipment. Errors in the construction phase will be reduced, thus increasing efficiency and reducing the cost of production.

Constructing a Model

Once a pattern has been developed, the next step is to construct the first model or prototype of the device. This step allows the client and the OT or OTA to discuss and experiment with changes in the design. This first model should be viewed as flexible and malleable, as well as experimental. At this point, the shape of the pattern can be changed, new materials can be tried, and dimensions can be altered.

Redesign After Trials

After any necessary redesign, the client begins to use the piece of equipment. Some new problems may arise at this stage that inform the client and OT personnel of changes that may need to be made. Only through a longer period of trial use can all of the client's needs in regard to use of an adaptive device become completely clear. In trial use, a piece of equipment is repeatedly used in order to ensure its effectiveness.

Fabricating Assistive Technology Devices

Materials

This chapter does not present a complete list of materials and their characteristics for use in fabricating adaptive equipment; however, the following characteristics are examples of those that should be considered when evaluating or selecting materials:

- Softness and pliability of shape—Necessary for pillows, slings, positioning equipment. Use cloth, canvas, or webbing; lamb's wool or "moleskin" for surface coverage; styrofoam pellets, cotton baton, foam rubber, or polyfoam for fillers.
- Resilience and pliability of shape—Needed for positioning devices. Use splinting materials such as Orthoplast (Johnson & Johnson, New Brunswick, NJ), tri-wall, acetate film, leather, rubber, or vinyl.
- Strength, solidity, and weight—Needed for laptrays, wheelchair arm supports, stabilizing equipment. Use wood, metal, hard plastics, or formica.

Tools

The materials chosen will determine the tools required to fabricate any piece of equipment. For example, cloth requires scissors and a sewing machine; splinting materials require scissors and a heating device; and the use of wood, metal, or plastic requires hand tools or power shop equipment during the construction process. The availability of tools and the OT's or OTA's skill in using tools contributes to the quality of the finished product.

Finishing

The final step in the construction of equipment is finishing. This step is of primary importance when one considers the emotional impact of equipment use for some clients. Rough or sharp surfaces and edges need to be sanded and rounded. Extraneous threads and uneven seams need to be trimmed and repaired. Finishes such as polyurethane varnish or nontoxic paint need to be applied to wooden objects. Colors selected may be neutral to de-emphasize the equipment or bright and colorful to make equipment more attractive. The work of finishing adaptive equipment, like making furniture for a home, merits fine workmanship with attention to important details so that the product is both professional and attractive.

Presentation of Constructed Equipment

Whether or not the use of the designed and constructed adaptive equipment has been part of the collaboration process, the OT or OTA should review the following information with the client when it is completed:

- Purpose
- Uses
- Limitations
- Care and maintenance
- Any precautions

Even a young child needs to know that the stabilizing pillow "helps you sit better or longer" (see Figure 32-2). The adult should know that the half-lapboard shown in Figure 32-4 places his or her affected arm in view to improve body awareness, control swelling, and prevent injury to an arm that lacks sensation. This review of the purposes of the equipment encourages proper use and, therefore, greater likelihood of its success. If the adaptive device is to be applied by another individual (nurse, aide, teacher, or parent), the details of proper application and positioning must be presented to avoid any discomfort to the client and to ensure safe use. On hospital and rehabilitation center departments, in classrooms, and in other community settings where several people assist the individual with equipment use, the placement of a diagram or picture of the equipment properly set up can be attached to the device as a helpful reference.

Documentation of Effectiveness of Design

The final step when constructing an assistive technology device is to follow up, checking with the modification of the device or improvement of its design for optimal function. If a particular device is used by many people, all of them should be followed and the fulfillment of the original purpose of the equipment validated with every individual. Questions such as the following can then be asked:

- How many individuals have used the device?
- For what length of time?
- How successfully did it fulfill its purpose?
- Should any modifications be made?

Compilation of this information will inform the OTA and OT who design and construct assistive technology whether the equipment's purpose is confirmed. If the equipment is also accepted and used by several clients, it may be timely to share this information with other OTs and OTAs through professional publication in journals and newsletters, as the examples provided in this chapter demonstrate. It is even possible to consider pursuing presentation to companies who manufacture adaptive equipment so that it becomes easily and commercially available.

Summary

Construction of assistive technology is addressed within the whole continuum of selection, design, and construction that is a part of the OT process of problem solving and clinical reasoning. A definition of adaptive equipment and assistive technology is given, together with significant historical uses of such devices. The role of the OT/OTA team was presented to inform the reader of the areas of supervision, collaboration, and independent work. Principles are delineated for determining need, selecting, designing, fabricating, presenting the device to the user, and follow-up. Important precautions and safety measures are stressed. Examples of well-constructed adaptive equipment are used to illustrate important considerations.

LEARNING ACTIVITIES

1. Describe the clinical reasoning process used in the selection of adaptive equipment.

2. Study the characteristics of well-constructed adaptive equipment. Working with a classmate or peer, view at least 5 pieces of adaptive equipment constructed by OTs or OTAs (visit clinics and use journal/magazine articles). Determine which characteristics are present and which are not.

3. Construct one of the pieces of adaptive equipment presented in this chapter.

4. Role play the process of instruction involved in presenting a piece of adaptive equipment to a client.

5. Design a piece of adaptive equipment for a problem seen during your clinic observations. First, look over equipment catalogs to see if there is any equipment commercially available to meet the client's need.

REFERENCES

American Occupational Therapy Association. (1999). *OT roles*. Bethesda, MD: Author.

American Occupational Therapy Association. (2002). Occupational therapy practice framework: Domain and process. *American Journal of Occupational Therapy, 56*, 609-639.

American Occupational Therapy Association. (2004). *The reference manual of official documents of the american occupational therapy association 10th ed*. Bethesda, MD: Author.

Chandler, D., & Knackert, B. (1997). Positioners for wheelchairs in long-term care facilities. *American Journal of Occupational Therapy, 51*, 921-924.

Cowan, M. K. (1988). Pillow helps keep young OT clients "stabilized." *OT Week, 2*(19), 5.

Duncan, S. (1986). Brief or new: Knitting device for bilateral upper extremity amputee. *American Journal of Occupational Therapy, 40*, 637-638.

Finlayson, M., & Havixbeck, K. (1992). A post-discharge study on the use of assistive devices. *Canadian Journal of Occupational Therapy, 59*, 201-207.

Gitlin, L. N., & Burgh, D. (1995). Issuing assistive devices to older patients in rehabilitation: An exploratory study. *American Journal of Occupational Therapy, 49*, 994-1000.

Hague, G. (1988). Brief or new: Makeup board for women with quadriplegia. *American Journal of Occupational Therapy, 42*, 253-255.

Monfort, K., & Case-Smith, J. (1997). The effects of a neonatal positioner on scapular rotation. *American Journal of Occupational Therapy, 51*, 378-384.

Neville-Jan, A., Piersol, C. V., Kielhofner, G., & Davis, K. (1993). Adaptive equipment: A study of utilization after discharge. *OT in Health Care, 8*(4), 3-18.

Schemm, R. L., & Gitlin, L. N. (1998). How OTs teach older patients to use bathing devices in rehabilitation. *American Journal of Occupational Therapy, 52*, 276-282.

Scoggin, A. E., & Parks, K. M. (1997). Latex sensitivity in children with spina bifida: Implications for occupational therapy practitioners. *American Journal of Occupational Therapy, 51*, 608-611.

Stark, S., (2004). Removing environmental barriers in the homes of older adults with disabilities improves occupational performance. *Occupational Therapy Journal of Research, 24*, 32-39.

von Funk, M. (1989). Positioning device has multiple benefits for patients. *Advance for Occupational Therapists, 13*, 13.

Walsh, M. (1987). Brief or new: Half-lapboard for hemiplegic patients. *American Journal of Occupational Therapy, 41*, 533-535.

Watson, D., & Wilson, S. (2003) *Task analysis: An individual population approach* (2nd ed.). Bethesda, MD: American Occupational Therapy Association.

Key Concepts

- Biomechanical model of practice: The treatment approach that deals with increasing strength, endurance, and ROM.
- Purpose and type of splints: The classification of splints according to their design and intended outcome.
- Biomechanical and anatomical principles of splinting: The use of splints to improve strength, ROM, and function of the hand through the selective application of force.
- Assessment: The process to determine if the client is a good candidate for a splint and what type of splint is appropriate for his or her particular problem.
- Fabrication techniques: Steps in splint construction.
- Client education: Process to ensure that the client understands the purpose of the splint, wearing schedule, and precautions.
- Follow-up procedures: Scheduled appointment to reassess for fit, comfort, progress, and need for adjustments.

Essential Vocabulary

bony prominence: Area where bone is close to the skin surface.
dynamic splint: Splint that has moveable components.
effects of force: The effect that materials have upon bone and tissue.
functional position: Ideal position of the hand and wrist for effective prehension.
palmar arches: Natural curves in the palm created by the structure of joints, ligaments, and muscles.
prehension: To use the hand to hold or manipulate objects.
splint: External device used to treat extremity problems.
static splint: Splint that immobilizes and has no moving parts.
thermoplastic: Plastic-based material that is soft and pliable when warmed and hard when cooled.

Chapter 33

BASIC SPLINTING

Jaclyn West-Frasier, MA, OTR

INTRODUCTION

The human hand is an amazing tool that sets us apart from other animals on this planet. We use our hands while still in the womb and continue throughout our lifespan. Our hands allow us to explore the environment, communicate through gestures and touch, and create through such forms as art and architecture. Our hands are powerful enough to grasp a 100-pound barbell but gentle enough to wipe a tear from a child's cheek. On any given day an individual may use his or her hands to comb his or her hair, communicate by keyboard, greet someone with a handshake, or turn the pages of a novel.

OT practitioners are concerned with the individual's ability to successfully perform ADL, work activities, and leisure or play activities. The human hand plays an integral role in occupational performance and any impairment of the hand will affect function. OTs use the technology of UE splinting as one of the methods to restore or improve hand function. This chapter will provide basic information on hand splinting, including history, description of splints, principles of splinting, assessment, techniques of fabrication, and special considerations.

HISTORY

Splinting is a technology that has been used by OT practitioners for decades. The theoretical basis for splinting is derived from the biomechanical model of practice. OT practitioners apply the biomechanical model to those individuals who have limitations in movement, strength, and endurance that interfere with successful performance of occupational tasks. Biomechanical components of functional movement include joint ROM, muscle strength, and endurance. Intervention through this model can be described by 3 approaches:

1. Prevention of deformity through programs of ROM and positioning, which may include the use of static or dynamic splints.
2. Restoration of lost function through programs that gradually increase the demand for movement, strength, and endurance until the desired level of function is achieved.

3. Compensation for permanent or prolonged limitations through programs that involve altering procedures or methods to accomplish desired tasks, or using devices attached to the body or placed in the environment to assist with task performance (Kielhofner, 1992).

Splinting is a valuable tool the OT may use to help prevent or minimize deformity, correct impairment, and restore or improve function in the upper extremities. The process of splinting does require an in-depth understanding of normal hand function, pathologies that can limit hand function, and the biomechanical principles involved in splint design. Incorrect use of splinting principles can have a negative impact on the final outcome and actually create additional deformities and further loss of function. To develop basic splinting skills, the OTA should work closely with the OT. As the OTA grows in expertise, he or she can work more independently in the design and fabrication of splints. OTAs with a desire to become proficient in splinting should also participate in continuing education opportunities.

BASIC CONCEPTS

Purpose of Splints

Splints are external devices that are applied to treat UE and LE problems that result from injury, disease processes, birth defects, or the aging process (Fess & Kiel, 1998). Splints may serve one or more of the following functions:

- Promote healing through support, restriction of movement, or immobilization.
- Correct or prevent deformity.
- Provide or assist motion.
- Base upon which to attach an assistive device.

The ultimate goal of a splinting program is to improve or restore UE function, which allows the individual to regain independence in daily activities and resume occupational roles (Fess & Kiel, 1998). Samples of splint functions are presented in the following examples.

A surgeon may refer a patient to OT for splinting after carpal tunnel repair. The OT may provide a rigid lightweight splint that immobilizes the wrist but allows finger movement. The wrist splint protects the hand during the healing process but allows the individual to perform low stress activities. An individual with hemiplegia from a CVA may be provided with a resting hand splint to prevent loss of ROM and formation of contractures. The same splint may serve to protect the hand from injury if sensory loss occurred as a result of the stroke. An individual with weak extensors of the fingers after an injury may be provided with a splint that uses springs to assist the fingers to straighten after he or she releases an object. This splint will allow the individual to effectively use the hand during daily activities and at the same time maintain ROM. An individual with a SCI may wear a positioning hand splint that also allows for the attachment of assistive devices such as eating utensils or hygiene implements. He or she is not able to grasp an object due to loss of muscle function, but the splint attachment allows him or her to independently feed him- or herself and perform hygiene activities.

Types of Splints

The materials used for splint construction have increased in variety. In the early years, OTs used plaster cast material or high temperature plastic to construct their splints. The use of high temperature plastics involved the creation of a plaster mold of the client's extremity. The splint material was heated in an oven to reach moldable consistency and then draped to conform to the mold of the individual's body part. This process was expensive, time-consuming, and hazardous to the therapist who had to work with the highly heated material.

Low temperature plastics were introduced several decades ago. The therapist heats the material in hot water to soften, and then cools to a temperature tolerated by the client. The material is then draped and molded directly to the client's extremity. Today, therapists may select from a wide assortment of materials and splint designs. Therapists are able to create custom splints by creating a pattern and fabricating the piece with materials of their choice. Splints can be ordered already precut in common patterns that can be heated and molded to the individual patient. Prefabricated or ready-made splints can be ordered through a catalog. Prefabricated splints are made from a variety of materials such as high temperature plastic, low temperature plastics, and fabric such as neoprene and knit elastics. The therapist measures the client and orders the proper size splint (Fess & Kiel, 1998).

The types of splints can be categorized as follows:

- A static splint immobilizes a joint or part of extremity. The purpose of a static splint is to rest or protect during healing, reduce pain, or prevent contracture. An example of a static splint is a resting hand splint (Figure 33-1).

- A dynamic splint provides one or more of the following: increases PROM, assists with AROM, or substitutes for lost motion. A dynamic splint usually has a static base upon which a moveable component has been added. The moveable component may consist of elastic, rubber bands, or springs (Belkin & Yasunda, 2001). An example of a dynamic splint is a dynamic MP flexion splint (Figure 33-2).

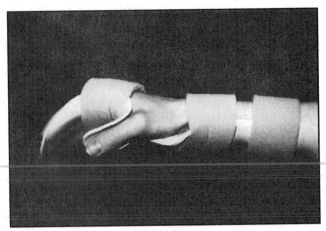

Figure 33-1. Resting hand splint.

PRINCIPLES OF SPLINTING

Hand Function

Hand function is dependent upon the interplay between bony structures, muscles and ligaments, blood supply, nerve supply, and mobility of the skin. The hand and wrist complex contains 27 bones. There are 19 bones distal to the carpals and 19 joints that make up the hand complex. The hand consists of 5 digits: 4 fingers and 1 thumb. Each digit has a CMC joint and a MCP joint. The fingers also have 2 interphalangeal (IP) joints, while the thumb has 1. The function of the CMC joints of the fingers is to allow cupping of the palm. The palmar arches allow the hand to conform to the shape of the object being held. The MCP joints, carpal joints, and associated muscles and ligaments form the palmar arches. They can be visualized across the width of the palm and down the length of the palm (Figure 33-3). The palmar arches also allow the fingers to be positioned for prehension activities (Levangie & Norkin, 2001).

Prehension involves the grasping or holding of an object between any 2 surfaces of the hand. There are infinite grip combinations, but research has identified classifications for various grips. A simple way to conceptualize grips is to consider either a power grip or precision handling (Levangie & Norkin, 2001). Power grip is a strong forceful flexion of all fingers to hold an object securely. An example of a strong power grip is holding tightly to a rope during a tug-of-war game. Precision handling is the placement of an object between fingers or finger and thumb. Picking up a raisin with thumb and index finger is an example of precision handling.

Placement of the hand for grasp activities is dependent upon intact wrist function. The optimal position of the wrist and fingers for effective hand function is referred to as the functional position (Figure 33-4). The functional position is as follows:

- Wrist in 20 degrees of extension and 10 degrees of ulnar deviation.

- Fingers flexed 45 degrees at the MCPs, 30 degrees at PIPs and 20 degrees at DIPs.

- Thumb abducted.

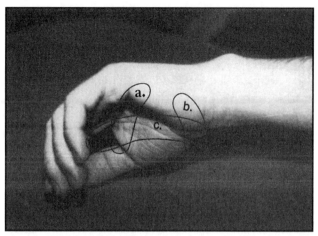

Figure 33-3. Arches of the hand. A. Distal transverse arch. B. Proximal transverse arch. C. Longitudinal arch.

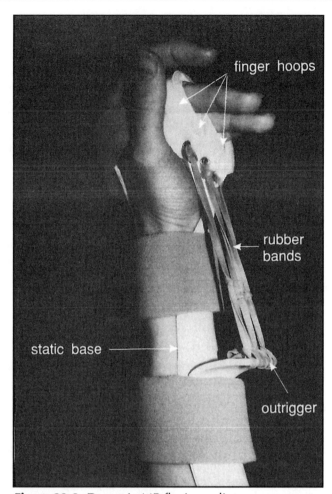

Figure 33-2. Dynamic MP flexion splint.

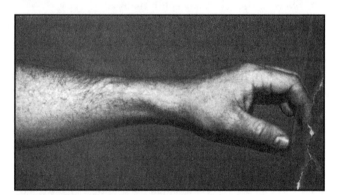

Figure 33-4. Functional position of the hand.

In this position, finger flexion occurs with the least amount of effort and the muscle tension in the hand is balanced (Fess & Kiel, 1998). When a resting hand splint is constructed, the therapist often chooses to splint the hand in the functional position.

Mechanical Principles

Mechanics deals with the effect of force. Muscles supply force in the hand. That force is transmitted to the ligaments and joints, which produces motion. Splints also apply force, which means they provide a degree of stress to structures they contact. Force from the splint should be sufficient to prevent contracture

and increase ROM but not cause damage. Undesirable effects of too much force from a splint may be damage to skin or underlying structures of ligaments, muscles, and joints. The amount of force to prevent contracture should be just enough to hold the joints in the end of range position (Belkin & Yasunda, 2001). Force should be applied at the appropriate angle of pull and must be carefully calibrated. A gauge is available to measure the force applied. Rubberbands and springs need to be checked frequently and adjusted to apply the desired amount of force and direction of pull to the joint. A well-designed, well-contoured splint will minimize stress from pressure and be tolerated much better by the client.

Design Principles

Before deciding which splint to make for the individual, several factors need to be considered. Consideration must be given toward the design of a splint program that is practical for the individual but also meets the specific needs of his or her condition. The therapist should try to answer the following questions before making a final decision on splint design:
- Does the client understand his or her condition and how he or she may benefit from a splint program?
- Is the individual likely to comply with the program?
- Will he or she perceive that the splint program interferes with his or her independence or ability to participate in daily activities?
- Is he or she self-conscious of being seen wearing a splint?
- Is he or she motivated toward recovery?
- Is he or she so motivated that he or she may overdo the specified program?
- Is he or she able to apply and remove the splint?
- If unable to do so, is there a motivated caregiver who can assist in this process?
- Will he or she follow a splint schedule?
- Does he or she have the cognitive abilities to fully understand and follow through with the program?

- Will he or she leave the splint on too long and be at risk for skin irritation or edema?
- Will he or she wear the splint long enough to produce desired results?
- Does he or she have other conditions that place him or her at risk for injury such as fragile skin or impaired sensation?

The therapist must consider the primary deficits of the hand and what splint type is most appropriate for treatment, taking into consideration the individual's characteristics of bony structures, scars, skin condition, any alterations in sensation, or other conditions (Fess & Kiel, 1998). The therapist will provide the most appropriate splint for the client's condition. However, if the therapist does not obtain answers to the above questions and take the time to thoroughly educate the client on the benefits of the splint, the splint will not be worn and outcomes will not be achieved. The therapist should design an individualized splint program that incorporates the client's perception of their situation and their personal goals for recovery.

ASSESSMENT

Typically, the splint program is part of the client's overall treatment. The client may also be involved in a program of ROM, therapeutic exercise, and graded activities. He or she may be following through on a home program of ROM, exercises, and ADL tasks designed to improve hand function. The therapist's initial evaluation would have consisted of obtaining information on occupational roles and performance, the perceived impact of the injury or disease process on activity performance, and client's goals for recovery. Additional areas evaluated would be ROM, muscle strength, and UE gross and fine motor coordination. The therapist would have obtained information on medical diagnoses, precautions, activity restrictions, and specific splint orders from the doctor if issued. The therapist would also ask if the patient has known allergies to splinting materials such as plastics, neoprene, or latex. The OT will consider results of all assessments prior to making a final decision on splint design for the individual. Once the splint is fabricated, the OT will provide frequent reassessment to evaluate effectiveness of the program and to determine if revisions should be made to the splint or the program.

The OTA may contribute to the initial evaluation by obtaining measures of ROM, grip and pinch strength, and administering standardized evaluations such as the 9-hole peg test. The OTA may be the professional working most often with the client and will need to check with him or her for any problems or concerns with the personalized splint program. The OTA will provide information to the OT to assist with the re-evaluation process. Under the supervision of the OT, the OTA may be making revisions to the splint or the splint program and monitoring the client's progress.

FABRICATION

Once a decision is made on splint design, the therapist will either fabricate a custom splint or provide the individual with the proper fitting prefabricated splint. One of the easiest custom splints for the beginner to fabricate is the resting hand splint. Instructions on fabricating a resting hand splint will be given in the following sections. Much can be learned by observing an experienced therapist as he or she creates a splint. Not all of the details of the fabrication process can be represented in written form.

Materials

Organize the work area to promote efficiency as well as comfort for the client. The client should sit at a sturdy table so he or she can rest his or her forearms on the table surface. Assemble the following items on a nearby work surface:

- Electric fry hand with temperature control
- Splint heat gun with a funnel
- Utility knife
- Curved blade scissors and straight blade scissors
- Clean towels
- Compression wrap
- 2-inch stockinet
- Paper and pencil for pattern
- Awl
- Tongs
- Soup ladle
- Sheet of thermoplastic splint material
- 1-inch sticky-back Velcro (Velcro USA Inc., Manchester, NH) hook
- Either one half-Velcro loop or similar strapping material such as Velfoam (WBC Industries, Westfield, NJ) (Figure 33-5)
- Cold spray or cool water

Pattern

Use paper and pencil to trace a pattern for the client's hand. Paper towel works well, as it is flexible and thus easier to check the fit directly on the client's arm and hand. Trace around the contours of the hand as shown in Figure 33-6, leaving extra margins so that the splint will fall midline along the arm and hand. It is better to err on the side of caution and have excess material that can be trimmed versus creating a splint that is too small and not useable. Cut the pattern out and try it on the patient; this allows you to inspect the dimensions of the splint. A forearm-based splint should extend two-thirds of the way up the arm toward the elbow. The client should be able to bend his or her elbow unhampered by the splint. If the length of the

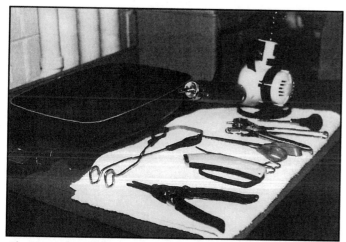

Figure 33-5. Splint construction tools.

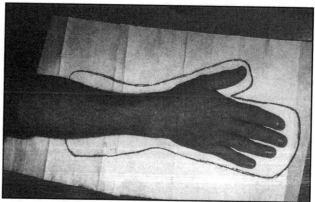

Figure 33-6. Making a pattern.

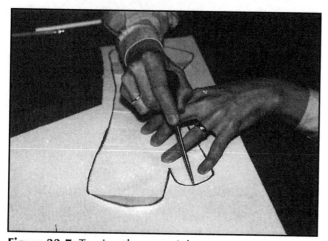

Figure 33-7. Tracing the material.

guides on the types of splint material available and recommended uses. Examples include Sammons Preston Rolyan and North Coast Medical.

Take the paper pattern and trace the pattern onto the sheet of material using an awl (Figure 33-7). Some splint materials can be marked with a pencil or pen, but the pen marks cannot be removed and will affect the looks of the final product. An awl will mark but not be obvious in the finished splint. Rough cut the pattern from the splint sheet. Rough cutting is cutting around the pattern but outside of the pattern lines using a blade or heavy duty splint scissors as shown in Figure 33-8.

Heating the Material

Each material will have manufacturer instructions that will tell you at what temperature the material should be heated and how much working time you have before the material cools and resumes its rigid properties. Orthoplast and San-Splint are both heated at 160°F and will take 1 to 2 minutes to soften and become moldable (Figure 33-9). Working time is approximately 3 to 5 minutes. Once the material has softened, use tongs to remove the splint pan and place on a clean towel. Lightly pat to remove water. Use scissors to cut out pattern on the lines (Figure 33-10). Make sure that all ends are rounded versus angled. A curved blade scissors will help to neatly cut the web space in the pattern.

Forming to Client

Allow the material to cool so that it can be placed on the skin and tolerated by the client. It is advisable to take a length of 2-inch stockinet and apply to the client's forearm, especially if he or she is unusually sensitive to heat. Have the client touch the splint material and let you know if it is a temperature he or she can tolerate. If you allow it to cool too much, that will limit the amount of time you have to mold the material.

As the material is cooling, have the client place his or her hand into the functional position. It may help to have him or her rest the arm on a pillow so that the arm is supported in an elevated position. It is important that he or she is comfortable and relaxed during this procedure so you get an accurate fit. A beginner will do better to first place the material onto a supinat-

splint is too short, pressure is not evenly distributed and pressure areas on the skin may be created. With the pattern placed on the client, you should make sure that it is long enough to extend partially beyond the end of the fingers and thumb, and evenly one-third to one-half up the sides of the forearm. Creating a correct paper pattern and sizing it on the client saves time and avoids errors during the fabrication process.

Preparing the Material for Fitting

A beginner should choose a more durable splint material such as Orthoplast or San-Splint (Sammons Preston Rolyan, Bolingbrook, IL). Orthoplast, which can take heavy handling, will not become marked from fingerprints and will not become overstretched. It is a plastic material with a rubber component, which gives it memory; it will return to its former shape after being stretched. It can also be reheated several times if you are not satisfied with your first attempt. It can be easily spot heated to correct or revise parts of the splint. Orthoplast has a maximum resistance to stretch and is ideal to use in larger splints for the elbow, shoulder, LE, and trunk. Materials such as Polyform (Sammons Preston Rolyan, Bolingbrook, IL) have a minimum resistance to stretch, conform easily to contours, and are ideal for hand and wrist splints. Refer to therapy supply catalogs for

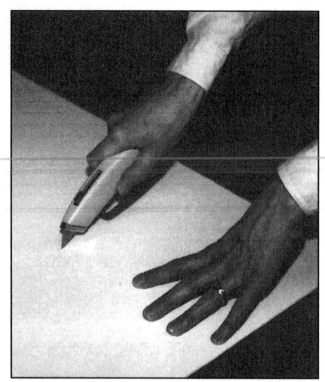

Figure 33-8. Rough cutting the splint.

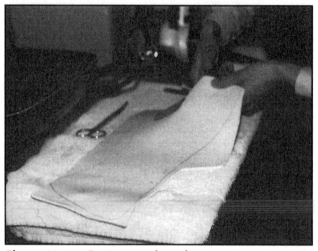

Figure 33-10. Cutting out the splint.

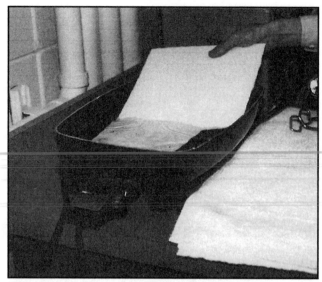

Figure 33-9. Heating the material.

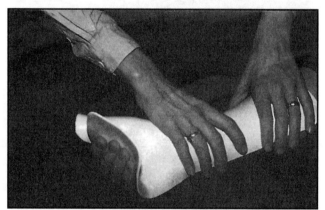

Figure 33-11. Placing the warmed material on the client.

then form the palmar aspect of the splint. With client maintaining the functional position, gently press the material up into the palmar arches so that the palmar aspect of the splint replicates the arches of the hand. Finally, shape the material to flex the fingers and abduct the thumb. Once satisfied on basic fit, gently flare up sides of splint along the ulnar and radial aspect of the hand. Ask client to maintain the functional position until the splint material has cooled.

Checking the Fit

Remove the compression wrap and check alignment of the splint a final time. While it is still slightly warm, some adjustments may be made. For instance, the splint may be too tight on the forearm edges due to pressure from the compression wrap. Gently stretch the splint away from the forearm. Also make sure that the splint is not placing pressure over the bony prominence of the wrist (Figure 33-13). Likewise, check for pressure over the heads of the MCP joints, dorsal surface of PIP joints, base of the thenar eminence, and the proximal and distal aspects of the splint. Gently stretch the material away from the skin to create a bubble of material over the bony landmarks. Use a pencil or

ed forearm and have the assistance of gravity to help mold the material. First make sure that the splint is lined up evenly on the forearm and that the material is correctly positioned in the web space (Figure 33-11). The next step is to loosely apply a compression wrap to secure the material to the contours of the forearm (Figure 33-12). If you are concerned with the client's ability to tolerate this procedure, you can speed up the setting of the material by using a compression wrap dipped first in cold water. Once the forearm is wrapped, have the client pronate the arm. If you complete the splint with forearm supinated, the fit may not be correct. Once pronated, realign the splint material if needed so that it comes up evenly on each side of the forearm. Check the wrist to make sure it is extended to 20 degrees and ulnarly deviated to 10 degrees. Check the web space for fit and

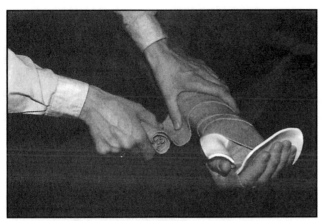

Figure 33-12. Wrapping with elastic bandage.

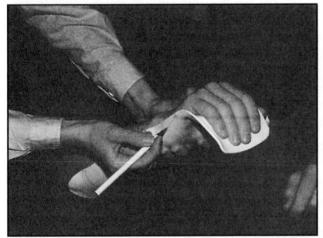

Figure 33-14. Marking the splint before trimming the excess.

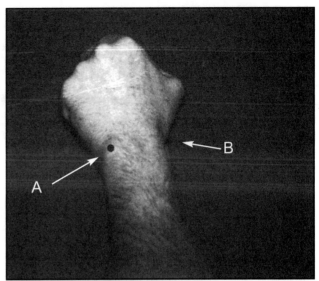

Figure 33-13. Bony prominences. A. Ulnar styloid. B. Radial styloid.

pen to mark areas of the splint that need further trimming (Figure 33-14). Gently remove the splint from the client's arm. To speed up the final set and not risk losing the contours during handling, run the splint under cold water or apply cold spray.

Final Adjustments

Check all edges of the splint for smoothness. If the edges are not smooth, they can create areas of pressure or irritation to the skin. Edges can be finished several ways. You can dip the edges of the splint in hot water to heat again to moldable consistency. It is difficult to heat the edges of the web space by dipping as you may lose the shape of the web space. Using a ladle or heat gun with nozzle will help apply heat only to the areas you need heated. Use sharp splint scissors to slightly trim edges. Orthoplast, if cut hot, will finish with a smooth edge. You can also roll your edges back slightly to create a rounded edge; this will also add to the stability of the splint. Roll back or slightly flare the proximal end of the forearm piece for added comfort for the wearer.

Have the client try the splint on for a final fitting. Check for areas where the splint is too tight against the skin or bony prominence. Also make sure the splint does not fit loosely because it will slide or migrate on the arm and hand and cause

friction irritation. Complete all necessary revisions before applying the strapping material.

Fasteners

Once you are satisfied with the fit, it is time to create the mechanism to fasten the splint to the extremity. Typically, a resting hand splint is fastened at 3 points: proximal forearm, wrist, and over the PIPs. This method of fastening will provide that the splint will not migrate and that gentle pressure is applied to help maintain the desired position. Strapping should be as wide as possible to decrease the amount of pressure on the skin. Strapping material can be purchased in rolls or premade straps may be purchased in packages.

Adhere the straps to the splint (Figure 33-15). This is commonly done using sticky-back Velcro hook. Trim the straps to fit and use your scissors to round the edges for comfort and to prevent fraying (Figure 33-16). For splints that require greater durability, the straps may be fastened with metal rivets.

Trial Wearing Period

It is highly recommended that you arrange to have the client don and doff the splint for the first time in your presence. Once the splint is properly donned, have the client perform a simple ADL task or functional UE activity. Check the client's perception of comfort and fit during performance and upon completion of the activity. Remove the splint and check for any reddened skin, which indicates an area of pressure. Make necessary adjustments of the splint to eliminate those pressure areas.

Client Education

The client should understand the rationale for the splint program, be able to apply and remove the splint independently, and demonstrate understanding of the care of the splint and the wearing schedule. They should also be instructed on wearing precautions. The client or client's caregivers need to be able to

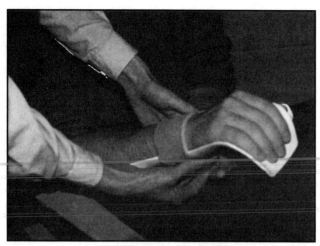

Figure 33-15. Adhering the straps to the splint.

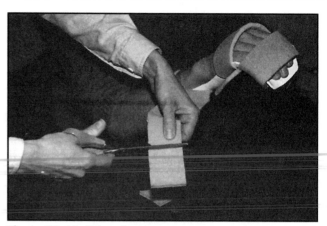

Figure 33-16. Trimming straps.

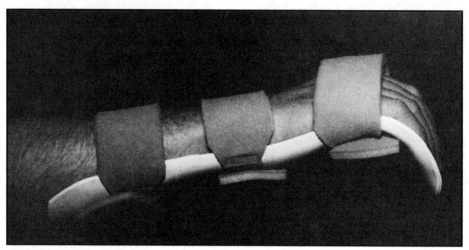

Figure 33-17. Completed resting hand splint.

monitor for pain, reddened areas, blisters, swelling, or rashes and immediately report problems to the therapist. He or she should stop wearing the splint until the therapist corrects the cause of the problem. The client should be instructed verbally and be provided with written instructions on wearing schedule, care of splint, and precautions. The client or client's caregiver should demonstrate to the therapist the application and removal of the splint. He or she should be encouraged to report back to the therapist any problems or concerns with the splint program so that needed adjustments may be made. After providing a splint, the therapist should arrange a time for a follow-up appointment to review client's tolerance to the program.

Some minor suggestions to increase comfort include wearing stockinet to absorb perspiration or lightly powdering the splint with cornstarch prior to application. If the client reports excess perspiration, a hole punch can be used to punch holes in the material or a perforated splinting material can be used. It is helpful to provide the client with extra straps or stockinet should they misplace or lose these items.

Once both therapist and client are satisfied with comfort and fit of the splint, and upon completion of client or caregiver instructions, the splint is ready to be issued to the client (Figure 33-17).

Follow-Up

It is the responsibility of the OT to provide follow up to a client who has received a splint and placed on a splint program. If the splint is one aspect of the therapy program, follow-up can easily be incorporated into later treatment sessions. If the client was referred for the sole purpose of splinting, then formal appointments should be made for follow up. The nature and severity of the condition and the individual needs of the client will determine the frequency of follow-up appointments and the interval between visits. The purpose of the visit is to check on fit of the splint, discuss any problems with the splint program, his or her success and compliance to the program, and to check for progress. The therapist may spend time problem solving with the client on issues that are affecting compliance. If fit and comfort are issues, the therapist will make modifications to the splint and advise the client on further strategies to increase comfort. The therapist will also take time to review information on splint program, exercise, graded activities, and the client's performance in occupational tasks. As the client demonstrates progress, the splint can be revised to obtain further gains and the exercise and the activity program upgraded to obtain additional progress. The initial wearing schedule may need to be

EVIDENCE-BASED TREATMENT STRATEGIES

Treatment Strategies	Authors
Background on evidence-based practice in splinting	Fess, 2002; Jansen, 2002
Correct or prevent deformity	Ball & Nanchahal, 2002; Glascow, Wilton, & Tooth, 2003; Li-Tsang, Hung, & Mak, 2002; Prosser, 1996
Restore or improve function	Banta, 1994; DiPasquale-Lehnerz, 1994; O'Connor, Marshall, & Massy-Westropp, 2003; Walker, Metzler, Cifu, & Swartz, 2000
Promote healing/decrease pain	Callinan & Mathiowetz, 1996; Fess & McCollum, 1998; Klein, 2003; Maddy & Meyerdierks, 1997; Mercer & Davis, 1995
Provide or assist motion	Hannah & Hudak, 2001; Lightbody, 1994

adjusted to accommodate to work schedules, self-care, and leisure activities. If the splint is interfering with performance of desired activities such as self-care, the therapist may be able to offer suggestions on adapting activities or the splint schedule to meet the activity needs of the client as well as the rehabilitative needs of his or her UE.

SUMMARY

This chapter presented basic information on splinting including purpose, biomechanical and anatomical principles, assessment, design, fabrication, and follow-up. The purpose of a splint is to maintain, improve, or restore function through the external application of force. The final outcome of a splint program is the improvement of UE function to allow independent performance of daily activities and satisfactory execution of occupational roles.

The experienced OTA will be able to design and fabricate basic static splints, monitor effectiveness of the program, and perform needed revisions; all with minimal supervision from the OT. The OTA who is a novice splinter can gain experience through observing and assisting the OT. OTAs can develop advanced skills by attending relevant workshops, working with OTs who are experienced splinters or certified hand therapists, and working in a setting that provides frequent opportunities to splint.

LEARNING ACTIVITIES

1. Work with another classmate to construct a resting hand splint for each other. Follow the procedures of creating a pattern, fabrication, trial wearing period, and client education on precautions. Then discuss how each of you felt in your roles as OTA and client.

2. Wear your splint for 1-hour periods during each of the following activities: self-care, vocational or home management, leisure, and the first hour after you go to bed. The wearing schedule will total 4 hours within a 24-hour period. Then discuss your experience in relationship to the impact the splint had on your occupational performance, your physical and emotional responses to the wearing experience, and reactions from others.

3. Interview your partner to find out what problems or issues he or she identified during his or her splint-wearing experience. Then attempt to revise the wearing schedule to continue 4 hours (nonsequential) of splint-wearing time per day that has the least negative impact on your occupational roles.

4. Design a client handout for your partner that specifies the wearing schedule from number 3 above and precautions.

5. Design a splint that is useful but also "really cool" to an 11-year-old girl or 9-year-old boy.

ACKNOWLEDGMENT

The author wishes to express appreciation to Cynthia L. Vennix, OTR/CHT for time spent in review for final chapter revisions.

REFERENCES

Ball, C., & Nanchahal, J. (2002). The use of splinting as a non-surgical treatment for Dupuytren's disease: A pilot study. *British Journal of Hand Therapy, 7,* 76-78.

Banta, C. (1994). A prospective, nonrandomized study of iontophoresis, wrist-splinting, and anti-inflammatory medication in the treatment of early-mild carpal tunnel syndrome. *Journal of Occupational Medicine, 36,* 166-168.

Belkin, J., & Yasunda, L. (2001). Orthotics. In L. Pedretti (Ed.), *Occupational therapy: Practice skills for physical dysfunction* (5th ed., pp. 529-566). St. Louis, MO: Mosby.

Callinan, N., & Mathiowetz, V. (1996). Soft versus hard resting hand splints in rheumatoid arthritis: Pain relief, preference, and compliance. *American Journal of Occupational Therapy, 50,* 347-353.

DiPasquale-Lehnerz, P. (1994). Orthotic intervention for development of hand function with C-6 quadriplegia. *American Journal of Occupational Therapy, 48,* 138-144.

Fess, E. (2002). A history of splinting: To understand the present, view the past. *Journal of Hand Therapy, 15*, 97-132.

Fess, E., & Kiel, J. (1998). Neuromuscular treatment: Upper extremity splinting. In M. Neistadt & E. Crepeau (Eds.), *Willard and Spackman's occupational therapy* (9th ed., pp. 406-421). Philadelphia: Lippincott, Williams & Wilkins.

Fess, E., & McCollum, M. (1998). The influence of splinting on healing tissues. *Journal of Hand Therapy, 11*, 157-161.

Glascow, C., Wilton, J., & Tooth, L. (2003). Optimal daily total end range time for contracture: Resolution in hand splinting. *Journal of Hand Therapy, 16*, 207-218.

Hannah, S., & Hudak, P. (2001). Splinting and radial nerve palsy: A single-subject experiment. *Journal of Hand Therapy, 14*, 195-201.

Jansen, C. (2002). Outcomes, treatment effectiveness, efficacy, and evidence-based practice: Examples from the world of splinting. *Journal of Hand Therapy, 15*, 136-143.

Kielhofner, G. (1992). *Conceptual foundations of occupational therapy* (2nd ed.). Philadelphia, PA: F. A. Davis.

Klein, L. (2003). Early active motion tendon protocol using one splint. *Journal of Hand Therapy, 16*, 199-206.

Levangie, P. K., & Norkin, C. C. (2001). *Joint structure and function: A comprehensive analysis* (3rd ed.). Philadelphia, PA: F. A. Davis.

Lightbody, S. (1994). Dynamic pronation splint in high level spinal cord injury: A case study. *Australian Occupational Therapy Journal, 41*, 83-85.

Li-Tsang, C., Hung, L., & Mak, A. (2002). The effect of corrective splinting on flexion contracture of rheumatoid fingers. *Journal of Hand Therapy, 15*, 185-191.

Maddy, L., & Meyerdierks, E. (1997). Dynamic extension assist splinting of acute central slip lacerations. *Journal of Hand Therapy, 10*, 206-212.

Mercer, C., & Davis, M. (1995). A survey of the uses and benefits of prefabricated wrist and thumb supports. *British Journal of Therapy and Rehabilitation, 2*, 599-603.

O'Connor, D., Marshall, S., & Massy-Westropp, N. (2003). Non-surgical treatment (other than steroid injection) for carpal tunnel syndrome. Cochrane Database System Reviews, 2003(1), CD003219. Abstract retrieved 11/25/03 from the CINAHL database.

Prosser, R. (1996). Splinting in the management of proximal interphalangeal joint flexion contracture. *Journal of Hand Therapy, 9*, 378-386.

Walker, W., Metzler, M., Cifu, D., & Swartz, Z. (2000). Neutral wrist splinting in carpal tunnel syndrome: A comparison of night-only versus full-time wear instructions. *Archives of Physical Medicine and Rehabilitation, 81*, 424-429.

Key Concepts

- Health: A state of complete physical, mental, cognitive, and social wellness.
- Health promotion: Growth and development to foster soundness of body, mind, and spirit.

Essential Vocabulary

Americans with Disabilities Act of 1990: Public law that guarantees disabled citizens access to work and public services.

ergonomics: Study of movement to accomplish tasks.

lifestyle redesign: Assisting clients in examining how occupations contribute to healthy or unhealthy states and customizing change.

WELLNESS AND
HEALTH PROMOTION

Karen Sladyk, PhD, OTR, FAOTA

INTRODUCTION

Not too long ago, lack of information made it nearly impossible to choose healthy lifestyles. In television commercials of the 1950s, some medical doctors recommended smoking cigarettes as a way to reduce stress and lose weight. With today's overload of information on health, consumers have to wade through volumes of often conflicting information to find healthy lifestyles. OT can help with this process (Gourley, 2000).

The WHO defines health as "a state of complete physical, mental, and social well-being" (1986). The National Wellness Association adds spiritual and intellectual components to the definition (Ratner, Johnson, & Jeffery, 1998). Health is not just the absence of sickness or disease. The concept of health becomes different for each individual, as the definition is inherently unique to different people and cultures.

OT is no longer just for those with a diagnosis. Health promotion is for those at risk of losing good health (Moyers, 1999). OT can provide a unique aspect to health promotion because of our understanding of occupation and daily living. Occupation is a natural format for health promotion because of its individuality. Health promotion is assisting ourselves and others in growth and development of sound body, mind, and spirit (Bowen, 1999). OT can use concepts of lifestyle redesign to assist clients individually, in groups, or whole communities in finding balance in their lives (Moyers, 1999).

Lifestyle redesign is a new concept in OT that involves customizing a person's routines of daily living to maximize health and satisfaction (Gourley, 2000). This process of redesign takes on many different facets and is specific to the needs of each individual. What might be identified as helpful to one person might be anxiety provoking to another. For example, computer ergonomics and managing the information highway is enjoyable to some, while expressing a talent in a craft is enjoyable to others. The key to lifestyle redesign is individual design.

The Department of Occupational Science and Occupational Therapy at the University of Southern California has opened a Center for Occupation and Lifestyle Redesign that focuses on community-based practice, education, and research. Based on OT founder George Barton's 1914 Consolation House, this new community center of 6,000 square feet includes innovative programs for the people of the neighborhood including gardening, computer analysis, culturally-focused activities, and crafts as occupation. Each program has a research component that allows faculty and students to study the importance of occupations on health (Gourley, 2000).

AREAS FOR HEALTH PROMOTION IN OCCUPATIONAL THERAPY

The concept of health promotion in practice is not new to OT practice. As OTAs, the well-being of the whole client has always been a focus of treatment. As people become more sophisticated about healthy lifestyles, opportunities for health promotion intervention have increased.

As this new and emerging area of practice is developing, new areas of practice are developing daily. This section introduces possible areas of practice for OT practitioners. Generally, the OTA would want to begin to integrate these areas into practice before specializing in health promotion. As community-based practice increases, so do the opportunities to include health promotion in practice.

Americans With Disabilities Act Consulting

The ADA (1990) changed the face of the public's understanding of people with disabilities as productive, healthy people. Industries, businesses, public offices, and other services are eager to comply with the act in an effort to service all people in their community. OT practitioners are potential resources for ADA consulting because of their knowledge of occupation, adaptation, and activity analysis. Practitioners interested in this can begin with a copy of the ADA and read about specific issues in their state (Fontana, 1999). As this law is constantly refined and defined because of litigation, it is important for the practitioner to remain current on all aspects of the law.

Assisted Living

A new housing alternative for the older adult, assisted living provides people with independence and support in a warm community setting (Smith, 1999). Since assisted living programs are significantly lower in costs over skilled nursing facilities, this area of housing options is getting much attention lately. Regulation of this area is moving forward to ensure that these sites provide quality programs.

OT has not been automatically included in this arena but has great potential for helping people stay in assisted living programs. OT in assisted living centers can include fall prevention, energy conservation, health education, and social opportunities. OT practitioners must market themselves to assisted living administrators who generally have a business education instead of a health education (Smith, 1999). Practitioners interested in this area need to monitor state laws and regulations to ensure opportunities for OT. As a member benefit, AOTA monitors state laws and can assist in promoting OT in this new area (Smith, 1999).

Community Redesign

Community and business leaders are often confused in trying to meet the needs of citizens within their community. Opportunities exist for OT practitioners to improve community situations for well people. Moyers (2000) reported unique OTs who were employed to improve quality of life within whole communities. For example, an OT helped her community redesign the transit system to be less exhausting for senior citizens, and an OT worked with a packaging company to design packages that were easy to open. Other opportunities could include playground design or writing business manuals for homeowners.

Community Wellness Programs

Every community has some type of adult education program typically set up in the evenings at local schools or churches. These programs include computer training, crafts, exercise, and educational programs. Most of these programs are eager for new classes to be developed and openly invite potential teachers to develop new programs. As OT practitioners have training in teaching and learning, it is a logical progression that they could develop exciting programs for well people in the community. Opportunities include stress management, time management, role management, protecting your back and joints, helping your teen adjust to adult roles, and living with a person with a disability. The list of potential programs for community education is endless. Just look at the list in the Practice Framework (AOTA, 2002) and you can begin to see the potential for health promotion in community education for both adults and children.

Ergonomics

The OT practitioner's understanding of anatomy, activity analysis, and movement provides the background for helping others utilize the workplace tools more effectively. Typically, ergonomics is an area that a practitioner enters after advanced training and work experience. Industry is particularly interested in specialists who can help their employees remain well and injury free (Fontana, 1999; O'Connor, 2000). Specialists in this area utilize the occupational performance areas of the Practice Framework (AOTA, 2002) to facilitate success in the work performance area. As in the assisted living arena, ergonomics require the practitioner to advocate OT to business leaders. As with any consulting position, your employer might have different concerns and motivations for having ergonomic training available to employees. For example, rests from repetitive actions might reduce injuries but also slow production (O'Connor, 2000).

Home and Private Consultant

Several opportunities are available in the private sector. Often individual people are looking for guidance concerning specific issues in their home or work life (Jacobs, 2000) (e.g., evaluating a home for safety concerns for an elderly couple or coaching a person who is up for a big promotion and nervous about the interview). Other opportunities exist such as consulting with a professional woman who is now on complete bed rest for the remainder of her pregnancy and missing her professional relationships from work or designing home gyms for specific families. Since OT is concerned with the job of living, consulting opportunities abound but are often untapped.

Spirituality and Hope

The depth of spirituality is in each activity we perform, for it adds richness to our lives (Peloquin, 1997). Acknowledging and understanding the role of spirituality in living a healthy life is currently of interest in OT (Christiansen, 1997). Spirituality can be used in health promotion as well as in rehabilitation. Spirituality work can be effective in both group and individual sessions. OT's role in spirituality is highlighted in different ways, including goal setting/attainment, occupational change, or life history (Spencer, Davidson, & White, 1997). First, practitioners can help clients utilize their spirituality by imagining the possibilities or evaluating the future through goal setting and goal attainment. Second, practitioners emphasize hope with the anticipated change over time. Third, the usefulness of narratives in telling life stories as therapy has been documented as an effective tool (Spencer et al., 1997).

GETTING STARTED

The first step in specializing in health promotion involves learning as much as possible about a specific problem and the need for service in that area. The OT practitioners may initially see health promotion opportunities as part of their regular work environment. Gaining experience in smaller health promotion opportunities will lead to confidence in large projects.

Initial opportunities in health promotion can include the following:

- Promote lifestyle redesign within your work environment during OT month (April).

- Make a pamphlet for health promotion that addresses the specific needs of your current patient population. Design a second pamphlet that addresses needs of family and friends.

- Take a skill you are using in your current practice and bring it to a community adult education program. Teach a class in stress reduction at the local adult education program or teach a class on spirituality and healing at your church.

- Notify a local public school that you are willing to organize a health fair for the children. Design a class where you teach health promotion concepts to the children. Let the children design a poster on good health for the health fair.

- Offer to do free ergonomic evaluations for friends and family members. When your experience increases, offer the same service at work.

- Offer a class on fall prevention to a local senior citizen center. Repeat the class at an assisted living center. Invite administrators to attend the class.

Once the OT practitioner has experience, it may be time to consider an entrepreneurial business. This is not new to OT, as OTs and OTAs have been designing equipment, giving seminars, and consulting for years. Sorensen (1999) recommends developing business skills, being focused, and testing your ideas. OT practitioners are naturally good at developing and testing ideas because that is part of the OT process. Often lacking are the business skills. Taylor (1999) recommends beginning with the Internal Revenue Service (IRS) for information that clarifies employee relationships from independent contractors. Further assistance should be sought from business professionals familiar with national, state, and local laws.

LEARNING ACTIVITIES

1. Visit a senior center or day care to assess wellness needs. Develop a wellness program that can be carried out by an OTA team. Implement the program for one semester.

2. Offer free work place evaluations to faculty and staff at your college. Visit the work site and write a paper addressing possible improvements.

3. Develop a pamphlet for dealing with the stresses of college. Produce and distribute the information on campus or with the assistance of the academic development center. Follow up by leading a stress reduction group.

REFERENCES

Americans with Disabilities Act. (1990). Public Law 101-336, 42 U.S.C. 12101.

American Occupational Therapy Association. (2002). The occupational therapy practice framework: Domain and process. *American Journal of Occupational Therapy, 56,* 609-633.

Bowen, J. E. (1999). Health promotion in the new millennium. *OT Practice, 20,* 14-18.

Christiansen, C. (1997). Acknowledging a spiritual dimension in OT practice. *American Journal of Occupational Therapy, 51,* 169-172.

Fontana, P. A. (1999). Pushing the envelope: Entering the industrial arena. *OT Practice, 20,* 20-22.

Gourley, M. (2000). Center for occupational therapy and lifestyle redesign. *OT Practice, 8,* 18-19.

Jacobs, K. (2000). Under renovation: Incorporating change. President's Keynote Address, 80th Annual AOTA Conference and Exposition, Seattle, WA; April 2.

Moyers, P. (1999). *The guide to occupational therapy practice.* Bethesda, MD: American Occupational Therapy Association.

Moyers, P. (2000). Promoting practice and the profession: Integrating the guide to OT practice. NEOTEC Conference, University of Hartford, CT, June 14.

O'Connor, S. M. (2000). OTs and office ergonomics consulting. *OT Practice, 8,* 12-16.

Peloquin, S. (1997). The spiritual depth of occupation: Making worlds and making meaning. *American Journal of Occupational Therapy, 51,* 167-168.

Ratner, P., Johnson, J., & Jeffery, B. (1998). Examining emotional, physical, social, and spiritual health determinates of self-rated health status. *American Journal of Health Promotion, 12,* 275-282.

Smith, K. (1999). States move forward with assisted living regulation. *OT Practice, 20,* 8.

Sorensen, J. (1999). Entrepreneurs: The spirit of OT. *OT Practice, 4*(3), 27-29.

Spencer, J., Davidson, H., & White, V. (1997). Helping clients develop hopes for the future. *American Journal of Occupational Therapy, 51,* 191-198.

Taylor, L. D. (1999). Twenty tips for employees and independent contractors. *OT Practice, 20,* 12-13.

World Health Organization. (1986). A discussion document on the concept and principles of health promotion. *Health Promotion, 1,* 73-78.

Key Concepts

- Life Skills Program: An educationally-based treatment program to help participants develop skills required for competent role performance.
- Stressful life event: An event that causes changes in and demands readjustment of an average person's normal routine.

Essential Vocabulary

hardiness: Personal characteristics that function to resist succumbing to the negative effects of dealing with stressful life events.

resilience: Characteristics and skills such as autonomy, competence, and problem solving that help an individual bounce back from adverse situations.

LIFE SKILLS

Denise Rotert, MA, OTR and Frank E. Gainer, MHS, OTR, FAOTA

INTRODUCTION

Why is it that some individuals cope with adverse circumstances better than others? It often seems like a mystery how some people can thrive under adversity. But it really isn't a mystery. Many individuals bounce back from stressful life events when they are armed with appropriate life skills. Individuals with at-risk behaviors can become resistant to negative outcomes if OTs and OTAs address and incorporate a program that accentuates positive self-concept, competent performance of daily living skills, and effective interpersonal relationships. The goal is to empower individuals at risk to reshape and mold a new way of living through the teaching of life skills.

RESILIENCE

Resilience is showing up as a concept in diverse areas such as business, health care, sports, education, religion, and the public media. Researchers are demonstrating how the skills and abilities of resilient people will help them to be more productive, happier, and healthier when faced with change, stress, and pressure of daily living.

Through a model called the Circle of Courage, the acquisition of life skills will enable a person to transcend from "at risk" to "resilient" (Brendtro, Brokenleg, & Van Bockern, 1990). This model is based on the Native American medicine wheel and is composed of 4 values: belonging, mastery, independence, and generosity. The Circle of Courage addresses empowerment and wholeness when the 4 come together to close the circle.

Belonging

The value of belonging is a universal need. Many individuals lack the significant skills that promote belonging, including the following actions: saying "hi," calling others by name, complimenting, touching, calling a friend, listening, and apologizing (Curwin & Mendler, 1988). "Those most alienated have virtually abandoned the pursuit of belonging and became guarded, lonely, distrustful, and unattached" (Brendtro & Brokenleg,

1993, p. 5). For example, Paul, a 14-year-old male who was a youth at risk, never received the appropriate supports to live a purposeful life. He was unwanted and unbonded. His unstable family life consisted of a father who committed suicide and a mother who herself was without support and needed parenting skills (Brendtro, 1997). He formed attachments to nurturing teachers as a substitute, but lost those attachments and his dedication to being a student due to moving. As a result, he increasingly felt outcast, bullied, and alienated. He became labeled as a troublemaker (Brendtro, 1997).

Mastery

The value of mastery is another component that will close part of the circle. Larson (1996) identified mastery as a belief in one's ability to successfully complete tasks that, in turn, can act as a motivator for behavior. OT may enhance mastery within an individual by nurturing success, identifying achievements, highlighting the positive, and modeling basic social skills. The goals of the Circle of Courage are to "develop cognitive, physical, social and spiritual competence" (Brendtro & Brokenleg, 1993, p. 8), which parallel the goals of OT. The youth at risk, mentioned in the previous paragraph, illustrates how he was not a master in any domain. His roles as student, son, and brother did not give him a sense of mastery and, as a result, at age 12, delinquent behavior began with stealing a piece of beef jerky from a store.

Independence

Individuals will be courageous if they develop a sense of independence. Independence can be referred to as personal power or autonomy and is an essential need in the lives of individuals. Power, as Larson (1996) describes it, allows the individual to make choices in his or her behaviors and activities that will lead him or her to happiness. It is taking an active role in one's destiny. OT may emphasize choice, problem solving, mediation, and leadership in order to accentuate an internal locus of control in which individuals are influential in their destiny. Powerlessness or a lack of independence may lead to rebellious and aggressive behaviors. In the youth's case from above, the rebellious act of stealing a piece of beef jerky led to a crime that would change the course of his whole life. He and a 17-year-old friend kidnapped, robbed, and murdered a cab driver. His "friend" played the role of being the father Paul never had, which resulted in the youth's inability to make prudent decisions. The deceptive older youth gave Paul a sense of belonging and, in turn, Paul made negative choices that resulted in living a life behind bars without the possibility of parole.

Generosity

The final component that makes a person resilient is the value termed *generosity*. "Unless the natural desire of children to help others is nourished, they fail to develop a sense of their own value and become absorbed in an empty, self-centered existence" (Brendtro & Brokenleg, 1993, p. 10). It is essential for OT personnel to give their clients an opportunity to show that they are needed and of value to other individuals. Through generosity, a life becomes purposeful. If it is not nurtured, one becomes a person at risk with a broken circle. Therapists may suggest volunteering to enhance responsibility, self-esteem, moral development, and commitment to democratic values (Brendtro & Brokenleg, 1993, p. 10). The youth described above will be challenged to create ways he can exhibit generosity in prison, but hopefully he will still find purpose in his life. His story is an extreme example, but illustrates that when the Circle of Courage is broken, feelings of alienation, inadequacy, and dependence result. The appropriate teaching and modeling of life skills may have resulted in this youth making positive choices to avoid prison and embrace a life full of freedom. His story can educate others that the human spirit is vulnerable.

HARDINESS

The term *hardiness* is used to describe individuals who do not develop and seem to be more resistant to predicted illnesses as a result of stressful life events (Kobasa, 1979). Hardiness is described as "a constellation of personality characteristics that function as a resistance resource in the encounter with stressful life events" (Kobasa, Maddi, & Kahn, 1982, p. 168). It is a difference that distinguishes persons who have a high degree of stress without falling ill from those that do fall ill when experiencing similar levels of stress. A life event is considered stressful if it "causes changes in, and demands readjustment of an average person's normal routine" (Kobasa et al., 1982, p. 2). In addition, Kobasa related that stressful life events can provide opportunities for potential growth (Kobasa et al., 1982).

The concept of hardiness includes 3 characteristics that were common and exhibited by a group of executives who had low incidents of stress-related illness. Those characteristics are commitment, control, and challenge (Kobasa et al., 1982, p. 168).

Commitment

Commitment is the ability to feel deeply involved in or committed to the activities of their lives (Kobasa, 1979, p. 3). A feeling of commitment to work, play, socialization, and self-care will be the focus of interest by OT.

Control

Control is the belief that they can control or influence the events of their experience (Kobasa, 1979, p. 3). The purview of OT is to assist an individual to take charge of his or her life, actions, and decisions.

Challenge

Challenge is the anticipation of change as an exciting challenge to further development (Kobasa, 1979, p. 3). Change is stressful and OT can help individuals to be creative and manage their reactions to that change.

Woven within the Kobasa et al.'s 3 "Cs" is the idea of interpersonal relationships, which could be considered as the fourth "C" of connection: an involvement with others. OT has long addressed interpersonal relationships for support and feedback.

Hardiness can be applied to areas of performance of work, play, and self-care. An individual with high hardiness can solve problems, adapt, and be creative in order that life events that may be stressful do not necessarily result in illness.

LIFE SKILLS DEVELOPMENT GROUPS

The Life Skills Development Groups were developed by 2 OTs in the U.S. Army in the 1970s. These groups were designed to treat acutely ill, psychiatric patients and included structured group tasks that were planned to assist the patient in development of adaptive behaviors.

The Life Skills Development Group was described as:
> …an educational approach to health development; however, the focus was not on what was taught but on the process of learning to satisfy one's needs in responsible ways. What the learner did was more important than what the teacher taught. (Thomes and Bajema, 1983, p. 40)

They were organized around 3 content areas, which included values clarification, competency training, and information classes. The groups started with values clarification since that was seen as a way to integrate group members quickly. Since the focus in the groups was on the tasks, members' participation was enhanced without the pressure seen in purely discussion groups. Competency training included the practice of skills related to "work, socialization, use of free time and self-maintenance" (Thomes & Bajema, 1983, p. 35). Role playing was used within the group along with the hospital setting and within the surrounding community. Information classes provided factual information furnished by the group facilitators or by speakers who may have been invited to speak on a specific area of expertise.

The Life Skills Development Groups were based on the idea that developing and practicing adaptive behaviors in "simulated, staged or actual life settings" (Thomes & Bajema, 1983, p. 44) will help the patient take those behaviors from the hospital setting into other areas of life. A key element was the modeling of behaviors by the group facilitators. Thomes and Bajema (1983, p. 47) stated that the "group is an action group, not a discussion group."

Description of the Program

A Life Skills Program is an educationally-based treatment program to help participants develop skills required for competent role performance. The program described here is based on the concepts of resilience, hardiness, and the Life Skills Development Group.

The Life Skills Program can be used as a prevention or intervention tool. As a preventive measure, having a systematic approach to increase someone's hardiness and resilience and then to add an integration of skills/behaviors for healthy living will increase the likelihood that a person will not only survive but thrive through a variety of challenging life events. As an intervention tool, the elements of the Life Skills Program can be used with substance abuse, psychiatric, rehabilitation, developmental disabilities—almost any age or diagnosis.

Participants in the Life Skills Program are given the opportunity to practice adaptive behaviors, take risks in trying new behaviors, and receive constructive criticism. The program utilizes groups but can be modified for use with individuals and can be applied with residential or hospitalized patients or with individuals in outpatient or community-based treatment programs. The program is flexible in how it is structured and how the specific activities are selected to meet the needs of each participant as well as the group. It is experiential in nature, uses paper/pencil activities, and may also include community exploration, problem solving, role playing, and interpersonal communication. Participants need to be active, organized, and have boundaries in order to benefit from the program. The intent of the Life Skills Program is not to provide answers but to give participants the tools to help them solve the problems of living (current and future).

Elements of the Program

- Stress management and relaxation: Seeking and trying new behaviors gives participants some adaptive skills for use in potential stress situations.
- Values clarification: Having an understanding of those things that are important will help the participants to have a better understanding of themselves.
- Goal setting and future planning: Developing a systematic way to pursue future goals helps participants to focus on objectives and troubleshoot potential barriers.
- Decision making and problem solving: Identifying problem areas and looking at alternative solutions helps the participant to broaden his or her options.

- Leisure interests: Exploring activities that will tap participants' interests will support an adaptive lifestyle.
- Time management: Being able to schedule, plan, and effectively utilize time will encourage health and discourage stress.
- Social skills and interaction: Learning effective communications skills along with skills for interacting with others will give participants a better chance for establishing meaningful relationships.
- Assertiveness: Standing up for one's rights, values, and interests will increase the likelihood that one's needs will be met.
- Anger management: Learning to take charge of anger will prevent anger from getting out of control.
- Self-concept: Having a sense of self-identity and self-esteem will assist participants to take more risks and be more adaptive.

See samples of goal-setting and decision-making activity plans in Table 35-1.

The educational sessions are sequenced to build one upon another or to stand alone, depending upon the population to be served. The structure of the group can allow for an individual to enter the program at any point and then participate through the entire series of educational sessions. There are typically a couple of days between sessions to allow participants to carry out assignments or to seek outside information if needed.

The facilitators of the Life Skills groups should have experience and interest in group dynamics and leadership skills. The ideal leadership situation would be to have cofacilitator teams with an OT and an OTA.

CASE STORY

John Rogers is a 21-year-old white male who is in his junior year at a midwestern college. He is currently working toward his Bachelor's degree with a Major in Education and a Minor in Psychology. He has begun to experience some uncomfortable anxiety during the last several months. There have been a couple of things that have been weighing on his mind and have begun to effect his ability to concentrate. These things include:

- He is not sure about his major or minor and whether or not these subjects will allow him to find a fulfilling job after graduation.
- He has begun to question his sexual orientation. He is finding that he is attracted to other males, which frightens him because of the implications it will have on his future plans and the reaction of his family members.

John had planned out his life following graduation, when he was going to go back to his small home town, get a job as a teacher, get married, and have a large family. This has been the expectation for as long as he can remember. He is the youngest of 5 children and his 2 older brothers and 2 older sisters are married, have children, and all live within an hour of their parents. They all seem happy to him but this does not seem to be the life that he finds meaningful.

Table 35-1

Samples of Goal-Setting and Decision-Making Activity Plans

Facilitator Instructions

Objective: To help participants identify and plan for ways to reach their personal goals.

What facilitators do:

1. Provide participants with worksheets to complete.
2. Explain the task.
3. Insure that each participant understands the task. Provide examples if necessary.
4. Assist participants in completion of the task by asking questions that might stimulate their thinking or formulate their goal statements.
5. Encourage group discussion and feedback after participants have had time to complete the task.
6. Model appropriate behaviors in writing goals, giving feedback, and discussing ideas.
7. Ask questions that will help participants to clarify their own goals.

Materials needed:
- Goal setting worksheets
- Pencils/pens

Decision Making

Objective: To identify a decision that needs to be made within the next 3 months.

Task instructions:

1. Pass out a 3 x 5 card to each participant.
2. On one side of the card, write a decision that you need to make within the next 3 months.
3. On the opposite side of the card, list 3 possible alternative decisions.
4. Each participant, in turn, will share his or her decision with the group along with the possible alternatives.
5. Group members are asked to verbally vote for the best alternative and to give the reason for their vote.

What facilitators do:

1. Pass out a 3 x 5 card to each participant.
2. Provide instructions for the task.
3. Stimulate the discussion portion of the task.

Materials needed:
- 3 x 5 cards
- Pencils/pens

John belongs to a fraternity and lives in the fraternity house. He is friends with all of the other guys in the house, and he has developed a close relationship with one guy in particular. They share many of their feelings and whenever the two of them are together there is an electricity between them that he cannot explain. John has never talked to his friend, Tim, about the feelings he has been experiencing about other men, especially him. John has been involved with females in the past, but those relationships never lasted more than a couple months.

All of these concerns have caused John to experience difficulty sleeping at night, a loss of appetite, difficulty focusing on his assignments, and being somewhat short and curt with his friends. John did a recent student teaching practicum and he found himself easily irritated by some of the adolescent behavior.

Tim suggested that John might want to go to the Student Health Center and talk to a professional about what was going on. John followed up on this suggestion and met with a coun-selor at the Student Health Center. The counselor realized that what John was experiencing was something normal for his age group. He was not suicidal, did not need inpatient hospitalization, and did not require any psychotropic medications. The counselor referred John to the Community Mental Health Center, which includes a Life Skills Program that allows individuals to focus on specific areas that were causing them anxiety or concern and to develop skills for living their lives.

The primary facilitator of the Life Skills Program was an OT who has an OTA as an assistant. The OT completed a comprehensive interview in order to evaluate the areas in which John was having difficulty in order to recommend the most appropriate track. The evaluation was directed at John's education/work history, family support and other social support, current living environment, goal inventory, time inventory, and a self-assessment of problem areas. The OTA was available to assist John with completing a pen and paper assessment in the form of a questionnaire that consisted of guiding questions on the above identified areas. The OT then reviewed the questionnaire with John and asked probing questions that allowed John to expand on his written answers.

It was agreed with John that he would benefit from addressing the following:

- Goal setting and future planning to help him get a handle on what he wants to do with his life.
- Social skills and interaction to gain support and information with others who are questioning their sexual orientation and are in various stages of the process of coming out.
- Values clarification to assist him in identifying what is now important to him at this stage in his life.
- Stress management and relaxation in order to learn his response to stress and how he can cope with it in order to minimize the disruption caused to his life.

Treatment Implementation and Goals

John was placed into the following Life Skills Program groups and the goals for each group were as follows:

Goal Setting and Future Planning

- Goal: John will complete a vocational inventory assessment in order to identify possible career alternatives.
- Goal: John will identify personal goals and establish a plan of action for achievement of those goals.

Social Skills and Interaction

- Goal: John will discuss with his friend Tim the issues that are ongoing in his life in order to obtain the support of his best friend.

Values Clarification

- Goal: John will attend the college's Gay and Lesbian Student Association weekly meetings in order to educate himself, further explore, and obtain support during his coming out process.

Stress Management and Relaxation

- Goal: John will complete a stress inventory and identify realistic coping mechanisms for his identified stressors.

John was involved in the Life Skills Program for 8 weeks. He responded well to the groups and accomplished the following:

Goal Setting and Future Planning

He completed a vocational inventory and found that his strongest interests were in a helping profession. Upon further exploration, he decided that he would complete his Bachelor's degree in Education with a minor in Psychology and then pursue a Master's degree in Social Work. He felt this would give him a variety of options when he graduates. He completed the goal setting activity worksheet (Figure 35-1), which outlined the process for goal achievement.

Social Skills and Interaction

With the group's encouragement, John discussed the issues that he has been addressing with Tim. Tim stated that he was

not gay, but he wanted to remain John's best friend and he was very supportive of John as he struggled to deal with these ongoing issues.

Values Clarification

John identified that it is important to him to share his news with his family so he has begun to work on how and when to do that. In addition, he attended the weekly meetings of the college's Gay and Lesbian Student Association and has found them to be a great support system. He has begun dating one of the other members.

Stress Management and Relaxation

John completed a stress inventory and learned more about the physiological reaction that his body undergoes when he is under stress. He learned various coping mechanisms to include relaxation techniques.

John felt that he had benefited significantly from the various Life Skills Program groups with which he was involved. He found it very informative to hear what other people were experiencing and how they coped with various issues in their lives. He also found the education component helpful and the ideas generated could be carried over into his current situation.

CLINICAL PROBLEM SOLVING

Since the principles and elements of the Life Skills Program can be used with a diverse population (clients/patients) of virtually all ages and with a variety of needs, there is not only one way to organize the experiential sessions. Following are some mini case studies that can be used to stimulate creative ways to address those needs. How might you plan a Life Skills Program for each of these individuals? How would you facilitate a group with these individuals? What might be indicators that each one of these individuals is increasing his or her resilience, hardiness, and life skills?

- Allison was just promoted in an up and coming business. She is excited about the opportunity, but would be required to relocate to a large city away from her family. This is the first time that she would not be close to her family members. She is worried that she cannot do it on her own. She is scared and wonders if the promotion is worth it.
- Leroy has been seen in OT for rehabilitation of his right dominant hand following laceration of his flexor tendons. He sustained the injury in a fight with his brother-in-law. He has a history of fighting and states that he is not able to control his anger.
- James knew his parents would eventually get divorced. During his second semester at college, he received a phone call that his father was moving out. He contemplates how his life will change and hates the thought that his family life is unstable and uncertain.
- Madeline moved to town after her husband died and she was clearly not able to continue managing the family farm. When she lived on the farm, she spent all of her time doing household chores in support of the workers

---

Goal Setting

Write down 5 goals that you would like to accomplish within the next 4 years.
1.
2.
3.
4.
5.

Copy the one that is the most important to you.

List 3 barriers that might get in the way:
1.
2.
3.

List 3 helpers that might help you get past the barriers:
1.
2.
3.

Write 5 steps to get to your most important goal:
1.
2.
3.
4.
5.

Figure 35-1. Goal setting activity worksheet.

such as cooking, cleaning, and washing. She identifies her only friends as her husband and the farmhands.

LEARNING ACTIVITIES

1. Lead a group on goal setting specific to your personal lives.
2. Present a project on spirituality as related to life skills.
3. Before lecture begins, list all the ways you have learned "life skills."

REFERENCES

Ackerson, B. J. (2000). Factors influencing life satisfaction in psychiatric rehabilitation. *Psychiatric Rehabilitation Journal, 23*(3), 253-261.

Baum, C. M., & Law, M. (1997). Occupational therapy practice: Focusing on occupational performance. *American Journal of Occupational Therapy, 51*(4), 277-288.

Brendtro, L. (1997). Mending broken spirits of youth. *Reclaiming Children and Youth: Journal of Emotional and Behavioral Problems, 5*(4), 197-202.

Brendtro, L., & Brokenleg, M. (1993). Beyond the curriculum of control. *Reclaiming Children and Youth: Journal of Emotional and Behavioral Problems, 1*(4), 5-11.

Brendtro, L., Brokenleg, M., & Van Bockern, S. (1990). *Reclaiming youth at risk: Our hope for the future.* Bloomington, IN: National Education Service.

Burleigh, S. A., Farber, R. S., & Gillard, M. (1998). Community integration and life satisfaction after traumatic brain injury: Long-term findings. *American Journal of Occupational Therapy, 52*(1), 45-52.

Christiansen, C. H. (1999). Defining lives: Occupation as identity: An essay on competence, coherence, and the creation of meaning. The 1999 Eleanor Clarke Slagle Lecture. *American Journal of Occupational Therapy, 53*(6), 547-558.

Curwin, R., & Mendler, A. (1988). *Discipline with dignity.* Alexandria, VA: Association for Supervision and Curriculum Development.

Gahnstrom-Strandqvist, K., Liukko, K., & Tham, K. (2003). The meaning of the working cooperative for persons with long-term mental illness: A phenomenological study. *American Journal of Occupational Therapy, 57*(3), 262-272.

Hull, J. B. (1998). The association of engagement in meaningful roles and life satisfaction in older adults after physical rehabilitation. Master's thesis.

Johnson, M. T. (1987). Occupational therapists and teaching of cognitive behavioral skills. *Occupational Therapy in Mental Health, 7*(3), 69-81.

EVIDENCE-BASED TREATMENT STRATEGIES

Treatment Strategies	Authors
Normalizing process	Gahnstrom-Strandqvist, Liukko, & Tham, 2003
Life coaching	Yousey, 2001
Leisure	Klasson & MacRae, 1985; Lloyd, King, Lampe, & McDougall, 2001; Schlien & Ray, 1997
Life satisfaction	Ackerson, 2000; Burleigh, Farber, & Gillard, 1998; Hull, 1998; Larsson & Branholm, 1996; Yerxa & Baum, 1986
Life skills including skill development in goal setting, assertiveness, problem solving, independent living skills, coping, stress management, prevocational, self-care, value clarification, and interpersonal skills	Ackerson, 2000; Christiansen, 1999; Johnson, 1987; Jones & McColl, 1991; Keller & Hayes, 1998; Klasson & MacRae, 1985; Kniepmann & Flanagan, 1995; Knis, 1995; Saunders, Sayer, & Goodale, 1999; Schlien & Ray, 1997; Thomes & Bajema, 1983; Waid, 1993; Watson & Thomes, 1983; Yerxa, 1998, 2000
Cognitive-behavioral therapy	Johnson, 1987
Locus of control	Yerxa & Baum, 1986
View of self	Gahnstrom-Strandqvist et al., 2003; Kniepmann & Flanagan, 1995
Mastery	Ackerson, 2000
Identity	Christiansen, 1999
Life activities and life-long learning	Baum & Law, 1997; Larsson & Branholm, 1996; Schlien & Ray, 1997
Competency	Thomes & Bajema, 1983

Jones, E. J., & McColl, M. A. (1991). Development and evaluation of an interactional life skills group for offenders. *Occupational Therapy Journal of Research, 11*(2), 80-92.

Keller, S., & Hayes, R. (1998). The relationship between the Allen Cognitive Level Test and the Life Skills Profile. *American Journal of Occupational Therapy, 52*(10), 851-856.

Klasson, E. M., & MacRae, A. (1985). A university-based occupational therapy clinic for chronic schizophrenics. *Occupational Therapy in Mental Health, 5*(2), 1-11.

Kniepmann, K., & Flanagan, J. (1995). Violence prevention for children and families. Conference Abstracts and Resources. American Occupational Therapy Association.

Knis, L. L. (1995). Coping skills: The play's the thing. *OT Week, 9*(35), 18-19.

Kobasa, S. C. (1979). Stressful life events, personality, and health: An inquiry into hardiness. *Journal of Personality and Social Psychology, 37,* 1-11.

Kobasa, S. C., Maddi, S. R., & Kahn, S. (1982). Hardiness and health: A prospective study. *Journal of Personality and Social Psychology, 42,* 168-177.

Larson, S. (1996). Meeting needs of youthful offenders through the spiritual dimension. *Reclaiming Children and Youth: Journal of Emotional and Behavioral Problems, 5*(3), 167-172.

Larsson, M., & Branholm, I. B. (1996). An approach to goal-planning in occupational therapy and rehabilitation. *Scandinavian Journal of Occupational Therapy, 3*(1), 14-19.

Lloyd, C., King, R., Lampe, J., & McDougall, S. (2001). The leisure satisfaction of people with psychiatric disabilities. *Psychiatric Rehabilitation Journal, 25*(2), 107-113.

Saunders, I., Sayer, M., & Goodale, A. (1999). The relationship between playfulness and coping in preschool children: A pilot study. *American Journal of Occupational Therapy, 53*(2), 221-226.

Schlien, S. J., & Ray, M. T. (1997). Leisure education for a quality transition to adulthood. *Journal of Vocational Rehabilitation, 8*(2), 155-169.

Thomes, L. J., & Bajema, S. L. (1983). The life skills development program: A history, overview and update. *Occupational Therapy in Mental Health, 3*(2), 35-48.

Waid, K. M. (1993). An occupational therapy perspective in the treatment of multiple personality disorder. *American Journal of Occupational Therapy, 47*(10), 872-876.

Watson, M. R., & Thomes, L. J. (1983). Project ABLE: A model for management of stress in the Army soldier. *Occupational Therapy in Mental Health, 3*(2), 55-61.

Yerxa, E. J. (1998). Health and the human spirit for occupation. *American Journal of Occupational Therapy, 52*(6), 412-418.

Yerxa, E. J. (2000). Occupational science: A renaissance of service to humankind through knowledge. *Occupational Therapy International, 7*(2), 87-98.

Yerxa, E. J., & Baum, C. (1986). Engagement in daily occupations and life satisfaction among people with spinal cord injuries. *Occupational Therapy Journal of Research, 6*(5), 271-283.

Yousey, J. R. (2001). Life coaching: A one-on-one approach to changing lives. *OT Practice, 6*(1), 11-14.

Key Concepts

- Activities of daily living (ADL): Encompass a client's entire life span.
- Client choice: Each individual client determines the importance of BADL and IADL.
- Level of function: Can range from independent to moderate assistance to dependent.
- Performance skills: Formal and informal evaluations and assessments will determine performance skill areas.
- Documentation: Must be thorough and show functional significance.
- Client-centered care: Facilitation of client-centered care occurs with a global perspective and team approach.

Essential Vocabulary

alternative living environment: Skilled nursing facility, assisted living facility, or group home type setting to which a client may be discharged.

mobile arm support (MAS) or upper limb orthotic system (ULOS): An adaptive device, usually attached to a client's wheelchair, utilized for assistance with self-feeding and grooming.

tetraplegia: Formerly referred to as quadriplegia; paralysis of all extremities and trunk.

Chapter 36

ACTIVITIES OF DAILY LIVING

Corina Hall, MS, OTR

INTRODUCTION

Activities of daily living, or ADL as they are most commonly referred to in OT, encompass one's entire life span and living situation. From birth to later age, a person must always complete some sort of ADL task. In the newborn, it is feeding; in the child, it is basic self-care, school, and play; in the teenager, it may definitely be self-care and grooming, school, leisure, and possibly work; in the adult, it may be self-care, sexual expression, parenting, working, leisure, and care- giving; and in elderly, it can be self-care, productivity, and leisure pursuits. But what does all this mean? It means that from birth to death we, as individuals, are constantly engaging in ADL, in other words... *life*. To illustrate this, consider these scenarios.

Simone, a 37-year-old accountant and mother of a newborn son, suddenly has a left cerebral hemispheric stroke that leaves her dominant side hemiplegic and expressively aphasic. How will she complete her basic self-care needs and those emergent to her son? How will she fulfill her multiple roles in life? Josef, a 66-year-old retired business owner, falls off the ladder while painting and breaks his hip and wrist. What is this active man to do now that he is nonweight-bearing and unable to complete any functional mobility? Monika, a 75-year-old greenhouse volunteer and grandmother of 6, has been forgetting to lock her front door on a regular basis, turning on the stove and not returning to it, and has become increasingly disheveled over the past 6 months. Is it safe for her to live alone? How can OT impact these 3 very different scenarios? Why are ADL so important?

OCCUPATIONAL THERAPY FRAMEWORK

Before discussion can begin on ADL, we must first incorporate our new professional document, the *Occupational Therapy Practice Framework: Domain and Process* (AOTA, 2002). This document has been published in order to describe areas of the profession's focus and actions and to delineate the process of OT evaluation, intervention, and outcomes as related to OT's role

to incorporate the use of occupation (AOTA, 2003). The area of ADL is described in the domain section under a broader heading of Performance in Areas of Occupation. The 7 performance areas listed in the domain section include ADL (or BADL), IADL, education, work, play, leisure, and social participation. For the purpose of this chapter, we will only be focusing on BADL and IADL.

The *Occupational Therapy Practice Framework* (AOTA, 2003) defines ADL as "activities that are oriented toward taking care of one's own body" (p. 33). The *Occupational Therapy Practice Framework* goes on to describe various ADL tasks, including bathing/showering, bowel and bladder management, dressing, eating, feeding, functional mobility, personal device care, personal hygiene and grooming, sexual activity, sleep/rest, and toilet hygiene. All of these areas are specifically defined in the *Occupational Therapy Practice Framework* and will not be defined in this chapter. IADL is defined as "activities that are oriented toward interacting with the environment and that are often complex—generally optional in nature" (p. 34). IADL encompass care of others, care of pets, child rearing, communication device use, community mobility, financial management, health management and maintenance, meal preparation and cleanup, safety procedures and emergency responses, and shopping. Table 36-1 indicates ADL and IADL areas.

MEASURING INDEPENDENCE IN ACTIVITIES OF DAILY LIVING

Before we further discuss ADL, one must first look at a measurement of level of independence, meaning at what level of assistance are clients functioning with regards to ADL/IADL. In this chapter, we will be utilizing a nationally recognized measure of level of independence known as the Functional Independence Measure or FIM (University of Buffalo Foundation Activities, Inc. [UBFA], 2002). The FIM is an instrument that utilizes a 7-level rating scale ranging from independent to dependent. A score of 7 for a task denotes complete independence, completed safely and within a reasonable amount of time. This client does so without any modifications

---

Table 36-1

Activities of Daily Living

ADL Areas	IADL Areas
Self-Care	**Home Management**
Bathing/showering	Meal preparation
Dressing	Shopping
Grooming	Cleaning
Toileting	Laundry
Eating	Child care
Personal hygiene	
Functional Mobility	**Community Management**
Bed mobility	Money management
Transfers to functional surfaces	Public transportation
Wheelchair mobility	Driving
Work/school	
Communication	**Environmental Safety**
Writing	Fire safety
Computer	911 call
Telephone/cellular telephone	Dangerous situation awareness
Sexual Expression	**Health Management**
Physical	Medication management
Verbal	Health risk knowledge
Virtual	Appointment scheduling

Adapted from American Occupational Therapy Association. (2002). *The reference manual of the official documents of the American Occupational Therapy Association, Inc* (9th ed.). Bethesda, MD: Author.

---

or assistive devices. A score of 6 denotes modified independence in which the activity requires an assistive device, the activity takes more than reasonable amount of time, or the action involves safety considerations. A score of 5 or lower on the scale indicates the need for an assistant or help in some way. A 5 indicates supervision or setup. The client requires no more assistance than standby, cuing, or coaxing without physical contact, or the helper sets up any needed items or applies orthoses or adaptive devices. A score of 4 for a given task indicates minimum assistance in which the client completes greater than 75% of a given activity. A score of 3 denotes moderate assistance in which the client performs 50% to 74% of a given task, while a 2 indicates maximum assistance in which the client completes 25% to 49% of task. A score of 1 signifies total assistance in which the client performs less than 25% of an activity (UBFA, 2002).

These measures will be seen throughout evaluations, progress reports, monthly reports, and/or discharge documentation on a regular basis; thus, it is necessary to familiarize practitioners with these common definitions/levels of independence. The grading of level of function has a tremendous impact on outcomes, discharge disposition, and level of assistance required by a client. For example, if a client is maximum assistance with bathing and transfers and lives alone, barriers to discharge are going to be quite different than a client who is functioning at a modified independence level or even a set-up level. Levels of function and their accuracy of measurement are also of great significance to third-party payer sources such as Medicare, Medicaid, and health maintenance organizations (HMOs) because they may only reimburse for services up until a certain level of independence. For example, if a client is at a supervision level at a rehabilitation center but has assistance at home from a family member, that client may be denied further rehabilitation services because the level of independence and support system indicates rehabilitation services are no longer indicated.

ACTIVITIES OF DAILY LIVING EVALUATION

There are multiple types of ADL/IADL evaluations that an OT or OTA may be involved in administering. There are evaluations for basic self-care areas, evaluations of UE, cognitive evaluations, visual/perceptual evaluations, evaluations for communication abilities, home evaluations, driving evaluations, work site evaluations, and wheelchair evaluations. One of the purposes of this chapter is to familiarize the OT practitioner with understanding the information presented on these evaluations and not so much the completion of it. The general purpose of an evaluation, specifically an ADL evaluation, is to gather client significant data related to specific life tasks and roles. Evaluations can be formally or informally completed. Figure 36-1 represents one of many OT evaluations and encompasses all major performance areas. With an emphasis on shortened length of stay at any health care facility, an evaluation must be completed as quickly as possible.

A practitioner must learn to balance observation, interview, and any formal testing with regards to the evaluation, with collaboration of client-centered goals, treatment intervention/planning, and discharge outcomes, and do so in an efficient manner. Observation and actual client task performance are 2 of the most reliable ways to achieve a level of independence score for a client. Observation and task performance will detect safety issues the client may have, allow for determination of underlying physical or cognitive deficits that decrease a client's level of independence, allow for determination of underlying visual/perceptual deficits that may require formal testing, and are the most accurate indicators of level of function in a client. Client interview is also a good evaluation of ADL; however, clients with cognitive or mental health deficits may not give reliable, accurate information. Follow-up with interdisciplinary team members and/or family may be indicated. An evaluation determines specific causes of performance deficits, including decreased strength, decreased ROM, fluctuating muscle tone, decreased endurance, increased pain, joint weightbearing restrictions/orthopedic restrictions, cognitive/psychosocial deficits, and/or incoordination. Observation of a client presents the practitioners with a clearer picture of overall deficits and allows for smooth transition of treatment intervention/planning and goal setting. Observation of performance may also give indication to treatment approaches, potential adaptive devices, splinting needs, and discharge planning that will be required to achieve functional outcomes set.

There are a number of formalized ADL evaluations to select from that allow for formalized scoring after administration. Although formal evaluations may take a longer period of time to complete, they have the ability to supply the practitioner with psychometric properties that increase the reliability and validity of the results. Often these evaluations provide standardized norms or final scores that make discharge planning easier, especially if the treatment team has conflicting opinions or if litigation is an issue. Formalized ADL evaluations may include the Milwaukee Evaluation of Daily Living Skills (MEDLS), the Kohlman Evaluation of Living Skills (KELS), the Functional Status Index (FSI), and the Klein-Bell ADL Scale (Christiansen & Matuska, 2004).

TREATMENT APPROACHES/ PLANNING INTERVENTION

A collaborative approach should be followed when completing treatment planning and intervention. The most important collaborative process involves the OT practitioner and the client. We will use the term *client* in this chapter to mean not just the patient, but any persons involved with that patient. This can range from spouse and family member to caregivers, friends, neighbors, parents, etc. The second collaboration process is between all disciplines that make up the rehabilitation team and can include PT, speech therapy, recreational therapy, social worker, case manager, doctor, nursing, dietician, etc. The third collaboration process is to explore a client's needs, support system, and resources prior to intervention, as these may dictate treatment intervention (Christiansen & Matuska, 2004).

There are multiple approaches that an OT practitioner can utilize during the treatment planning and intervention stage when collaborating to increase a client's ADL status. This section will first discuss those approaches, followed with planning and intervention strategies.

Remediation or rehabilitative strategies involve incorporating motor, cognitive, or sensory techniques to partially or fully restore the specific causes related to decreased performance with ADL tasks. An example of this would be a client with Guillain-Barré syndrome, who presents to the OT practitioner with decreased UE dressing secondary to muscular weakness. The remediation approach would involve muscle strengthening with hopes of follow-through with increased independence in the dressing task. Techniques and treatment theories that arise from neuroscience, biomechanics, and/or motor control are included in remediation strategies (Christiansen & Matuska, 2004). A balance of the 2 approaches should be utilized to maximize a client's ability to meet outcome objectives and goals.

Compensatory strategies involve the client's ability to perform an ADL task within his or her current capabilities or relearn new techniques for accomplishing ADL goals (e.g., learning one-handed dressing techniques after a stroke). Compensatory strategies also may involve manipulation of a client's environment in order to successfully accomplish a task despite any limitations in ability. An example of this might be installing an environmental control unit for household electrical appliances such as lights, television, computer, etc. With this modification, a client with tetraplegia is able to access his or her home with voice commands or head/eye movements. Another example of compensatory strategies with regards to manipulation involves routine and set-up of environment in such a way that a client with schizophrenia is able to accurately perform basic ADL. With a structured environment and routine organization, this client can consistently complete tasks with minimal interruption of a task. A third type of compensatory strategy is the use of adaptive devices to facilitate the ADL process. This can be a product already designed or a creative device fabricated by the OT practitioner. For example, a client having hand tremors secondary to PD may increase independence with self-feeding with weighted utensils. The last compensatory strategy involves any ADL task to be completed by a family member, caregiver, home health aide, personal care attendant, or any other designated, trained member of a client's environment. As OT practitioners, we must remember that the client's perception of independence related to ADL may not be the same as others, thus collaboration with the client is a first priority in treatment planning and intervention (Christiansen & Matuska, 2004).

Corina Hall Rehab Institute
Occupational Therapy Evaluation

Patient Name	
Patient Age	Male/Female
Date of Admission	Date of Referral
Diagnosis	
Onset of Illness	

Past Medical History ______

Current Life Roles ______

Precautions ______

Current Living Situation ______

Support System ______

KEY

1 - Total Assistance/Dependent	*4 - Minimal Assistance/Contact Guard Assistance*	*7 - Indepent*
2 - Maximum Assistance	*5 - Supervision/Verbal Cues*	*TBA = To be assessed*
3 - Moderate Assistance	*6 - Modified Independence*	*N/A = Not applicable*

BASIC DAILY LIVING SKILLS

	Status *(see key above)*	Transfer Type *(circle one)*	Comments *(Include DME/Adaptive Devices)*
Feeding			
Grooming			
UE Dressing			
LE Dressing			
Bathing			
Toiletting			
Bed Mobility			
Bed/Chair/Wheelchair transfer		SPT Ambulatory Dependent Lift	
Toilet Transfer		SPT Ambulatory Dependent Lift	
Tub/Shower Transfer		SPT Ambulatory Dependent Lift	
Car/SUV/Van Transfer		SPT Ambulatory Dependent Lift	
Other			

INSTRUMENTAL DAILY LIVING SKILLS		Comments
Meal Preparation		
Homemaking		
School/Work Skills		
Community Skills		
Leisure Skills		
Other		

Figure 36-1A. Sample occupational therapy evaluation.

Treatment planning and intervention involves effective communication between not only interdisciplinary team members and the client, but also between OT practitioners.

Performance Skills Specific for Activities of Daily Living

Treatment approaches will vary with specific performance deficit areas and specific diagnoses. The next section of this chapter will focus on these specific ADL treatment techniques and principles. Keep in mind that clients are separate individu-

UPPER EXTREMITY EVALUATION   Hand Dominance: Right Left

ROM, Muscle
Strenth, Tone   _____
                  _____
                  _____
                  _____

Gross Motor/Fine
Motor Coordination _____
                  _____
                  _____

Sensation   _____
                  _____

Pain   _____

ENDURANCE LEVEL   _____

**WHEELCHAIR
SEATING AND
POSITIONING**   _____
                  _____
                  _____

COGNITIVE STATUS _____
                  _____
                  _____

**VISUAL /
PERCEPTUAL
STATUS**   _____
                  _____
                  _____

PATIENT GOALS   _____
                  _____

TREATMENT GOALS   **TREATMENT GOALS**
SHORT TERM   *LONG TERM*

_____   _____
_____   _____
_____   _____
_____   _____

Goals/Treatment Plan were/were not discussed with and were/were not understood by patient

**BARRIERS TO
DISCHARGE**   _____
                  _____

TREATMENT PLAN
_____ Patient to be placed on Occupational Therapy Program
_____ Patient educated for independent treatment program/to be monitored
_____ Discharge patient with no further OT Services at this time/re-consult as necessary

_____   _____
Therapist's signature   *Date*

Figure 36-1B. Sample occupational therapy evaluation.

als, and remedies that work well for one client may not work for another, even though they may have similar presentations or diagnoses.

Muscle Weakness and Activities of Daily Living

As an OT practitioner, one must first recognize the cause of the muscle weakness and whether or not it is temporary or permanent. In clients with complete spinal cord injuries, it is a generalization that one can maintain current muscle strength in innervated areas; however, in muscles innervated above the level of injury, there may not be any strength recovery. A compensatory approach may be utilized in this scenario. A client with Guillain-Barré syndrome has the good potential to regain muscle strength lost and thus a combination of remediation and compensatory strategies should be utilized.

Another factor to consider in muscle weakness is the exhausting effort it may take a client to complete ADL tasks. Energy conservation techniques should be incorporated to facilitate ease of task and decrease expenditure of current muscle strength. Some diagnoses, such as MS, have exacerbations of decreased strength, and energy conservation, as well as adaptive devices, may need to be utilized. Let us take a look at more specific ADL tasks with relation to muscle weakness and adaptive equipment.

Dressing

Long-handled devices can be utilized for energy conservation, while larger fitting clothing, slip-on type shoes or placement of elastic shoelaces, sock aids, and replacing fasteners on shirts with Velcro or zippers can all be utilized to assist a client with dressing tasks. Remember the location where a client completes dressing can also decrease need for full muscle strength. For example, completing lower body dressing in bed allows the client to utilize rolling side-to side to hike underwear and pants over hips. Figure 36-2 depicts adaptive dressing devices.

Feeding

MAS or ULOS may be used for proximal UE support during feeding task, or upper extremities may be supported on a raised table surface in order to achieve support. However, clients may resist this type of equipment. Light-weight utensils, dorsal wrist supports with universal cuffs, built-up handles, plate guards, scoop dishes, bi-handled cups, and straws are just a few of the adapted devices available for clients with weakened hand/grip strength.

Grooming

Adaptive devices and environmental adaptations can be utilized to facilitate independence in grooming with the client having muscle weakness. Suction cup denture brushes, electric toothbrushes, large capped toothpaste, and curved-bar holders have been made for assistance with razors, hairbrushes, and make-up items. Grooming devices such as a hair dryer can be mounted on a wall. Also remember that grooming tasks do not have to be completed standing up at the sink, and a seated position is a great way to incorporate energy conservation.

Transfers

Bath and shower seats are available in all shapes and sizes to promote energy conservation in transfers and in bathing. Bed canes or rails can be utilized to increase independence with bed mobility, while decreased amount of strength and energy needed to complete this task. A wheelchair, manual or power, may be indicated for functional mobility. Bedside or rolling commodes may be utilized to facilitate independence with toilet transfer and toileting during periods of decreased strength.

Home Management

There are multiple types of environmental control units that require only eye gaze, head movements, or voice commands to utilize. For people with tetraplegia, this allows increased independence within their home living area. Clients can also be educated on, and can practice, incorporating work simplification techniques, which will lead to decreased energy required to complete home as well as childcare or work tasks (Pedretti & Early, 2001; Trombly & Radomski, 2002).

Incoordination and Activities of Daily Living

As an OT practitioner, one must again distinguish a cause for incoordination in one or both hands. Are tremors or shakiness the targeting problem or is there generalized muscle weakness in the hand? A variety of CNS disorders, including PD, TBI, MS, and even medication side effects, can result in incoordination. Another factor of incoordination to consider is changes that occur in the hands secondary to arthritis. In this scenario, lack of coordination would stem from skeletal changes that have occurred in the hands, thus decreasing abilities in the hand. We will discuss arthritis and ADL in more depth when discussing ADL and lack of ROM. A basic consideration with clients who present with incoordination is the premise of stabilization. By stabilizing an object, such as a shirt, or stabilizing proximal body parts, such as forearms on a table, there is an increased chance of success with fine motor tasks.

Dressing

Large-handled, weighted dressing aids such as button hooks; pull on pants, skirts, or shorts with elastic waist bands; slip-on shoes or placement of elastic shoelaces; sports bras or camisoles; pullovers; and T-shirts prevent needing to complete buttons, or keeping shirts fastened and donning/doffing overhead. Keep in mind that dressing from bed or chair will give support to client to enhance functional performance.

Feeding

It is important to make self-feeding safe for clients with decreased coordination. We must also keep in mind any social ramifications encountered when feeding becomes messy due to lack of control in the hands. To assist clients in self-feeding, utilize a nonskid surface for plate to rest upon, scoop dishes or plate guards, weighted utensils, straws, and handled mugs to increase effectiveness and independence.

Grooming

Weighted wrist cuffs may be helpful to assist the patient with performing grooming tasks such as brushing teeth, combing hair, shaving, and/or makeup application. Electrical appliances, such as shavers and toothbrushes, may increase stability in the hands, along with suction brushes for dental and nail care. Bath mittens for bathing combined with soap-on-a-rope can facilitate safe and effective bathing.

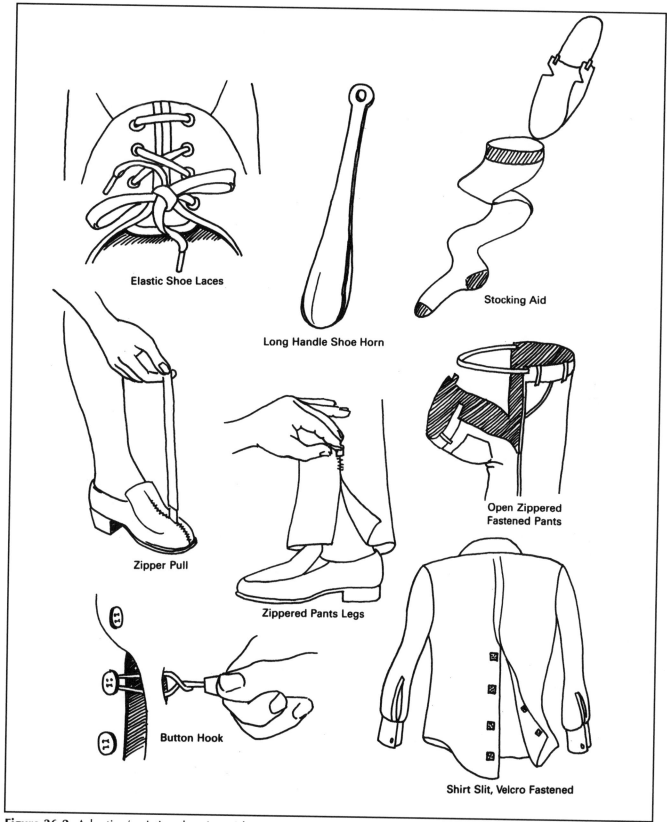

Elastic Shoe Laces

Long Handle Shoe Horn

Stocking Aid

Zipper Pull

Zippered Pants Legs

Open Zippered Fastened Pants

Button Hook

Shirt Slit, Velcro Fastened

Figure 36-2. Adaptive/assistive dressing aids.

Transfers

Mobility devices and ambulation aids are utilized dependent upon the severity of incoordination in a client. Adaptive devices such as raised toilet seats, commodes, bath seats, and grab bars can increase independence with a client while placing them at minimal risk for safety. A wheelchair may be indicated if clients are at increased risk for falls secondary to decreased coordination.

Home Management

Adaptations can be made to promote independence throughout the home in clients who present with decreased coordination. Large handles may be placed on all appliances, doorknobs, and electronic equipment utilized by a client. Frequently utilized items in the kitchen and bathroom should be stored within easy reach. Unbreakable dishes, spill-proof mugs, and large-handled, weighted utensils can be purchased for facilitation of independence during meal preparation and feeding. Nonskid mats or surfaces are helpful for stabilizing any objects on kitchen and bathroom counter tops. Figure 36-3 depicts adaptive homemaking devices.

Decreased Range of Motion and Activities of Daily Living

A lack of ROM can occur in any UE joint; however, the most frequently encountered are the shoulder and hand. Involved in these 2 joints are reach and grasp and thus these are the 2 areas most affected when there is a temporary or permanent loss of ROM. Lost ROM can be a result of UE trauma/surgery, arthritis and arthritic changes that have occurred within anatomical structures, or perhaps edema has caused a temporary loss in ROM. In all areas of ADL, adaptation is a key step toward independence.

Dressing

Long-handled devices such as reachers, dressing sticks, sock aids, elastic shoelaces, and shoe horns can be utilized to compensate for decreased reach to lower extremities and for joint protection techniques in hands. Built-up handles on button-hooks and zipper pulls will facilitate any UE clothing items. Adding elastic or Velcro to sleeves eliminates fastenings on shirts, jackets, and coats. Clients may want to utilize clothing that is a bit larger than their normal size, which can also facilitate independence with dressing tasks.

Feeding

Eating utensils may require adaptive handles in order to increase independence with clients and decreased grasp. Lengthened or angled utensils can be used separately or in conjunction with universal cuffs and facilitate ease of self-feeding. A plate guard or scoop dish can also assist with eating.

Grooming

Long handles or large grips placed on combs, hair brushes, razors, makeup, and toothbrushes can assist clients with decreased reach or grasp. Adaptive devices are available to place on aerosol spray cans, toothpaste, and hair care items to allow for ease of use with decreased grip and ROM.

Transfers

In addition to the aforementioned adaptive devices such as raised toilet seats, bath seats, etc., grab bars and a hand-held shower head can make bathing and transferring safely possible for clients with limited ROM and grasp. When assistive devices are necessary for ambulation, ambulatory aids can be adapted by building up cane or walker handles and wheelchair rims or by applying platforms to ease use of hands for UE support during functional ambulation. When limited ROM affects the client's ability to negotiate steps, a stair glide may be an option to increase independence within the home and to access all areas, even when limitations may exist.

Homemaking

Many of the adaptations that we have discussed can also be put into practice with clients who present with ROM limitations. Joint protection techniques are recommended in those clients presenting with arthritis. Eliminating bending and excessive reaching are the goals to be accomplished to increase independence with homemaking tasks. Strive for creating and educating clients on long-handled, lightweight appliances, and modify the environment to allow for limitations (Pedretti & Early, 2001; Trombly & Radomski, 2002).

Hemiplegia and Activities of Daily Living

ADL among clients with weakness was discussed earlier, but we will now spend some time discussing ADL with clients who have hemiplegia as a result of a CVA (i.e., stroke) or TBI. In clients' presenting with hemiplegia, the primary focus of ADL is on one-handed, compensatory techniques. The practitioner must also take into account that clients with hemiplegia have the potential of having decreased visual skills, decreased cognition, and decreased speech abilities to varying degrees of severity.

Dressing

There are multiple techniques for completing UE and LE dressing using a one-handed technique. The basic premise is that a client puts on, or dons, clothing items on the affected extremity first and then proceeds with the sound side. When taking off, or doffing, clothing, a client undresses the sound side first and then completes the affected side. This rule need not apply with socks and shoes. Adaptive devices such as elastic shoelaces, sock aids, and shoehorns may be utilized if the client has the cognitive capabilities of learning the use of new objects. Due to the potential for decreased balance, dressing may be completed with increased safety at a seated chair level or seated in bed level.

Feeding

A client may utilize a one-handed rocker knife for cutting items safely, along with using a plate guard or scoop dish to accommodate self-feeding.

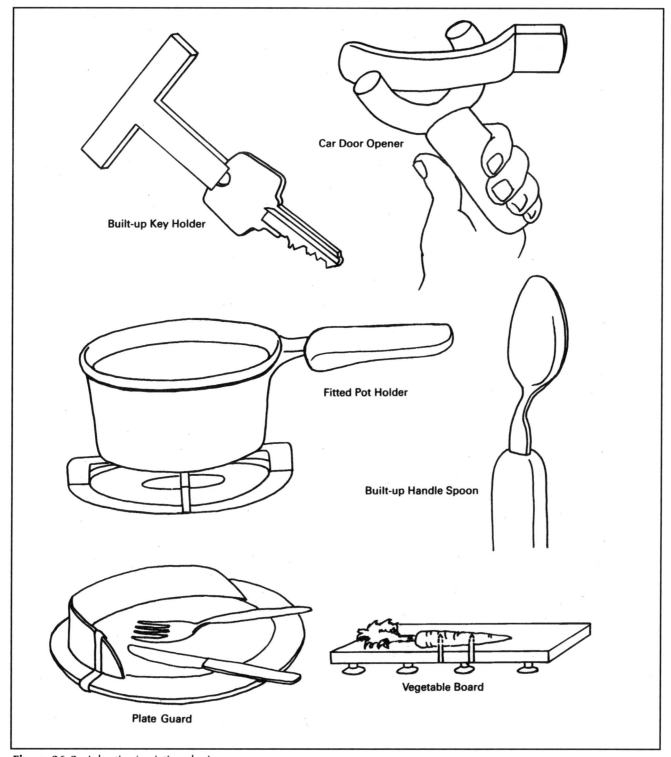

Figure 36-3. Adaptive/assistive devices.

Grooming

One-handed techniques are utilized to open items such as toothpaste, mouth wash, deodorant, and all other grooming or personal items that a client applies. When balance is a factor, allow the client to complete grooming tasks in a seated position to increase safety and decrease risk for falls. Take heed that a client may require assistance with thoroughness if visual neglect is an issue.

Transfers

Adaptive devices will be dependent upon a client's level of function. Bathroom equipment may be utilized when balance, strength, and cognition are limiting factors. Family or caregiver training may be required for household transfer and equipment usage if a client is functioning at a lower level. Wheelchair or ambulation devices may also be required for the client. Safe positioning of the hemiplegic extremity should be a focus during transfer scenarios to prevent further injury.

Homemaking

One-handed techniques need to be incorporated into homemaking skills during the treatment session. Adaptive devices such as one-handed can openers, mixers, and other utensils are available to facilitate independence. Suction cups or nonskid mats should be utilized for effective stabilization of any items utilized during functional homemaking tasks (Pedretti & Early, 2001; Trombly & Radomski, 2002).

Wheelchair Level Activities of Daily Living

A major consideration for clients whose primary mode of mobility will be at a wheelchair level, be it a manual or power wheelchair, is environmental modifications. Home environments are designed for an upright individual, so careful deliberation must be made to allow for wheelchair accommodations within a client's living situation. The OT practitioner should complete home evaluations as soon as possible in order to facilitate changes that are required within a client's setting. As an OT practitioner, you must keep in mind that client or family members may not accommodate recommendations, and alternative living environments may be indicated.

Dressing

For a person with paraplegia and low-level tetraplegia, lower body dressing is usually completed in bed in order to accommodate any balance issues. Upper body dressing can be completed in bed or from the wheelchair, depending on sitting balance and ability to tolerate upright positions. Long-handled utensils may be utilized to facilitate increased ease for lower body dressing. For high-level tetraplegics, dressing may not be a goal of the client, and in such a case caregiver or family training must occur to increase awareness of techniques and safety issues.

Feeding

Feeding status will be dependent upon physical status. A client with paraplegia should have no deficits with self-feeding from a wheelchair level unless other limitations are present. Please refer to decreased muscle strength section for further adaptations with regards to feeding. Environmental adaptations may need to be made in order to allow access to the table, with awareness of clearance of wheelchair.

Grooming

Grooming status will be dependent upon physical status. A client with paraplegia should have no deficits with grooming from a wheelchair level unless other limitations are present. Please refer to decreased muscle strength section for further adaptations with regards to grooming. Environmental adaptations may need to be made in order to allow access to sink with awareness of clearance and maneuverability of wheelchair within bathroom setting.

Transfers

Adaptive devices for transfers are again dependent upon the client's level of function. A rolling shower chair or bath bench may be required to facilitate safe and effective transfers into the bathroom area. A hospital bed or rails may be indicated to facilitate independence with bed mobility and positioning. A formal wheelchair evaluation must occur with an OT practitioner to provide options for the best seating and positioning, best mobility adaptations, and accurate fit for each individual client.

Home Management

After a thorough home assessment is completed, recommendations should be made with regards to having everything in a client's environment accessible from wheelchair level. Education and training should be provided to the client with regards to compensatory techniques when accessibility is not an option in one's living environment. Remodeling may be indicated, in which case collaboration with an architect or contractor may be beneficial.

Cognitive and Psychosocial Issues and Activities of Daily Living

Multiple cognitive areas and psychological issues will impact ADL and daily functioning. Diagnoses such as TBI or CVA may cause decreased cognitive areas, including memory, attention, planning, initiation, organization, insight, problem solving, and safety awareness. Other diagnoses such as Alzheimer's or dementia can impact memory and awareness. Developmental disorders such as CP or mental retardation (MR) impact learning abilities as well as cognition. Mental health disorders such as schizophrenia, depression, and bipolar disorder may cause positive or negative symptoms, along with pharmacological side effects, that impact performance of ADL (Hansen & Atchison, 1999). A comprehensive cognitive evaluation must be completed to provide the OT practitioner with a global understanding of a client's overall status and ability to learn in order to best facilitate plan of treatment for ADL remediation. An understanding of cognitive deficits will allow for client, family, and/or caregiver education with regards to safety and verbal cues required to increase independence.

In all areas of ADL, including dressing, feeding, grooming, transfers, and homemaking, a key goal is safety for the client and caregiver. Basic ADL tasks may need to be organized in simplistic fashion, and verbal cues, or prompting, may be required for accurate and safe completion of tasks.

DOCUMENTATION OF PERFORMANCE AND PROGRESS

Thorough documentation is a key concept in a world that is driven by lawsuits. At any time, a colleague, supervisor, administrator, third-party payer source, or attorney can review the practitioner's notes. Our own association, the AOTA, outlines and discusses fundamental elements of documentation in their manual of official documents (AOTA, 2002). Clearly all performance must be documented, but along with client performance, an OT practitioner must document subjective findings; education completed with client, family, caregiver, and/or nursing staff; and a response to the education provided. Also take note that how the education is completed, be it via demonstration, written material, or verbal guidance, must be documented. Remember, education should occur daily in treatment sessions; thus, it is an important part of any documentation. Figure 36-4 depicts a daily progress note with all components necessary for a complete progress report. Documentation requirements will vary depending on the type of facility in which you are employed; however, there are regulatory agencies, such as CARF or JCAHO, who set guidelines for standards of documentation. Along with daily progress, one must also continually re-evaluate, albeit informally, client goals and barriers to discharge as treatment progresses. This truly allows for client-centered care and a continuity that is required in today's health care system.

CLINICAL REASONING

Figures 36-5A and 36-5B are examples of initial evaluations you have just received from an OT practitioner. Review the record as if you were the treating OTA. What are the strengths? Is there anything missing? What are pertinent pieces of information you can extract from this evaluation? What are things that need to be added to this evaluation? A treatment plan would include education for joint protection and labor saving strategies to be incorporated into basic ADL areas such as dressing and bed mobility. UE and LE strengthening via transfer training, standing tolerance, and actual homemaking tasks to increase endurance and increased independence in transfer skills, and client goal of meal preparation. Figure 36-6 depicts what a progress note would look like following a treatment session with this client. Is it clear to you as an outside treatment provider? What should be done next?

SUMMARY

ADL certainly do cover one's entire lifespan and can be essential components of our client's goals as they face adversity with a temporary or permanent disability. ADL are major areas that will be addressed by the OT practitioner. An evaluation consisting of interview and client performance of tasks will give the OT practitioner a global perspective of a client and will allow for collaboration of client-centered treatment and client-centered goals to occur. A focus of OT intervention and educa-

tion is to maximize clients potential for functional performance tasks through retraining and/or adaptive devices. Thorough documentation of our services must not be overlooked or taken lightly and must always utilize a client-centered focus to retain the future of OT services.

LEARNING ACTIVITIES

1. List 4 major areas of BADL.
2. List 4 major areas of IADL.
3. List at least 3 self-care tasks, 3 communication tasks, and 3 functional mobility tasks.
4. List at least 3 home management tasks, 3 community living tasks, and 3 health management tasks.
5. Review an adaptive equipment catalog and choose 10 adaptive devices used for personal hygiene and grooming for a person with right CVA. Consider the cost in the choice of these devices.
6. Demonstrate the use of 3 adaptive dressing devices mentioned in this chapter.
7. Teach another person to don and doff a full-sleeve shirt using one hand.

REFERENCES

American Occupational Therapy Association. (2002). *The reference manual of the official documents of the American Occupational Therapy Association, Inc* (9th ed.). Bethesda, MD: Author.

American Occupational Therapy Association. (2003). *Occupational therapy practice framework: Domain and process.* Bethesda, MD: Author.

Atwood, S. M., Holm, M. B., & James, A. (1994). Activities of daily living capabilities and values of long-term care facility residents. *American Journal of Occupational Therapy, 48,* 710-716.

Barger II, A., Funkhouser, K. B., Gravitz, T. L., Jusko, H. A., Lokke, S. L., McCullen, L. M., et al. (2000). Potential variable affecting the use of reachers by the elderly. *Physical and Occupational Therapy in Geriatrics, 17,* 51-82.

Brandt, A. (2001). The power of independence. *Rehabilitation Management, 14,* 54,56,58.

Calderon, K. S. (2001). Making the connection between depression and activity levels among the oldest-old: A measure of life satisfaction. *Activities, Adaptation & Aging, 25,* 59-73.

Christiansen, C., & Matuska, K. (2004). *Ways of living: Self-care strategies for special needs* (3rd ed.). Bethesda, MD: American Occupational Therapy Association.

Cooke, K. Z., Fisher, A. G., Mayberry, W., & Oakley, F. (2000). Differences in activities of daily living process skills of persons with and without alzheimer's disease. *Occupational Therapy Journal of Research, 20,* 87-105.

Goverover, Y,. & Hinojosa, J. (2002). Categorization and deductive reasoning: predictors of instrumental activity of daily living performance in adults with brain injury. *American Journal of Occupational Therapy, 56,* 509-516.

Hansen, R., & Atchison, B. (1999). *Conditions in occupational therapy: Effect on occupational performance* (2nd ed.). Philadelphia, PA: Lippincott, Williams & Wilkins.

The Burke Rehabilitation Hospital

Inpatient Therapy Daily Notes

Date: 01/14/2004

Service Date/Time: 1/14/2004 3:11:00PM
INPATIENT OCCUPATIONAL THERAPY ORTHOPEDIC DAILY NOTE

DIAGNOSIS: S/P BILAT TKR's

WEIGHT BEARING STATUS: (B) LE- is weight bearing as tolerated .

TREATMENT/INTERVENTION:
Bed Mobility: From a standard bed patient performed sit to supine independently and leg lifter and patient performed supine to sit independently and leg lifter .

Transfers:
WHEELCHAIR: Patient performed an ambulatory transfer using a cane to a manual wheelchair with contact guard .
TOILET: Patient performed an ambulatory transfer using a cane to a standard toilet with RTS with arms with contact guard .
TUB/SHOWER: Patient performed an ambulatory transfer using a cane to the tub with grab bars and with a tub safety rail with moderate assistance .
TUB/SHOWER: Patient performed an ambulatory transfer using a cane to the tub with grab bars and with a tub safety rail with minimal assistance .
BED/MAT: Patient performed an ambulatory transfer using a cane to a standard bed with contact guard .
BED/MAT: Patient performed an ambulatory transfer using a cane to a mat with contact guard .
Comment: Pt. required vcs for cane management.

Education: Education in bed transfers, toilet/commode transfers, tub/shower transfers, wheelchair transfers, was provided to the patient who demonstrated knowledge and carryover.

Therapeutic Exercise: Seated EOM, pt. performed 5 minutes AROM exercises with BLE positioning on a bolster to increase flexion/extension for increased ROM and thereby improved transfers. Prior to therex pt. required mod. A to complete tub transfer, after therex, pt. required min A, OT observes improved knee flexion after therex.

DME: Pt. to decide if she wants to get tub safety rail and grab bar.

TOTAL TREATMENT TIME: 45 minutes

TREATMENT RENDERED:
OT Self Care/Home Management (ADL, homemaking)

TREATMENT PLAN: Continue with current treatment plan. Continue OT services for:
-- car transfer
-- light homemaking
-- tub transfer
-- lower body dressing

Electronically Signed by: Raimondi, Sue, OT\L
Note Written and Signed on: 01/14/2004

Figure 36-4. A daily progress note with all components necessary for a complete progress report. (Reproduced with permission of The Burke Rehabilitation Hospital, White Plains, NY.)

Corina Hall Rehab Institute
Occupational Therapy Evaluation

Patient Name	Simone
Patient Age	37 Male/(Female)
Date of Admission 2/14/04	Date of Referral 2/14/04
Diagnosis	(L)CVA; (R) hemiplegia
Onset of Illness	2/7/04

Past Medical History No significant PMH: Full term birth unremarkable

Current Life Roles Works PT as an accountant for major corp. Married ē 1 son: age 3. Daily routine is childcare, household duties including finances. Enjoys sports/family

Precautions at risk for falls; on coumadin

Current Living Situation lives in single family home, 3 steps to enter, 12 steps to 2nd floor. Bedroom/master bath 2nd floor; 1/2 ba. downstairs.

Support System husband/family/friends all supportive;

KEY

1 - Total Assistance/Dependent	4 - Minimal Assistance/Contact Guard Assistance	7 - Indepent
2 - Maximum Assistance	5 - Supervision/Verbal Cues	TBA = To be assessed
3 - Moderate Assistance	6 - Modified Independence	N/A = Not applicable

BASIC DAILY LIVING SKILLS

	Status (see key above)	Transfer Type (circle one)	Comments (Include DME/Adaptive Devices)
Feeding	5		Requires assist ē set up
Grooming	4		Seated; assist ē setup
UE Dressing	4		bra/T-shirt
LE Dressing	3		donned all LE garments
Bathing	2		seated level
Toiletting	3		
Bed Mobility	4		Verbal cues for technique
Bed/Chair/Wheelchair transfer	3	(SPT) Ambulatory Dependent Lift	—
Toilet Transfer	3	(SPT) Ambulatory Dependent Lift	raised toilet seat ē arms
Tub/Shower Transfer	2	(SPT) Ambulatory Dependent Lift	tub transfer bench
Car/SUV/Van Transfer	TBA	SPT Ambulatory Dependent Lift	
Other			

INSTRUMENTAL DAILY LIVING SKILLS

		Comments
Meal Preparation	TBA	Husband reports that patient completes all IADL's on a regular basis.
Homemaking		
School/Work Skills		
Community Skills		
Leisure Skills		
Other		

Figure 36-5A1. Examples of initial evaluations.

UPPER EXTREMITY EVALUATION   Hand Dominance: Right / Left

ROM, Muscle Strenth, Tone
Ⓛ UE WNL for AROM, Muscle strength + tone. Ⓡ UE presents c̄ full AROM throughout. Generalized 3/5 muscle strength; slightly increased to in elbow flexors and wrist fixors

Gross Motor/Fine Motor Coordination
WNL Ⓛ UE; Ⓡ hand presents c̄ decreased accuracy for tip pinch, opposition, placement and translation. No tremors noted. Able to utilize Ⓡ UE as gross assist.

Sensation
WNL for light touch, sharp/dull in Ⓑ UE. Decreased proprioception and kinesthesia in Ⓡ hand.

Pain
Per patient report no pain at this time.

ENDURANCE LEVEL
Fair for initial eval. as evidenced by reported fatigue p̄ evaluation.

WHEELCHAIR SEATING AND POSITIONING
Pt. fitted in standard w/c c̄ 18×16 Jay 2 cushion and Jay 2 tall back in order to promote symmetrical sitting, upright trunk + chest, facilitation of increased trunk support.

COGNITIVE STATUS
Patient alert, O × 3, noted word finding deficits; No internal/external distraction. Able to follow 2 step verbal directions; LTM appears intact as evidence by good historian. Further formal assessment indicated.

VISUAL / PERCEPTUAL STATUS
Acuity; saccades and tracking appear WFL. Pt. wears corrective lenses for distance. No neglect noted during functional evaluation. Further assessment indicated.

PATIENT GOALS
"I want to be able to play outside with my son."
"I want to be able to put in my contact lenses."

TREATMENT GOALS
SHORT TERM
Patient will complete bed mobility c̄ Ⓢ/VC's.
Patient will perform SPT c̄ CGA + DME.
Patient to complete grooming c̄ Ⓢ in standing.
Patient to complete UE/LE c̄ Ⓢ/VC's.
Patient to complete simple meal prep. c̄ min Ⓐ.
Goals/Treatment Plan (were) / were not discussed with and (were) / were not understood by patient

TREATMENT GOALS
LONG TERM
Ⓘ c̄ basic ADL's
Ⓢ c̄ IADL's
Ⓘ c̄ all surface transfers

BARRIERS TO DISCHARGE
↓ transfer abilities; limited dressing ability; limited childcare abilities; limited homemaking skills;

TREATMENT PLAN
✓ Patient to be placed on Occupational Therapy Program
___ Patient educated for independent treatment program/to be monitored
___ Discharge patient with no further OT Services at this time/re-consult as necessary

_____ Jzell OTR/L_____   02/14/04.
Therapist's signature   Date

Figure 36-5A2. Examples of initial evaluations.

The Burke Rehabilitation Hospital

Inpatient Occupational Therapy

Date: 01/10/2004

Service Date/Time: 1/10/2004 1:24:00PM

INPATIENT OCCUPATIONAL THERAPY
ORTHOPEDIC INITIAL EVALUATION

DIAGNOSIS: S/P BILAT TKR's
Weight Bearing Status: (B) LE- is weight bearing as tolerated .
-- Pt. states that she lives with her husand who can be very helpful with meal preparation and her 2 daughters live nearby whom will assist with laundry. Pt. states that her daily routine consists of sleeping late, performing meal preparation and enjoying time with her husband. Pt. reports that she had shingles 3 years ago which left her with neuralgia over the L lateral aspect of her trunk which is "quite painful", pt.is on medication to relieve the pain.

FUNCTIONAL STATUS:
BASIC ACTIVITIES OF DAILY LIVING:
Clothing Acquisition: Patient   is dependent on others to provide clothing prior to dressing.
Upper Body Dressing

Shirt	Set-up Help Only

Upper Body Dressing FIM Score: 5
Upper Body Dressing Status after Intervention/Education: Supervision
Lower Body Dressing

Underpants	Moderate Assistance
Pants	Moderate Assistance
TEDS	Dependent
Shoes	Maximum Assistance

Assistive Devices Used: none
Lower Body Dressing FIM Score: 2
Lower Body Dressing Status after Intervention/Education: Supervision – pt. issued reacher, LHSH and elastic shoelaces with good understanding.
Bed Mobility:

Activity	Assistance	Cues
Rolling to the Right	Minimal Assist.	Verbal cues for technique and Tactile cues for technique
Rolling to the Left	Minimal Assist	Verbal cues for technique and Tactile cues for technique
Supine to Sit	Moderate Assist	Verbal cues for technique
Sit to Supine	Moderate Assist	Verbal cues for technique

Overall status using following intervention and education (including any precautions i.e. THP) Minimal Assistance -- Pt. issued leg lifter and demonstrated ability to perform sit <--> supine with min A/vcs.

Transfers:
DME used prior to admission: tub safety rail, cane(s),
Additional DME owned (but not used PTA): RTS with arms,
Bed/Mat:

> **Surface:**Standard Bed
> **Level of Assistance:** Mod Assist
> **Method:** Ambulatory with RW
> **DME :** none

Wheelchair:

> **Surface:** Manual W/C
> **Level of Assistance:** Contact Guard
> **Method:** Ambulatory with RW

Figure 36-5B. Examples of initial evaluations. (Reproduced with permission of The Burke Rehabilitation Hospital, White Plains, NY.)

The Burke Rehabilitation Hospital

Inpatient Therapy Daily Notes

Date: 01/14/2004

Service Date/Time: 1/14/2004 3:11:00PM
INPATIENT OCCUPATIONAL THERAPY
ORTHOPEDIC DAILY NOTE

DIAGNOSIS: S/P BILAT TKR's

WEIGHT BEARING STATUS: (B) LE- is weight bearing as tolerated .

TREATMENT/INTERVENTION:
Bed Mobility: From a standard bed patient performed sit to supine independently and leg lifter and patient performed supine to sit independently and leg lifter .

Transfers:
 WHEELCHAIR: Patient performed an ambulatory transfer using a cane to a manual wheelchair with contact guard .
 TOILET: Patient performed an ambulatory transfer using a cane to a standard toilet with RTS with arms with contact guard .
 TUB/SHOWER: Patient performed an ambulatory transfer using a cane to the tub with grab bars and with a tub safety rail with moderate assistance .
 TUB/SHOWER: Patient performed an ambulatory transfer using a cane to the tub with grab bars and with a tub safety rail with minimal assistance .
 BED/MAT: Patient performed an ambulatory transfer using a cane to a standard bed with contact guard .
 BED/MAT: Patient performed an ambulatory transfer using a cane to a mat with contact guard .
 Comment: Pt. required vcs for cane management.

Education: Education in bed transfers, toilet/commode transfers, tub/shower transfers, wheelchair transfers, was provided to the patient who demonstrated knowledge and carryover.

Therapeutic Exercise: Seated EOM, pt. performed 5 minutes AROM exercises with BLE positioning on a bolster to increase flexion/extension for increased ROM and thereby improved transfers. Prior to therex pt. required mod. A to complete tub transfer, after therex, pt. required min A, OT observes improved knee flexion after therex.

DME: Pt. to decide if she wants to get tub safety rail and grab bar.

TOTAL TREATMENT TIME: 45 minutes

TREATMENT RENDERED:
OT Self Care/Home Management (ADL, homemaking)

TREATMENT PLAN: Continue with current treatment plan. Continue OT services for:
-- car transfer
-- light homemaking
-- tub transfer
-- lower body dressing

Electronically Signed by: Raimondi, Sue, OT\L
Note Written and Signed on: 01/14/2004

Figure 36-6. A progress note following a treatment session with a client. (Reproduced with permission of The Burke Rehabilitation Hospital, White Plains, NY.)

EVIDENCE-BASED TREATMENT STRATEGIES

Treatment Strategies	Authors
Hemiplegia	Koltin & Rosen, 1996; Mayer, 2000
Wheelchair ADL	Brandt, 2001; Reid, Angus, McKeever, & Miller, 2003
Adaptive devices	Barger II et al., 2000; Kling, Persson, & Gardulf, 2002; Klinger & Spaulding, 2001; Lund & Nygard, 2003; Mann, Hurren, & Tomita, 1995; Tyson & Strong, 1990
Depression	Calderon, 2001
Aging and ADL	Atwood, Holm, & James, 1994; Kraskowsky & Finlayson, 2001
Alzheimer's disease and ADL	Cooke, Fisher, Mayberry, & Oakley, 2000; Rogers, 2003; Venable & Mitchell, 1991
Brain injury	Goverover & Hinojosa, 2002
Teens/young adults	Healy & Rigby, 1999; Kellegrew, 1998
Quality of life	Stineman, Wechsler, Ross, & Maislin, 2003
ADL assessments	Rogers, Gwinn, & Holm, 2001
Fatigue and ADL	Mathiowetz, Matuska, & Murphy, 2001; Vanage, Gilbertson, & Mathiowetz, 2003

Healy, H., & Rigby, P. (1999). Promoting independence for teens and young adults with physical disabilities. *Canadian Journal of Occupational Therapy, 66,* 240-249.

Kellegrew, D. H. (1998). Creating opportunities for occupation: An intervention to promote self-care independence of young children with special needs. *American Journal of Occupational Therapy, 52,* 457-465.

Kling, C., Persson, A., & Gardulf, A. (2002). The ADL ability and use of technical aids in persons with late effects of polio. American Journal of Occupational Therapy, 56, 457-461.

Klinger, L. & Spaulding, S. J. (2001). Occupational therapy treatment of chronic pain and use of assistive devices in older adults. *Topics in Geriatric Rehabilitation, 16,* 34-44.

Koltin, S. E., & Rosen, H. S. (1996). Hemiplegia and feeding: An occupational therapy approach to upper extremity management. *Topics in Stroke Rehabilitation, 3,* 69-86.

Kraskowsky, L. H., & Finlayson, M. (2001). Factors affecting older adults' use of adaptive equipment: Review of literature. *American Journal of Occupational Therapy, 55,* 303-310.

Lund, M. L. & Nygard, L. (2003). Incorporating or resisting assistive devices: different approaches to achieving a desired self-image. *OTJR: Occupation, Participation and Health, 23,* 67-75.

Mann, W. C., Hurren, D., & Tomita, M. (1995). Assistive devices used by hone-based elderly persons with arthritis. American Journal of Occupational Therapy, 48, 810-820.

Mathiowetz, V., Matuska, K. M., & Murphy, M. E. (2001). Efficacy of energy conservation course for persons with multiple sclerosis. *Archives of Physical Medicine and Rehabilitation, 82,* 449-456.

Mayer, T. K. (2000). One-handed in a two-handed world. *Topics in Stroke Rehabilitation, 7,* 50-56.

Pedretti, L. W., & Early, M. B. (2001). *Occupational therapy: Practice skills for physical dysfunction* (5th ed.). St. Louis, MO: Mosby Company.

Reid, D., Angus, J., McKeever, P., & Miller, K.L. (2003) Home is where their wheels are: Experiences of women wheelchair users. American Journal of Occupational Therapy, 57, 186-195.

Rogers, J. C. (2003). Understanding Alzheimer disease: From diagnosis to rehabilitation. *Physical and Occupational Therapy in Geriatrics, 20,* 103-123.

Rogers, J. C., Gwinn, S. M. G., & Holm, M. B. (2001). Comparing act ivies of daily living assessment instruments: FIM, MDS, OASIS, MDS-PAC. *Physical and Occupational Therapy in Geriatrics, 18,* 1-25.

Stineman, M., Wechsler, B., Ross, R., & Maislin, G. (2003). A method of measuring quality of life through subjective weighting of functional status. *Archives of Physical Medicine and Rehabilitation, 81,* 515-522.

Trombly, C. A., & Radomski, M. V. (2002). *Occupational therapy for physical dysfunction* (5th ed.). Philadelphia, PA: Lippincott, Williams & Wilkins.

Tyson, R. & Strong, J. (1990). Adaptive equipment: its effectiveness for people with chronic lower back pain. *Occupational Therapy Journal of Research, 10,* 111-121.

University of Buffalo Foundation Activities, Inc. (2002). *IRF-PAI training manual.* Buffalo, NY: UB Foundation Activities, Inc.

Vanage, S. M., Gilbertson, K. K., & Mathiowetz, V. (2003). Effects of energy conservation course on fatigue impact for persons with progressive multiple sclerosis. *American Journal of Occupational Therapy, 57,* 315-323.

Venable, S. D., & Mitchell, M. M. (1991). Temporal adaptation and performance of daily living activities in persons with alzheimer's disease. *Physical and Occupational Therapy in Geriatrics, 9,* 31-49.

The Burke Rehabilitation Hospital

Inpatient Occupational Therapy

Date: 01/10/2004

DME: w/c cushion

Bed/Chair/Wheelchair Transfer FIM Score: 3

Toilet:
                    Surface: Standard
Toilet Transfer FIM Score: 0 -- N/A secondary to pain and decreased ROM in BLE, pt. reports pain 7-8/10

Tub/Shower:
                    Surface: Tub
                    Tub/Shower Transfer FIM Score: Tub Transfer: 0 -- N/A secondary to pain 7-8/10.

Social Interaction: FIM/SOCIAL INTERACTION: 7; Patient interacts and participates appropriately with staff and others.
Problem Solving: FIM/PROBLEM SOLVING: 5; Patient requires help to solve basic routine problems only when stressed (less than 10% of the time) and needs help to solve complex/abstract problems.
Memory: FIM/MEMORY: 7; The patient recognizes people frequently encountered, remembers daily routines, and follow directions without the need for repetition.

OBJECTIVE:
Upper Extremity Function: UE function is WNL.

Wheelchair Mobility/ Management -
 A manual wheelchair is used for mobility. Patient requires minimal assistance to propel 150 feet in the wheelchair. The patient requires supervision/verbal cues with brakes, and requires physical assistance with leg rests, .

TREATMENT GOALS:
Short Term:
BED MOBILITY GOAL:
Patient will perform supine to sit, sit to supine,   independently with assistive devices.

BADL GOAL:
Patient will perform lower body dressing,   with supervision and/or verbal cues

TRANSFER GOAL:
Patient will perform transfers with appropriate mobility device and DME/assistive devices as needed.
Patient will perform transfers to hospital bed, toilet, and arm chair,   independently.
Pt. will perform car transfer with supervision.

Treatment Outcome (Long Term Goals):
Patient will perform the following activities with good adherence to precautions, and use of appropriate mobility device, DME and/or assistive devices.

BED MOBILITY GOAL:
Patient will perform all position changes   independently.

BADL GOAL:
Patient will perform all dressing tasks and clothing acquisition   independently with assistive devices.

IADL Goal:
Patient will perform light meal prep,   independently with increased time and effort.

Real record 36-1A. (Reproduced with permission of The Burke Rehabilitation Hospital, White Plains, NY.)

The Burke Rehabilitation Hospital

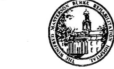

Inpatient Occupational Therapy

Date: 01/10/2004

TRANSFER GOAL:
Patient will perform transfer to bed, toilet, chair,   independently.
Patient will perform transfer to tub/shower, car   with supervision and/or verbal cues.

HEP GOAL:
Patient will perform home exercise program of AROM exercises strengthening exercises   independently.

Patient to perform community re-entry visit at an ambulatory level in hospaialt/community (as appropriate) with supervision.

IMPRESSION/ASSESSMENT:

Patient is a 75 year old F admitted to Burke Rehabilitation Hospital with a diagnosis of S/P BILAT TKR's . Patient presents to occupational therapy with primary impairments of: decreased coordination, postural deviations, decreased endurance/stamina, decreased strength, decreased balance, pain, edema, decreased ROM, . These problems impact independence and safety in the following functional activities: basic activities of daily living, instrumental activities of daily living, bed mobility/transitional movements, transfers, ambulatory mobility, community re-entry skills, leisure activities, . These impairments and functional limitations have resulted in patient's inability to participate in the roles of: self caregiver homemaker, active family member, participant in social activities, participant in leisure activities, . Patient requires inpatient skilled occupational therapy services to address the above noted deficit areas and to maximize safety and minimize burden of care.

Barriers:
Limited Transfer skills Limited dressing ability Limited homemaking ability

Treatment Plan:
OT Therapeutic Activities to Improve Functional Performance
OT Self Care/Home Management (ADL, homemaking)
OT Community Reentry Visit
OT Wheelchair Management
OT Therapeutic Procedure - Group Session
OT Therapeutic Procedure - Therapeutic Exercises
OT Hot Packs/Cold Packs
OT Patient/Family Education (not hands on)
OT Supplies
OT Charting
OT Community/Work Reintegration

Frequency: Individual 5x/wk. and Group 6x/wk.

Goals / treatment plan were discussed with and understood by patient .

Treatment Time:
Session 1: 45 minutes

Treatment Rendered:
 OT Initial Evaluation

Electronically Signed by: Raimondi, Sue, OT\L

Note Written and Signed on: 01/10/2004

Real record 36-1B. (Reproduced with permission of The Burke Rehabilitation Hospital, White Plains, NY.)

Key Concepts

- Legislation and regulation: The implementation of laws, rules, and regulations that impact the practice of work.
- Job analysis: A structured process that identifies the physical/functional aspects of work.
- Functional testing: An evaluation of an individual's physical ability to perform selected work-related tasks.
- Goal setting related to return to work: Designing programs with goals that match the physical abilities of the worker to the functional requirements of the job.
- Intervention plan: A plan that identifies problems and determines goals for the purpose of returning the individual to work.
- Work simulation: Actual or simulated work activity that matches the critical demands of a given job.
- Communication with work re-entry team: A process used to focus all stakeholders on the return to work plan.

Essential Vocabulary

cumulative trauma disorders: A group of work-related musculoskeletal and peripheral nerve disorders associated with highly repetitive tasks and/or forceful activity.

ergonomics: The application of scientific information concerning human beings to the design of objects, systems, and environments for human use. It is the science of matching the job to the worker and the product to the user.

functional capacity evaluation: A systematic evaluation of an individual's physical capacities and functional abilities related to the performance of work movements.

graded activities and work tasks: Those activities and tasks in which the duration, weights, heights, forces, and frequency are increased as the worker's physical abilities increase.

occupational rehabilitation: A structured program that uses exercise, education, aerobic conditioning, and actual or simulated work tasks to increase an individual's functional capacities for safe and productive return to work.

reasonable accommodation: Any change in the work environment or the way work is customarily performed that enables a qualified individual with a disability equal employment opportunity.

WORK INJURY ACTIVITIES

Barbara Larson, MA, OTR, FAOTA

INTRODUCTION

"Work 200 years ago was everyone's responsibility, a direct, positive effort to better one's lot in life and to improve the collective society" (Bing, 1989, p. 3).

Maurer (1979), in a 2-year study of the unemployed, concluded that work continues to be a fundamental human need and provides not just a livelihood, but also an essential passage into human community.

Fundamental to the profession of OT is the concept of work (Jacobs, 1995). Work is a performance area of occupation; it has specific activity demands and requires certain performance skills (AOTA, 2001). A worker's performance skills must meet the activity demands of a given job. When there is a change in the worker's status, be it physical, psychological, or sociocultural, engagement in the occupation of work is affected (Rice & Luster, 2002).

Physical changes stemming from injuries or illnesses could be traumatic or a result of neuromusculoskeletal disorders (Hegman & Moore, 1998). Psychological events could be triggered by family or work stress. Sociocultural issues such as age discrimination could displace a worker (Rice & Luster, 2002). Neurological, sensory, or other changes related to aging could affect a worker's safety and productivity (Larson, 2001). This chapter will explore work activities for individuals who can no longer meet the requirements of their job.

OCCUPATIONAL THERAPISTS' UNIQUE ROLE IN THE RETURN-TO-WORK PROCESS

OT practitioners possess characteristics gained from their education and clinical experience that make them uniquely suited for a major role in the rehabilitation of persons with work-related injuries (Ellexson, 1985). These characteristics help the OT practitioner identify and address behaviors that may hinder the individual's ability to benefit from the return to work process (Rice & Luster, 2002). The OT practitioner uses clinical reasoning skills in designing intervention programs to improve occupational performance (Moyers, 1999). These clinical reasoning skills are supported by knowledge of the disease process, an understanding of the manifestations of psychosocial behavior, and a recognition of the complexities of current reimbursement systems.

RETURN TO WORK

The primary role of the OT practitioner in providing services to the injured worker is evaluating functional performance as compared with job requirements (Rice & Luster, 2002). When evaluating the worker, the OT practitioner must consider all factors that influence the performance of actual job tasks. This includes worker's abilities, skills, neurobehavioral factors, physical health and fitness, cognition, psychological and emotional well-being, and the environment in which the job exists (Christiansen & Baum, 1997).

Evidence has shown that early intervention is crucial to a successful program outcome (King, 1998). As a result, the focus of occupational rehabilitation is on early intervention and early return to work programs. Ongoing, timely communication among all stakeholders in the return to work process is an important part of early intervention strategies. King (1998, p. 262) identified the following as programs that fall within the domain of occupational rehabilitation:

- Functional job analysis
- Functional capacity evaluations
- Physical reconditioning
- Worker retraining
- Return-to-work transitioning
- Ergonomic program development and job modification
- Modified duty assignments
- Work-injury prevention education
- Workstation modifications
- On-site rehabilitation services

Evaluation of the injured worker includes identifying what is important and meaningful to the client related to work. The data gathering process for this information will include identifying the worker's priorities and desired outcomes that will lead to engagement in the occupation of work (AOTA, 2002). Determining if the occupational skills of the individual are intact or if his or her ability for adaptation is compromised is an important part of OT evaluation (Kielhofner, 2002).

Functional testing provides the information necessary to help make determinations on physical work ability. The worker may have deficits in strength, ROM, flexibility, or endurance that prevent him or her from being able to perform critical job demands. A Functional Capacity Evaluation (FCE) of physical and cognitive abilities can provide baseline information for formulating an intervention plan (Rice & Luster, 2002). The recommendations from a FCE provide an employer with the information needed to make accurate, timely return-to-work decisions (Isernhagen, 1995). Matching the FCE results to the actual job is important in the return-to-work process. In order to obtain accurate, valid information about job functions and related physical demands, the OT practitioner may find it necessary to visit the job site. Analysis methods will vary depending on the purpose and complexity of the job in question. The analysis may involve a walk through and observation of the tasks performed by the worker. In a more in-depth analysis, physical job requirements are measured and documented and potential ergonomic stressors identified (Isernhagen, 1995).

Analyzing work is a critical component of all phases of intervention and should include the assessment of a person's suitability for work. With this process, the match between the worker and the work is maximized (Bohr, 1998). Combining information about the worker's abilities and deficits and information from the job site visit is important when designing a return-to-work program.

An occupational rehabilitation program may be necessary to address deficits identified in the evaluation to prepare the worker for the transition to work. The program should be individualized and include exercises to address strength, ROM, and flexibility deficits; cardiovascular conditioning exercises; graded work activities designed to simulate actual work tasks; and education in proper body mechanics and safe work techniques (Darphin, 1995). The OT practitioner must address changes in the worker's performance patterns that may have occurred since he or she has been off work (AOTA, 2002). Acceptance by coworkers and establishing work routines will be as important as having the physical abilities to perform the job. To make a successful work transition, the individual must have the skills to adapt to the role of worker (Kielhofner, 2002).

The program must be goal directed and requires motivation and active participation by the worker (King, 1998). If the goal is not attainable due to residual problems from an individual's injury, illness, or disability, the OT practitioner informs the appropriate individuals (i.e., physician, case manager, employer), who in turn, will make the necessary decisions for the employee's well-being.

As the program progresses, the OT practitioner provides the physician with information regarding an individual's readiness for work. In most states, it is the physician who makes the final decision for release to work. The OT and OTA, through evaluation and intervention, help maximize a safe and productive transition from the occupational rehabilitation setting to the workplace.

The focus of the occupational rehabilitation program is away from a purely biomechanical approach and emphasizes a collaborative structure among all parties involved in the return-to-work process (King, 1998). The program could take place in a clinical setting, at the workplace, or a combination of both.

FRAMES OF REFERENCE/ MODELS OF PRACTICE

OT practitioners often find the biomechanical frame of reference and the Model of Human Occupation helpful in guiding intervention for the employee who is recovering from work-related illness or injury.

The biomechanical frame of reference is used to structure intervention for individuals with functional limitations due to impairments in body structures and body functions (James, 2003). These impairments include decreased strength, flexibility, ROM, and endurance. In using the biomechanical model, the OT practitioner is concerned with restoring the functional motion necessary to sustain occupational performance (Kielhofner, 2004). The OT practitioner selects activities that are directed toward the individual's physical deficits. Compensatory and/or modification techniques in the form of job modifications may be necessary if the worker is unable to perform the critical demands of his or her job (AOTA, 2002).

The Model of Human Occupation can be used by the therapist to guide the worker in a direction that enhances self-esteem, supports worker behavior, and maintains worker identity. "Problems encountered in volition, habituation, performance capacity and the environment may all contribute to the individual becoming disengaged from his or her occupations" (Barrett & Kielhofner, 2003, p. 216) The worker, when engaged in actual activity that replicates work and is meaningful and relevant to him or her, can benefit from therapy and achieve change. By gaining competency in social roles and achieving successful role performance, the worker acquires the ability to put his or her efforts toward regaining the physical capacities necessary to return to work (Kielhofner, 2002).

It is important to note the biomechanical frame of reference alone is narrowly focused. Clients with biomechanical impairments may have other deficits not addressed in the biomechanical approach (James, 2003). The integration of the biomechanical frame of reference with the Model of Human Occupation provides a holistic framework in which to address the total needs of the worker (James, 2003).

Regulatory Considerations

To be effective in the treatment of the industrial worker, OT practitioners must be aware of laws and regulations affecting both workers and employers. The laws that have the greatest impact on OT practitioners providing services to injured workers and employers are the ADA, Workers' compensation, and the Occupational Health and Safety Act (OSHA).

Americans With Disabilities Act

The ADA was passed in 1990. The ADA prohibits the exclusion of individuals with physical or mental disabilities from jobs, services, activities, or benefits (Kornblau & Ellexson, 1995). Employers are required to provide reasonable accommodations to those individuals protected by the ADA. Reasonable accommodation as defined by the ADA includes any change in the work environment or the way work is customarily performed that enables an individual with a disability to enjoy equal employment opportunity (Kornblau & Ellexson, 1995). The OT and OTA may be involved in assisting the employer design reasonable accommodations for individuals with disabilities.

Workers' Compensation

Workers' compensation laws are a product of the 20th century. The workers' compensation system protects the rights of workers with illnesses or injuries sustained on the job. Workers' compensation pays wage replacement and medical costs for the worker. Although each state workers' compensation law is different in its administration, interpretation, and benefit level, states do share some common principles (Ellexson, 1985).

Workers' compensation is a major cost to employers. The average employer pays 2% to 3% of payroll for workers' compensation insurance (Larson, 1995). The OT practitioner through timely, efficient, effective service can have a positive impact on reducing workers' compensation costs incurred by the employer.

Occupational Safety and Health Administration

The U.S. Congress established OSHA in 1970. As defined in legislation, P. L. 91-596, the mission of the Occupational Safety and Health Act of 1970 is to assure, so far as possible, every working man and woman in the nation has safe and healthful working conditions. It is up to the employer to enforce the standards set by OSHA. Refusal to do so can result in significant fines and reprimands. OTs often work with employers on ergonomics and safety issues related to OSHA compliance.

Occupational Therapist/Occupational Therapy Assistant Collaboration

By developing a collaborative relationship, the OT and OTA use and combine their unique skills to deliver efficient, effective OT services (Glanz & Richman, 1997). The OT and OTA can have a positive impact on the individual who has had work interrupted by injury or illness. The OT focuses on problem identification, problem analysis, and the designing of appropriate evaluations and interventions for problem solution. The OTA focuses on carrying out the intervention plan, including reporting and documenting client responses, participation, and progress toward goals. The OT/OTA team addresses both the physical and psychosocial issues affecting the worker's ability to function on the job and participate in work. Each has a role that requires timely communication between each other and with members of the return-to-work team (Glanz & Richman, 1997). The return-to-work team includes many individuals, the most important being the worker. Actual team participants will vary depending on the needs of the individual worker. Team members may include the following:

- Health care providers, including the physician, OT, and OTA.
- Representatives of the employer, including human resource personnel, the occupational health nurse, safety manager, union representative, and department supervisor.
- A rehabilitation consultant or case manager who may be representing the insurance company.
- The insurer or representative thereof.

Depending on the needs of the individual, a psychologist or vocational evaluator may be part of the team. In striving to achieve the best outcome for the worker, the OT and OTA may also interact with engineers, ergonomists, architects, vocational specialists, and attorneys. The different backgrounds of the OT and OTA will provide the opportunity for each to gain insight into and mutually share perceptions about a worker's community, culture, values, and work behaviors (Grady, 1995).

CASE STUDY 1

Background Information

John is a 42-year-old auto mechanic who has worked for the same employer for 14 years. John sustained a right shoulder injury when reaching overhead to remove a transmission from a car. John was seen by a physician and referred to a therapist for treatment of his shoulder. Following his acute therapy program, John continued to report pain and discomfort in his right shoulder.

Evaluation

John was referred to the occupational rehabilitation department for an FCE to determine his ability to perform the work tasks related to his job as an auto mechanic. The OT performed the FCE. The results of the FCE outlined John's current physical abilities and limitations. John showed no deficits in his ability to walk, stand, or sit. He was able to perform low positional activities such as kneeling, crouching, and squatting. John showed decreased physical capacities in the following areas: floor to waist lift was limited to 30#, working with the right arm overhead could only be done occasionally, and push and pull was limited to 30# of force for 20 feet.

At the request of the OT, the OTA visited the work site to determine the physical job demands of the auto mechanic position. From her job analysis, the job demands were identified as follows:

- Lifting: (Frequently) lifts car, truck, and van tires 20# to 50#, up to 125# (rarely) from ground to chest level when removing or replacing tires on vehicles (assistance is available when lifting above 50#).
- Push/Pull: (Occasionally) Moving tire racks about 25 feet, from inside garage to outside. 50# of force is required to push or pull the racks.

- Reaching/Elevated Work: (Frequently) A 32" horizontal reach is required to work under hood of vehicles. A vertical overhead reach is required to work underneath vehicles that are positioned on the hoist.

Intervention Planning

Based on the results of the FCE and the job analysis, it was determined John would benefit from an occupational rehabilitation program. The OT developed the intervention plan from the results of the FCE and the job analysis information received from the OTA. The program would address John's deficits in right UE strength and endurance and the functional work tasks of lift, push, pull, and overhead work. The long-term goal of the program was return to work at his previous job in 2 to 3 weeks.

John would start in the clinic 5 days per week at 4 hours per day. After 2 weeks, he would return to work full time and alternate between modified duty and his regular job. A week transition would be allowed to return to full time on his previous job. The program goals included the following:

- Education on safe lifting and body mechanics when handling tires, tools, and equipment and when performing other auto mechanic job duties.
- Cardiovascular conditioning, including exercise bike, upper body ergometer, and walking program, to increase endurance to perform job tasks for 8 hours.
- Continuation of the graded exercise program started in acute therapy to increase strength and flexibility in the right shoulder.
- Work simulation activities, including lifting tires from ground to chest level as when removing or replacing tires on vehicles, reaching overhead while using tools to simulate working on cars, pushing and pulling carts to simulate moving the tire racks in and out of the building.

The OTA, under the supervision of the OT, carried out the intervention plan. The exercises, cardiovascular conditioning, and work simulation activities were graded to achieve the return-to-work goals in 3 weeks.

The OT re-evaluated John's physical status at the end of week 1 and adjusted the program based on his physical capacities and functional status. The OTA implemented the changes as directed by the OT. Based on John's progress, the OTA was able to increase the amount of time spent on work simulation tasks.

The employer was contacted by the OT to discuss ergonomic considerations related to the overhead reaching and static postures required for vehicle maintenance. One of the changes made was to have longer sockets made for some of the wrenches. This would minimize the reaching distance when loosening or attaching nuts and bolts. A second change was to suspend the air hoses from the ceiling rather than having the mechanics hold them up while working on a vehicle. This minimized the static loading of the arms and shoulders while working in the overhead position.

Work Transition

Following week 2, the OT reassessed John's physical capacities. Based on his progress, John was released to return to work by his physician. Prior to actual return to the job, the OT, OTA, rehabilitation consultant, employer, and John met at the workplace to make sure the work transition plan was clearly understood by all parties. John would spend his first week at work alternating 4 hours of modified duty with 4 hours of regular duty. The modified duty included sweeping, cleaning tasks, and processing customer work orders. The regular duty included performing safety checks and maintenance on cars, light trucks, and vans. Prior to John returning to work, the employer had made the ergonomic changes discussed with the OT.

Program Discontinuation

The OTA made a job site visit the first week to monitor John's transition from modified duty to the regular job. The OTA made sure John was using the techniques he had learned and practiced in the occupational rehabilitation program to complete his work tasks. She also observed the ergonomic changes made by the employer. After 2 weeks of transition back at work, John was able to perform his previous job on a full-time basis. He returned to his regular job and was discharged from the occupational rehabilitation program.

Clinical Reasoning

Two weeks after John returned to work, his employer called the OT. John was refusing to follow his return-to-work recommendations. John told the employer he did not think his return-to-work program was any good. The OT talked with the OTA to find out if John had raised any of these issues during his return-to-work program. The OTA stated John had not voiced any concerns. The OT arranged a meeting at the work site with John, his employer, herself, and the OTA. John was given the opportunity to express his concerns. The OT did not dwell on why he did not bring up these concerns during the program. The OT focused the interaction with John and his employer on concerns related to the work setting. While it was important for John to express his concerns, it was equally important for him to take responsibility for his part of the return-to-work plan. The discussion at the meeting was directed toward John's transition to work. In the future, if John identified areas of concern related to his recommendations, he would tell his employer. He and the employer would develop a plan to address the issue. If there were changes in the job tasks, equipment, or work methods, the employer would contact the OT to (1) assess the changes and (2) make sure John was working within his physical abilities using good ergonomic principles.

CASE STUDY 2

Background Information

Mary worked as a financial planner for a large brokerage firm. She had recently been diagnosed with MS. At about the time of Mary's diagnosis, her company was planning a project to remodel all employee offices. The human resource director was concerned that Mary's office be remodeled to accommodate the physical changes she might experience depending on the progression of her MS. The human resource director contacted an OT she had worked with in the past. The OT was asked to meet with the office design architect to discuss the office blueprints. The OT was also asked to meet with Mary to make sure both her current and future needs were considered with the workstation redesign. The OT met with the architect to review blueprints of the proposed workstation and made specific recommendations. The OTA interviewed Mary and reviewed work simplification and energy conservation techniques related to both the placement of office equipment and performance of specific work tasks. The OT and OTA identified employee and work site issues and made recommendations to the employer. Employee and work site issues and recommendations include the following:

1. Proper Sitting
   - Employee and Work Site Issues. The existing chair does not fit properly. The chair arms are too high, not adjustable, and require the employee to hike up her shoulders to use them. The lumbar support is fixed and does not allow individual adjustment.
   - Recommendations. When selecting a chair, consider the following chair characteristics:
     - ○ The ease with which the height can be adjusted.
     - ○ Whether the seated position can be changed easily.
     - ○ The type of support provided by the seat pan and back rest.
     - ○ The adjustability of the angle formed between the seat pan and backrest.
     - ○ The lumbar support of the chair.
     - ○ The base of support and if the chair swivels.
     - ○ Material and padding that make up the chair.

2. Leg/Chair Clearance
   - Employee and Work Site Issues. Blueprints of the work counter were reviewed regarding leg clearance when using an office chair and allowing enough leg clearance for eventual wheelchair use.
   - Recommendations. The supports that hold up the counter will be designed to maximize leg clearance and movement both for office chairs and wheelchair use.

3. Computer Work Area
   - Employee and Work Site Issues. The computer will be positioned in a corner with an under-the-counter keyboard. According to the architect, the under-the-counter keyboard is adjustable and has an attached mouse holder.
   - Recommendations. Make sure adequate knee clearance exists with the under-the-counter keyboard and mouse holder. With this corner arrangement, enough space will exist that the work area could be modified in the future to allow Mary to rest her arms on the counter top to provide more upper arm, shoulder, and forearm support when using the keyboard.

4. Work Area
   - Employee and Work Site Issues. The employee wanted the work area designed with enough space so work papers could be left on the desk.
   - Recommendations. The workstation will be designed in a U shape to allow 2 corner work areas: one for the computer and keyboard and one for writing tasks and projects.

(5) Lighting
   - Employee and Work Site Issues. The employee would like task lighting as well as overhead lighting.
   - Recommendations. The lighting set-up will allow counter height switches to adjust the overhead lighting, and space and wiring for individual desk lamps for task lighting.

(6) Energy Conservation/Work Simplification
   - Employee and Work Site Issues. The work area should be set up to minimize energy output to achieve work tasks. The employee stated she often gets fatigued walking out to the printer.
   - Recommendations. Counters will allow both writing and computer work without having to put away papers. Space for a printer will be factored into workstation design.

Upon completion of the report, the OT and OTA met with the human resource director and the employee to make sure there was a clear understanding of the recommendations. The meeting also validated the feasibility of the recommendations. The human resource director will stay in contact with the OT and told the employee to bring to her attention any issues she felt could be addressed by OT.

Clinical Reasoning

One week following the meeting, the OT received a call from the human resource director. The human resource director had just been informed of budget cuts in the dollars allocated for office remodeling. The OT was asked to prioritize Mary's needs since the project was being scaled back. The OT developed a plan and met with the human resource director and Mary. The following was determined as a result of the meeting:

- A new chair was an immediate priority, as the existing chair did not fit properly.
- The current work area needed temporary changes to allow space for both computer work and tasks requiring desk space. This would address issues related to energy conservation and work simplification.
- The above work areas would be temporary. At the suggestion of the OT, Mary's office was first on the remodeling

EVIDENCE-BASED TREATMENT STRATEGIES

Treatment Strategies	Authors
Identify changes in worker status affecting work performance	Christiansen & Baum, 1997; Hegman & Moore, 1998; Larson, 2001; Rice & Luster, 2002
Early intervention for return to work	King, 1998
Functional testing	Isernhagen, 1995; Rice & Luster, 2002
Identifying physical job demands	Bohr, 1998; Isernhagen, 1995
Role performance, concept of work, improving occupational performance	Barrett & Kielhofner, 2003; Christiansen & Baum, 1997; Jacobs, 1995; Kielhofner, 2002; King, 1998; Moyers, 1999
Increase physical abilities of worker	Darphin, 1995; James, 2003
Keep worker active and involved in return to work program	Barrett & Kielhofner, 2003; James, 2003; King, 1998
Regulation	Kornblau & Ellexson, 1995

schedule. If Mary's condition changed and it became necessary for her to use a wheelchair, remodeling would be done immediately.

The OTA would work with Mary on the fitting of a new office chair and assist with the temporary changes and accommodations to her workstation.

LEARNING ACTIVITIES

1. Follow the case rulings that come down through the courts related to the ADA.
2. Look up the Job Accommodation Network on the Internet and become familiar with its purpose and activities.
3. Go to an industrial trade show and become familiar with the equipment, tools, and terminology used in different industries.
4. Identify additional work simulation tasks for the auto mechanic related to his specific job tasks that you could use in an occupational rehabilitation program.
5. Working with a peer, brainstorm to develop a list of additional energy conservation activities for a person with MS who works in an office.
6. Follow the OSHA as it works to secure passage of Ergonomic Guidelines through the United States Congress.
7. Talk with a vocational specialist and find out how they use information from a FCE to assist in placing individuals who may have physical, cognitive, or psychosocial deficits in work settings.
8. Interview an architect and find out how he or she approaches designing facilities for individuals with disabilities.

REFERENCES

American Occupational Therapy Association. (2002). Occupational therapy practice framework: Domain and process. *American Journal of Occupational Therapy, 56,* 609-639.

Barrett, L., & Kielhofner, G. (2003). Theories derived from occupational behavior perspectives. In E. B. Crepeau, E. S. Cohn, & B. A. Schell (Eds.), *Willard & Spackman's occupational therapy* (10th ed., pp. 209-219). Philadelphia, PA: Lippincott, Williams and Wilkins.

Bing, R. K. (1989). Work is a four-letter word! A historical perspective. In S. Hertfleder & C. Gwin (Eds.), *Work in progress: Occupational therapy in work programs.* Rockville, MD: American Occupational Therapy Association.

Bohr, P. C. (1998). Work analysis. In P. M. King (Ed.), *Source book of occupational rehabilitation* (pp. 229-245). New York: Plenum Press.

Christiansen, C., & Baum, C., (1997). Person-environment-occupational performance: A conceptual model for practice. In C. Christiansen & C. Baum (Eds.), *Occupational therapy: Enabling functioning and well-being* (pp. 47-70). Thorofare, NJ: SLACK Incorporated.

Darphin, L. (1995). Work-hardening and work-conditioning perspectives. In S. J. Isernhagen (Ed.), *The comprehensive guide to work injury management* (pp. 443-462). Gaithersburg, MD: Aspen.

Ellexson, M. T. (1985). *The unique role of occupational therapy in industry. Work related programs in occupational therapy.* Binghamton, NY: Haworth Press.

Glanz, C. H., & Richman, N. (1997). OTR-COTA collaboration in home health: Roles and supervisory issues. *American Journal of Occupational Therapy, 51*(6), 446-457.

Grady, A. P. (1995). Building inclusive community: A challenge for occupational therapy. 1994 Eleanor Clarke Slagle Lecture. *American Journal of Occupational Therapy, 49,* 300-310.

Hegman, K. T., & Moore, S. J. (1998). Common neuromusculoskeletal disorders. In P. M. King (Ed.), *Sourcebook of occupational rehabilitation* (pp. 19-41). New York: Plenum Press.

Isernhagen, S. J. (1995). Contemporary issues in functional capacity evaluation. In S. J. Isernhagen (Ed.), *The comprehensive guide to work injury management* (pp. 410-429). Gaithersburg, MD: Aspen.

Jacobs, K. (1995). Preparing for return to work. In C. A. Trombly (Ed.), *Occupational therapy for physical dysfunction* (4th ed.). Baltimore, MD: Williams & Wilkins.

James, A. B. (2003). Biomechanical frame of reference. In E. B. Crepeau, E. B. Cohn, & B. A. Boyt Schell (Eds.), *Willard and Spackman's occupational therapy* (pp. 240-242). Philadelphia, PA: Lippincott, Williams & Wilkins.

Kielhofner, G. (2002). *Model of human occupation: Theory and application* (3rd ed.). Baltimore, MD: Lippincott, Williams and Wilkins.

Kielhofner, G. (2004). *Conceptual foundations of occupational therapy* (3rd ed.). Philadelphia, PA: F. A. Davis.

King, P. M. (1998). Work hardening and work conditioning. In P. M. King (Ed), *Sourcebook of occupational rehabilitation* (pp. 257-273). New York: Plenum Press.

Kornblau, B. L., & Ellexson, M. T. (1995). Reasonable accommodation and the Americans with Disabilities Act. In S. J. Isernhagen (Ed.), *The comprehensive guide to work injury management* (pp. 781-795). Gaithersburg, MD: Aspen.

Larson, B. L. (1995). Work rehabilitation. The importance of networking with the employer to achieve successful outcomes. In S. J. Isernhagen (Ed.), *The comprehensive guide to work injury management* (pp. 483-497). Gaithersburg, MD: Aspen.

Larson, B. L. (2001). The aging worker. *Work, 16*(1), 67-68.

Maurer, H. (1979). *Not working: An oral history of the unemployed.* New York: Holt, Rhinehart & Winston.

Moyers, P. A. (1999.) The guide to occupational therapy practice. *American Journal of Occupational Therapy, 53*(3), 247-322.

Rice, V. J., & Luster, S. (2002). Restoring competence for the worker role. In C. A. Trombley & M. V. Radomski (Eds.), *Occupational therapy for physical dysfunction* (5th ed., pp. 715-744). Baltimore, MD: Lippincott, Williams and Wilkins.

MANAGEMENT AND PRACTICE ISSUES

Key Concepts

- Effect size (ES): The strength or power of the relationship between 2 variables.
- Ethics: Character and morals of the profession and its practitioners.
- Evidence-based practice (EBP): Using the available research information to make the best decision in day-to day practice.
- ICIDH-2: *International Classification of Impairment, Disabilities, and Handicaps.*
- p-value (p): A statistical calculation that is associated with the power of significance of the data.
- Quantitative: Studies related to the statistical analysis of numerical values.
- Qualitative: Studies related to attributes in observation, interviews, and/or groups.
- Statistical significance: The chance that the results are not due to error.

Essential Vocabulary

abstract: A summary of the article or paper.

adaptive: Flexible; ability to adjust to change.

ADHD: Attention deficit hyperactivity disorder.

analysis of variance (ANOVA): Statistical data that are used to measure differences.

cohorts: A study that follows one or more groups, one of which has a defined condition.

competence: Ability to independently apply basic skills and knowledge with good clinical reasoning, judgment, and ethics.

context: Environment.

cost-effectiveness: The best use of available resources, equipment, and personnel.

data: Any numerical value that is used in research. Data should be communicated as "data are."

domain: Area.

efficacy: Effectiveness.

frequency: A numerical count of each occurrence.

FIM: Functional Independence Measure is a tool used to measure the outcome of a patient's performance.

historical: A record of past events.

mean: The average of a set of numbers that is derived by dividing the sum of all the scores by the number of values.

median: Middle score in the range of all the values.

meta-analysis: Literature reviews that provide statistical analysis of the research studies in attempts to integrate the findings.

mode: The most common or frequent score.

multiple sclerosis (MS): A chronic disabling disease that affects the CNS.

occupational performance areas: Activities of daily living, work, play, and leisure.

principles: A combination of emotional and thoughtful qualities.

randomized clinical trials (RCTs): The participants are randomly assigned to the study groups.

range: The difference between the highest and lowest scores.

reliability: The consistency, regularity, and uniformity of a measurement.

sample: A segment, part, or example of a population.

sensory integration (SI): Treatment to enhance the development of basic SI processing using vestibular, tactile, proprioceptive, and other somatosensory input to elicit adaptive responses as needed for gross and fine motor abilities, behavior, language, and sensorimotor functioning.

standard deviation: How scores relate to the average scores.

theoretical: Educated, organized point of view.

variability: How scores differ from each other.

variance: The score of variability that describes differences.

Evidence-Based Practice

Paula Wright, MS, OTR

Ongoing health care changes at both the federal and state level have had a significant impact on how health care is provided. Changes in reimbursement have caused insurance providers to require more efficient and effective therapy services. Some insurance providers quote what they have determined to be the evidence to health care providers when authorizing evaluation and/or treatment. All OT practitioners should be armed with the ability to provide evidence for why a specific treatment is chosen. Supplying the evidence for practice to both the consumer and the insurance provider can reinforce the value and meaning of the foundation of our profession.

What Is Evidence-Based Practice?

Sackett, Richardson, Rosenberg, and Haynes (1997) describe the growth of evidence-based medicine (EBM) from the middle of the 19th century when decisions regarding the care of patients was based on the best, currently available evidence. The authors further describe EBM as a never-ending process of gathering appropriate clinical evidence from clinically relevant research to enable accurate, efficient, and safe decisions about patient care. Tickle-Degnen introduced the Evidence-Based Practice Forum in 1999. OT practitioners are using evidence to determine the best practice, like a toolbox, to aid in clinical reasoning, and are more able to inform consumers of the efficiency, cost effectiveness, benefit, and safety of therapeutic techniques (Abreu, Peloquin, & Ottenbacher, 1998). The concept of the toolbox, however, should not be misunderstood as a cookbook.

EBP is an integrated combination of both clinical, external evidence and clinical expertise. The clinical, external evidence can provide information both quantitative and/or qualitative, but this evidence alone can never replace the knowledge and skilled analysis of this information by the practitioner. It is the practitioner that must interpret the information and decide if it is applicable and meaningful to the specific patient and patient-related question.

Both RCTs and meta-analysis are the most powerful and highly respected forms of research. EBP is not restricted to RCTs and meta-analysis. RCTs are experiments that are controlled. Participants in the study are randomly assigned to 1 of 2 groups. One group receives the intervention that is being questioned, and the other group receives a standard intervention or no intervention at all. A meta-analysis is a scientific method of gathering a variety of research studies on a similar topic and doing statistical analysis to interpret, compare, and summarize the quantitative findings. A meta-analysis is viewed as one of the strongest types of evidence with the most objective data. Abreu (2002) comments that a meta-analysis that is limited to RCT is noted to be the most powerful evidence that is easily generalized to clinical practice. The "power" of a study is determined statistically by having the right number of participants in the study for the data gathered to show a significant change from pre- to post-test or a significant difference in a comparison with a treatment group. As OT practitioners, our debt to our clients is in obtaining the best current evidence that can answer the question at hand. The permission from and the choices of the health care consumer are essential in laying out the plan for the individual patient (Abreu, 2002). Today's health care consumers are clever and have an awareness of resources and practical issues. OT practitioners will need to be prepared to share their knowledge, expertise, and the evidence with the consumer. What will you say when asked, "What is the evidence for what you do?"

Why Should You Become an Evidence-Based Practitioner?

Holm (2003, pp. 9-11) outlines the reasons as follows:
10. It sounds impressive.
9. Your team will be impressed.
8. Your patients will be impressed.
7. Everyone is doing it.
6. You want to know what your students are talking about.
5. You want to be reimbursed.

4. You want to be a competent practitioner.

3. You want to be a scientific practitioner.

2. You want to be an ethical practitioner.

1. You want the best outcome for your clients.

Historically, the evidence in OT has been passed down from clinician to clinician (Abreu & Chang, 2002). OT practitioners, over our course of history as a profession, have used a broad spectrum of evidence to guide our practice. This spectrum of evidence is a combination of multiple sources: evaluation data, patient preferences, clinical beliefs, traditional knowledge, and opinions and/or theories of experts and research. The American Occupational Therapy Code of Ethics (AOTA, 2002a) demonstrates our commitment as a profession to performing our clinical practice based on accurate and current information, thus providing the right services and performing these services correctly. The guiding principles in our code of ethics are outlined in principle 3B and 4B as follows:

> Principle 3B. "Occupational therapy practitioners shall fully inform the service recipient of the nature, risks, and potential outcomes of any intervention" (AOTA, 2002a, p. 122).

> Principle 4B. "Occupational therapy practitioners shall critically examine and keep current with emerging knowledge relevant to their practice so they may perform their duties on the basis of accurate information" (AOTA, 2002a, p. 123).

HOW DO YOU BECOME AN EVIDENCE-BASED PRACTITIONER?

Abreu (2002) described 4 EBP steps:

1. Framing the question
2. Searching, sorting, and making sense of the evidence
3. Communicating the findings
4. Re-evaluation of the evidence

To best understand this process, this chapter will review the first 3 steps.

Framing the Question

The question may be related to any topic or area concerning the care of your patients. It can be a problem, intervention, or the comparison of the effectiveness of treatment techniques. As clinicians, our goal is to put together the best treatment plan that maximizes the patient's ability to benefit and achieve the best outcome. Try to describe the client or group that requires intervention in your question. The client may be a specific patient and the group could be a diagnostic category. Use your knowledge from previous experience to select the intervention to be investigated.

Examples of research questions that have been reviewed in the literature are presented here for your review. It is important for you to take the time to review the actual text article, as the information or end results may or may not be meaningful to your individual patients.

- Stroke: Does rehabilitation affect outcome? This was questioned in an article authored by Lehmann et al. (1975) from the department of rehabilitation medicine at the University of Washington School of Medicine. The data gathered and analyzed from this study made several valuable findings.

  1. From admission to discharge, there is a significant gain in functional levels of self-feeding, dressing, bowel and bladder elimination, walking, transfer activities, and mobility.

  2. The same significant difference was demonstrated for all functional tasks from admission to follow-up with the exception of eating. Eating showed a decline in ability from discharge to follow-up. The majority of the patients chose to have assistance with cutting their meat rather than doing it themselves. Otherwise, they were able to self-feed independently.

  3. The authors acknowledged in their literature review that the majority of spontaneous recovery of function occurs during the first 6 months, and any additional gains can be attributed to learning from the therapy interventions in rehabilitation at even a year afterward.

  4. In an analysis of costs, the data obtained in this study indicated that the cost to society for maintaining stroke victims is less when rehabilitation techniques had been provided.

- In a meta-analysis of research on SI treatment, Vargas and Camilli (1999) questioned whether the existing research studies support the effectiveness of using SI approaches. The authors reviewed 27 research articles that were published from 1972. A significant difference was seen between ESs in earlier (ES .60) versus more recent studies (ES .03) of SI treatment when compared to no treatment. The authors also noted that SI treatment was found to be equal to alternative, psychoeducational, or motoric interventions.

- Is there an effect of verbal instruction on functional reach in persons with and without CVA? In a repeated measure study designed by the researchers at Boston University (Fasoli, Trombly, Tickle-Degnen, & Verfaellie, 2002), the data reinforced that patients benefit from the use of simple verbal instructions regarding the following: visual attention to the objects, encouragement to think about the natural properties of the object (size, shape, etc.), and the sensation of moving the extremity while engaged in occupational tasks that involve reaching.

- Is there a relationship between ICIDH-2 domains of body systems, functional outcomes, and participation in daily life activities in a community context? This question was addressed by Spencer et al. (2002). This article is a representation of a combined quantitative and qualitative research method. Although the findings are discussed later in this chapter, the data demonstrate that functional outcomes are strongly influenced by patient choices and the availability of support in the community.

- What is the theoretical frame of reference that supports a top-down approach to intervention that includes task specific intervention and cognitive approaches? Gentile (1992) is a clinical expert in the field of movement science. This author approached the framework for treatment from a movement science perspective. This theory supports the occupational therapy practitioner as an active problem solver with the ability to facilitate ways to help patients achieve functional goals by using a model of skill acquisition and adaptive behaviors.

Okay, so there are 4 questions that have been asked. What's next? You now search and sort through the multitude of literature available to determine the best information. This will require a critical review of the literature and the ability to rank each review based on established criteria.

Searching, Sorting, and Making Sense of the Evidence

In order to determine the best current practices for the care of patients, we must be able to search, sort, select, and summarize the information presented. The Internet has opened our access to an abundant supply of information. Some databases are public databases and provide free access to users, such as PubMed (www.pubmed.nl), Cochrane (www.cochrane.org), Google (www.google.com), or the Agency for Health Care Policy and Research (AHCPR) (www.ahrq.gov). Other databases, such as Cumulative Index to Nursing & Allied Health (CINAHL) (www.cinahl.com) or MEDLINE, require access codes through subscriptions that are available to individuals or through affiliation with a university or library. MEDLINE is a recognized source of a wide range of literature from the United States National Library of Medicine. OTseeker (Occupational Therapy Systematic Evaluation of Evidence) is available at www.otseeker.com and is freely available. It currently contains abstracts of systematic reviews and ratings of RCTs that are specifically applicable to the practice of occupational therapy. Access to the AOTA, Wilma West Library, and OT Search is now available online through AOTA for an additional subscription rate.

In addition, articles from professional peer reviewed journals typically provide excellent sources of research studies. Examples of such journals include, but are not limited to, the following: *American Journal of Occupational Therapy* (AJOT), the *Journal of American Medical Association* (JAMA), the *Archives of Physical Medicine and Rehabilitation, Developmental and Behavioral Pediatrics,* the *Journal of Pediatrics, Journal of Abnormal Child Psychology, Australian Journal of Occupational Therapy, Journal of Learning Disabilities,* the *New England Journal of Medicine, OTJR: Occupation, Participation and Health, Journal of Rehabilitation Medicine, Journal of Hand Surgery, Journal of Gerontology, Medical Sciences, Journal of Neurology, American Journal of Mental Deficiency,* and *Developmental Medicine and Child Neurology.* Researchers must be careful in selecting Internet sources, making sure they are scholarly information and not postings made by parties with nonscholarly interests.

Sorting the research can be overwhelming and seemingly complex unless one understands that research evidence is already categorized and ranked based on the strength or power of the research design, randomization of participants in the study, and the clinical significance of the research findings.

Abreu (2002) and Holm (2001) outlined the 5 levels of evidence for EBP. This hierarchy should help the practitioner to select the best current available evidence in the literature. If you, the busy OT practitioner, devote your precious reading time to the selection of patient specific searches and critique, you will be able to incorporate the best evidence into your practice.

Table 38-1 is adapted from descriptions by Liberman and Scheer (2002), Law (2002), and Sackett et al. (1997).

Let's look at an example of a study from each of the levels, using articles that may be beneficial to the current practice of OT.

Level I Evidence

This is systematic review of well-designed RCT. In a meta-analysis of studies involving 44 articles, Trombly and Ma (2002) and Ma and Trombly (2002) synthesized the combined research findings regarding the impact on restoration of function for those who had experienced a stroke. The organized review concluded that the practice of OT effectively improves participation and activity following stroke. Homemaking activities were noted to result in more significant improvement in thinking and reasoning skills in comparison to pencil and paper drills and tasks that focused purely on ignored space and movement of the opposite extremity into the ignored space. What does this mean to the OT practitioner? The authors' concluded based on the data that coordinated movement improved when OT interventions used the following:

- Written and pictorial examples of movement exercises.
- Activities using meaningful functional objects as goals.
- Treatment sessions including specific functional goals for practicing movement.
- Activities that included simultaneous but independent arm movement.
- Imaginative thinking about the use of the affected limb.

The authors further noted that research of inhibitory splinting yielded no significant findings. These findings seemingly support the foundation of "occupation" as the core to the practice of OT treatment with this particular population. These findings support the client-centered framework approaches that are outlined in the *Occupational Therapy Practice Framework* (AOTA, 2002b). Trombly and Ma (2002) and Ma and Trombly (2002) concluded that the treatment and approaches used by OT practitioners that are task-oriented, based in activity analysis, engage the client in meaningful occupations and promote positive self-image are, in general, effective in the remediation of clients who have experienced a stroke. They deducted, however, that no specific treatment approach has been sufficiently researched and ongoing research is required to contribute to this body of knowledge.

Table 38-1

Levels of Evidence for Occupational Therapy Literature—Research Reviews

Level	Definition of Evidence
I	Systematic RCTs, meta-analysis, adequate sample size
II	Non-RCTs with a minimum of 2 groups; small sample size
III	Non-RCTs with at least 1 treatment group; longitudinal studies; pre- and posttest; cohort; case studies
IV	Evidence based on opinions of experts or respected authorities; well-designed nonexperimental studies; single-subject design; may be descriptive studies; literary publications of expert panels
V	Expressed opinions of individuals who have written and reviewed guidelines based on their clinical or theoretic experience and/or knowledge
NA	Narratives, case reports
	Sample Size Criteria
A	$n \geq 20$ participants per condition ($\geq$ means, equal to or greater than)
B	$n \leq 20$ participants per condition ($\leq$ means, equal to or less than)

Level II Evidence

This is strong evidence that is obtained from a minimum of one RCT. Rahman, Thomas, and Rice (2002) studied 42 women and 9 men who were 60 years old or older. The participants in this study were randomly assigned to 1 of 4 groups. The study was designed to use traditional tools that we use in practice: dynamometer and a pinch meter to measure grip and pinch strength. The specific amount of force, in pounds of pressure, needed to open common household containers was measured. Statistical relationships between measurements were obtained. The containers used for the study were described by the authors as squeeze bottles, prescription medicine bottles, large prescription bottles, over-the-counter medicine bottles, and an aerosol pump spray bottle with trigger. Containers were determined by the investigators to require various patterns of grip and manipulation, such as dual pinch, push-down and rotation, alignment of arrows as markers to pop-off the lid, and depression of button by thumb and index finger in trigger motion. This study was noted to be a replication of one previously conducted by Rice, Meyer, Walker, and Fisk in 1998 (Rice, Leonard, & Carter, 1998). The results of the recent study, on average, did not demonstrate significant relationships between grip strength, pinch strength, and forces to open and operate containers. The findings indicated that men tended to use greater force, in pound of pressure, than women on 2 out of the 6 containers.

The trend suggested that elderly persons tend to expend more energy than their younger participants in the earlier study. The article provides useful statistical information on the normal range in scores with minimal and maximal ranges, as well as standard deviations for each container. This may be useful infor-

mation to an OT practitioner in determining the level of weakness that an elderly person would need to demonstrate in order to be unable to open specific containers. It is important to keep in mind that the participants in the study were considered to be well elderly persons with no notable strength deficits for their ages. It is thereby hypothesized by the authors that elderly persons with hand strength deficits would require a higher proportion of their maximum strength in order to open containers. This study supported other studies that noted that decreased hand strength with the normal aging processes are related to decreased success at functional occupational performances that require dexterity and/or strength.

Level III Evidence

This level evidence is the result of non-RCTs, single group prepost, cohort, or longitudinal studies. A cohort is a group that has been exposed to a similar situation. This could be a diagnostic category or a disease process, such as PD, bipolar disorder, or AIDS. Several studies have been chosen as examples for this level of evidence.

The first is a brief report by Schultheis, Garay, Millis, and DeLuca (2002). The researchers reviewed a 5-year period of time of incidents of MVCs and motor vehicle violations amongst drivers with a diagnosis of MS, when cognitive impairment is noted to be present. The study participants included 27 persons with MS and 17 well individuals. All participants were free of assistive driving devices; were able to walk independently 25 feet, in equal to or less than 20 seconds; and had been driving continuously with current state licenses during the 5 years of the study. Neuropsychological tests, adult intelligence tests, and perceptual motor tests were used to measure cognitive functioning. The driving records of all the participants were also reviewed. The results showed a statistically significant relationship (p = .0013) between the incidence of MVCs and the well individuals (control group). The study group with MS and cognitive impairment demonstrated a significantly greater incidence of one or more crashes in comparison with the group of participants without cognitive impairment (p = .01) and the control group (p = .01). Interestingly, there was no statistical significance between the groups of participants with MS, without cognitive impairment when compared to the well individuals (control group). It is important to note that the MS group in the study were those without physical limitations. The results of this study tend to suggest, with a 99% level of confidence, that persons without physical limitation but with cognitive impairments, as a component of a diagnosis with MS, demonstrate a higher incidence of MVCs. In addition, there was no significant relationship between the group and motor vehicle violations. This suggests that cognitive deficits in those individuals with MS were at a greater risk for MVCs than those without cognitive deficits. Although this study has its limitations in sample size and lack of inclusion of person with MS with physical limitations, it represents one of the first studies of this clinical group in relationship to driving performance based on the department of motor vehicle records of crashes and violations. Although the ability to drive provides an individual with a sense of an independent lifestyle, it also presents a significant safety risk for both society and the individuals if there is the presence of cognitive impairment and MS. These findings support the need for clinical comprehensive driving assessments and the potential for the implementation of OT treatment strategies for persons with MS.

The second example involves a study by Rasmussen and Gillberg (2000). The authors conducted a controlled, longitudinal, community-based study on the outcome of 55 subjects at 22 years of age who had a diagnosis of ADHD with/or without a diagnosis of developmental coordination disorder (DCD). This report covers a 15-year period of time from initial assessment with unmedicated children with diagnoses of ADHD and DCD. There were a total of 101 participants (62 males and 39 females). Fifty-five were identified as index cases, ADHD with DCD group (42 male and 13 female). Index cases, in this study, refer to the study group. The comparison group consisted of 46 individuals (20 male and 26 female). All participants were recruited from a general population and examined by researchers who were unaware of the diagnoses of any of the participants.

Thirty-nine of the index group had combinations of problems: deficits in attention, motor control, and perception. A poor outcome was seen in 58% of the study group and 13% of the control group with a level of significance of p < .001. The most severe participants with ADHD and DCD and the small group with DCD had the worse outcomes at 69% and 80%, respectively. Poor outcome, at the conclusion of the 15-year study, was associated with 8 of the participants being diagnosed with autism spectrum disorder and 3 others with psychiatric disorders. In addition, 24% in the index group and 4% in the control group had issues with alcohol abuse with a level of significance of p < .02. These findings were also associated with the abused usage of other controlled substances. Eight or 19% of the index group had committed criminal offenses. There were personality disorders in 33% of index and in 7% of control group at the p < .01 level of significance. Antisocial personality disorder was the most frequent diagnosis in the ADHD group with 15% of the index and 2% of the control group at the p < .06 level of significance.

Severe inattention was described in 44% of the index group and 7% of the control group at a p < .001 level of significance. It is important to note that 49% of the index cases and 9% of the participants in the control group had a diagnosis of ADHD at 22 years of age at the p < .001 level of significance. A tic disorder was noted in 16 (29%) of the index group and 3 (7%) of the control group at a p < .01 level of significance. Eleven percent of the index group and none of the control group were on sick pension programs secondary to neuropsychiatric problems. Eighty percent of the index group and 26% of the control group had completed less than 12 years in school; 5 (38%) had attended classrooms for the mentally retarded for more than 1 year even though they had no diagnosis of mental retardation. One participant (2%) attended a university. Fourteen disorders were noted in 3 participants of the index group who were unable to read or write at all at 22 years of age. Fifty-eight percent of the index group and 15% of the control group had reading/writing disorders at a p < .001 level of significance.

In the most severe ADHD with DCD participants of the index group, 77% demonstrated reduced reading speed, whereas in the moderate ADHD with DCD group, the outcome for this category was 44%. The DCD-only group had reading/writing problems at a rate that was consistent with the ADHD with DCD group. The ADHD-only group, however, performed better than the control group.

So, what do all these numbers mean? This study provides valid information since none of the participants were on medications or received treatment in a clinic over the course of the 15-year study. Recent community-based studies of children in Sweden demonstrated a positive relationship with ADHD in childhood and neuropsychiatric disorders in their early adult years. Limitation to the study includes a small sample size. The authors hypothesize that the frequency of combined ADHD and DCD may be a negative prognostic indicator in children with ADHD for poor psychosocial functioning and psychiatric issues in adulthood. The authors support a need to learn about the long-term outcome of children diagnosed with ADHD with DCD.

In this article review, the p-value has been noted in reference to the level of significance. p-value is a statistical calculation that is associated with the statistical significance of the effect of the study. Generally speaking, p-values of p that are greater than .05 may have a low level of significance if the sample size is small. On the other hand, a p-value of p that is less than .05 may have the power to detect a significant level of confidence in the outcome of the study. In other words, a p-value that is less than or equal to .05 may be reported to have 95% level of confidence that the relationship found between the 2 variables in the study were significant. In reading any research-related article, the p-value may lead to different conclusions about the effectiveness of a clinical intervention. In these situations, the wisdom and experience of the clinician reading the article is required to use clinical reasoning in their decision-making process as to whether the information reviewed is applicable and relevant to their patient. Another meaningful statistical variable is ES. This numerical value indicates the strength or power of the relationship between 2 variables. ES does not mean a cause-and-effect relationship. Take a moment to look back to the example in the Framing the Question section on p. 474. The second example on SI treatment indicated a significant difference between ESs in earlier (ES .60) versus more recent studies (ES .03) of SI treatment when compared to no treatment. This may be translated to say that the meta-analysis by Vargas and Camilli (1999) found that overall the earlier research studies demonstrated a significant effect in comparison to the later studies on the use of SI treatment versus no treatment at all.

A third and final example of a Level III article is one in which the researchers used both qualitative and quantitative methods in their research design. Spencer et al. (2002) conducted a study using the ICIDH-2 to measure the body functions and structure; ability to perform functional tasks; the performance of daily activities in the social context of home, neighborhood, and community; and the environmental influences of participation in daily life activities. Seventeen African-American elderly persons, who were 58 to 93 years of age, with an average age of 73, were followed for 6 months after hospitalization for acute conditions. All participants, self-identified as African American or black, had been judged clinically to have the cognitive abilities to be interviewed and had available Functional Independence Measure (FIM) scores. All participants were chosen based on the potential of this particular population to illustrate adaptive processes that may differ from other elderly persons.

The authors noted strong family relationships, role flexibility, and religious affiliations as aspects of the families of these participants to adapt to physical disabilities. In the hospital, 16 out of 17 participants showed improvements in scores and 1 showed a decline. The findings from the functional outcomes (FIM) scores from discharge to follow-up in the community demonstrated the participants' ability to perform self-care tasks outside of the unfamiliar hospital environment. In addition, the participants, when seen in the community, demonstrated their ability to make choices about how things got done, including assistance from others. Postdischarge, 11 participants demonstrated improved FIM scores and 6 declined.

The researchers grouped the participants based on their patterns of participation in activity. The groups were described as:

- Primary home-centered, self-care.
- Home-centered, self-care, and household activities.
- Home-neighborhood and community self-care, household, and leisure.

The importance of ADL skills in the lives of elderly persons is considered to be diverse and indicates the need for outcomes that correlate to the patient's value preferences. The participants in this study made choices and trade offs in terms of time and energy expenditure on activities, their medical status, and availability of resources as to what was meaningful and of value to them in the context of their home, neighborhood, and community. The participants who returned to their prior level of functioning in the home environment also had a history of adaptability, coping skills, and spiritual faith. The participants who did not return to their prior level of activities had more serious health issues, a history of depression, and tended to blame external factors for their current difficulties. Although this study was a small sample size, it does support visiting elderly in their own contexts to assess functional abilities, rather than relying on observations and interviews in unfamiliar acute care settings.

Level IV Evidence

This level of evidence includes evidence based on opinions of experts or respected authorities, well-designed nonexperimental studies, single subject design, descriptive studies, and literary publications of expert panels. Although the lowest level of evidence, this type of research can provide valid foundations for treatment when reviewed carefully. In a single subject design study by Kamil and Correia (1990), the use of a dynamic elbow flexion splint for infants born with arthrogryposis multiplex congenital (AMC) was explored. These infants are born with severe combinations of contractures of shoulder adductors, shoulder internal rotators, and elbow extensors. The fabrication, application, and management of the dynamic flexion splint are described by the authors, with directions for use, by other clinicians included in the text article. The multiple joint contractures are attributed to an unknown etiology, but possibly related to in utero abnormal positioning; muscle involvement, as well as ligament and joint disorder.

The splint was applied to a 7-day-old female with elbows positioned at 20 degrees hyperextension with passive correction noted to be 20 degrees of flexion. Treatment for the infant in this study included gentle stretching and serial splinting. Splints were initially applied 12 hours a day. At 6 months of age, the splints were replaced with bivalve, long arm elbow flexion splints. By 8 months of age, passive elbow flexion increased to 70 degrees; at 9 months, 80 degrees; and at 12 months, 100 degrees with splint wearing noted for 2 1.5 hour blocks of time each day. The authors report an increase in the infant's functional use of the splint during daily activities as a positive functional outcome of this particular intervention.

This article described a single subject research design that evaluates the effectiveness of the use of a specific treatment technique. It is speculated that there was good compliance with the splint program from the infant's caregivers, which undoubtedly significantly contributed to the positive effects of this intervention. In a clinical setting, given an infant with a diagnosis of AMC, the benefit of serial splinting could be easily generalized given the splint fabrication abilities of the OT practitioner.

The aforementioned examples should guide the reader in being able to apply the research to his or her particular client population. Once the similarities and differences between his or her clients and the research participants have been determined, he or she will be better prepared to communicate the research findings to others. Johansson (1999) commented that OT practitioners must become accustomed to speaking the language of outcomes to others in order to demonstrate the efficacy of our services. Some suggestions in communication include the following (Johansson, 1999):

- The use of standardized assessments.
- Summarizing treatment sessions in progress notes in functional and measurable terms.
- In searching and sorting the literature, look for the best and most recent studies.
- Keep a "Research Index Card" for each article reviewed with notations or quotes from each study that pertains to your patient population or specific interventions.
- Adopt the evidence-based approaches into your repertoire of treatment.

Now that you have searched and sorted, how do you go about reading the EBP article? Figure 38-1 should assist you in this process.

Communicating the Findings

Now that you have reviewed the scholarly research, it is time to discuss your findings with your client. It is important to determine beforehand the consumer's level of understanding. Your communication with the clients and their families needs to be at a level, pace, and vocabulary that is consistent with their level. In today's health care environment, the use of an interpreter may be most beneficial for those consumers whose primary speaking language is different from yours. Although they may appear to speak and understand the language that you use, receiving the information and being able to asks questions in their primary language may minimize misunderstandings. Encourage the consumer to take the lead in the decision-making process, taking into consideration what is a value preference and most important to them. This will support your implementation of the *Occupational Therapy Practice Framework* (AOTA, 2002b) of having a client-centered approach. As outlined in our *Code of Ethics* (AOTA, 2002a), it is our responsibility to communicate the most valid and reliable methods to the consumer.

Tickle-Degnen (1998) described the following method to assist with the clinical reasoning when analyzing the significance of meta-analysis to your client population:

- Summarize the information.
- Discuss possible outcomes of participation or nonparticipation in treatment.
- Validate inclusion in decision-making process using numerical interpretations to enhance understanding.
- Refrain from using professional jargon.
- Make information individualized to your patient.
- If true, state that the evidence may be weak and why.
- Discuss the cost and benefit of participating or not participating in OT.

New research is continuously being published that is more accessible and can be used to improve our practice and credibility. The time has come for us to actively evaluate whether the interventions that we choose are simply based on our personal preferences or are the best choices for the functional outcomes of our clients. Should EBP play a role in your professional career? Of course it should. Hopefully, this chapter has assisted your thinking process to implement this efficiently and effectively in your busy life. The challenge will always be your ability to synthesize your clinical expertise with the current best evidence from systematic reviews of the professional literature.

The AOTA has recognized the climate of the health care arena and strives to assist the OT practitioner to improve the quality of services, access to OT outcome literature, and the importance to demonstrate the value of OT interventions. The AOTA national office is dedicated to providing the practitioner with access to OT outcome literature and has introduced what is known as AOTA's Evidence-Based Literature Review Project. This is one reason why your membership dues are so important to the advancement of the OT profession. Members can learn more by accessing the AOTA Web site at www.aota.org. The EBP link contains a series of briefs that are easy to read and summarizes articles that have been preselected from the professional literature and reviewed by experts in the field. The briefs are noted to report on primarily Level I and Level II research studies. Resources and links are provided to assist the clinician with the search process. The initial briefs scheduled to be available on the Web site are related to stroke, traumatic brain injury, MS, and PD. The AOTA, your state association, and other professional organizations are offering evidence-based continuing education courses or workshops. There are multiple avenues available to you and resources at your fingertips to assist with your pursuit of putting evidence into the practice of OT. The authors of the treatment techniques sections of this book have provided evidence-based treatment strategies that are easy to understand. You are encouraged to review these strategies and make note of the articles that are outlined in the evidence-based treatment strategies. Table 38-2 provides you with evidence-based journal articles related to EBP in OT.

SUMMARY

It is much easier in today's age of the Internet to search for current and relevant studies related to patient care and the practice of OT. Do not let this be your only source of information. It is critical for you to review the actual text of professional and peer-reviewed articles. Use your knowledge and clinical reasoning skills to determine the potential usefulness and value of the information to your patient population. Remember that decisions should be made based on this information, not only because it made good sense, but because it was what the patient wanted. In that way, your services will be client centered. In Figure 38-2, a model of clinical reasoning in EBP is presented with the emphasis of keeping the client as the primary focus in occupational performance and the outcome of the participation in the environment, home, school, community, etc. If you keep in mind the value of providing the right services and doing the right things, you will be well on your way to putting evidence into the practice of OT.

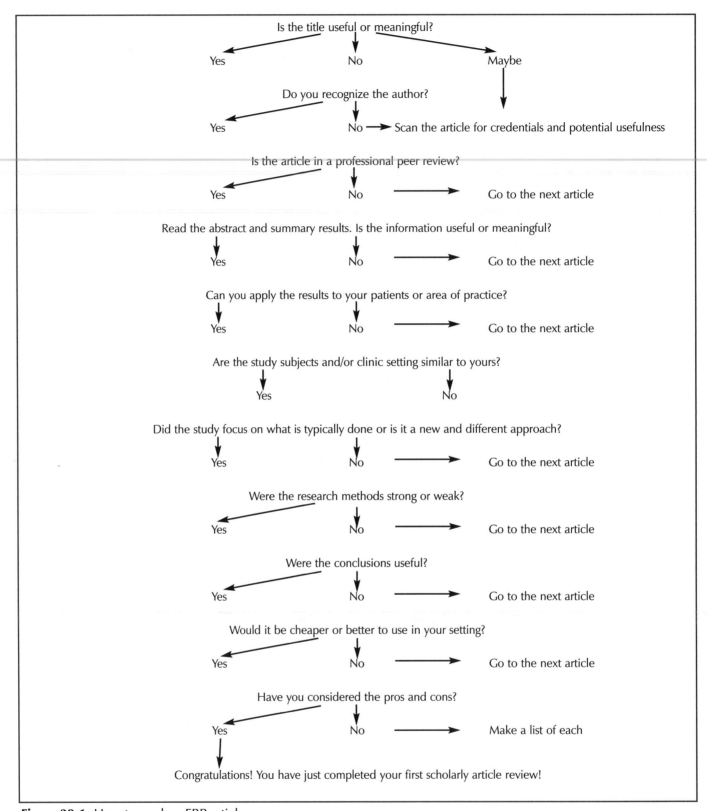

Figure 38-1. How to read an EBP article.

Table 38-2

Evidence-Based Treatment Strategies

Topic	Article
Therapist's perceptions	Dubouloz, Egan, Vallerand, & von Zweck, 1999; Dysart & Tomlin, 2002
Qualitative research to inform clients	Hammell, 2001
Purposeful activity	Lin, Wu, Tickle-Degnen, & Coster, 1997
Communication outcomes	Tickle-Degnen, 1998
Cochrane review: experience of 3 occupational therapists	Gervais, Poirier, Iterson, Egan, & Tickle-Degnen, 2002
Treatment planning	Tickle-Degnen, 1998
Therapeutic relationship	Tickle-Degnen, 2002
Measurement of treatment effectiveness	Davies & Gavin, 1999
Use of EBP, day to day	Ilott, 2003; Tickle-Degnen, 1999, 2000
AOTA's EBP literature review project	Liberman & Scheer, 2002

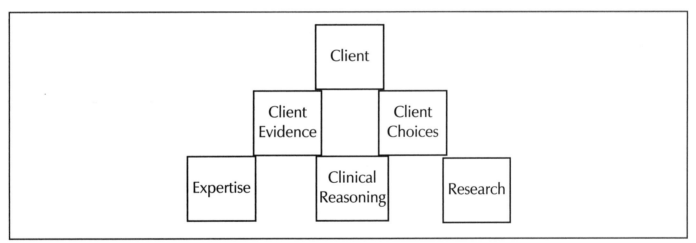

Figure 38-2. Model of clinical reasoning in EBP.

LEARNING ACTIVITIES

1. Conduct your own literature search on a topic of your choice. Begin a file system for personal use or establish a file system that other students can share in the library or OT office.

2. Find a piece of media that supports an undocumented science claim—infomercials or print material claiming instant weight loss, herbal "detoxifying" drinks, or other issues. Investigate the claims using evidence-based research.

3. Cruise the Internet looking for information or ads that are not evidence based.

REFERENCES

Abreu, B. C., & Chang, P. F. (2002). Getting started in evidence-based practice. American Occupational Therapy Association Continuing Education Article. October, CE-1 to CE-7.

Abreu, B. C., Peloquin, S. M., & Ottenbacher, K. (1998). Competence in scientific inquiry and research. American Journal of Occupational Therapy, 52, 751-759.

American Occupational Therapy Association. (2002a). Occupational therapy code of ethics. In The Reference Manual of the Official Documents (9th ed.). Bethesda, MD: Author.

American Occupational Therapy Association. (2002b). Occupational therapy practice framework: Domain & process. In The Reference Manual of the Official Documents (9th ed.). Bethesda, MD: Author.

Davies, P. L., & Gavin, W. J. (1999). Measurement issues in treatment effectiveness studies. *American Journal of Occupational Therapy, 53*(4), 363-372.

Dubouloz, C. J., Egan, M., Vallerand, J., & von Zweck, C. (1999). Occupational therapists' perception of evidence-based practice. *American Journal of Occupational Therapy, 53*, 445-458.

Dysart, A. M., & Tomlin, G. S. (2002). Factors related to evidence-based practice among U.S. occupational therapy clinicians. *American Journal of Occupational Therapy, 56*, 275-284.

Fasoli, S. E., Trombly, C. A., Tickle-Degnen, L., & Verfaellie, M. H. (2002). Effects of instructions on functional reach in persons with and without cerebrovascular accident. *American Journal of Occupational Therapy, 56*(4), 380-390.

Gentile, A. M. (1992). Movement disorders in children. *Medical Sport Science, 6*, 31-40.

Gervais, I. S., Poirier, A., Van Iterson, L., Egan, M., & Tickle-Degnen, L. (2002). Evidence-based practice forum. Attempting to use a cochrane review: Experience of three occupational therapists. *American Journal of Occupational Therapy, 56*(1), 110-113.

Hammell, K. W. (2001). Using qualitative research to inform the client-centered evidence-based practice of occupational therapy. *British Journal of Occupational Therapy, 64*, 228-234.

Holm, M. B. (2001). The 2000 Eleanor Clarke Slagle lecture. Our mandate for the new millennium: Evidence-based practice. *American Journal of Occupational Therapy, 54*, 575-585.

Holm, M. B. (2003). Top 10 reasons for becoming an evidence-based practitioner. *Occupational Therapy Practice, 8*(3), 9-11.

Ilott, I. (2003). Challenging the rhetoric and reality: Only an individual and systematic approach will work for evidence-based occupational therapy. *American Journal of Occupational Therapy, 57*(3), 351-354.

Johansson, C. (1999). Evidence-based therapy: The proof is in the science. *OT Week, July*, 8-9.

Kamil, N. I., & Correia, A. M. (1990). A dynamic elbow flexion splint for an infant with arthrogryposis. *American Journal of Occupational Therapy, 44*(5), 460-461.

Law, M. (2002). *Evidence-based rehabilitation: A guide to practice.* Thorofare, NJ: SLACK Incorporated.

Lehmann, J. F., DeLateur, B. J., Fowler, R. S., Warren, C. G., Arnhold, R., Schertzer, G., et al. (1975). Stroke: Does rehabilitation affect outcome? *Archives of Physical Medical Rehabilitation, 56*(9), 375-382.

Liberman, D., & Scheer, J. (2002). Evidence-based practice forum. AOTA's evidence-based literature review project: An overview. *American Journal of Occupational Therapy, 56*, 344-349.

Lin, K., Wu, C., Tickle-Degnen, L. & Coster, W. (1997). Enhancing occupational performance through occupationally embedded exercise: A meta-analytic review. *Occupational Therapy Journal of Research, 17*, 25-47.

Ma, H., & Trombly, C. A. (2002). A synthesis of the effects of occupational therapy for persons with stroke, part II. Remediation of impairments. *American Journal of Occupational Therapy, 56*, 260-274.

Rahman, N., Thomas, J. J., & Rice, M. S. (2002). The relationship between hand strength and the forces used to access containers by well elderly persons. *American Journal of Occupational Therapy, 56*, 78-85.

Rasmussen, P., & Gillberg, C. (2000). Natural outcome of ADHD with developmental coordination disorder at age 22 years; A controlled, longitudinal, community-based study. *Journal of the American Academy of Child and Adolescent Psychiatry, 11*, 1424-1431.

Rice, M. S., Leonard, C., & Carter, M. (1998). Grip strengths and required forces in accessing everyday containers in a normal population. *American Journal of Occupational Therapy, 52*, 621-626.

Sackett, D. L., Richardson, W. S., Rosenberg, W., & Haynes, R. B. (1997). *Evidence-based medicine. How to practice & teach ebm.* London: Churchill Livingstone.

Schultheis, M. T., Garay, E., Millis, S. R., & DeLuca, J. (2002). Motor vehicle crashes and violations among drivers with multiple sclerosis. *Archives of Physical Medicine and Rehabilitation, 83*, 1175-1178.

Spencer, J., Hersch, G., Shelton, M., Ripple, J., Spencer, C., Dyer, C. B., et al. (2002). Functional outcomes and daily life activities of African American elders after hospitalization. *American Journal of Occupational Therapy, 56*(2), 149-159.

Tickle-Degnen, L. (1998). Communicating with clients about treatment outcomes: The use of meta-analytic evidence in collaborative treatment planning. *American Journal of Occupational Therapy, 52*(7), 526-530.

Tickle-Degnen, L. (1999). Evidence-based practice forum. Organizing, evaluating, and using evidence in occupational therapy. *American Journal of Occupational Therapy, 53*, 537-539.

Tickle-Degnen, L. (2000). Evidence-based practice forum. What is the best evidence to use in practice? *American Journal of Occupational Therapy, 54*(2), 218-221.

Tickle-Degnen, L. (2002). Evidence-based practice forum. Client-centered practice, therapeutic relationship, and the use of research evidence. *American Journal of Occupational Therapy, 56*(4), 470-474.

Trombly, C. A., & Ma, H. (2002). A synthesis of the effects of occupational therapy for persons with stroke, part 1: Restoration of roles, tasks and activities. *American Journal Occupational Therapy, 56*, 250-259.

Vargas, S., & Camilli, G. (1999). A meta-analysis of research on sensory integration treatment. *American Journal of Occupational Therapy, 53*, 189-198.

SUGGESTED READINGS

Abreu, B. C., & Chang, P. F. (2002). Getting started in evidence-based practice. American Occupational Therapy Association Continuing Education Article. October, CE-1 to CE-7.

Holm, M. B. (2001). The 2000 Eleanor Clarke Slagle lecture. Our mandate for the new millennium: Evidence-based practice. *American Journal of Occupational Therapy, 54*, 575-585.

Law, M. (2002). *Evidence-based rehabilitation: A guide to practice.* Thorofare, NJ: SLACK Incorporated.

Key Concepts

- Research is the science and art of asking meaningful questions and finding credible and defensible answers to those questions.
- Important roles that research plays in OT include expanding the knowledge and skills base of educators and practitioners, providing justification for clinical decisions, and fueling healthy debate essential to the continued advancement of the profession.
- OTAs can integrate research strategies into their daily practice to enhance client care and their own professional development.

Essential Vocabulary

applied research: Seeks to find answers to questions that have practical applications in real world conditions.

empirical research: Involves making observations and collecting data about people and their environments.

problem statement: Describes real-life circumstances that are problematic for individuals, groups, or settings.

qualitative approach to research: Uses methods that identify, collect, and analyze data in non-numerical formats, such as words and pictures.

quantitative approach to research: Uses methods that measure, collect, and analyze data in numerical formats.

reliable measurements: In quantitative research, they are consistent and accurate.

research question: Guides research efforts so that the outcomes can be used to help alleviate the problem.

theoretical research: Involves synthesizing ideas, formulating concepts, and making predictions.

trustworthiness criteria: In qualitative research, are used to determine the credibility and applicability of results.

valid measurements: In quantitative research, they actually represent what they are supposed to represent.

UNDERSTANDING RESEARCH

Sandy Bell, PhD, PT

INTRODUCTION

Monday morning. With coffee in hand, June Ortez, OTA, rushed to make it to the rehab facility's medical library by 8. She and her supervisor, Dela Greene, OT, had arranged their schedules so that they could spend the first hour of the day looking up information about a new drug to treat persons with Alzheimer's disease. The previous Friday, Dela had completed an evaluation of a new patient, Mr. Chang, who was taking this drug. The admitting physician had explained to Dela that this patient was one of the first for whom she had prescribed the drug and she was anxious to see how Mr. Chang progressed in his OT.

As they got started, June posed the question, "I wonder what Mr. Chang's physical and cognitive functions will be like after taking the medication and what type of OT treatments will be best for him?" Using one of the library's computers, June and Dela started out by conducting a search using the name of the drug. The library's medical journal collection had 2 of the articles that came up in their search. Dela made a photocopy of each article and began to read over them. On the computer, June passed by the links for chat rooms and support groups. She looked up the author of one of the articles and that led her to the Web site for a medical center in Arizona. Here she found that the author was the medical director of a well-respected memory clinic associated with the center. June was excited to see that the clinic had posted information about the drug as well as rehab strategies developed by OTs who worked with patients during the clinical trials at the clinic. June printed this information and shared it with Dela.

They learned that the drug was particularly effective in improving both short-term and procedural memory during the mid stages of Alzheimer's disease, and in clinical trials, persons on the drug were able to perform ADL they had previously lost. Together, June and Dela reviewed the rehab strategies and identified a few activities they would try with Mr. Chang later that day. Dela knew that it might be a year or two before anything about the drug and implications for treatment would appear in any of the OT journals. She planned to call the OT at the clinic in Arizona listed as the author of the rehab protocols to find out more information. June offered to keep a journal about her work with Mr. Chang to supplement the chart documentation where she would record in more detail her observations of

his physical and cognitive functions, moods, and interactions with his family and the medical staff.

At 8:55 June and Dela left the library to start their patient visits for the day. June felt particularly energized—perhaps it was the coffee!

If you had asked June, she may not have told you that she started her day doing research, but that's just what she did. This scenario is just one of several that illustrate the opportunities an OTA has to engage in research during the course of his or her professional activities.

WHAT IS RESEARCH?

At its most fundamental level, research is the asking of questions and finding of answers. Though asking questions and finding answers are an everyday occurrence, the ways in which one goes about these activities determines the extent to which they qualify as research. Research involves the systematic, mindful, and disciplined use of techniques to formulate questions that are meaningful and answers that are defensible. Additionally, research has its own set of ethical considerations and means of communicating ideas and findings. Where differences and distinctions emerge in research are the specific objectives for engaging in research, the methods used to pose questions and find answers, and in the nature of the outcomes or products of research efforts.

APPLICATIONS OF RESEARCH IN OCCUPATIONAL THERAPY

You can gain a good appreciation for the variety of goals, methods, and products of research by looking at the many applications of research in the OT profession. The adoption of EBP has brought research to the forefront of OT practice. In EBP, practitioners locate, review, and interpret research literature related to a specific patient problem to gather evidence to support their clinical decisions (Holm, 2001). In the scenario above, June and Dela were engaged in the beginning stages of

EBP. In clinical settings, OTs and OTAs can participate in case studies—collecting data to provide in-depth descriptions of an individual's history and condition, response to treatment, as well as personal and environmental factors (Portney & Watkins, 1993). June's use of a detailed journal to record her observations of Mr. Chang's response to various treatment strategies is an example of data that may be collected in a clinical case study.

In academic settings, OT faculty, as well as students, often engage in research projects—providing much of the "evidence" in EBP. Faculty may receive grant monies to support a research agenda that may involve many studies over the course of many years. Often, faculty researchers present at conferences and publish in professional journals, sharing their insights, methods, and findings with their constituents in OT and other rehab professionals. Research conducted by masters and doctoral students also plays an important role in contributing to the knowledge base in OT.

In addition to participating in the review of literature for EBP and in collecting data for a case study, OTAs can engage in identifying problems of practice that are in need of study, assessing client satisfaction or quality assurance outcomes, and exploring the theoretical or historical basis for specific intervention practices (Sladyk, 2003). As demonstrated by June and Dela in the above scenario, research activities can form the basis for collaboration between an OTA and his or her OT supervisor, as well as with other health care team members.

Frequently, a distinction is made between being a research consumer and being a research practitioner (Royeen, 1997). This division is useful for distinguishing between persons who characteristically conduct research studies from persons who characteristically use or apply research findings but do not conduct research studies themselves. Historically, clinicians in patient care settings have resigned themselves to the role of research consumer and professionals in academic settings have assumed the role of research practitioner or producer. Yet, this distinction should not preclude a practicing OTA or OT from engaging in research. Indeed, engaging in research involves both being a critical consumer of the research conducted by others and applying the knowledge gained to design and conduct one's own investigations on both small and large scales. In the following sections, you will be introduced to many key concepts about the fundamentals of research. This chapter can serve as an initial resource, an invitation to explore the possibilities of research with peers, instructors, supervisors, and mentors during the course of your OT education and practice.

BASIC, APPLIED, AND ACTION RESEARCH

Research is classified in different ways. One way is by the overall objectives of the research endeavor. This classification of research has 3 levels: basic, applied, and action.

- In basic research, the objectives are to discover new knowledge and to find out how things work or what they are made of. Individuals who study the cellular structure of scar tissue or how the brain functions when processing sensory stimuli are conducting basic research.

- In applied research, the objectives are to find answers to practical problems or to test the findings of basic research under real world conditions. Most of the research engaged in by OTs, OTAs, and other rehab professionals is of this type. A team of therapists in a school district who examine the relationship between family structure and student compliance with home routines are conducting applied research. A doctoral candidate comparing cognitive function among persons with different types of sensory deficits is also conducting applied research.

- In action research, the objectives are to document and improve the quality of individual practice or the functions of an organization in a specific setting (Johnson, 2002). Action research is conducted by practitioners in their own work settings. It involves a cyclical process of identifying a problem, planning a solution, putting the plan into action, assessing the outcomes, and using the outcomes to further refine the problem. Whereas the outcomes of basic and applied research are commonly generalized to other settings, the outcomes of action research are used only in the setting in which the data were collected. Home care therapists testing out a plan to increase the efficiency with which they complete new patient intake evaluations are conducting action research when they systematically observe and measure the impact of the plan and use the information to further explore ways to increase intake efficiency.

EMPIRICAL AND THEORETICAL RESEARCH

Up to this point in the chapter, most of the examples of research have involved making observations and collecting data. Research of this type is empirical research. Empirical means knowledge based on information gained from experience or from observations using the senses. When people think of research, they commonly think of empirical research, and this is the type of research on which EBP is focused. However, there is a different and equally important type of research that explores ideas rather than people or things: theoretical research.

Theoretical research generates new knowledge using cognitive processes to analyze and synthesize ideas and information. The ideas and information may come from a variety of sources, including books, articles, conversations with others, and individual observations and experiences. Theoretical researchers organize and build upon the ideas in ways that enable greater understanding in a particular field. The outcome or product of theoretical research is a theory that can be used to examine known relationships and predict future relationships. Maslow's Hierarchy of Needs is an example of a theory that has been used in the field of OT for nearly 50 years to better understand human development and motivation (Leary, 2001).

The research base for any profession such as OT includes both empirical and theoretical research. Though they are distinct from each other, empirical and theoretical research are closely intertwined, with each type of research serving as the

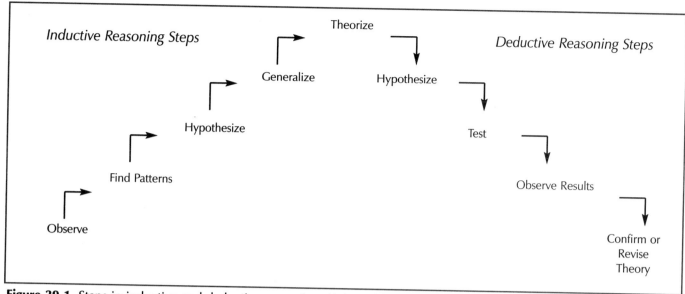

Figure 39-1. Steps in inductive and deductive reasoning. (Adapted from Trochim, W. M. K. [2001]. *The research methods knowledge base* [2nd ed., pp. 17-18]. Cincinnati: Atomic Dog Publishing.)

starting point for the other. Empirical research is often dedicated to testing a theory in real world situations, and theoretical research often uses results from empirical studies to generate new ideas.

Inductive and Deductive Reasoning

As stated earlier, research—whether empirical or theoretical—involves a systematic and disciplined approach to asking questions and finding answers. Researchers commonly use 2 different logistical strategies to complete their investigations and explorations: deductive reasoning and inductive reasoning. Deductive reasoning starts with a theory or hypothesis and proceeds to test it under specific circumstances to see if holds true. For example, using Maslow's Hierarchy of Needs as a theoretical base, a therapist may hypothesize or deduce that, in general, teenagers with psychiatric disorders are primarily motivated by needs for self-esteem and belonging. The therapist may test this hypothesis by measuring teenaged clients' perceptions of needs and evaluating the effectiveness of interventions designed to support self-esteem and peer acceptance.

Whereas deductive reasoning involves starting with generalizations and observing to see if they hold true under specific circumstances, inductive reasoning involves starting with specific observations and using them as a basis for generalizations or constructing theories (Portney & Watkins, 1993). Suppose the therapist in the previous paragraph started by observing that teenagers with psychiatric diagnoses with whom he works tend to be preoccupied with the need for feeling accepted by one's peers and struggling with feelings of self-doubt. He may discover that his observations are consistent with Maslow's theory of Hierarchy of Needs and generalize that all teenagers, with or without a clinical diagnosis, tend to be preoccupied with needs for self-esteem and acceptance.

Researchers can use both deductive and inductive reasoning processes to complete empirical and theoretical research efforts. Just as empirical and theoretical research are closely intertwined, so too are deductive and inductive reasoning. Figure 39-1 illustrates the steps in each type of reasoning. Each strategy only accounts for half of the ways individuals go about asking questions and finding answers; together, they enable a systematic, disciplined, and complete means to discovery.

Getting Started: The Research Problem and Research Question

As you can see, research plays a variety of roles in the field of OT. Because a great deal of the research conducted and reviewed by OT students and professionals is applied and empirical, this type of research will be the focus for an overview of processes involved in starting a research study.

Define the Problem

This first step, defining the problem that your study will address, is perhaps the most important. Completing a research endeavor requires a fair amount of deliberation, time, and resources so it should be worth doing. That is, it should be directed at improving knowledge, understanding, or practice in an area about which you and others are concerned. The problem should be stated so that it describes the actual experiences of individuals, groups, or settings that it impacts.

Here is an example of a problem statement:

- After finger joint replacement, individuals can experience finger flexor muscle contractures if they do not maintain both PROM and AROM, which can lead to functional limitations in ADL.

Notice how this statement describes the problem not only in terms of tissue impairment, but also in terms of its significance for individuals at the functional level. Often, novice researchers neglect to answer the "so what?" question when defining a problem. They describe the immediate circumstances that are problematic (e.g., flexor contractures after finger joint surgery), yet not include why the circumstances are problematic (e.g., contractures can lead to limitations in ADL).

Here is an example of an incomplete problem statement:

- Faculty in OT degree programs commonly lack the resources and supports needed to publish in scholarly journals.

Here is the complete problem statement, which addresses the "So what?" question:

- Faculty in OT degree programs commonly lack the resources and supports needed to publish in scholarly journals, which can result in their not earning tenure and high turnover rates among program faculty.

Once you have identified the problem on which you will focus your research study, the next step is to formulate a specific question that will guide your efforts.

State the Research Question

Most often, a research problem represents a broad area of concern, and you will not be able to address every aspect of a problem in a single study. A research question serves to narrow your focus to specific aspects of a problem that are most significant to you. Invariably, one problem can spawn many questions. Related to the problem above about the risk of finger flexor contractures after surgery and subsequent functional limitations in ADL, one researcher may ask, "What treatment strategy is more effective in maintaining PROM after finger joint replacement surgery, passive stretching of the finger and wrist flexors or passive mobilization of surrounding joints?" Another researcher may be more interested to find out, "Is there a relationship between the type of replacement joint used in surgery and the incidence of flexor contractures?" And yet a third researcher may ask, "Among persons over the age of 80, what factors characterize individual's perceptions of their ability to perform ADL after finger joint replacement surgery and how do their perceptions compare to those of family members?" After posing the research question, each researcher would proceed to design and carry out a study to answer that question. As you can imagine, with regards to the 3 research questions above, each study would be quite different from the other 2.

After posing the research question, the next task for researchers is selecting methods to identify, collect, and analyze data that they can use to formulate an answer to the question. The answer becomes the basis for interventions to alleviate the original problem. Selecting the best methods to answer a research question can be a challenge. The next section presents an overview of the methods from which a researcher can choose and factors that influence selecting one method over another.

Introduction to Quantitative and Qualitative Research

As previously mentioned, much of the research conducted and reviewed by OT students and professionals is applied and empirical (i.e., its objective is to improve practice through the collection and analysis of data). Data are information about attributes or characteristics of something that are of interest to researchers. Examples of types of information researchers may want to know about include individuals' age, gender, level of education, perceptions about functional goals or pain levels, and environmental circumstances, such as work demands and family structure. Data that are represented in numerical form are called quantitative data; data that are represented in non-numerical form, such as written descriptions or pictures, are called qualitative data.

Researchers generally use 1 of 2 general approaches to answer their research questions. The approach is based on the type of data that they plan to collect and analyze. A quantitative approach uses methods that can define, measure, collect, and analyze data in numerical formats. A qualitative approach uses methods that can identify, collect, and analyze data that exist in non-numerical formats. Both quantitative and qualitative studies start with defining the problem and posing the research question. From this point on, the 2 approaches differ in many important ways.

Quantitative Research Concepts, Methods, and Designs

Variables and Their Operational Definitions

After defining the problem and posing the research question, researchers using quantitative methods must decide exactly what type of information they need in order to answer the research question. First, they must define the attribute, trait, or characteristic they need to know about. An attribute, trait, or characteristic is called a variable. By definition, a variable is any attribute that can vary among individuals, objects, or settings (Fraenkel & Wallen, 2000). Client age, gender, diagnosis, and cognitive status are common variables of interest to researchers in clinical settings. With respect to the 3 sample research questions presented in the previous section, PROM, type of joint replacement, and perceptions of ability to perform ADLs are all variables.

Because many studies can use the same variable (e.g., many studies include client age as a variable), researchers must describe exactly what a variable represents and how they plan to measure it in their own study. This description is known as an operational definition. According to Portney and Watkins

(1993), "Operational definitions clarify terms by explaining how they are observed or measured, including the delineation of tools and procedures used to obtain those measurements. The operational definition should be sufficiently detailed that another researcher could replicate the procedure or condition" (p. 98). With regards to an operational definition for the variable client age, one researcher may define it as "age in years at the time of last birthday," while another researcher may define it more precisely as "age in number of years and months" (for example, 70 years versus 70 years and 3 months).

Instruments

Implied in an operational definition of a variable is how that variable will be measured. An instrument is used to measure a variable. The nature of the variable will determine the type of instrument to be used. Some variables, such as height, weight, and ROM have pre-established instruments readily available (e.g., a body scale for weight or a goniometer for ROM). Other variables, particularly those reflecting individual perceptions and values under specific circumstances, may require researchers to develop instruments specific for their own studies. For example, the researcher who wanted to measure client and family members' perceptions of the client's ability to perform ADL after finger joint replacement surgery might develop a questionnaire to measure these perceptions. The questionnaire may ask individuals to rate on a scale of 0 to 10 (where 0 = totally dependent on another person and 10 = totally independent) the extent to which the client could independently perform 12 different ADL requiring various types of finger dexterity and strength.

Valid and Reliable Measurements

Because quantitative studies rely on numerical values for data, researchers need to be very confident that the values they obtained from their instruments are valid (i.e., they actually represent what they are supposed to represent) and reliable (i.e., they will remain consistent and free from error). A goniometer may represent a valid measure of finger joint ROM; it does measure what it is designed to measure. However, if the measures are taken sometimes with the wrist in neutral and other times with the wrist in extension, the values will be inconsistent from one measurement to the next, and therefore unreliable. Conversely, measurement values can be invalid yet reliable. Suppose the researcher who wanted to measure perceptions of a client's ability to perform ADL asked clients to record their heart rate with an electronic device each time they completed an activity. The record of heart rate values obtained from the device would most likely be very reliable, yet the values would not be a valid representation of perceived independence. In the first instance, the measures of joint ROM were valid yet not reliable, and in the second instance, the heart rate values were reliable yet not valid. Researchers should strive to make sure the numbers they obtain in a quantitative study are both valid and reliable representations of the variables they wish to measure.

Sampling

The numbers in a quantitative study can describe attributes of individuals, groups, organizations, or clinical settings. These are sources of data in a study and represent the study sample. The members of a sample, also known as subjects, participants, or units of study, are selected from a larger population. Often, one of the primary objectives of quantitative research is to find out about attributes and relationships in a sample and generalize the findings to the population from which it was selected. Including every patient who ever had finger joint replacement surgery in a study of the comparative benefits of 2 treatment strategies to maintain joint ROM would be impractical, if not impossible. The researcher selects a manageable sample of patients to participate in the study, and at the same time hopes that the findings will be applicable to and benefit many current and future patients who undergo this type of surgery.

Researchers use a variety of strategies to select participants in quantitative studies; some strategies enable generalizing the findings of the sample to the population better than others do. In random sampling, where each member of the population has an equal chance of being selected for the study, the characteristics of the sample are most likely to represent those of the population. With random sampling, researchers maximize the chances that the ways in which subjects respond to a specific treatment, for example, are similar to the ways members of the whole population would respond.

In contrast, nonrandom sampling involves selecting participants from a population because they have specific characteristics. Researchers may select participants out of convenience because they are readily available (a convenience sample) or deliberately select participants based on specific criteria (purposive sample). Researchers often use convenience or purposive sampling knowing that they will be limited in the extent to which they can generalize their findings to others who did not participate in the study.

Following is an illustration of the differences between random and nonrandom convenience sampling. First, the researcher comparing the benefits of 2 treatment strategies to maintain joint ROM after finger joint replacement surgery may work with a surgeon who is very supportive of the study and arrange to have the surgeon provide an information sheet to his patients about volunteering for the study. At the end of the study, the researcher would have a lot of information about how this surgeon's patients responded to the 2 treatments but could not generalize the findings to the patients of other surgeons. On the other hand, the researcher could arrange to receive lists of all the patients who had undergone finger joint replacement surgery performed by surgeons from a variety of medical teaching facilities and randomly select patients on the lists to contact and invite to participate in the study. Using this sampling strategy, the researcher could generalize, with relative confidence, the findings to a larger population of persons who have undergone finger joint replacement surgery.

Sample Size

In addition to the way in which participants are selected for a study, randomly or nonrandomly, the number of participants selected also impacts the extent to which researchers can generalize their findings. In general, the more participants in a sample, the greater the chances the sample characteristics reflect those in the population (for studies using random sampling) or in the pool of potential participants (for studies using nonrandom sampling). Because numbers are used for data in quantitative research, researchers must analyze the data using statistics. Statistics is the science of using numbers to answer questions. Though a discussion of statistical analyses is beyond the scope of this chapter, you should keep in mind 3 things about sample size and statistical tests:

1. Sample size directly affects the outcomes of a statistical test; the more participants, the more accurate the test outcomes.

2. The more variables a researcher includes in a statistical test, the more participants needed to ensure that the test outcome is accurate.

3. The less reliable the scores from an instrument used to measure a variable, the more participants needed to ensure that the statistical test outcome is accurate.

Frequently, logistics and resources such as time, money, space, and personnel determine the number of participants in a study. The ways in which a researcher tries to gather a sample, however, can also impact the final sample size. Sometimes researchers go about sampling in a haphazard manner. They may use ineffective ways of informing potential participants about the study. Or, researchers may be overly "pushy" in recruiting efforts and lose potential volunteers because they do not feel comfortable. Later in the chapter, more details about recruiting participants will be covered in the discussion of ethical issues in research.

Quantitative Research Designs

A description of some of the more common ways quantitative research studies are designed will help illustrate many of the concepts and methods covered in this section. The first distinction made in the actual design of a study is whether it is experimental, quasi-experimental, or nonexperimental.

Experimental

Experimental designs seek to identify, with as much confidence as possible, "a cause-and-effect relationship between a particular action or condition (the independent variable) and an observed response (the dependent variable)" (Portney & Watkins, 1993, p. 125). Experimental designs always use random selection of participants from a population and, if groups are involved, random assignment of participants to groups.

The double-blind randomized control-group pretest-post-test design is considered the "gold standard" in medical research and commonly used to measure the effects of new drugs or treatments before they are approved for routine practice. In this type of study, participants are randomly selected from a population and then randomly assigned to either a group that will receive the treatment (treatment group) or a group that will not receive the treatment (control group). In many studies of this type, the control group receives a placebo treatment. The status of all participants is measured prior to their receiving any treatment or placebo and then again after receiving the treatment or placebo and the outcomes of the two groups are compared. If the treatment group status has improved more than the control group's, the researchers can be highly confident that the difference was due to the treatment. The double-blind component in this design refers to the fact that neither the treatment providers nor the participants in the study know if they are part of the treatment group or the placebo group. These types of studies may have many hundreds of participants in them and be repeated at a variety of facilities around the country before a new treatment is approved for routine practice.

Quasi-Experimental

True experimental design studies are an important resource for EBP in OT. Unfortunately, they require a great deal of resources that often exceed those available to researchers in academic and clinical settings. In these settings, when researchers cannot meet the requirements of randomized participant selection and/or use of control groups, they design quasi-experimental studies. Quasi-experimental studies may seek to compare differences between two or more groups under different conditions or examine the response of one group to one or more conditions (Portney & Watkins, 1993; Royeen, 1997). These studies can also serve as important resources in EBP. An example of a quasi-experimental design is the study described above of the researcher who used a convenience sample of patients from one surgeon to assess the benefits of two treatment strategies to maintain joint ROM after finger joint replacement surgery.

Nonexperimental

Quite frequently, researchers do not wish to determine a cause and effect or compare outcomes under different conditions, but rather they seek to describe the nature of variables or explore relationships among variables in specific populations or under specific circumstances. Studies of this type are nonexperimental studies. Though they have limited utility in making EBP decisions, nonexperimental studies are valuable in establishing a foundation of knowledge on which quasi-experimental and experimental studies are based (Portney & Watkins, 1993).

Two common nonexperimental designs are descriptive and correlational. In descriptive quantitative studies, researchers collect numerical data, often on a variety of variables, which they use to describe characteristics of specific individuals, groups, organizations, or conditions. For example, a researcher interested in describing cognitive development among children diagnosed with postpartum onset of CP would use a descriptive study design.

In correlational studies, "researchers investigate possible relationships among variables without trying to influence those variables" (Fraenkel & Wallen, 2000, p. 359). A correlation represents a relationship between 2 characteristics (e.g., the relationship between grip strength and age). A correlation can be positive, meaning that as the values on one variable go up so do the values on the other variable. The correlation between age and grip strength among children is positive. Conversely, the correlation between age and grip strength among adults is negative because as adults increase in age, their grip strength tends to decline. Similar to descriptive studies, correlational studies can only describe the nature and extent of relationships among variables, they cannot determine whether one variable caused an effect in another. Regardless, correlational studies play an important role in contributing to the clinical knowledge base because they identify tendencies and trends and help practitioners make associations among what may seem like an array of unrelated signs and symptoms when working with clients.

Single-Subject and Case Study Designs

An overview of quantitative research designs common to OT and other health care fields would not be complete without a discussion of 2 additional designs: the single-subject experimental design and the case study nonexperimental design. Single-subject experimental studies involve only one purposefully selected case or subject. Though researchers are not concerned with generalizing results to other cases, the design is considered experimental because it allows for making determinations of cause and effect. First, a baseline set of data on variables of interests is established after taking measures on multiple occasions. Measurements continue as the study progresses into the intervention phase where the subject is exposed to a carefully designed treatment or intervention. Data from the baseline phase is compared to data from the intervention phase to see if any changes have occurred. The intervention is then removed and measures continue to see if the changes return to baseline levels. A variation on this design is to include a second intervention after the second baseline phase to make sure that any changes that occurred after the first intervention were not an accident or just due to chance. If researchers find a consistent change in status after each intervention and change back toward baseline levels when the intervention is removed, they can be very confident that the intervention was the cause of the observed changes.

Like the single-subject experimental design, the case study nonexperimental design also involves just one subject. "Typically, case studies involve the in-depth description of an individual's condition or response to treatment; however, case studies can also focus on a group, institution, or other social unit, such as particular school, community, or family" (Portney & Watkins, 1993, p. 234). The subjects selected for case study often represent new, unique, or noteworthy circumstances. They provide opportunities for researchers and practitioners to share what they have learned from intensive study of just one case. The data collected about a case can be both numerical (e.g., records of heart rate, blood pressure, and frequencies in performing activities) as well as non-numerical (e.g., written observation notes, photographs, and samples of products created by the subject). When case studies include non-numerical data, they crossover into the domain of qualitative research, which is the focus of the next section.

Qualitative Research Concepts, Methods, and Designs

In quantitative studies, researchers seek to answer questions that can be answered with numbers, such as "How much of X is there?" "How often does Y occur?" "What happens to X when I do Y?" "How does X compare to Y?" or "What is the relationship between X and Y?" In qualitative studies, researchers pose questions that need to be answered with words or visual displays—questions such as, "What is it like for a child to live in a foster home?" "How do clinical instructors decide what type of feedback to provide students during fieldwork?" or "How do therapists learn a new patient charting system?" A key challenge for researchers is to design a study and select methods that best answer their research questions. Figure 39-2 illustrates the steps involved in conducting both quantitative and qualitative studies. As you can see, both approaches start with defining the problem and posing the research question and end with reporting results, making conclusions, and making recommendations. The central parts of each process, the design and methods, are different because the research questions posed in quantitative and qualitative studies are different.

Qualitative research is always nonexperimental. Its purpose is to describe and record, as accurately as possible, individual or group lived experiences, behaviors, processes, perspectives, and/or values. Organizational functioning or cultural phenomena may also be the focus of qualitative research (Strauss & Corbin, 1998). Qualitative researchers rarely purposefully introduce an intervention to an individual or group. Sometimes, they may participate in group or social functions (a role known as participant-observer), yet most often they try to observe and collect information in ways that have a minimal impact on participants or environments under study.

Sampling and Sample Size

In qualitative research studies, researchers use purposeful sampling to select the individual, group, and/or social setting that will provide the richest source of data and enable a thorough and credible answer to the research question. Marshall and Rossman (1999) state that a "realistic" site for data collection is one where:

> …(a) entry is possible; (b) there is a high probability that a rich mix of the processes, people, programs, interactions, and structures of interest are present; (c) the researcher is likely to be able to build trusting relations with the participants in the study; and (d) data quality and credibility of the study are reasonable assured. (p. 69)

The number of participants in qualitative studies is usually much smaller than in quantitative studies. As discussed earlier, in quantitative studies, the more participants the greater the likelihood that the sample is an accurate reflection of the population from which it came, and the more confident researchers can be in generalizing the results of statistical tests from the

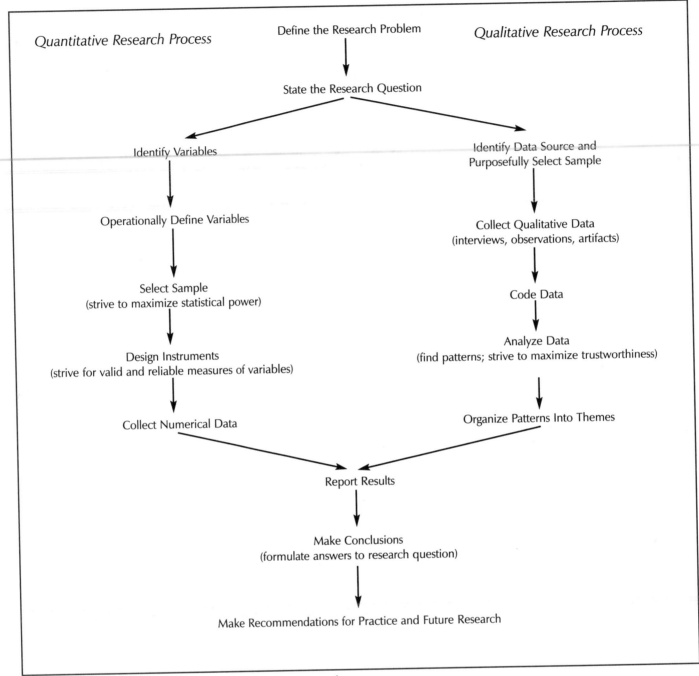

Figure 39-2. Steps in quantitative and qualitative research.

sample to the population. In qualitative studies, researchers are not concerned with statistics and generalizing their findings to a larger population. They seek small samples with specific qualities, rather than samples with a good deal of quantity. For example, a researcher may design a study to answer the question, "How do clinical instructors decide what type of feedback to provide students during fieldwork?" and invite just 6 to 10 instructors to participate in the study. To explore whether instructors perceive that their decisions about student feedback are influenced by the setting in which they work, the research may purposefully select 2 or 3 instructors from large teaching hospitals, 2 or 3 instructors from outpatient behavioral clinics, and 2 or 3 instructors from home care or school settings.

Data Collection

Because data in qualitative studies differ from data in quantitative studies, methods researchers use to collect data differ considerably. In quantitative studies, researchers define the variables they wish to measure and then strive to measure them using instruments that will provide valid and reliable results. In qualitative studies, often the researcher does not know what he or she will find. Variables are not defined prior to collecting data; rather characteristics of participants or environments are labeled and defined after the data have been collected and analyzed.

Typically, data collection in qualitative research involves using a variety of methods and gathering data from a variety of sources. Because qualitative researchers do not use instruments and statistics to tell them how valid and reliable their data are, they try to ensure that their data are accurate by using a series of checks and double checks. The process is akin to that used by a police officer investigating an auto accident—he or she may interview 3 or 4 different individuals who witnessed the accident from different perspectives in order to piece together a whole picture of what happened. This process of using at least 3 different sources of data to get an accurate account of a phenomenon is known as *triangulation* (Portney & Watkins, 1993).

Some of the most common methods of data collection in qualitative studies are interview, observation, and review of artifacts. Interviews may be structured, semistructured, or unstructured depending on the extent to which the questions are determined ahead of time and whether or not the questions need to be presented in a set sequence. Usually researchers audiotape record interviews and then transcribe what was said so that it can be reviewed many times during data analysis. Researchers may use an individual interview format to gather the perspectives of individual participants or choose a focus-group interview format to collect perceptions of a group of individuals. Focus groups are an effective way to capture the dynamics that may be at play in a group. Often, interactions among group members trigger ideas, emotions, or behaviors that would not be apparent in an individual interview.

Qualitative researchers also rely on observation to collect data. Observation is the best method to use when researchers want to document the behavior of individuals or groups in familiar or unfamiliar settings. Researchers usually record their observations in writing as field notes, though sometimes they record their observations in the field and transcribe them later. Field notes are "detailed, non-judgmental, concrete descriptions of what has been observed" (Marshall & Rossman, 1999, p. 107). Qualitative researchers recognize that their presence may affect the behavior they observe in others and that their own preferences and biases may affect how they conduct their observations. For this reason, researchers try to observe and record in a reflective journal their own actions and reactions during their data collection experiences. The journal becomes a valuable reference during data analysis, when researchers strive to acknowledge how their own biases may affect the process of understanding the data.

A third source of data in qualitative studies is artifacts. Artifacts are tangible objects that represent expressions of underlying values, beliefs, perspectives, skills, or knowledge held by individuals or groups. Some examples of artifacts include personal journals, drawings, crafts, Web sites, assignments submitted by students, internal memos in an organization, training manuals, and evaluation forms. The list is practically endless, and researchers must carefully choose artifacts that contribute meaningful data and help answer the research question. In the study of how clinical instructors decide what type of feedback to provide students during fieldwork, the researcher may examine student performance evaluation forms completed by instructors at the middle and end of their students' fieldwork experience. The clinical instructor manual provided by the academic institution as well as copies of any department or facility-wide policies that pertain to employee responsibilities and behaviors while in the role of clinical instructor may also be valuable artifacts for review.

Data Analysis

Analysis of qualitative data is a complex process of reviewing, organizing, comparing, and contrasting the data many times until researchers are satisfied that the meanings, perspectives, attitudes, and relationships underlying the data have been accurately identified. The process is largely inductive, meaning researchers start with specific observations and end with hypotheses or broader generalizations about the meaning of the data. Initially, researchers code the data into categories and subcategories. If a statement made by one participant is similar to that made by another, these 2 statements would be coded into the same category. At first, the volume of data in a qualitative study can seem insurmountable, but through methodical analysis, researchers can find recurrent patterns, or themes, in the data that become the basis for formulating an answer to the research question (Marshall & Rossman, 1999). For example, in analyzing the data about how clinical instructors decide what type of feedback to provide students during fieldwork, the researcher may find that the majority of instructors mentioned that they gave feedback to students modeled after the ways they received it when they were students. This category of data becomes the basis of a theme that the researcher can use to answer the research question. This theme may be one of many that together make up a complete answer to the question.

Trustworthiness

Whether conducting a qualitative or quantitative study, researchers strive to ensure that their results are an accurate reflection of what was actually present or occurred at the time data were collected. In quantitative studies, the rigor of a study is assessed by the validity and reliability of the data and the precision of the statistical tests used to analyze the data. In qualitative studies, the rigor of a study is assessed by a different, yet equally rigorous set of criteria, known as trustworthiness criteria.

The 4 types of trustworthiness criteria are credibility, dependability, confirmability, and transferability (Trochim, 2001). Like quantitative studies, the criteria pertain to both the data collection and data analysis phases of a study.

1. Credibility refers to the extent to which the data reflect what researchers actually observed, heard, read, or otherwise perceived. Some strategies that researchers use to ensure their data are credible include:

   o Member checking (asking participants to review the data and provide feedback about its accuracy)

   o Triangulation (collecting and cross-referencing data from multiple sources)

   o Peer debriefing (sharing interpretations of the data with a colleague not associated with the study for feedback about whether the interpretations seem plausible)

2. Dependability refers to the extent to which results would be comparable if the study was repeated with similar participants and in similar contexts. Researchers leave an audit trail (i.e., a complete documentation of methods and procedures) to ensure that another researcher could replicate the study.

3. Confirmability refers to the extent to which the results are free from the researcher's own biases, values, and assumptions and can be confirmed by others. Researchers establish confirmability in many of the same ways as they establish credibility.

4. Transferability refers to the extent to which the results can be transferred, or generalized, to persons and settings outside the study. Researchers provide a "thick description" of their methods, data, and results so that consumers of the research can decide for themselves the extent to which they feel the findings are applicable to their own circumstances.

Qualitative Research Designs

Similar to quantitative research, researchers use a variety of approaches and designs in qualitative research. Three common designs are phenomenology, ethnography, and case study. Phenomenological studies seek to understand individual experiences and the meanings people make of their experiences. Portney and Watkins (1993) provide an excellent example of a phenomenological study:

> For instance, therapists could investigate the phenomenon of "fear of falling" in elderly individuals. The true depth of the dimensions of feelings, thoughts, and behaviors that are part of this phenomenon can be investigated only by questioning and observing the individual who has experienced falls as well as those who interact with that individual. (p. 239)

The objective of ethnographic studies is to describe an intact cultural group in its natural setting. Researchers characteristically immerse themselves in the culture for prolonged periods in order to obtain an accurate and complete description of the social relationships, roles, and forces that shape the culture (Portney & Watkins, 1993; Royeen, 1997). For example, an ethnographic approach would be appropriate to understand how different cultures treat members of their society who have physical or mental disabilities.

Lastly, the case study design is used in qualitative research to understand the experiences of one specific individual, group, or context. Similar to the quantitative approach to case study, the qualitative approach involves intensive observation and data collection. Case studies are a way of telling the "story" of one individual or case to enable insight into the experiences of others.

In the opening scenario of the chapter, June Ortez, OTA and Dela Greene, OT are poised to embark on a case study of Mr. Chang. Mr. Chang presents the opportunity to better understand, both quantitatively and qualitatively, the effects of the new medication for persons with Alzheimer's disease. The "rip-

ple effects" of any improvements in Mr. Chang's cognitive abilities on his and his caretakers' lived experiences, feelings, and expectations cannot be adequately captured using quantitative measures alone. With the approval of the patient, family, and medical facility, June and Dela could supplement performance measures for Mr. Chang with detailed interviews of family members and hospital staff and conduct follow-up interviews and observations in the home after discharge. With the support of their employer, and perhaps in consultation with colleagues from an academic program, June and Dela may find themselves at the next national conference sharing the outcomes of their case study of Mr. Chang to the benefit of other therapists and their clients far beyond the scope of their own facility.

PROTECTION OF RIGHTS FOR HUMAN SUBJECTS

This chapter concludes with a discussion of ethical considerations in research, with a focus on the rights of human subjects in research and how they are protected. In the preceding sections, many examples of research studies used to illustrate key concepts included participants or subjects. The scenarios reflect real life situations and they would not be complete without mentioning that all of the participants were willing volunteers who had full understanding of what their participation entailed, gave their consent before any data were collected, and had all information collected about them kept in strict confidence. These conditions of participation—volunteerism, informed consent, and confidentiality—are basic rights of individuals who participate in any type of research.

Code of Federal Regulations Title 45 Public Welfare: Part 46 Protection of Human Subjects

The protection of human subjects in research is a federally mandated and regulated right of citizenship in the United States (Title 45, 1991). The Office for Human Research Protections (OHRP) in the Department of Health and Human Services (DHHS) is responsible for oversight of this regulation. The regulation "applies to all research involving human subjects conducted, supported or otherwise subject to regulation by any Federal Department or Agency . . ." (Title 45, 1991, p. 3). Nearly every public or private health care facility and educational institution is in someway federally regulated, and therefore any studies involving human subjects conducted by members of the organization must comply with the regulation. The first step in the process is to determine if a study actually qualifies as research.

Is it Research?

Health care facilities and academic institutions collect and manage a great deal of data about members of their organizations, job applicants, clients, customers, and vendors. For example, in order to maintain accreditation, hospitals must complete regular assessments of patient satisfaction, employee skills, and quality control efforts. Academic institutions conduct evaluations of programs, using data about student outcomes and preferences, to determine if programs are viable. When data about individuals are collected and analyzed solely for the purposes of assessing the internal functions of an organization, as in the case of program evaluation and quality assurance studies, the activities do not qualify as research involving human subjects. Title 45 Part 46 (1991) defines research as "a systematic investigation, including research development, testing and evaluation, designed to develop or contribute to generalizable knowledge" (p. 6). To determine if your activities qualify as research, ask yourself if you intend to collect information about individuals that can be used by others to further understanding about a problem or phenomenon that extends beyond the boundaries of your organization. If you answer yes, then most likely your activities qualify as research.

The Institutional Review Board

Title 45 Part 46 (1991) requires that any facility or institution covered by this policy provide written assurance to the DHHS that it will comply with the regulations and that it will establish an Institutional Review Board (IRB) with at least 5 members to oversee all research conducted at the facility. The IRB is also responsible for making determinations about whether a study, such as an employee satisfaction survey, does not qualify as research and can be exempt from further IRB review. Persons planning to conduct a research study involving human subjects must complete and submit a proposal to the IRB and wait for its approval before collecting any data. The proposal asks researchers to describe in detail the methods they plan to use to recruit and select subjects, collect data, manage data after it has been collected, and report results. Studies in which participants are at minimal risk, such as quantitative studies using questionnaires or surveys and qualitative studies using interviews and observations, usually receive an expedited review by 1 or 2 members of the IRB. Studies in which participants may be at risk of physical or psychological injury, such as those where blood samples are taken or where individuals receive medication, are required to have a full review involving all members of the IRB. If a proposal is deemed exempt by the IRB, the researchers can proceed with the study without any further review. Proposals for studies that receive an expedited or full review need to be reviewed by the IRB annually or anytime any major changes are made to the study methods.

Recruiting Subjects

In both expedited and full reviews, the IRB is most concerned with how participants will be treated throughout the entire research study, from the recruitment phase all the way to reporting results and storage of data after completion of the study. First, the recruitment strategies must not coerce, threaten, or discriminate against potential participants in any way. Privacy rights must not be violated in the process of obtaining names or information about individuals. Potential participants must receive information about why they are being asked to participate in a study and what their involvement will entail.

Individuals who choose not to volunteer for a study must not be penalized or have services to which they are entitled withheld.

Informed Consent

After an individual indicates an initial interest in participating in a study, he or she must give informed consent to become a subject. If a study is low risk and the data can never be linked to particular subjects (as in the case of an anonymous survey), individuals can give their consent to participate orally after reviewing an information sheet about the study. If a study is designed such that researchers can link specific data to a specific subject, as is the case with most clinical and qualitative studies, subjects must give their informed consent in writing by signing an informed consent form. In either circumstance, information about the study must be provided in language understandable to the subject and include the following basic elements of informed consent outlined in Title 45 Part 46 (1991, pp. 13-15):

- An explanation of the purpose of the research and the expected duration of a subject's participation.
- A description of the procedures and any foreseeable risks or benefits to the subject.
- Disclosure of any alternative procedures or courses of treatment that may be available to the subject.
- An explanation of the extent to which confidentiality of information about the subject will be maintained.
- Information about whom the subject can contact for answers to questions about his or her rights as a human subject.
- A statement that participation is voluntary and that the subject may withdraw from the study at any time without penalty.

Confidentiality and Anonymity

Sometimes, researchers collect data from participants in a study and never know the identity of the participant who is the source of a particular piece of data. In studies of this sort, the data are said to be anonymous. Examples include studies in which a participant fills out a questionnaire without putting his or her name on it or where researchers use a pre-established database as the source of their data such as the U.S. Census.

In studies where researchers know the identity of participants and any piece of data can be linked to the individual it represents, the identity of all participants must be kept confidential. This means that researchers must not disclose the fact that a particular individual participated in a study or report the data and results in ways that could enable linking the information to a specific subject. In quantitative studies, researchers commonly replace participant names with subject code numbers and report the data in aggregate, presenting the average profile of a group and not the profile of specific individuals in the group. In qualitative studies, where researchers often report exact comments made by individual participants, they replace the participant names with pseudonyms to maintain subject confidentiality.

Ethics in Research

Being an ethical researcher is quite similar to being an ethical health care provider and professional. Maintaining subject confidentiality is not that different from maintaining client or patient confidentiality. Like clients who entrust their care to you, subjects in a study consent to participate with the understanding that you will treat them with respect, do them no harm (physically or psychologically), keep your word, and protect their safety. The *Code of Ethics* (AOTA, 2000) is a resource for dealing with ethical dilemmas during the course of your professional activities. The *Code of Ethics* can be supplemented with *The Belmont Report: Ethical Principles and Guidelines for the Protection of Human Subjects in Research* produced by U.S. Department of Health, Education, and Welfare (1979) for additional guidance on identifying and managing ethical issues while conducting research.

SUMMARY

OTs and OTAs can use research as a means to better understand problems in practice and education and to identify meaningful and effective ways to alleviate them. Theoretical research can serve as the foundation for empirical studies of new ideas and techniques, and the outcomes of empirical studies can provide the fuel for expanding theory. Quantitative and qualitative approaches to applied empirical research are commonly employed in the field of OT. The outcomes of well-executed, experimental quantitative studies provide much of the basis for EBP. Nonexperimental qualitative studies also play an important role in the profession by uncovering the unique perceptions, needs, and experiences of persons with whom we work. Regardless of the approach used to conduct a study, when human subjects are involved, their rights must be protected. This chapter provides a starting point for exploring the possibilities of research and integrating it into your educational and professional work.

LEARNING ACTIVITIES

1. In small groups, design a research study involving an occupation or issue of importance to college students.

2. Invite the librarian to class to talk about resources available to OT students at your school.

3. Design surveys that you think are clear and then get feedback from different groups of people to confirm or repute the clarity of the survey.

4. Investigate what clinical practitioners want in research and what projects they may be participating in. Ask about quality assurance projects at their site.

5. Survey OT practitioners about their fears in doing research.

REFERENCES

American Occupational Therapy Association. (2000). OT Code of Ethics 2000 (online). Retrieved January 25, 2005, from http://www.aota.org/members/ area2/links/LINK03.asp

Fraenkel, J. R., & Wallen, N. E. (2000). *How to design and evaluate research in education* (4th ed.). Boston: McGraw-Hill.

Holm, M. B. (2001). Our mandate for the new millennium: Evidence-based practice, 2000 Eleanor Clarke Slagle lecture. *American Journal of Occupational Therapy, 54,* 574-585.

Johnson, A. P. (2002). *A short guide to action research.* Boston: Allyn & Bacon.

Leary, C. A. (2001). Human development. In K. Sladyk & S. E. Ryan (Eds.), *Ryan's occupational therapy assistant: Principles, practice issues, and techniques* (3rd ed., pp. 39-44). Thorofare, NJ: SLACK Incorporated.

Marshall, C., & Rossman, G. B. (1999) *Designing qualitative research* (3rd ed.). Thousand Oaks, CA: Sage.

Portney, L. G., & Watkins, M. P. (1993). *Foundations of clinical research: Applications to practice.* Norwalk, CT: Appleton & Lange.

Royeen, C. B. (1997). *A research primer in occupational and physical therapy.* Bethesda, MD: American Occupational Therapy Association.

Sladyk, K. (2003). Research. In K. Sladyk (Ed.), *OT study cards in a box* (2nd ed., pp. 12-1-12-32). Thorofare, NJ: SLACK Incorporated.

Strauss, A., & Corbin, J. (1998). *Basics of qualitative research* (2nd ed.). Thousand Oaks, CA: Sage.

Title 45 Code of Federal Regulations, Public Welfare: Part 46 Protection of Human Subjects, 56 Fed. Reg. 28003 (June 18, 1991). Retrieved January 25, 2005, from http://ohrp.osophs.dhhs.gov/humansubjects/guidance /45cfr45.htm

Trochim, W. M. K. (2001). *The research methods knowledge base* (2nd ed.). Cincinnati: Atomic Dog Publishing.

U.S. Department of Health, Education, and Welfare. (1979). The Belmont Report: Ethical principles and guidelines for the protection of human subjects in research. Retrieved January 25, 2005, from http://ohrp.osophs.dhhs.gov/humansubjects/guidance/Belmont.htm.

Key Concepts

- Confidentiality: A person's information is protected and not disclosed without permission.
- Documentation: A legally binding, written form of communication among health care providers and payers.
- Medicare: A government health care insurance program for people over 65 and those with disabilities. The largest reimbursement system for OT services.

Essential Vocabulary

assessment: Specific tools and measures used in evaluation.

discharge process: Planning begins at admission to improve quality treatment.

progress note: A legal document that reports treatment progress or lack of progress for a client.

SOAP note: A method to structure a progress note.

third-party payer: An insurance or contract program responsible for paying for OT services.

treatment plan: A legal document that outlines the plan of treatment for a client.

DOCUMENTATION

Karen Sladyk, PhD, OTR, FAOTA

Ask any OTA or OT what they dislike the most about their job and they may tell you the documentation. Although often talked about in a negative manner, documentation is one of the most important skills an OTA can develop. Documentation is the means by which we communicate our treatment to other health professionals and third-party payers. In addition, documentation is often used to demonstrate quality care of our consumers. Needless to say, documentation is an important aspect of our practice. It is important that OTAs develop documentation skills early and continue to refine the skills throughout their careers. This chapter will address both the basic treatment plan and treatment notes.

AMERICAN OCCUPATIONAL THERAPY ASSOCIATION OFFICIAL DOCUMENTS THAT SUPPORT THE DOCUMENTATION PROCESS

The AOTA provides several documents that help OT practitioners succeed in documentation including:

- *Occupational Therapy Practice Framework: Domain and Process* (AOTA, 2002)
- *Guidelines for Documentation of Occupational Therapy* (AOTA, 2003)
- *Standards of Practice for Occupational Therapy* (AOTA, 1998)
- *Occupational Therapy Code of Ethics* (AOTA, 2000).

Being a member of AOTA provides excellent services for addressing your documentation questions, especially in the always-changing rules of Medicare reimbursement. AOTA counts on members to document the effectiveness of OT services so AOTA can affect national policy (Metzler, 2004) and advocate for further funding on Capitol Hill. In turn, AOTA notifies members of reimbursement changes through its Web site, publications, and conferences.

ROLE OF THE *OCCUPATIONAL THERAPY PRACTICE FRAMEWORK* IN DOCUMENTATION

The *Practice Framework* (AOTA, 2002) is covered in detail in Chapter 5; however, it is reviewed as it relates to documentation here. The *Practice Framework* can be helpful in structuring a documentation system as it was designed to provide language to the practice of OT. Especially useful are the areas of occupational performance (ADL, education, work, leisure) in guiding assessment and intervention and therefore documentation. In addition, the *Practice Framework* uses language more common in international health care and is not limited to the language of a medical model. Skills required to be successful (motor, cognitive, social) in the performance of occupation are not strictly defined in the document but can be used in documentation of patient's progress when describing occupational performance.

CONFIDENTIALITY

No discussion of documentation would be complete without first addressing the importance of client confidentiality. The *Occupational Therapy Code of Ethics* (AOTA, 2000), standard three, protects information about a client from being shared with anyone outside the treatment team. In addition, HIPAA regulations (Health and Human Services, 2004) provide legal ramifications if patient confidentiality is broken. This includes bringing notes home that identify the patient, talking about a resident in the elevator, or sharing interesting stories with identifying information with family and friends. An OTA must work hard to make sure patient confidentiality is protected at all times.

Table 40-1

Steps to Writing a Treatment Plan

- Develop a list of problems and behavioral indicators, consider a frame of reference.
- Identify assets and prioritize the problem list.
- Develop goals and objectives that are clear and measurable.
- Design activities that are meaningful to the person.
- Identify expected outcomes and discharge criteria.

COMPONENTS OF DOCUMENTATION

Documentation benefits the patient, reimbursement agencies, treatment providers, and the profession (Lloyd, 2004). Documentation provides a written history to evaluation, intervention, and outcomes of treatment (AOTA, 2002). Documentation components include:

- Client information
- Occupational profile
- Assessments used and the results
- Treatment plan with goals and objectives
- Progress reports
- Discharge planning
- Transition plan to other service settings
- Outcome or discontinuation reports (Acquaviva, 1998; AOTA, 2003)

Effective documentation (Lloyd, 2004) is clear and concise while explaining the need for skilled intervention. In addition, the documentation explains the practitioner's clinical reasoning but avoids jargon or theory unfamiliar to other health care providers. As documentation is legally binding, practitioners must note changes in client functioning and interpretation of data. Outcomes must be measurable and functional (Lloyd, 2004).

MEDICARE

Medicare is the largest funding source for OT services and has special rules and policies in place to maximize client recovery while maintaining low costs (Lemke, 2004). While the OTA will not likely deal directly with Medicare, it is important to understand how the reimbursement system works.

Medicare is a health care insurance program funded by the government of the United States for people over age 65 and those with disabilities. The Centers for Medicare and Medicaid Services (CMS) is the governmental agency that oversees the program and interprets the laws developed by Congress. The government does not reimburse facilities or providers directly but uses carriers or fiscal intermediaries to oversee the billing process.

Medicare uses a coding system (CPT) to bill, and only approved codes are reimbursed. Funding is typically related to the patient's Rehabilitation Utilization Group (RUG) based on the data or assessment results of the Minimum Data Set (MDS). Patients require physician certification that services are medically necessary with reason for intervention and time required. Documentation of client progress and the facility's compliance to all policies is necessary for avoiding Medicare denials of reimbursement (Lemke, 2004).

OTHER FUNDING SOURCES

While Medicare is the largest provider of reimbursement of OT services, many more third-party payers are available to OT consumers including private health care insurance, CHAMPUS for uniformed services, workers' compensation, IDEA for disabled students, Section 504 of the rehabilitation act, state agencies, grant programs, and private pay (Thomas, 1998). Each program requires its own documentation system. For example, a public school student receiving OT services will require an IEP, while an adult returning to work after an injury and using a grant for adapting his car will require different documentation. Some agencies funded by state agencies, such as a clubhouse program for people with schizophrenia, may require only minimal client documentation but focus on client successes in the community. Inpatient hospitalization programs generally have traditional documentation of assessment, intervention, and discharge planning. The fundamentals of documentation are addressed in the next sections.

TREATMENT PLAN

A treatment plan is likely to be the first formal piece of documentation an OTA is likely to write. Both the OTA and OT participate in the treatment evaluation and the resulting treatment plan but the OT is ultimately responsible for the treatment plan. After the evaluations have been completed, a comprehensive treatment plan must be documented.

Each facility has established its own method for documenting a treatment plan. Some facilities have developed critical pathways that dictate the treatment plan, reducing the documentation needs. Generally, a treatment plan includes problems, assets, goals/objectives, treatments, and outcomes/discharge criteria (Table 40-1).

Table 40-2

Linking Problems to Behaviors

Problem	Behavioral Indicator
Poor personal grooming	Does not shave or shower
Poor coping skills	Does not get out of bed until 10:30, cries
Provider role in family disrupted	Wants to work, feels embarrassed
Lack of enjoyment	Feels sad, does not like fishing, isolates self

---

Step One—Developing a Problem List and Behavioral Indicators

The first step in writing an OT treatment plan is to establish a list of problems the patient is facing and show behavioral evidence that these are problems. To do this, the OTA should review the *Practice Framework* (AOTA, 2002) and make a written list of potential problems. Consider the following case story:

Jim is a 40-year-old male who has recently lost his management job due to downsizing of his workplace. Initially, he was happy to be laid off because he had the opportunity to look for a job he "really wanted" and catch up on reading. Lately, he has been disappointed because job offers are not coming in like he thought. His unemployment support will be ending soon (6 weeks) and Jim has become depressed. He does not get out of bed until 10:30 am and has not been showering or shaving. His wife has found him crying in his home office with the lights off. His wife further reports that he sits around all day doing nothing and does not even enjoy his hobby of fishing with his teenage son. Jim reports he is upset that he can no longer support his family and only wishes for a job. He says he is not suicidal but states he is an embarrassment to his family. His wife and son deny he is an embarrassment and have been very supportive of his job search.

Jim is having problems in work, ADL, and leisure (Table 40-2).

Step Two—Prioritizing the List With Patient Assets

As with many patients, the OT and OTA are likely to identify more problems than can be realistically addressed during treatment. Therefore, the therapist must set a priority list of problems to be addressed. To do this, identifying patient assets helps to prioritize treatment problems. In the case of Jim, he has several assets to draw on including:

- He has a good work history with management skills.
- He has a supportive wife and son.
- He has a history of good ADL and leisure skills.
- Although ending soon, he currently has unemployment support.

In developing a priority list of treatment problems for any patient, the issue of safety is always placed first. In this case, Jim is not suicidal and safety is not an issue. Looking at his problem list, the following prioritization might be successful:

- Poor coping skills
- Family role disturbance
- Lack of enjoyment
- Poor grooming

Poor coping skills is placed first because of its impact in all areas of work, ADL, and leisure. Poor grooming is placed last because it is impacted by the other problems, and Jim has a history of being successful in grooming prior to his recent depression. Looking at his list of assets also supports this priority list in that Jim appears to have support but is not utilizing the support to help him cope.

Step Three—Developing Goals and Objectives

The next step is to develop realistic goals and objectives for Jim to meet prior to his discharge. Considerations in developing goals and objectives include analyzing the type of facility in which the patient is being treated, the expected discharge plans, and the limits of his third-party payer. Most important are the patient's goals. In Jim's case, he is being treated in a day treatment program for professionals. He spends late afternoons and evenings in his home and will return home after his discharge. Jim's third-party payer has agreed to cover 30 days of day treatment and because of the current financial strain, Jim is unable to pay for services beyond the initial 30 days. Jim states that his only goal is to return to work and be the breadwinner of the family.

To guide the development of the goals, objectives, and treatment techniques, the OT must consider a frame of reference. In Jim's case, several frames of reference could be appropriate, including the Model of Human Occupation, cognitive-behavioral, or psychodynamic. Choosing a frame of reference depends on your knowledge of the frames, the frames the facility uses, and the resources of the program. In Jim's case, the facility uses a cognitive-behavioral approach because the program is for professionals with generally high levels of education and the stay is generally limited to 30 days. Several other frames of reference, including occupational performance theories, would be equally successful.

Writing goals and objectives for a treatment plan is a difficult task. Changes in laws and review organizations have lead to the requirement that goals and objectives must be individualized and clearly measurable. Each goal and objective must be so clear that any professional reviewing the record would have an understanding of what is expected of the patient. Several methods have been developed to teach students how to write measurable goals. All these methods lead to successful goal writing. It is not unusual to have different OT faculty teach you different methods.

The goals and objectives are written in the same way but the goal is the end product of several objectives. Think of goals and objectives as a staircase. The goal is written on the top step. Several objectives will lead to the final goal. Objectives may need to be adjusted as the patient moves through treatment but the ultimate goal is the patient's highest functioning. Consider the following steps toward living a healthy lifestyle:

- Goal: Eat healthy and exercise daily
  - ○ Obj #1 Talk to others who eat healthy and exercise daily
  - ○ Obj 2# Plan 1 healthy meal, call local health club
  - ○ Obj #3 Eat 1 healthy meal, walk 15 minutes daily
  - ○ Obj #4 Eat 2 healthy meals, exercise 20 minutes daily

In this chapter, we will use the ABCD method for writing goals and objectives. The ABCD method uses the following system for developing clear, measurable goals and objectives:

- Audience
- Behavior
- Condition
- Degree

The audience of the goal is the patient. The behavior is what is expected of the patient. The condition is the specific details, rules, or bounties of the behavior. Lastly, the degree is when the behavior is completed. Each problem on the treatment plan must have a goal and set of objectives. So in Jim's case (four problems), four sets of goals and matching objectives would be developed by the OT and OTA in the final treatment plan. First, consider the following goal for the problem of coping skills:

Within 30 days, Jim will verbally list 3 coping strategies for dealing with his depression using 1 strategy each day for the last 10 days.

Audience	Jim
Behavior	Verbally list 3 coping strategies
Condition	Use 1 strategy for the last 10 days
Degree	Within 30 days

An appropriate first step to reaching this goal would be an objective that has Jim finding out what coping skills are. Consider the following objective: Within 7 days, Jim will attend 3 coping skills groups, making a list of coping skills in a journal.

Audience	Jim
Behavior	Attend 3 coping skills group
Condition	List skills in journal
Degree	Within 7 days

Step Four—Designing Activities

OT uses activities to improve function in their patients. The next step in the treatment plan is to design specific activities to meet the individual goals and objectives of the patient. One

problem that students often have when developing a treatment plan is to jump right into the treatment before laying the groundwork. When this happens, the results are an activity that the therapist wants to do, not an activity that has meaning or function to the patient.

Before developing activities for your patient, review the individual problems, assets, goals, and objectives. Ask yourself, "Will this be meaningful to my patient?" Return to the case story of Jim. His first problem involves coping skills, and goal is for him to identify and use coping skills. His family is trying to be supportive but at this time Jim is not using them for support. He is trying to carry the burden of unemployment himself. Jim has been referred to a coping skills group where other people are dealing with the same issues. The nature of a group means that some of the members are dealing with coping better than Jim and some are not. OT practitioners can use these different levels to be therapeutic. For example, Jim's first objective is to identify coping skills. The therapist could simply read a list of coping skills to the group members but this would not be meaningful to Jim. Instead, the therapist asks Jim to develop a survey of coping skills and to survey both patients and staff on the use of coping skills. This allows Jim to use his management skills. After the survey is done, Jim begins to develop a journal where he can keep the results. Because Jim enjoyed reading, he may be interested in journaling. Even if he does not keep journaling after his discharge, he may find the written record of his survey helpful later.

Step Five—Outcomes/Discharge Planning

The last step in developing and documenting a treatment plan is to set the criteria that the patient will need to be discharged and return to life outside of your program. This may be a difficult step for a novice OTA. Many ask, "How can I predict how my patient will look at discharge if I don't even know him or her yet?" With experience, this task will become easier. The reality is that discharge planning should start the moment the patient is admitted. This allows for effective and efficient treatment to be started from the beginning. Discharge planning can always be adjusted along the way but having an outcome vision from the beginning will allow the treatment to be focused from the start.

In Jim's case, the discharge plan was clear from the beginning. He would return home after the 30 days of day treatment. Community outpatient visits once a week or unemployment self-help groups might be appropriate referrals and are likely to be investigated by a social worker on the team with input from OT. The treatment team feels that Jim's outcome criteria, including his ability to maintain his ADL independently, returning enjoyment of his leisure hobbies, and ability to return to actively seeking employment, are attainable in 30 days. Besides OT and social work mentioned above, Jim has access to a medical doctor for medication, a clinical psychologist for insight therapy, a therapeutic recreation specialist for practicing his hobbies, and a nurse for medication education and case management. Together, the treatment team develops the outcome criteria and discharge plans using input from all team members including OT.

Date _____

S: "I feel relief that I'm here in this coping skills group. I did not know there were other people that felt the same way I did."

O: Jim attended 3 coping skills groups this week and was seen for 2 individual sessions of 45 minutes each.

A: Jim was initially hesitant to join the coping skills group and needed an individual session to be convinced to try the group. He was encouraged to talk to his case manager about the group and agreed to try it once. Once in group, he became relaxed and began to actively participate. He was asked to develop a survey on coping skills used by others and is in the process of collecting his data. Jim has made friends in the group and has been seen socializing with them outside of group time. Although his affect remains depressed, he was seen smiling when talking about his projects. No evidence of suicidal ideation or psychomotor retardation was noted. First week objective was partially met.

P: Jim will continue to gather his data for his surveys. He will report the results to the group and document the results in his journal.

Karen Sladyk, OTR/L

Figure 40-1. Example of a SOAP note after the first week of treatment.

Summary

This chapter has provided an outline for writing a basic OT treatment plan. Multidisciplinary treatment plans are routine in practice with OT contributing a part. Before you can write a multidisciplinary treatment plan, you must master a basic OT plan. The steps include identifying problems, identifying assets, prioritizing problems, setting goals and objectives, developing treatment activities, and setting outcome criteria and discharge plans. Several case stories will follow the end of this chapter to practice writing a treatment plan. The following section will address documentation after the initial treatment plan.

PROGRESS NOTE WRITING

After writing a treatment plan, the OT practitioner begins treatment and must document progress or lack of progress in the facility record. Just like treatment plans, each facility has developed policies on note writing that meets the needs of laws and review organizations. There are many different types or styles of note writing. In this section of the chapter, you will learn the basics of a SOAP note and a narrative note.

SOAP Note

The SOAP format is well established in the medical field but less used in community or educational systems. SOAP is an acronym for:

Subjective, Objective, Assessment, Plan

The benefit of a SOAP note is that it provides a structure that all disciplines can use and understand. This consistency between disciplines allows for a quick review of the record for trends and patterns in patient behavior or treatment progress.

The note begins with a subjective statement from the patient that is interesting because it reflects current functioning as seen by the patient. The objective data follow. This includes how many times the patient was seen, what type of activities were done, and any other specific, measurable data. The assessment section includes the writer's interpretation of data and assessment of goals or objectives. Lastly, the plan section includes the next step for the patient (Borcherding & Kappel, 2002).

Returning to the case story of Jim, a SOAP note after the first week of treatment might look like the example in Figure 40-1.

Narrative Note

A narrative note allows for more flexibility than the SOAP note but does not have the structure that some practitioners like. In a narrative note, the writer is responsible for including all the data in a smooth, flowing, descriptive note. Generally, the writer begins with objective information such as attendance and participation in treatment, then follows with interpretive information such as patient reaction. Finally, a review of objectives met and plans for the next treatment sessions are included. The SOAP format can be easily converted to a narrative format by switching the subjective and objective sections and leaving out the headings. A narrative note for Jim might look the example in Figure 40-2.

DOCUMENTING PROGRESS

The first step in writing any type of note is to gather the appropriate data. Be sure you have dates of attendance, information about participation, whether objectives were met, and future plans. The best way to get good at writing notes is to write a lot and to get feedback on your notes. Generally, this will happen during fieldwork. In-class assignments might also include note writing. Like writing objectives, teachers teach note writing in many different ways. Although this may be frustrating as you try to master one style of note writing, remember that learning many different styles will improve the flexibility of your thinking.

Sometimes the best way to see how to write a note is to look at how not to write a note. The narrative note in Figure 40-3 is full of problems.

Let us review the many errors in this note. First, grammar and spelling are serious issues. It is assumed that college educated people will have notes free of grammar and spelling errors. Before you pass in a note, check for grammar and spelling errors. An occasional error is part of being human but ask yourself, "What am I saying about my clinical thinking when I enter this note in the record?" Remember, all your written work is a reflec-

Date _____

Jim attended 3 coping skills groups this week and was seen for 2 individual sessions of 45 minutes each. He stated, "I feel relief that I'm here in this coping skills group. I did not know there were other people that felt the same way I did."

Jim was initially hesitant to join the coping skills group and needed an individual session to be convinced to try the group. He was encouraged to talk to his case manager about the group and agreed to try it once. Once in group, he became relaxed and began to actively participate. He was asked to develop a survey on coping skills used by others and is in the process of collecting his data. Jim has made friends in the group and has been seen socializing with them outside of group time. Although his affect remains depressed, he was seen smiling when talking about his projects. No evidence of suicidal ideation or psychomotor retardation was noted. First week objective was partially met.

The plan will have Jim continue to gather his data for his surveys, report the results to the group, and document the results in his journal.

Karen Sladyk, OTR/L

Figure 40-2. Example of a narrative note.

Date: _____

Jim came to group all the time this week. He made a survey, a journal, a college, a junk sculpture, and a god's eye for his wife. He didn't want to come to group at the start and had to be talked to and then saw his case manager and then came. He said he didn't want to do this stuff and wouldn't get anything out of it and didn't see the point anyway. When he came he was very depressed but did smile some. The plan is to encourage Jim to attend and to have Jim make an ashetray and a leather key chane.

I. M. Wayoff, OTR/L

Figure 40-3. Example of a narrative note full of problems.

tion of you. Project the image of a hardworking, competent OTA (Borcherding & Kappel, 2002; Sladyk, 1997).

One other major problem in this note is the endless list of tasks the patient completed. As you likely know, the profession of OT is not widely known or understood by many people, including other health professionals. When a note focuses on the things a patient made instead of how he or she responded to treatment, it appears that the OT department is nothing more than people who keep patients busy all day. As an OT practitioner, it is your responsibility to help other professionals understand how activity improves function. The focus of a note should be on function, not on what the patient made (Borcherding & Kappel, 2002; Sladyk, 1997). See Table 40-3 for other helpful hints for treatment plan writing, note writing, and general college assignment writing.

Summary

Note writing can be a simple task after you have mastered the basic format and the specific facility rules. Use the treatment plan as a starting place to write a progress note. Comment on both subjective and objective data. Interpret the data and make a plan for the future. Make sure your notes are free of grammar and spelling errors. Follow the helpful hints in Table 40-3 for problem-free progress notes.

SKILL APPLICATION

The best way to master treatment plan writing and progress note writing is to practice. Use the following case stories to practice writing a basic OT treatment plan and progress note. For a more realistic case story, use a patient that you have observed in fieldwork or a more detailed case story provided to you by your teacher.

1. The worksheet outline in Figure 40-4 can be helpful in organizing an assignment for OT school. Use the *Practice Framework* (AOTA, 2002) when identifying problems.

Kathy Smith—Depression

Kathy Smith is a 44-year-old female who began to suffer from major depression 3 weeks ago on the anniversary of her best friend's accidental death. She lives in a 2-story house with her husband and 15-year-old son. She is currently on a medical leave from her job as a deli clerk at a local supermarket. Although Mrs. Smith worked outside the home, she felt it was important to see her son off to school each morning and was home just after her son returned from school. Prior to her depression, Mrs. Smith led an active social life. She and her husband played tennis with other couples and she enjoyed going out for coffee and chatting with girlfriends.

Table 40-3

Helpful Hints

- Check all data for correctness: Make sure everything from the date to the treatment results are accurately reported.
- Be spelling error free: Spelling errors project an image of an uneducated professional. Carry a dictionary with you at all times. If unsure of a spelling, consider a different word.
- Use professional language: Avoid street terms. "We had to stop her from talking" becomes "Patient was tangential and required maximum limit setting."
- Tell how the patient functioned: Avoid endless lists of projects the patient made.
- The PLAN must be the patient's: Many practitioners make the mistake of writing what they plan to do in the plan section of a note. The plan must be the patient's not the therapist's. No good: "The therapist will increase ROM 10 degrees." Instead use: "Patient will gain 10 degrees ROM."
- Stay in one tense: Do not jump tense such as: is, was, are, and were. Past tense is preferred.
- Write in the third person: Do not use I. Call yourself the OT or OTA.
- No contractions: No didn't, shouldn't, wouldn't. In college level professional work, write out both words.
- No run on sentences: A sentence should have only one "and," with no more than 2 thoughts. If you have more than 2 thoughts, make a new sentence.
- No vague words: No very, a lot, some, many. These words have different meanings to different people. Tell exactly how much and do not use these words at all.
- Do not blacken out a mistake: If you make an error, put one line through the error and write "error" next to it. Black marks look like you are trying to hide something.
- Do not use white-out on a mistake: If you make an error, put one line through the error and write "error" next to it. White-out looks like you are trying to hide something.
- Never use another patient's name in a record: This breaks confidentially rules. Some facilities will allow you to use initials but check before you write.
- Sign the note legibly: Review organizations will cite you if they cannot read your signature.

Mrs. Smith was hospitalized for 15 days for depression at a local hospital and received OT services twice daily during her stay. Since her discharge from the hospital, she has been living at home with her husband and son. Mrs. Smith has been receiving therapy services at a local outpatient mental health center where you are a student. During the day, Mrs. Smith has her sister with her until it is time for therapy; however, her sister is from out of state and will be returning home in 2 weeks. Mrs. Smith's OT is your fieldwork supervisor and you have been assigned to her treatment.

Current status:
- Chief complaint: "I have no energy to do anything"
- Motor activity: Slow and lethargic, ambulatory.
- Speech: Slow, low volume, no hearing impairment.
- Mood and affect: Mood is sad, affect is sometimes sad, sometimes flat, or sometimes agitated. Endurance for activity depends on other therapy scheduled.
- Thought: Content of thought is around friend's death and what death was like for friend. Denies suicidal thoughts or plans. Is easily distracted from conversations or tasks and is easily confused in situations outside of her home.
- Perception: During in-patient hospitalization, she did hear her friend's voice calling to her, however this stopped with medication and she is not experiencing this currently.
- Appearance: Neat and clean.

- Intellectual functioning:
  - Orientation: Oriented x3, however, slow and needs time to process questions.
  - Fund of knowledge: Bright woman with 2 years of college.
  - Abstract: Can abstract if given time, however, needs to be refocused to thought.
- ADL: Sister sets everything out and helps her get ready for her appointments. Appetite is poor.
- Insight and judgment: Aware of her depression and has expressed an interest in getting well,; however, has had a difficult time making changes in her behavior.

The recreational therapist has just brought Mrs. Smith into your waiting area after her recreation therapy evaluation. The therapist tells you to look out because "Kathy is a little cranky today." You greet Mrs. Smith and begin to explain what you were thinking about working on in treatment. Mrs. Smith looks at you and says "whatever" in a monotone voice.

Bill Jones—Cerebrovascular Accident

Bill Jones is a 44-year-old male who suffered a CVA 4 weeks ago. He lives in a 2-story house with his wife and 16-year-old daughter. He is currently on a medical leave from his job as a department store manager. Although his job requires him to work long hours, Mr. Jones is a devoted father and makes breakfast for

---

Treatment Plan Practice Worksheet

Treatment Problems, Behavioral Indicators, Possible Frame of Reference:
   What are the problems and what evidence do you have to indicate these are problems?

Assets:

Prioritized Problems:
   Safety is always considered first.

Goals and Objectives:
   Audience, Behavior, Condition, Degree

Treatment Activities:
   Separate groups from individual activities

Outcomes/Discharge Plans:

Figure 40-4. Treatment plan practice worksheet.

his daughter each morning before she goes to school. Prior to his CVA, Mr. Jones led an active social life. He and his wife bowl and play tennis with other couples and he enjoyed drinking coffee while ice fishing with his "guy friends."

Mr. Jones was hospitalized for 15 days at a local hospital following his CVA and he received OT services twice daily during his stay. Since his discharge from the hospital, he has been living at home with his wife and daughter. His wife works full time to maintain the family's health insurance. Mr. Jones has been receiving therapy services at a local out-patient rehabilitation center where you are a student. During the day, Mr. Jones has a home health aide with him until it is time for therapy; however, he is only eligible for a home health aide for 6 more weeks. Mr. Jones's OT is your fieldwork supervisor and you have been assigned to his treatment.

Current status:

- ROM: Right is normal for AROM

    Left is normal for PROM
- Strength: Right is normal

    Left is flaccid; however, last MMT treatment showed trace movement
- Endurance: Fluctuates between 20 to 35 minutes depending on PT/OT schedule
- Sensation:
  - Proprioception: Right is normal. Left is impaired. However, left has improved since beginning outpatient therapy.
  - Hot/cold: Both left and right are normal.
  - Localization of tactile stimuli: Right is normal. Left is diminished on both anterior and posterior sides as well as diminished on left side of face.
  - Perception: Displays hemianopsia and constructional apraxia, normal receptive understanding.
  - Gross and fine motor: Right is normal but unable to assess left UE due to flaccidity. He walks with a quad cane (a stable, 4 legged cane).
- Affect: Sad or flat at times. Progressively becoming less cooperative during treatment. Sad when family visits or when he talks about his daughter.
- Oral functioning: Tends to choke on liquids, especially coffee, mouth drops, mild tongue lateralization from midline to right, he is able to speak.
- Daily living skills: Mild dressing apraxia, aide sets up meals and assists grooming and hygiene.

The physical therapist has just brought Mr. Jones into your waiting area after his PT evaluation. The therapist tells you to look out because "Bill is a little cranky today." You greet Mr. Jones and begin to explain what you were thinking about working on in treatment. Mr. Jones looks at you and says "whatever" in a monotone voice.

2. Note Writing Case Stories: The people in the case stories presented in the treatment planning section of this chapter have now completed 1 week of treatment under your care. Use the following information to write a SOAP progress note and a narrative progress note. Check the

first week information against what you know in the treatment plan. Include the date and sign the note with your name and credentials.

Kathy Smith—First Week of Treatment

Data collected:

Attendance: Three socialization groups, 5 relaxation groups, 2 evening family groups, and was seen for 5 short (15 min) individual sessions.

Affect: Varied between depressed (tearful) to sad but appropriate to the discussion. Expressed embarrassment to not being able to control crying during family group.

Attention to task: Fine with some verbal redirecting. In relaxation she said, "I really like these exercises because I can remember the good times with my friend without crying."

Motor activity and speech: Improved but still slow.

ADL: No changes in home life.

Bill Jones—First Week of Treatment

Data collected:

Attendance: One hour of individual OT treatment daily and 4 self range of motion groups.

Perception: Continues to display hemianopsia and constructional apraxia, normal receptive understanding.

Gross and fine motor: Right is normal. Left UE showing beginnings of tone. He walks with a quad cane (a stable, 4-legged cane).

Affect: Sad or flat at times. Progressively becoming less cooperative during treatment. Started to cry when he talks about his daughter. Counseling techniques were used and patient reported relief.

ADL: Choked on liquids when he rushed but was able to drink 2 oz of coffee. Stated he "was very proud and that was the best coffee he ever had."

---

3. Evaluate your note.

[ ] Data accurate
[ ] Spelling correct
[ ] Grammar correct
[ ] Used professional language
[ ] Focus on functioning
[ ] No contractions
[ ] Written in past tense
[ ] No run on sentences
[ ] No vague words
[ ] Plan is patient focused
[ ] No blackened words or white-out
[ ] Signed legibly

Web sites useful for documentation information concerning Medicare and HIPAA:

www.hhs.gov/ocr/hipaa for HIPPA information

http://cms.hhs.gov.medlearn/default.asp for Medicare information

www.cms.hhs.gov/forms for Medicare forms

The documentation samples of this chapter were previously published in Sladyk (1997).

LEARNING ACTIVITIES

1. Watch a TV show that has characters that might have disabilities. For example: on "Frasier," Miles is extremely anxious or on "Home Improvement," Tim has fine motor planning problems. Document an OT session using SOAP and narrative notes.

2. Write behavioral objectives for students in class. Ask for a volunteer who smokes. Have the class "decide" how she will quit smoking: cut down, cold turkey, or evasion therapy. Have the class write an objective for each week of a 6- to 8-week program.

REFERENCES

Acquaviva, J. D. (1998). *Effective documentation for occupational therapy.* Bethesda, MD: American Occupational Therapy Association.

American Occupational Therapy Association. (1998). Standards of practice for occupational therapy. *American Journal of Occupational Therapy, 52,* 866-869.

American Occupational Therapy Association. (2000). Occupational therapy code of ethics. *American Journal of Occupational Therapy, 54,* 614-616.

American Occupational Therapy Association. (2002). The occupational therapy practice framework: Domain and process. *American Journal of Occupational Therapy, 56,* 609-633.

American Occupational Therapy Association. (2003). Guidelines for documentation of occupational therapy. *American Journal of Occupational Therapy, 57,* 646-649.

Borcherding, S., & Kappel, C. (2002). *The OTA's guide to writing SOAP notes.* Thorofare, NJ: SLACK Incorporated.

United States Department of Health and Human Services. (2004). HIPPA regulations. Retrieved October 12, 2004, from http://www.hhs.gov/ocr/hipaa.

Lemke, L. (2004). Defensive documentation: Managing Medicare denials. *OT Practice, September 6,* 8-12.

Lloyd, L. S. (2004). Documenting for patients and payers. *OT Practice, July 12,* 6.

Metzler, C. A. (2004). Policy and politics in 2004. *OT Practice, March 8,* 7.

Sladyk, K. (1997). *OT student primer: A guide to college success.* Thorofare, NJ: SLACK Incorporated.

Thomas, V. J. (1998). Evolving health care systems: Payment for occupational therapy services. In J. D. Acquaviva (Ed.), *Effective documentation for occupational therapy.* Bethesda, MD: American Occupational Therapy Association.

Key Concepts

- Supervision: Process of providing guidance and direction to others.
- Service competence: Consistently demonstrated skills equivalent to a professional.

Essential Vocabulary

advanced-level practice: OT or OTA with 3 or more years experience and advanced skills in specialty areas.
entry-level practice: OT or OTA with less than 1 year experience.
intermediate-level practice: Competent entry-level skills practitioner with 1 to 3 years experience.

OCCUPATIONAL THERAPY ASSISTANT SUPERVISION

Sally E. Ryan, COTA, ROH, Retired and Karen Sladyk, PhD, OTR, FAOTA

INTRODUCTION

Throughout the history of the OTA, numerous questions have arisen regarding supervision issues. Questions continue about who supervises the OTA, under what circumstances, how frequently, and whether the supervision is close or general. Other questions concern who OTAs may supervise and the circumstances under which supervision may take place, as well as the experience necessary for assistants to provide supervision. This chapter discusses these issues and focuses on specific practice examples as well as guiding principles, patterns, and responsibilities of supervision. Utilization issues and related concerns will also be discussed. The importance of career enhancement opportunities is also emphasized.

Supervision may be defined as the process of providing guidance and direction to employees and others. It involves assuming responsibility for the actions of workers, students, volunteers, and others in carrying out the mission and goals of the unit, the department, or the system within a given organization. It also involves overseeing, managing, and providing leadership. Individuals who assume supervisory roles must possess strong interpersonal, intraprofessional, and management skills. They must exhibit the ability to be role models, mentors, instructors, problem-solvers, arbitrators, and evaluators. Successful supervisors are comfortable in their roles and are often characterized by their supervisees as effective, caring, and involved. They are attuned to individual needs and are committed to helping individuals achieve their full potential, resulting in exemplary delivery of services and high job satisfaction. Moreover, they are effective team builders who have a keen understanding of the many ways that technical and professional staff members provide complementary skills, and they create an environment in which collaboration is valued.

TERMINOLOGY

For the reader to have a good understanding of the many facets of supervision, it is important to know the meaning of the following terms and designations based on the official documents of the AOTA (AOTA, 2004).

- **Entry-level practice:** The OTA or registered OT who has less than 1 year of practice experience; the OTA is competent to deliver OT services, as stated in the AOTA entry-level role delineation, under the direction of an OT. Close supervision is required.

- **Intermediate-level practice:** The OTA or OT who has 1 to 3 years of practice experience and is competent to carry out entry-level tasks. The OTA exhibits skills to carry out a variety of ADL in treatment and may be developing additional, more advanced skills in a special interest area.

- **Advanced-level practice:** The OTA or OT who has 3 or more years of practice experience and has achieved the intermediate level. The OTA has demonstrated advanced level skills that may be clinical, educational, or administrative.

- **Close supervision:** Direct, on-site, daily contact.

- **General supervision:** Frequent, face-to-face meetings at the worksite and regular communication between the OT and the OTA by telephone, written documents, or electronic conference. According to Medicare guidelines, general supervision is initial direction and periodic inspection of the actual activity; however, the supervisor need not always be physically present or on the premises when the assistant is performing services. AOTA recommends that general supervision of the OTA should be used only after service competencies have been demonstrated to the supervising therapist. These authors also emphasize that contact by the OT may be less than daily but should be a minimum of 3 to 5 direct contact hours per week for the full-time OTA. Supervision time is prorated for the part-time OTA.

- **Service competence:** Implies that the OT and OTA can perform the same or equivalent tasks and obtain the same results. This assurance is necessary whenever an OT delegates tasks to an OTA.

- **OT aide:** Designation given to individuals who perform routine tasks in the OT department. Through on-the-job training, they learn skills in transporting patients, setting up treatment activities, maintaining supplies and equipment, and other related activities.

- Volunteer: Unpaid worker who assists with varying tasks in the department such as typing, filing, preparing bulletin boards, serving refreshments, maintaining the library, and shopping for patients (AOTA, 2004).

Guiding Principles and Patterns

The AOTA has suggested supervision guidelines for OTAs (AOTA, 2004). These documents summarize supervision of OTAs in typical practice settings but do not present information about assistants who practice as activities directors, educators, or in other nontraditional roles where they do not provide OT treatment services. The following principles and patterns of supervision were drawn from these sources.

Supervision Levels of Personnel

1. Entry-level OTAs require close supervision from an OT or intermediate- or advanced-level OTA for delivery of patient services. General supervision by an experienced OT or OTA is needed for management and administrative tasks. Entry-level OTAs should not have supervisory responsibilities.
2. Intermediate-level OTAs require general clinical supervision from an intermediate- or advanced-level OT. General supervision from an experienced OT or advanced-level OTA is needed for management and administration.
3. Intermediate-level OTAs may provide administrative supervision and clinical direction to entry-level OTAs and OTA Levels I and II fieldwork students. Intermediate-level OTAs may supervise aides and volunteers.
4. Advanced-level OTAs require general clinical supervision from an intermediate or advanced-level OT; general management supervision is provided by an experienced OT. Advanced-level OTAs provide administrative supervision and clinical direction to entry-level OTAs and OTA levels I and II fieldwork students, as well as supervise aides and volunteers (Schell, 1985).

Service Competency

1. It is the responsibility of the supervisor to establish the supervisee's level of service competency. A variety of methods, such as observation, videotaping, independent test-scoring, and cotreatment can be used.
2. Service competency is more easily established for frequently used procedures. Infrequently used procedures may require closer supervision.
3. It is suggested that the acceptable standard of agreement set by the OT to be met by the supervisees is 3 consecutive agreements before service competency has been established (AOTA, 2004).

Patient Condition

1. Regardless of the patient's condition, the OTA may not independently evaluate or initiate the treatment process prior to the OT's evaluation; however, the OTA may contribute to the evaluation process.
2. More supervision is required for the OTA who is working with a person whose condition is rapidly changing due to the need for frequent evaluation, re-evaluation, and treatment modifications.
3. Treatment techniques that require simultaneous re-evaluation of the treatment response are more appropriately performed by an OT.
4. The OTA requires close supervision in implementing a treatment program for the acutely ill individual due to the complex problems and the degree of change frequently seen.
5. The OTA may carry out treatment with a greater degree of independence for patients who are stable or nonacute, or who have a controlled condition.
6. It is the OTA's responsibility to report all changes in patient performance and any other pertinent facts to the supervising therapist (AOTA, 2004).

Regulations and Standards

1. It is the responsibility of every supervisor and supervisee to know and adhere to the supervisory and related regulations set forth by Medicare, Medicaid, and other third-party payers who provide reimbursement for OT services that the supervisor and supervisee carry out. For example, the Medicare guidelines for OT state that while the skills of a qualified OT are required to evaluate the patient's level of function and develop a plan of treatment, the implementation of the plan may also be carried out by a qualified OTA functioning under the general supervision of the qualified OT.
2. It is the responsibility of every supervisor and supervisee to know and adhere to the supervisory and related regulations set forth by Medicare, the JCAHO, and the CARF when working for institutions that fall under their jurisdiction.
3. It is the responsibility of every supervisor and supervisee providing OT services in a state that has regulatory laws, such as licensure, registration, or certification, to know and adhere to the supervisory and related regulations required by that state.
4. It is the responsibility of every supervisor and supervisee to know and adhere to the *Standards of Practice* (Appendix B) and the *Occupational Therapy Code of Ethics* (Appendix C) established by the AOTA (AOTA, 2004).

Table 41-1

Examples of Supervisor and Supervisee Roles

Supervisor	*Supervisee*
Provide orientation to the facility and program.	Participate in orientation activities.
Assess periodically level of competency.	Participate in competency assessment activities.
Define and assign specific responsibilities.	Carry out responsibilities effectively, seeking clarification if unsure.
Establish criteria for performance evaluation and timelines.	Discuss criteria and establish clear understanding of expectations.
Schedule formal and informal meetings to identify problems, needs, and concerns and to solicit ideas.	Participate regularly in meetings, openly and honestly discussing issues and providing feedback and ideas.
Give feedback relative to areas of future growth and skill.	Seek new knowledge and skills and set professional goals development, providing resources as needed.
Develop and modify job descriptions.	Recommend changes in job description.

General Employment

Because supervision is a collaborative process between the supervisor and the supervisee, it is extremely important for each individual to have a clear understanding of his or her respective responsibilities (Cohn, 1998). Examples of these responsibilities are shown in Table 41-1.

UTILIZATION OF PERSONNEL

Some OTs serving as supervisors are recognizing the need to utilize OTAs more effectively due to increased demand for services, budget constraints, and limited availability of personnel (Brooks, 1982). The term *cost-effective* means producing the best results in relation to dollars spent. In an article on calculating cost-effectiveness of OTAs, Dennis (1988) presents convincing data that supports the cost-effective assumption. Linroth and Boulay (1988) also stress the need for employing more OTAs in terms of increased productivity and cost-containment. Over the past 30 years, concern has been voiced regarding the underutilization of assistants. The pattern of employment seen in many OT departments confirms the problem. Recent changes in Medicare funding have left many OT departments confused about services and billing by OTs and OTAs. Some departments have responded by hiring only OTs, while others have continued to support OTAs. An interesting contrast is seen in the field of engineering, where it is not unusual for one professional engineer to supervise 6 technicians. Despite great strides, the OT profession needs to increase its efforts to provide a better balance of technical and professional personnel in the delivery of patient services.

The Army Medical Specialist Corps provides an example of effective utilization of assistants, as the ratio of OTAs to OTs in the majority of their clinics in the United States is quite high. It is also significant to note that military workloads and levels of productivity are considerably higher than those found in the civilian sector (R. Swift, 1991, personal correspondence). More utilization models and related patterns of supervision such as these are needed to allow the OT to provide more services to more patients.

Care must also be taken to ensure that OTAs are not overutilized. Failure to hire the proper level of personnel for the job requirements and to provide adequate supervision is unacceptable. OT services cannot be provided by an OTA who is not receiving OT supervision and must be discontinued (AOTA, 2004). Evert, in her 1992 Presidential address (Evert, 1993), provides a scenario that typifies the supervisory dilemmas faced by many OTAs when an OT is not available: the OTA must often refuse to treat the patient, even in the face of administrative pressure to do so.

CAREER OPPORTUNITIES

A good supervisor must provide opportunities for challenge, growth, and advancement for supervisees as vehicles for career enhancement. Strickland (1988) describes a career development planning model adopted by a large medical facility for employees in the OT department. Career ladders have been established that provide a variety of options for both OTs and OTAs, including development of adaptive equipment and techniques, professional writing, educational presentations, and development of new programs and projects. Opportunities such as these can be a shared collegial experience among OTs and

OTAs, which enhance day-to-day working relationships and, ultimately, job and career satisfaction.

Supervision Partnership

Supervision is often disliked by many people due to the unknowns that might come up in supervision meetings or negative experiences from the past. Students have likely had supervision from former jobs or faculty in OTA school and may have had mixed results. A common problem is over-interpreting the supervision feedback and personalizing the information, causing hurt feelings between the supervisor and supervisee. Each supervisor has his or her own style. Ideally, the supervisor is open-minded and prepared for the task of guiding the OTA in his or her professional development. Ideally, the supervisee wants feedback to grow professionally by improving procedural, interactive, and conditional skills.

Depending on the needs of the OTA and the department, formal supervision meetings should be set in a regular schedule. A new graduate with a supervising OT in the same immediate treatment area as the new OTA may require less formal supervision than a new graduate working in different areas of a large facility. A new graduate needs daily face-to-face contact with his or her supervisor. In addition, a formal weekly 30- to 60-minute meeting should be arranged. These meetings should be documented by the OT as supervision meetings. These notes may be needed at a later date to show progress in the OTA's professional development. Accreditation agencies such as JCAHO expect supervision to be documented, and cosigning notes is not considered supervision.

The supervisee should come to meetings with a prepared list of questions based on his or her caseload. The supervision meeting should begin with a review of issues from former meetings and an update on those issues. The supervisor should then ask about current issues. Together the supervisor and supervisee should develop a plan of action for dealing with the current issues. A timeline for reporting back on the current issues should be developed. The supervisor should assist the OTA in problem-solving and clinical reasoning. The supervisee should be prepared to actively participate in this process. The supervision process becomes nonproductive when the OTA simply asks, "What should I do?" with a problem, and the supervisor simply directs the answer. If appropriate, the supervisor may suggest helpful resources to further develop the OTA's professional development.

From time to time, there may be style differences between the supervisor and supervisee. This may develop when there is disagreement between different treatment approaches or disagreement on supervision approaches. Ideally, both parties can address the issues openly. The following are suggestions for dealing with problem supervision:

- The OTA's supervision needs are not being met—The OTA, using "I" statements, clarifies his or her needs. For example, "I need to meet with you at our regular scheduled time consistently because I feel uncomfortable with my current caseload. I understand we cannot meet today because of the important meeting, but I hope I can spend some time with you tomorrow morning." Notice how many "I" statements there are compared to "you" statements. "I" statements show that the OTA is taking personal responsibility and not insulting the supervisor with blame.

- The OTA's supervision is not being documented—Often the supervisor does not know that supervision must be documented. Remind the supervisor and if the problem does not resolve, ask if it is acceptable to document supervision yourself. These documentation notes are legal documents that can be requested by administration or outside agencies at any time. Ideally, supervision documentation will be used to document professional growth, including service competence, and be used for promotions and recommendations.

- The supervisor and supervisee have different styles—The OTA can ask that supervision styles be one of the topics of discussion for the next supervision meeting. If the supervisor's style is autocratic, the OTA can inform the supervisor that as a professional goal, he or she would like to participate in a supervision process that is more collaborative and reciprocal. If the OTA feels the supervisor's style is too open, that he or she cannot get the specific answers he or she needs, he or she can inform the supervisor that he or she would like to participate in professional conversations but to relieve her initial anxiety, he or she would like specific direction on this problem. Using "I" statements as discussed above are effective in dealing with different styles because they do not attack the style but only say, "I need something different."

Case Study

Sue is a recent graduate of an accredited OTA program and has been working for 11 months in a large skilled nursing facility with 60 beds of subacute rehabilitation. Most of her clients are orthopedic cases but she is starting to see more people with stroke and head injury. Although she never thought she would miss school and all the homework, she has been recently thinking about furthering her education to learn more about the clients she currently sees.

The staff of the OT department where Sue works usually gathers for lunch in the ADL kitchen. The 4 OTs and the 3 other OTAs all have different opinions of what Sue should do. Two OTs feel she should return to college to become an OT. Two OTs feel she should return to college and major in kinesiology or biology. The other OTAs have varying opinions about what continuing education she should do but agree she should not go back to college. To complicate things further, her family also has different opinions.

At supervision, Sue brings up the issue of conflicting advice about returning to school. Her supervisor, Lori, asks a few probing questions to find out what Sue has been thinking to this point. Lori then asks about the opinions Sue has been offered, and they discuss the possible reasons each person had in offering their specific advice. Sue comes to see that each opinion offered is a reflection of the things that person values. Lori asks Sue about short- and long-term goals. Sue says that she is interested in learning more about her clients with neurological impairments for now, but would like to teach a lab at the local community college OTA program "someday." Lori is familiar with the community college that Sue is talking about and shares her information about teaching there. Lori asks Sue to think about her goals and come up with a list of educational options that best fit her professional development goals. Lori tells Sue about the resources the facility can offer her for professional development.

At the next supervision meeting, Sue says she would like to return to school with the eventual goal of completing her BS in psychology. Sue believes that this major would allow her to best understand her neurological clients from both a science and art perspective. She addressed her long-term goal with her family, who agreed they would be supportive of her part-time study. For now, Sue wanted to learn about head injury as quickly as possible. Sue wanted to know if Lori could help with this short-term goal. Lori reinforced Sue's decision-making process and supported her long-term goal. Together they developed a plan to reach her short-term goal. First, Sue would be partnered with an OT with expertise in head injury. They would cotreat for 2 hours per week while Sue maintained her current caseload. Second, because Sue was a member of AOTA, she could participate in home-based, self-study material on cognition available to members. The facility would reimburse her costs if she presented an in-house inservice on what she learned as it related to her specific facility. This inservice would allow Sue to see if she liked the classroom teaching experience. If Sue was pleased with the inservice experience, the facility would offer the inservice free of charge to the community college students to give Sue further experience. Lastly, Sue would check the Internet for possible accredited college courses about head injury. Because the Internet is full of unreliable information, Sue and Lori agreed that the best approach for finding solid information about head injury treatment was to stick with an accredited college. Further, she may be able to transfer the Internet class as an elective in her BS program if the college offered regional accreditation.

Notice that Lori never gives Sue advice, but instead guides Sue to make her own choices and decisions.

SUMMARY

Supervision is a complex and dynamic process that involves a variety of skills and abilities. Ideally, it is a process of collaboration and reciprocation between the supervisor and the supervisee. It should be viewed as a partnership between professional and technical personnel.

Supervision is a process of providing guidance and direction to others. It involves assuming responsibility for workers and others in carrying out the mission and goals of the unit, the department, or the system within an organization. Knowledge of discipline-specific terminology and designations is necessary and provides a foundation for understanding OT supervision principles and patterns. These are delineated and discussed in terms of levels of personnel, service competency, patient condi-

tions, regulations and standards, and general employment. Examples of supervisor and supervisee responsibilities are stressed. Models for increased utilization of technical personnel that demonstrate increased delivery of services in a cost-effective manner are needed. These models should also emphasize ways that technical and professional personnel can be challenged and achieve career growth through varied options. Career enhancement opportunities are necessary to build relationships with workers and increase job and career satisfaction.

LEARNING ACTIVITIES

1. Conduct an informal interview with at least 3 supervisors and ask them to list their major responsibilities of their supervisees.

2. Conduct an informal interview with at least 3 supervisees and ask them to list their major responsibilities to their supervisor.

3. Compare the information obtained in items 1 and 2 with the information shown in Table 41-1, noting similarities and differences.

4. Role play the following scene with a peer: The OT supervisor has asked you to administer a structured assessment that you have only performed once before. You are feeling very uncomfortable about this request. What actions will you take? After the role play, seek feedback and suggestions from your peer.

5. Interview an OTA who has at least 1 year of experience. Determine in what career enhancement opportunities he or she is engaged. Determine the role of the supervisor in this plan.

REFERENCES

American Occupational Therapy Association. (2004). *Official documents of the AOTA*. Bethesda, MD: Author.

Brooks, B. (1982). OTA issues: Yesterday, today, and tomorrow. *American Journal of Occupational Therapy, 36*, 567-568.

Cohn, E. S. (1998). Interdisciplinary communication and supervision of personnel. In M. Neistadt & E. B. Crepeau (Eds.), *Willard & Spackman's OT*. Philadelphia, PA: Lippincott.

Dennis, M. (1988). Calculating cost effectiveness with the OTA. In J. A. Johnson (Ed.), *OTAs—Opportunities and challenges*. New York, NY: Haworth Press.

Evert, M. M. (1993). New president's address: Daily practice dilemmas. *American Journal of Occupational Therapy, 43*, 7-9.

Linroth, R., & Boulay, P. (1988). OTAs: Preparation for change. In J. A. Johnson (Ed.), *OTAs—Opportunities and challenges*. New York, NY: Haworth Press.

Schell, B. (1985). Guide to classification of OT personnel. *American Journal of Occupational Therapy, 39*, 803-810.

Strickland L. R. (1988). Career ladder development for OTAs. In J. A. Johnson (Ed.), *OTAs—Opportunities and challenges*. New York, NY: Haworth Press.

Key Concepts

- Activity director: A person responsible for organizing and implementing a variety of activities designed to meet the needs of a specific population.
- Activity program: Meeting the needs of a resident's healthy activity level.
- Resident: The Medicare description of a person living in a long-term care facility.

Essential Vocabulary

creative activities: Tasks that encourage expression.
democratic community activities: Opportunities to participate in the development of the community as a whole.
educational activities: Opportunities for lifelong learning.
leisure activities: Tasks for pleasure.
Omnibus Budget Reconciliation Act (OBRA): Law mandating reforms in nursing homes.
physical activities: Tasks using sensorimotor skills.
productive activities: Work substitute tasks.
social access activities: Tasks involving interaction.
spiritual activities: Religion- or spirituality-based tasks.

The Occupational Therapy Assistant as Activity Director

Sally E. Ryan, COTA, ROH, Retired and Karen Sladyk, PhD, OTR, FAOTA

Introduction

Without regard to where a person lives—their home, dorm housing, or a skilled nursing facility—people enjoy leisure. The concept of play has changed over history but in modern times people understand that play and leisure add value to one's life (McLean, Hurd, & Rogers, 2005). The choices in recreation vary from commercial products such as amusement parks to no-cost products such as taking a walk in a city park. Despite money and time constraints, people still seek play, leisure, and recreation in life. This is especially true of residents of skilled nursing homes, assistive living facilities, or congregate housing programs. These types of housing and services typically employ a person to coordinate a leisure activity program.

The position of activity director, coordinator, or supervisor is one for which the OTA is well qualified. With an educational background in human development throughout the lifespan, disabling conditions, the teaching/learning process, group dynamics, and activity analysis, as well as an understanding of every individual's need for purposeful, meaningful activity, the OTA is able to carry out activities programs of exceptional quality.

Activity directors are employed in a variety of settings, including community centers, large apartment and condominium complexes for the well and the disabled, group homes, halfway houses, institutions for people with mentally retarded or chronic mental illness, and long-term care settings for the elderly and others. Since a large number of OTAs are employed as activity directors in long-term care facilities, this chapter focuses on principles and applications for those settings. Although in many cases the majority of people residing in these facilities are elderly, a growing number of younger individuals are also residents. Whatever the site or the population, activity planning must meet the unique needs and interests of the consumer. Special measures must be taken to ensure that these individuals do not feel isolated due to age or residence. The activity director is often in a position to help develop these social partnerships.

Definitions

An activities program may be defined as an ongoing plan for providing meaningful activities, which is determined in relation to the individual needs and interests of those involved. Such programs are designed to provide a variety of opportunities for individuals to participate in activities, with the goal being to promote their physical, mental, and social well-being (American Therapeutic Recreation Association [ATRA], 1987; National Association of Activity Professionals [NAAP], 1990).

An activity director is employed by the facility and is directly responsible for planning, scheduling, implementing, documenting, managing, and evaluating an activities program. The term *resident* is used in keeping with the terminology adopted in the current Medicare and Medicaid standards for long-term care facilities (Health Care Financing Administration [HCFA], 1999). The program is designed with the overall goal of meeting the individual resident's needs for healthy activity that will aid in maintaining optimum levels of functioning and quality of life.

An activities consultant is a qualified individual who is employed by the facility to provide guidance to the activity director about all aspects of the activities program (ATRA, 1998). This person may also provide consultation to other staff members and departments as requested by administration. OTs, experienced OTAs, therapeutic recreation specialists, and social workers often provide consultative services.

Legislation and Regulations

The Department of Health and Human Services established the toughest requirements to date for Medicare and Medicaid programs in 1995 for long-term care facilities (HCFA, 1999), including specific regulations for activities departments and personnel. Complete copies of all regulations are available from state health/human services offices.

Many of the legislative improvements center around the Nursing Home Reform Amendments of the Omnibus Budget Reconciliation Act (OBRA) of 1987, which were designed to improve the standards of nursing homes "from the bottom up" and became law in 1990 (Saltz, 1990). Establishment of these amendments is an attempt to set minimum standards across the country for all nursing homes that receive federal aid. A database (HCFA, 1998) of the results of Medicare inspections of each nursing home in the United States is updated yearly on the Medicare Web site (www.medicare.gov). These standards address the following:

- Rights and quality of life
- Preadmission screening
- Assessment and quality of care
- Training of nurse's aides
- Annual resident review
- Facility survey and certification
- Enforcement

Experts have noted that the standards for resident assessment are one of the most important provisions of the law. Resident rights are free choice and freedom from chemical and physical restraints used for control, involuntary seclusion, discipline, or staff convenience (Saltz, 1990). Further, the new requirements mandate that individuals be assessed in terms of strengths as well as weaknesses, level of initiative and involvement, and personal preferences, with an emphasis on resident outcomes.

In addition to these federal regulations for skilled nursing facilities (SNFs) and intermediate care facilities (ICFs), most state health departments and licensing agencies have specific regulations for activities programs. The activity director must have a complete understanding of all of these regulations before initiating an activities program.

CAREER AND EDUCATIONAL INFORMATION

The ATRA (1998) shows the demand for activity staff to continue to grow in the new millennium. Activity staff should have training in physical, biological, and behavioral sciences. The activity department should be designed similar to other therapeutic departments in the facility. The director and all employees of the department must have a job description that specifically outlines all responsibilities and expectations. The following items should be included:

- Job title, supervisor, and supervisees.
- Qualifications, including formal education and training and any specialized training that might be required, such as recommendation, reality orientation and reminiscence techniques, cardiopulmonary resuscitation (CPR), and first aid.
- Licensure and/or certification requirements.
- Skills such as effective written communication, verbal communication, and related public relations activities.
- Required participation in continuing education and professional activities.
- Specific activities responsibilities, such as assessing individual resident activities needs; planning, scheduling, implementing, documenting, and evaluating the activities program. Definitive time lines should be included

(e.g., weekly, monthly, or quarterly).

- Participation in the care planning process, including specific requirements for attending meetings and frequency.
- Staff and volunteer recruitment, training, supervision, evaluation, and termination.
- Inservice education training responsibilities for staff and volunteers.
- Reports to be prepared and their frequency.
- Procurement and maintenance of supplies and equipment.
- Orientation activities for new employees and residents in the facility.
- Other responsibilities, such as coordinating a barber, beautician, and voting appointments.
- Methods and frequency of evaluation; conditions of probationary employment.

Job descriptions should be reviewed and modified as necessary, at least on an annual basis. Sample job descriptions for activity directors are often available from state health departments.

DEVELOPING AN ACTIVITIES PLAN

The first step in developing an activities plan is data collection about the likely participants. The medical record and the resident preadmission history will provide information regarding the primary and secondary diagnosis, precautions and limitations, physician's approval for activities participation, the resident's birthday, nationality, social history, and the name of a family contact (ATRA, 1991).

Another step in the data collection process is to determine the interests of the residents. A structured questionnaire or interview may be used to seek information in specific areas of activities. One method is to divide potential activities into the following 8 activity categories:

1. Physical
2. Social
3. Creative
4. Productive (work substitute)
5. Educational
6. Leisure
7. Spiritual
8. Democratic community activities

These are described further in Table 42-1.

Another method of categorizing activities is in terms of their potential to be supportive, provide maintenance, or provide empowerment. The following definitions are drawn from the NAAP's *Standards of Practice* (1990).

- Supportive activities promote a comfortable environment while providing stimulation or solace to those individuals who cannot benefit from either maintenance or empowerment activities. Such activities are usually provided to those individuals who may be severely cognitively or physically impaired or those unable to participate in a group program. Examples include providing soft back-

---

Table 42-1

Eight Activity Categories

1. Physical activities: These activities might include participation in exercise groups, sports, and games such as lawn bowling, shuffleboard, badminton, and daily walks.

2. Social access activities: Activities in this category include parties, picnics, meals at community restaurants, and tea time. The primary goal is to provide an opportunity for patients to interact socially. Family members should also be invited to some of these events.

3. Creative activities: Crafts, calligraphy, creative writing, and oil and watercolor painting are examples of creative activities. Such endeavors provide an outlet for creative expression, and although they often are presented in a group setting, socialization is not required.

4. Productive (work substitute) activities: Many people have a need to be engaged in a productive activity. Work on community service projects, such as flyer fundraising packets for the American Cancer Society or stuffing envelopes for a local charity, should be provided. Other work-related activities include writing and producing a daily newspaper, rolling bandages for the Red Cross, and baking items for a bazaar. Productive volunteer endeavors such as these allow the participants to continue to make a meaningful contribution to society.

5. Educational activities: Opportunities for lifelong learning are virtually endless. Photography clubs, music appreciation groups, and book review and discussion groups are examples. Individual activities, such as learning to speak a foreign language or to operate a computer, should also be included.

6. Leisure activities: Almost everyone needs time to read a good book, write letters, listen to the radio, or view a favorite television program. Quiet strolls in the park or just sitting on the patio observing and enjoying nature can be meaningful, refreshing pastimes.

7. Spiritual activities: Spiritual needs can be met in a variety of ways, such as participation in Bible study groups, a choir, or regularly scheduled religious services in the facility as well as the community. A missionary group often assists in fulfilling spiritual needs as well.

8. Democratic community activities: Living in a residential community affords members many opportunities to assume roles in determining the future of their community. These empowering activities include organizing forums for discussion and resolution of issues of mutual interest, forming a resident and state council to discuss problems and concerns and to establish policies, writing editorials for the facility newspaper, and organizing advice related to political and social issues that impact on the quality of life of the participants. Because they focus on opportunities for individuals to redevelop a sense of purpose in their lives, samples may be found under the categories of creative, productive, and democratic community activities, as well as others.

---

ground music; placing plants, pictures, and other colorful objects in the resident's room; and providing sensory stimulation.

- Maintenance activities provide the individual with opportunities to maintain physical, cognitive, social, spiritual, and emotional health. These areas are delineated under the 8 activity categories discussed in Table 42-1.

- Empowerment activities focus on the promotion of self-respect by providing opportunities for self-expression, choice, social responsibility, and personal responsibility. These activities differ from those designed to provide maintenance.

Whatever methods are used to categorize activities, it is important to ensure that every resident has an opportunity to participate in meaningful activities that are of interest and based on individual needs, strengths, and goals (ATRA, 1991). Activities that require decision-making should be emphasized as well, and resident collaboration should be a focus at every stage of treatment.

If potential participants fill out a questionnaire, an interview should also be arranged to verify and expand each resident's needs. If residents are reluctant to discuss items on a questionnaire, a more generalized approach may be used by asking open-ended questions such as:

- What activities did you enjoy before coming to the nursing home?

- What are some of the things you did during your spare time this week?

- If you were the activity director, what do you think would be an important activity to provide?

The interviewer should provide added cues as necessary to keep the responses to questions on target. Speaking with family members and other staff is also recommended to gain as much additional input as possible, especially if the resident is cognitively impaired or uncommunicative. Figure 42-1 provides an example of a form that may be used.

Once the data are gathered, the information must be tabulated and categorized and priorities established in terms of available staff, volunteers, space, existing supplies and equipment, community resources, and operating budget. For example, if the category of creative activities indicates that many residents are interested in arts and crafts, a general session should be scheduled daily. Perhaps a small number are interested in knitting. While they could participate in the general group, they may also enjoy forming a knitting club that meets once a week to work on a special project, such as knitting hats and mittens for a children's home or homeless people in the community.

Name _____ Room _____ Admit Date _____

Date of Birth _____ Age _____ Hometown _____

Marital Status _____ Children _____ Grandchildren _____ Great Grandchildren _____

Siblings _____ Do any live nearby? _____

Ethnic/Cultural Background _____

Languages Spoken _____ Religion _____

Education _____

Occupations _____

Work History _____

Registered Voter _____ Veteran _____ Branch of Service _____

Clubs and Organizations _____

Interests: (Code—S = small group; G = large group; I = individual)

Note: Interviewer should give examples in each category below.

- Physical activities _____

_____

- Social access activities _____

_____

- Creative activities _____

_____

- Productive activities _____

_____

- Educational activities _____

_____

- Leisure activities _____

_____

- Spiritual activities _____

_____

- Democratic community activities _____

_____

- Typical Day Profile _____

_____

- Typical Week Profile _____

_____

Life Goals

_____

_____

Previous Living Arrangement _____

Physician _____ Reason for Admission _____

Diagnosis _____ Functional Limitations/Strengths _____

Mobility _____ Vision _____

Hearing _____ Comprehension _____

Orientation _____ Behavior _____

Attention Span _____ Other _____

Contact Person _____ Phone _____

Address _____

Figure 42-1. Activity interest questionnaire, developed by S. E. Ryan, 1991.

Initial activity planning can best be accomplished by setting up a general grid calendar with days on the left, including Saturday and Sunday, and the 8 major categories of activities listed across the top. Enter the large group activities first—those in which residents indicated the greatest interest, such as crafts, movies, concerts, and games. Next, enter the small group activities, such as baking, gardening, and oil painting. Determine which of these activities the existing staff and volunteers can supervise, and identify additional needs. Be sure that necessary space, supplies, and equipment are available. Look for gaps in the plan and be creative about introducing new activities. It is also important to determine whether activities are primarily active or passive in terms of degree of participation. Every effort should be made to schedule out-of-building activities, such as picnics, shopping tours, and visits to zoos, so that residents maintain contact with the community. Some individuals will

---

Table 42-2

Activity Program Individualized Treatment Plan

- Problem/need: Few social contacts; rarely participates in any group activities.
- Capabilities/strengths: Articulate; knowledgeable about current events and sports.
- Activity goal: Participation in one small group event.
- Approach: Invite to current events group or sports group as a resource person; offer a choice and structure role to be as non-threatening as possible; stress that others are interested in the information that individual could share.

---

prefer not to join groups; therefore, time must be set aside for individual activity participation.

Activities needs cannot be totally met by a program that only schedules events Monday through Friday during the usual daytime working hours. Flexibility is necessary, and every effort should be made to provide some activities in the evenings and on weekends. Arrangements can usually be made for the assigned staff members to take compensatory time off during the regular workweek. The proposed activities plan should also be evaluated to ensure that at least some of the activities are held at a time when family members can participate, and efforts should be made to encourage them to do so.

Once the general grid plan is developed and staffing patterns are established, it is important to look at timing of the events. Consideration must be given to regularly scheduled activities such as meals, routine nursing care, physicians' rounds, OT or PT schedules, and visiting hours. These times are appropriate for the activity staff to document progress and complete department maintenance responsibilities.

Public Relations

Effective public relations are an important component of activity planning. When the final monthly plan is developed, it must be communicated as widely as possible. Copies should be provided to administration and all departments in the facility, as well as to each resident at least 7 days in advance. Large weekly posters should be made and posted in prominent locations throughout the building. Individual posters should also be made to advertise special events, such as a concert or a bazaar. If a public address system is available, use it to make daily announcements of forthcoming events. Flyers can be mailed to family members when events are scheduled in which they may participate. The community should also be informed through providing local newspapers with press releases of activities of interest, such as a resident's 100th birthday or an announcement of the individuals who received ribbons for their entries in the county fair.

Related Planning Principles

Activities planning must always occur at least 1 month in advance. Failure to do so will produce undo stress for the director, staff, and volunteers and will result in unmet resident activities needs. Even the most thorough planning will not be flawless. The activity director must have alternative plans to draw

upon when, for example, the high school band does not show up for a concert or a torrential rainstorm ruins picnic plans. Flexibility, adaptability, and resourcefulness are important attributes of the successful activity director.

Individual activity plans should be developed for every resident and be included in the total resident care plan. Problems and needs are identified and specific objectives are established along with methods for accomplishing the goals. Copies of both state and federal regulations should be obtained to be sure all required information is included. A brief example of a plan is provided in Table 42-2 (NAAP, 1990).

A confidential card system should be developed for each resident's individual activity plan. The resident's card should also have information on the primary and secondary diagnosis, limitations and precautions, physician's permission to participate in activities, birthdate, and other pertinent social history facts. Preferences should also be noted, such as small group versus large group participation and afternoon activities versus morning or evening activities. Locating the card system in a central but secure place, such as the activity department office, will allow all staff members convenient access to it. Additional information on patient care planning and specific activity plans appears in the section on Records and Reports (p. 522).

Implementing the Activities Program

Once initial planning has been completed, the activities program is implemented, often gradually over several weeks. As activities take place, the activity director must carefully monitor all aspects to ensure that the programming is effective in helping to meet residents' goals. The following items are of particular importance:

- General attendance and degree of participation.
- Adequacy of staff and volunteer coverage.
- Adequacy of space, furnishings, equipment, and supplies.
- Adequacy of lighting, ventilation, temperature control, and general safety.
- Effectiveness of communication with other departments.
- Timing in relation to other activities taking place in the facility.
- Specific ways to improve the activity and the degree of participation the next time it is presented.

Another helpful method is to break activities down into very specific activity components, particularly if they tend to take too much time or participation is less than expected. An example would be the weekly songfest. This activity is made up of at least 12 distinct parts:

1. Furniture arrangement.
2. Transportation for nonambulatory participants.
3. Introduction of song leader and pianist.
4. Distribution of song sheets.
5. Use of an overhead projector with enlarged words to songs.
6. Use of clapping and marching activities.
7. Distribution and use of rhythm instruments.
8. Playing "Name that Tune" game.
9. Collecting and storing supplies and equipment.
10. Returning nonambulatory residents to their units.
11. Rearranging furniture.
12. Documenting participation.

Keeping a clipboard close at hand is a good idea so that observations relative to the issue presented in the preceding sections may be recorded immediately. It is also important to seek critiques from participants, as well as staff members and volunteers. An activities planning committee should be established to review past events and make recommendations for future activities. Feedback should be incorporated into a regularly scheduled quality improvement plan.

Resident Motivation

A successful activity program involves much more than planning and carrying out a variety of activities. It must also include the creation of an atmosphere that is warm, friendly, caring, and as nonthreatening as possible; an atmosphere that offers decision-making opportunities and promotes independence; and an atmosphere in which residents are offered encouragement and support but are never coerced or forced to participate. These are very important motivational factors (Wlodkowski, 1990).

The main activity room should serve as a gathering spot for those who just want to get away from their room for a while. Space should be provided for people to observe the activities taking place, particularly new residents. Serving coffee and tea, within diet restrictions, is a method to comfortably include observers in the activities group. It encourages socialization and may increase motivation to become directly involved in the activity.

Motivation comes from within, but it can be enhanced by showing a genuine interest in the residents. Sometimes writing a short personal note to invite an individual to participate will be a motivating factor. Others will be motivated or drawn to activities because they can be assured of some degree of success and they feel "needed" by the other group members. For example, a person who is not interested in working on the mosaic mural in the dining room may be willing to spend hours sorting tile so that the others can work more efficiently.

RECORDS AND REPORTS

A system of regular documentation must be established in keeping with the requirements of federal, state, and facility regulations. The general categories of documentation include resident care plans, activity plans, activity notes, activity schedules, and participation records. The latter must be maintained for all group and one-to-one activities and should be a part of the resident's permanent record. Confidentiality must be maintained for all resident records and reports. Records should also be maintained for all staff members and volunteers, indicating hours worked as well as major responsibilities. Budget reports must be prepared regularly, and the administration of the facility may require monthly summary reports of the activities program, as well as an annual report. The activity director will also be responsible for developing and maintaining an activities policies and procedures manual. It is also advisable to keep records of supply needs and an inventory of equipment and furnishings.

Resident Care Plans

One of the main purposes of resident care planning is to assess needs and problems in a systematic way. Specific goals are established and methods are identified for accomplishing them. The resident care plan must be completed soon after admission and must include a comprehensive activity assessment. Comprehensive resident care plans promote a coordinated effort in providing medical as well as multidisciplinary services for the individual. Effective care planning must include the resident, the family, significant others, as well as the primary health care providers in the facility. Resident care plans must be reviewed and revised regularly. Medicare and Medicaid regulations require the use of a standardized assessment called the Resident Assessment System, which includes a minimum data set (MDS) to provide a framework for planning (AOTA, 1990). The activity assessment must reflect information from the MDS. After admission, the MDS is used as a means of updating the staff relative to the resident's status, particularly during times of change.

ACTIVITIES PLANS

Activities plans are developed, evaluated, and updated on a regular basis, usually monthly. They are a part of the resident's clinical record. The activity director must allocate specific blocks of time each week for this task to ensure that all plans are always up to date. To assist in this process, a system should be developed for staff and volunteers to share daily observations of individual residents. A notebook with a page for each resident is a simple way of collecting the information. A personal computer may also be used. An example of the way these observations might be written is shown in Figure 42-2. Whatever system is developed to share information, the activity director must be sure the documentation is secure and confidential.

12/5/04. Task: Mosaic flowerpot. Participation: Initially slow to begin but worked for 1 hour. Said he was nervous about being the current event group leader next week.

S. Basket, Volunteer

12/7/04. Task: Mosaic project. Participation: Mr. J not pleased with final results, stated it looks too "girly." He was able to problem solve by suggesting he give it to the nurse for the day room. Expressed interest in wood puzzle.

B. Melling, Activity Aide

Figure 42-2. Sample of recorded observations.

3/21/04. During the past week, Mr. Johnson participated in 9.5 hours of scheduled therapeutic recreation events. Mr. Johnson actively participated in woodworking activities every weekday morning for 1 hour. He frequently takes a nap after lunch but participated in the weekly photography club and the current events group in the afternoon. He was the discussion leader of the current events group on 2 occasions this week. He initially appeared nervous about this role, but reported he was pleased with his skills after several members complimented him. He also visited the library twice this week and stated that "reading is one of my greatest pleasures." When asked to take a leadership role in a new book club for both residents and staff, he was excited and agreed to be at the planning committee meeting next Monday. He is maintaining the level of activity noted last month.

Jane Doe, COTA, Activity Director

Figure 42-3. Sample activities note.

In addition to contributing to the activity plan, observation notes such as these will also assist the activity director in evaluating each resident's degree of progress in attaining goals.

Activities Notes

Activities notes (Figure 42-3) are included in the resident's clinical record and should be written by approved staff whenever change is noted or at least once a month. A good activity note should include a summary of the types of activities the person had been participating in, the frequency of participation, and the time involved. Notes should reflect maintenance, progress, or decline. Quotations may be used. All notes must be dated, written legibly in ink, and signed. Use of abbreviations should be avoided unless the facility has an approved list of abbreviations for use in records. Activity notes must be objective, accurate, and complete. They should relate directly to the activity plan and the total resident care plan.

Participation Records

Participation records should be maintained on a daily basis to provide an overall view of activity trends and fluctuations. Such records will reflect individual resident activity and inactivity. Further, these records are a barometer of interest in specific activities. Such records may also be used to provide justification for hiring additional staff members. Graph paper may be used to develop a simple participation recording form. The names of all residents are listed on the left-hand side and the different activities are listed across the top. To save space, use a coding system such as "C" = crafts, "B" = baking, and "G" = gardening. It is important to remember that if people come to the activity area and fall asleep, they have not participated and should not be listed on the participation record.

Activities Schedules

Activities schedules are generally the monthly calendar of events. These schedules should be filed, as they provide specific information on the variety of activities offered and when. The schedules may also be coded to indicate whether activities require active or passive participation and the number of staff members and volunteers that are needed for each activity. Review of past schedules is a great help in planning for future events.

Activities Reports

Summary reports of the activities program are written regularly as required by the administration and at least annually. A typical report might include information about the number of residents participating in the 8 major activity areas (physical, social, creative, productive, educational, diversional, spiritual, and democratic community) with a breakdown of individual and group activities. New or unique events may be highlighted. Budget information should be included in the categories of income, expenditures, and cash on hand. The number of staff and volunteers should be noted as well as consultation services received. Inservice training programs for staff and volunteers should be briefly described.

Policy and Procedure Manual

The activity director is responsible for developing, reviewing, and revising the departmental policy and procedure manual. A policy may be defined as a statement that describes how basic program objectives can be met. Policies are not subject to frequent change. Procedures are methods for carrying out the policy and are subject to modification as need arises. For example, the policy and procedures for conducting a birthday party might be written as shown in Figure 42-4.

Subject: Birthday parties.

Policy: A monthly birthday party shall be held in the facility.

Purpose: To honor all residents who are celebrating a birthday during that month.

Responsibility: The activity director shall be responsible for planning and carrying out the party.

Procedures:
1. Written invitations will be sent to all residents celebrating a birthday during a given month. Invitations will also be sent to family members.
2. The date, time, and location of the party will be advertised at least 2 weeks in advance. All residents and staff are invited.
3. Corsages and boutonnieres will be provided for those being honored.
4. Cake, ice cream, and beverages must be ordered from the dietary department at least 1 week in advance of the event. Provisions for those on special diets must be accommodated.
5. Prizes may be awarded to the youngest and the oldest residents who are celebrating their birthday.
6. Musical entertainment will be provided.

Figure 42-4. Policy and procedures for a birthday party.

STAFFING NEEDS

The literature yields little information on the topic of staffing requirements. The authors believe that the employment of one full-time activity director for every 50 to 60 residents should be an absolute minimum in skilled and intermediate care facilities. Individual state regulations and licensing agencies may specify other minimums for activity personnel. It should be kept in mind that providing a minimum number of activities personnel may not allow maximum services to be provided in meeting the residents' individual activity needs and enhancing their quality of life.

As more individuals become actively involved in the activities program and increased needs are identified, it may be necessary to increase the staff size. Before hiring additional personnel, a specific job description must be developed that includes most of the items described in the beginning of this chapter. Administration must approve all new staff positions. Plans and procedures must also be developed for orienting and evaluating new employees and providing for their continuing education.

Volunteers

Although volunteers are a most important asset to any activities program, they should never take the place of paid staff under any circumstances. Rather, they should be used to enhance the program.

Before a volunteer program is initiated, legal and insurance issues must be considered to ensure that adequate liability safeguards are provided. Volunteers should be recruited, screened, and trained using a developed protocol, as needs arise to assist in increasing the effectiveness of the program. They can often provide some of the extra services that personalize the program, particularly in relation to individual needs. Volunteers can carry out a variety of tasks including letter writing, resident and departmental shopping, leading songfests, teaching creative activities, and word processing. Volunteers may be recruited through facility posters, more formal advertising in church and synagogue bulletins, high school/college newspapers, and general announcements at neighborhood events. All volunteers must have specific job descriptions and hours. Volunteers should participate in an orientation and training program. Records of service need to be maintained on each volunteer for service awards, letters of recommendation, or hours required to meet some other need, such as college applications or scouting awards. It is important to recognize volunteers for their contributions at least annually. Certificates or pins should be presented at a special gathering in their honor.

PROGRAM MANAGEMENT

As a departmental manager, the activity director must develop systems and approaches that will provide for the most effective and efficient delivery of activities services to meet the goals of the residents, the department, and the health care facility. Failure to do so may result in decreased motivation and interest on the part of workers and participants.

It is the responsibility of the supervisor to develop and utilize objective tools, such as job descriptions and evaluation forms to measure employee performance. The supervisor should also encourage the staff to participate in self-evaluation activities on a regular basis (ATRA, 1993). Individual job performance goal setting should be a collaborative process between the supervisor and the supervisees. When specific deficits in performance are noted, the supervisor should be constructive in the criticism given by providing guidance, resources, and opportunities that will assist the worker in skill improvement.

Above all, an effective supervisor must be caring, honest, objective, be willing to carry "a fair share" of the workload, and be open in relationships. A person who provides a strong role model and demonstrates a sincere interest in the well-being of those he or she supervises is indeed effective.

Interdisciplinary Role

Most health care facilities view the activity director as a department head and an integral member of the health care team. The activity director should participate in all department head meetings and patient care planning conferences, as the delivery of effective activity services depends on cooperation from and coordination with a number of other departments. Efforts should be made to develop both structured and informal communication channels that will ensure quality resident care and the achievement of goals.

Continuing Education

We live in an age where change occurs very rapidly, particularly in our health care delivery systems. The activity director, in collaboration with administration, staff, and volunteers, and with necessary outside consultation, must identify the continuing education needs and develop a plan to meet these needs (ATRA, 1993). Such a plan must include the required financial support. For example, many facilities require all staff members and volunteers to take a first aid course, and some require specialized training in cardiopulmonary resuscitation (CPR). As residents' needs change, staff members may also need to be trained in the techniques of reality orientation, remotivation, and reminiscence therapy. The activity director and everyone involved in the delivery of activities services must be given opportunities to participate in continuing education courses and workshops to ensure that existing skills are maintained and new ones acquired. Continuing education is important to provide necessary activities services, to enhance those services, and to be responsive to the changing needs of the residents.

Financial Planning Role

The activity director is responsible for financial planning for the department and must have skills in developing and managing a budget. The main categories that must be considered in budgeting are salaries, nonexpendable equipment, expendable equipment and supplies, maintenance and repair, travel, and professional development. Projected income and cash-on-hand figures should also be included.

Salary

Salaries are generally the largest budget item. In planning, consideration must be given to actual salary amounts as well as postprobationary raises, merit and cost of living increases, overtime costs, and annual bonuses. Social security contributions, health care benefits, retirement plans, and life insurance costs must also be included. Consult with the human resource manager of the facility.

Nonexpendable Equipment

Purchases of major items, such as stereo systems, tables, and desks, are included in this category. Generally, this is equipment that is not "used up" and is expected to last 5 to 20 years. Before requesting new equipment, it is wise to check with other departments such as housekeeping to see if the needed items are in storage or available from another area of the facility.

Expendable Equipment and Supplies

This category of budget planning is likely to result in mistakes due to false assumptions or inaccurate information. The big problem lies in determining exactly what is "expendable." Generally, any item that is "used up" over a short period of time is considered expendable. According to the "Ryan Rule," "anything smaller than a large bread box, that is not bolted down, kept under lock and key, or constant surveillance is eventually expendable." Table looms, radios, coffeepots, and hand tools are among the items that frequently disappear. Office supplies, crafts, food, and day-to-day supplies are all expendables.

Interdepartmental Activities

Another aspect that makes budget planning difficult is "who pays for what" when several departments participate in an activity. For example, when a picnic is held in the park, is the cost of food charged to the dietary department or the activities department? If a nurse's aide is designated to assist with the activity, are the hours worked charged against the nursing budget or the activity budget? Matters such as these must be resolved with administration prior to the event. Once these questions have been answered, more accurate planning can occur. One method is to keep track of actual expenses for 3 months, multiply that amount by 4, and add at least 12% to cover inflation and margin of error.

Maintenance and Repair

Routine maintenance is required for sewing machines, powered woodworking tools, computers, and all audiovisual equipment. Departmental painting and redecorating may also be included in this category.

Travel

Expenses incurred for bus rentals for resident outings are generally the largest item in this category. If the facility has a vehicle for resident use, determine if any charges are made to your department. Reimbursement of employee and volunteer mileage for errands and shopping should also be covered in this budget category.

Professional Development

In light of the many rapid changes in health care policy, coupled with new research, legislation, and resulting changes in the provision of services, it is important for activity directors and activities personnel to have opportunities for professional development. Costs for continuing education courses and workshops, conventions, conferences, meetings, books, journals, related travel, and per diem costs are items that should be covered.

Income Sources

Cash donations, bazaar receipts, and bake sale proceeds are examples of income sources. The activity director must have a clear understanding of exactly what the administration expectations are for income-producing activities. Although some activities may be self-supporting in terms of revenue generated, it is an unreal expectation to believe an activity will generate enough income to cover expenses. Activities programs should never be forced to exploit resident endeavors to raise money.

Consultation

A consultant is a person who is employed by a facility on a contractual basis to provide indirect service. Consultants may be used to give information, assist in strategy development and problem resolution, to clarify issues, and to advise (AOTA, 1993). Typically, a consultant is employed by administration to provide services to a department or several departments in relation to specific concerns. Consultative services may be as short as a one-time visit or may extend over several months or years depending on the nature of the consultation required. It is important to understand that a consultant works "outside" the facility and brings expertise and an objective viewpoint to the facility.

The activity director might use a consultant to assist in providing information about and interpretation of federal and state regulations regarding activities programming. Other areas in which a consultant might offer assistance include continuing education and general community resources, activity suggestions for nonparticipating residents, establishing resident care planning goals, and suggesting ways to improve departmental management procedures. A consultant can also be a valuable resource for developing strategies for improved communication with another department or individual.

It is very important to note that when an OT is employed as a consultant it does not mean that OT services are being provided. Further clarification is found in the official position paper of the AOTA (1994) entitled *Position Paper: OT and Long-Term Services and Supports*.

Coordination of Occupational Therapy and Activities Services

In recent years, I have become increasingly concerned about the apparent "division" in some long-term care facilities that provide both activities and OT services. These services may not be coordinated and there may be little effort to reinforce the residents' goals from OT in the activity program. Informal observation and feedback from individuals working in the field present an interesting contrast in terms of "what is" and "what could be." A number of nursing homes and other long-term care facilities employ OTs and OTAs on a contractual basis to provide direct services under what is often viewed as a medical, rehabilitation model, frequently oriented primarily to physical dysfunction. The same facility may also employ OTAs to deliver activity services under a more holistic, humanistic, supportive, and maintenance model. Unfortunately, communication between the 2 services may be minimal. For example, a person with hemiparesis may be working on coordination activities in OT and an OTA in the activities department could reinforce treatment, but this coordination may not take place in many instances. It is imperative these efforts are coordinated and that the service providers critique their respective models and methods of service delivery to ensure maximum benefits to the recipients that are also cost-effective.

NEW MODEL FOR LONG-TERM CARE

The Lazarus Project provides a model that should be considered as a possible solution to the problems in long-term care facilities that extend beyond those discussed previously. The model outlines the politics of empowerment based on a community model of democratic governance where residents, staff, and administration participate equally in creating an environment that is responsive to all member needs, thus improving the quality of life for those residing in these facilities (Kari & Michels, 1991). The OTA serving as an activity director or a direct OT service provider can have a marked influence in bringing about the necessary changes in 2000 and beyond, using the innovative principles stressed in this important work.

The Lazarus Vision

It seems fitting to leave the reader with a vision for the future in which the profession can play a vital role. While members of other age groups may be served by nursing homes, the needs of the frail elderly deserve particular attention. Therefore, the vision statement from the Lazarus Project is shown in Figure 42-5 to provide a vehicle for study, reflection, and challenge, and a catalyst for implementing needed change (Kari & Michels, 1991).

SUMMARY

The role of the OTA as an activity director offers many challenges and opportunities. Skills in assessing activities needs, planning, implementing, documenting, managing, and evaluating programs are essential. An activity director must also have strong interpersonal, leadership, supervision, and management abilities. The need for qualified activities personnel in long-term care facilities for the elderly and others is increasing, and the educational background of OTAs provides them with excellent preparation for such positions; however, employment of an OTA or OT consultant does not mean that OT direct services are being provided.

Recent federal legislation is emphasized and provides a foundation for following topics. Discussion of specific documentation needs and financial and other management tasks provides the reader with basic information. Interdisciplinary roles and consultation are a focus as well. The need for coordination between activities services and OT services is addressed and culminates with a brief discussion of a model for service delivery in the 2000s and beyond and in which OTAs can play a vital part, regardless of their specific roles in the provision of long-term care services.

LEARNING ACTIVITIES

1. Visit a long-term care facility that has an activities program. Review the calendar of events and determine the variety of offerings in terms of the 8 major categories identified in Table 42-1.

The Lazarus Project Vision

The Lazarus Project believes that frail elders can be contributing members to society. It is through contribution that individuals exercise power and are able to live a life of meaning and dignity. Empowerment happens when communities are created—communities which govern themselves by drawing on the diverse strengths of members to address common problems.

The Lazarus Project believes this kind of community can be created in nursing home environments. This requires a broad, holistic understanding of health. This concept of health includes the ability to have authority in one's life, to shape one's environment, and to extend influence within a broader public world.

Aging is a public issue; it is not simply an individual experience. When people become older and more frail, their ability to be contributing members to society changes. In a society that measures worth in terms of contributions and influence, the loss of physical and cognitive capacity quickly defines frail elders as "a problem." One of the ways the public has chosen to address this "problem" is to separate itself from chronically ill and disabled elders by "institutionalizing" the aging.

The authors of the Lazarus Project believe that the focus on the medical and service missions of long-term care institutions views residents as incapacitated rather than as contributors. When this assumption becomes embedded in the institution's governing system, it can lead to a loss of power for all involved—the residents, the staff, administrators, and families. This loss of influence constrains an institution's ability to effectively respond to the problems of aging.

Figure 42-5. The Lazarus Project vision.

2. Practice using the form in the text as an interviewing guide with at least 3 people over age 70.
3. Assume that a group of 6 residents is interested in participating in a baking group. Plan this activity in detail, breaking it down into specific components.
4. Discuss the following question with a peer: "How does an activities program differ from an OT direct service program?"
5. Read the mission statement of the Lazarus Project. Discuss implications with a classmate.
6. Make a general grid of activities for the 8 categories listed in Table 42-1. Discuss staffing needs and budget requests to run this program for a facility of 45 elderly SNF residents. Repeat the same project for a group home for 10 people with mental retardation or 18 people with long-term, chronic schizophrenia.

ACKNOWLEDGMENTS

Appreciation is extended to Nancy Kari, MPH, OTR, and Peg Michels, MA, for sharing material from the Lazarus Project. Special thanks is also given to Shirley H. Carr, MA, OTR, FAOTA, for her critique and helpful comments and to Pamela Hayle, therapeutic activities programmer, for providing information and forms. Penny Boulet, COTA, is also acknowledged for providing resources.

REFERENCES

American Therapeutic Recreation Association. (1987). *Definition of therapeutic recreation*. Alexandria, VA: Author.

American Therapeutic Recreation Association. (1991). *Standards for the practice*. Alexandria, VA: Author.

American Therapeutic Recreation Association. (1993). *Standards for the practice of therapeutic recreation and self-assessment guide*. Alexandria, VA: Author.

American Therapeutic Recreation Association. (1998). *Career information*. Alexandria, VA: Author.

American Occupational Therapy Association. (1990). *Resident assessment system*. Rockville, MD: Author.

American Occupational Therapy Association. (1993). Occupational therapy roles. *American Journal of Occupational Therapy, 47*, 1087-1099.

American Occupational Therapy Association. (1994). Position paper: OT and long-term services and supports. *American Journal of Occupational Therapy, 48*, 1035-1036.

Healthcare Financing Administration. (1998). *Choosing a nursing home*. Washington, DC: Author. #HCFA-10121.

Healthcare Financing Administration. (1999). *HCFA fact sheet*. Washington, DC: HCFA Press Office.

Kari, N., & Michels, P. (1991). The Lazarus Project: A politics of empowerment. *American Journal of Occupational Therapy, 45*, 719-725.

McLean, D. D., Hurd, A. R., & Rogers, N. B. (2005). *Kraus' Recreation and leisure in modern society*. Sudbury, MA: Jones and Barlett Publishers.

National Association of Activity Professionals. (1990). *Standards of practice: Section A—Standards of care*. Washington, DC: Author.

Saltz, D. L. (1990). Celebration marks reform of nursing homes. *OT Week, 4*(41), 12-13.

Wlodkowski, R. J. (1990). *Enhancing adult motivation to learn*. San Francisco, CA: Jossey-Bass.

Key Concepts

- Ethics: Honesty, truthfulness, and morals.
- AOTA's *Occupational Therapy Code of Ethics* (2000): A pledge of high values and behaviors articulated through 7 identified principles and includes descriptions of expected standards of member behavior.

Essential Vocabulary

autonomy: Promoting self-determination.
beneficence: Doing good for others.
duty: Meeting one's responsibilities.
fidelity: Keeping your word.
justice: Complying with rules, laws, regulations, and policies.
nonmaleficence: Doing no harm.
normative ethics: Caring and influencing the quality of life of all members of society.
sanction: Disciplinary action taken against Code of Ethics violators.
veracity: Being truthful.

FUNCTIONAL ETHICS

S. Maggie Reitz, PhD, OTR, FAOTA

INTRODUCTION

The purpose of this chapter is for you, an OT student, to gain a working knowledge of functional ethics—the ability to apply knowledge of ethics to your day-to-day life in your current role as an OT student and as a future practitioner, educator, or researcher. This information will be especially helpful during your fieldwork experiences and your transition to the role of practitioner. However, additional training, ongoing reading, and self-study will be required for you to be an ethical, competent practitioner who is able to negotiate the complexities of today's practice arenas.

This chapter will introduce you to official professional documents, identify common ethical dilemmas and responses, and describe the profession's role in social and occupational justice as an example of normative ethics. A description of the AOTA's *Occupational Therapy Code of Ethics* (AOTA, 2000) is provided. Contrasts between professional and unethical behaviors are discussed. Problem behaviors not supported by the *Occupational Therapy Code of Ethics*, but sometimes exhibited by students, are identified. This section is followed by a brief discussion of dilemmas that practitioners may face. A practical method for analyzing and resolving ethical dilemmas is also presented. Finally, resources to assist the student in arriving at an appropriate response to ethical issues, including social injustice, are described.

LANGUAGE OF ETHICS

The language used to discuss ethics can initially be confusing and intimidating. However, after learning a few basic terms, the importance of ethics to the profession's credibility becomes apparent (Reitz, 1997). With additional study, this language can be used as a tool to advocate for your clients as well as social and occupational justice. The ethics vocabulary is extensive. Essential terms and basic definitions are included in this chapter. These definitions were developed from a variety of resources, predominantly the articles and glossary of the *Reference Guide to the Occupational Therapy Code of Ethics*

(Scott, 2003). The student is encouraged to review the glossary of terms in this guide for additional terms and definitions.

Ethics

What are ethics? If you were to ask this question of OT students or even random people on the street, you would receive a variety of responses. However, it would be easy to find common themes among the varied responses, including values such as honesty, truthfulness, morals, and doing the "right" thing. Ideals such as these are interwoven in the core values and attitudes identified by the profession of OT (AOTA, 1993). These core values and attitudes are essential to any discussion of OT ethics. They "are organized around seven basic concepts—altruism, equality, freedom, justice, dignity, truth, and prudence" (AOTA, 1993, p. 1085).

Mosey (1981) described ethics as being the analysis of voluntary human behavior that impacts others, "the institutions of the society, or the physical, mental, or the moral development of the individual" (p. 20). Scott (2003, p. 83) defines ethics as:

> ...a systematic view of rules of conduct that is grounded in philosophical principles and theory. The character and customs of societal values and norms that are assumed in a given cultural, professional, or institutional setting as ways of determining right and wrong.

It has also been described as the foundation of a society, as ethics provide guidance to its members regarding their relationships with others. The manner in which the ethical beliefs of a culture are carried out is of special importance to those who may be in danger of mistreatment due to age, illness, disability, or other possible areas of discrimination (e.g., gender, ethnicity, creed, lifestyle). Knowledge of the prevailing societal ethics and their congruence with your profession's Code of Ethics, especially as it relates to the disenfranchised, is part of your responsibility of being a future health care professional.

Nonmaleficence and Beneficence

The terms *nonmaleficence* and *beneficence* are used frequently in medicine and health. Nonmaleficence "is closely associated with the maxim… 'above all [or first] do no harm'" (Beauchamp & Childress, 2001, p. 113) and is "the duty to ensure that no harm is done" (Scott, 2003, p. 83). The term *beneficence* expands on the concept of doing no harm to also include seeking to prevent harm, removing harm, as well as doing or promoting good (Beauchamp & Childress, 2001). As a provider of OT services, you are duty bound to practice nonmaleficence and beneficence by doing good for others, providing beneficial services, and balancing risk and benefits while performing assessments and interventions (AOTA, 2003; Reitz, 1997).

In your role as an occupational student, an example of nonmaleficence would be refraining from offering health advice to fellow students or family members until you have sufficient training in order to prevent harm. An example of beneficence would be to report obstacles or malfunctioning automatic doors to ensure accessibility to buildings and emergency exits.

Duty, Veracity, and Fidelity

Although similar in meaning, these terms are not identical. "Duty is a broad term which includes the important behaviors of meeting one's responsibilities and performing one's work competently… this means completing the tasks required by your role as an OT student in a safe, ethical, and skilled manner" (Reitz, 1997, p. 248). As a student, you have a duty to follow academic integrity policies and be aware of program requirements. Veracity simply means to be truthful, while fidelity means being faithful or keeping your word. In health care, fidelity implies more than just keeping your word, but also that your behavior with clients and families is consistent with the values of loyalty and trust (Beauchamp & Childress, 2001).

CODE OF ETHICS

Mosey (1981) described the necessary criteria that distinguish a job from a profession. One of these criteria is a code of ethics. A profession and its code of ethics typically develop and evolve over time for various reasons, including forces of society. Mosey views a code of ethics as a "contract" between a profession and the society it serves. The earliest written form of a code for OT practitioners was entitled the "Pledge and Creed for Occupational Therapists" (Mosey, 1981). This document remained unchanged until 1977 (Mosey, 1981). Since 1977, the profession's code of ethics has continued to evolve, undergoing revisions in 1979, 1988, 1994, and 2000 (AOTA, 2000). This document is reviewed every 6 years, so another revision may occur in the near future.

The AOTA's *Occupational Therapy Code of Ethics* "is a public statement of the common set of values and principles used to promote and maintain high standards of behavior in occupational therapy" (AOTA, 2000, p. 614). Seven principles are included in the current version. These 7 principles center on the well-being of those who receive our services, confidentiality, competence, complying with laws and policies, the provision of accurate truthful information, and the fair treatment of colleagues and other professionals (AOTA, 2000). The principles contained in the code help clarify our core values and provide

guidance by showing their connection to the daily life of a student or practitioner. This document can be easily accessed and should be periodically reviewed by those to whom it applies, including educators, students, practitioners, administrators, consultants, entrepreneurs, and researchers who are members of AOTA (AOTA, 2003). The latest version of the *Occupational Therapy Code of Ethics* is available on-line by selecting "About AOTA," then "Occupational Therapy Code of Ethics 2000" from AOTA's homepage at the following address: www.aota.org.

When a student becomes a member of the AOTA, he or she commits to following the *Occupational Therapy Code of Ethics* and its Enforcement Procedures (Hansen, 2003a). The Enforcement Procedures for *Occupational Therapy Code of Ethics* (2002) appear in the *Reference Guide to the Occupational Therapy Code of Ethics* (AOTA, 2003). Although a student may not be a member of AOTA, the OT program in which he or she is enrolled may use this code of ethics as part of its student Code of Conduct. It is suggested that you determine which code or codes apply at your particular educational setting as well as those that may be specific to your state or geographical practice area. Although many State Regulatory Boards use AOTA's *Occupational Therapy Code of Ethics* as their standard of ethical behavior (Hansen, 2003a), others have their own language to address ethical conduct. Therefore, it is prudent to ensure that you understand which version is in effect and follow any and all applicable ethical codes.

PROFESSIONAL BEHAVIOR

A job becomes a profession once it has been recognized as such by a society (Mosey, 1981). The profession is then awarded certain privileges, such as status and autonomy. In return, however, the profession has a responsibility to serve that society in a competent and respectful manner. Professional behavior is necessary for all students and practitioners of a profession to uphold its responsibility to society. Professional conduct encompasses a wide array of behaviors that are important for success both in classroom and practice environments. Examples of professional behavior that are important factors in students' academic and clinical success include punctuality, enthusiasm, cooperation, communicating appropriately (both verbally and nonverbally), the ability to accept criticism, and being nonjudgmental.

Many OT educational programs have developed feedback mechanisms to encourage the development of these crucial behaviors among students. Kasar, Clark, Watson, and Pfister developed a form at the University of Scranton, which includes 10 items that address such topics as communication skills, initiation, and clinical reasoning. This form appears as an appendix in a textbook on professional behaviors (Kasar & Clark, 2000). It is a good tool for students and faculty to evaluate classroom behaviors that are linked to success in fieldwork and employment.

It is important for students to receive frequent feedback regarding the skills and behaviors they have successfully mastered, as well as those requiring additional work. The presence of unprofessional behavior indicates an area in which feedback is needed. Some examples of unprofessional behaviors include missing class, tardiness, failing to contribute your fair share to a group project, leaving trash in the classroom, leaving your cell phone on, and engaging in side conversations during class. Often students do not realize the impact of these behaviors on others. Many of the above-mentioned unacceptable behaviors are distracting to teachers as well as student peers. These behaviors are not tolerated during fieldwork placements or employment settings and should also not be tolerated in the academic setting. In addition, they are contrary to the values of nonmaleficence and beneficence.

UNETHICAL BEHAVIOR

Acting in a manner counter to the principles detailed in any ethical code or student code of conduct that applies to you is unethical behavior. Some students, at times, engage in unethical behavior. When confronted about these behaviors, they often express dismay and confusion, not understanding that their behavior is unacceptable and bothersome to others. They are, after all, not "bad" people. They mean no harm, and therefore often fail to see the "wrong" in what they have done. Upon further questioning, however, students behaving unprofessionally or unethically often admit they simply had not thought clearly about their behavior and had allowed the stress of school or other important life roles to cloud their judgment.

Problem behaviors vary in seriousness. The resulting consequences usually vary in direct proportion to the seriousness of the problem behavior. Behaviors described above as being unprofessional, such as engaging in side conversations during class, can be viewed as both unprofessional and unethical. They are viewed as unethical since the behavior is contrary to the core values of freedom and equality because the behavior disturbs the educational process of their peers. Regardless of how disruptive this particular behavior is viewed on a continuum of problem behaviors, it is far less serious than, for example, plagiarism. Plagiarism and other serious unethical behaviors will be discussed below.

PROBLEM STUDENT BEHAVIORS

It is important, as a preventive measure, to outline possible behaviors students may lapse into that can place them at risk for failure or expulsion from their OT educational program. This way you, as a student, can monitor your own behavior and develop appropriate behaviors and skills that are needed to be a competent student and future practitioner, educator, or researcher. The development of positive professional habits is easier and more rewarding than the difficult challenge of changing poor habits once they are ingrained. In addition, you should be aware of unprofessional and unethical behaviors in others and develop skills to appropriately confront peers who engage in such behaviors. It is also important to remember that as a member of an institution or organization, you may be obligated to report breaches of student conduct codes or the AOTA *Occupational Therapy Code of Ethics*.

A variety of problem behaviors are described below. This list is by no means exhaustive, but serves to illustrate inappropriate behaviors that are sometimes encountered by OT academic and clinical faculty. When a fellow student observes such behaviors, he or she should be aware that it is appropriate and necessary to confront the individual or individuals involved. This confrontation may not be easy. Help in analyzing the situation may be needed and is available from a number of sources identified later in this chapter. Although confronting unethical behavior is not easy, it ultimately benefits the individuals involved as well as the profession and society.

Some of the behaviors described below are blatantly unethical (e.g., plagiarism); these behaviors are on the very serious end of the continuum of unethical and unprofessional behaviors. Other behaviors, however, may be less obvious and could be argued as being nonissues by some individuals (e.g., misguided motivation to become an OT practitioner). These behaviors have been placed at the end of the list and are followed by a discussion of the associated ambiguity.

Confidentiality

As an OT student, you will have access to a variety of personal information about clients and their families. Depending on the size of your community and your fieldwork placement, you may know these people either directly or indirectly. The temptation to gossip can be strong but must be avoided. Telling "war stories" can help health professionals cope with the human suffering encountered during the process of assisting people in adapting to stressful circumstances. However, care must be exercised both in terms of to whom and where these stories are told. Be careful to maintain proper confidentiality and respect for clients.

Students should respect the confidentiality of information that is shared by peers and instructors in class. "Due to the nature of OT education, sometimes students and instructors have personal examples that are relevant to class discussions. This information should be respected and not used for gossip" (Reitz, 1997, p. 252). Confidentiality is required under Principle 3E of the AOTA *Occupational Therapy Code of Ethics*, which states: "Occupational therapy personnel shall protect all privileged, confidential forms of written, verbal, and electronic communication gained from educational, practice, research, and investigational activities unless otherwise mandated by local, state or federal regulations" (AOTA, 2000, p. 615).

Sexual/Dating Relationships

It is inappropriate for students to date their instructors, mentors, supervisors, clients, or client's family member. Most schools have policies that address this issue. Many professional ethical codes also prohibit this behavior either directly or indirectly. In some places, certain professions, such as psychologists, specify that such relationships are considered inappropriate even after the professional relationship has ended (State of Maryland, Title 10, 1992). Students should seek clarification of the prevailing code at their educational institution and within the regulatory body of their state or other applicable jurisdiction.

Dating and maintaining a sexual relationship with a client would be in violation of Principle 2A of the AOTA *Occupational Therapy Code of Ethics*. This principle states, "occupational therapy personnel shall maintain relationships that do not exploit the recipient of services sexually, physically, emotionally, financially, socially or in any other manner" (AOTA, 2000, p. 614). In addition, students should be aware that engaging "in a sexual relationship with a minor or patient with mental impairments would be breaching Principle 2A" (Kyler-Hutchison & Mah, 2003, p. 81). Participating in this type of behavior is also most likely a criminal act (Kyler-Hutchison & Mah, 2003).

Lack of Commitment to the Educational Process

Studies have reported a variety of reasons why students cheat, including "pressure to get high grades, parental pressure, a desire to excel, pressure to get a job, laziness, a lack of responsibility, a lack of character, poor self-image, a lack of pride in a job well done, and a lack of personal integrity" (McCabe, Treviño, & Butterfield, 2001, p. 228). Students in an OT program may cheat for similar reasons. For example, at times, students, for a variety of reasons, may be unaware of or lose sight of the importance of individual assignments and the purpose of those assignments relative to the goals of the overall curriculum. Sometimes this lack of awareness is of limited consequence. However, at other times it may lead students to dismiss assignments as "busy work" and cause them to use shortcuts that undermine the true goals of the assignments. These shortcuts often involve some sort of cheating. This cheating can take the form of re-working a friend's old paper and submitting it as original work, collaborating on an assignment that was supposed to be completed independently, making up data instead of collecting it, taking old papers or drafts of other students' work from the recycling bin or shared hard drive in a computer lab, or sharing answers during an exam.

All of these behaviors are serious and may result in equally serious consequences as determined by your specific OT educational program. They also show a lack of understanding and respect for the curriculum. Assignments are carefully crafted to ensure that each student develops the skills he or she needs to be a competent practitioner. Cheating, therefore, can negatively impact the development of skills necessary to be a competent practitioner. It is also inconsistent with the core values of justice and truth and Principles 4 through 6 of the AOTA *Occupational Therapy Code of Ethics*. The end result is that cheating shortchanges the student and the profession, but, most sadly, it is likely to hurt the future clients of those engaging in this behavior.

Appropriate Collaboration Versus Cheating

The faculty in OT educational programs are responsible for assisting in the development of OTs and OTAs through a variety of methods, including individual and group work. The faculty is also responsible for evaluating the academic performance of each student to determine his or her level of skill, knowledge, clinical reasoning, and readiness for fieldwork placement. Each student's individual and group work must be examined to properly conduct this ongoing evaluation. Faculty members complete this task in order to ensure that students receive the feedback necessary to develop into competent and ethical OT professionals.

Group activities and assignments are meaningful learning tools. However, it is important to remember that your study partners will not necessarily be there beside you as you treat patients in your future careers. You must each be able to function independently as competent therapists. Even when working with other team members, you must be capable of providing competent and thorough patient care independent of the skills of your colleagues. However, this independence does not mean that as an OT practitioner you are prohibited from seeking additional supervision or mentoring when needed. In fact, it is encouraged by Principles 4D and 4G of the AOTA *Occupational Therapy Code of Ethics*.

Plagiarism

In general, plagiarism is considered "unauthorized use of works or ideas from others without permission or proper credit. Using the 'intellectual property' of others without permission or proper credit constitutes theft, as would improper acquisition of physical property" (Pigg, 1989, p. 103). Most OT schools and publications follow the recommended style described in the most current *Publication Manual of the American Psychological Association* (APA, 2001), which is often referred to as the *APA Publication Manual*. The *APA Publication Manual* indicates that when paraphrasing is used, proper credit must be given to the original author or source. The manual also provides guidance and cautions such as being aware that if you quote a sizable passage from a source in addition to citing the source, you may need to contact the copyright holder for permission to use the material. In addition, techniques to cite electronic sources are reviewed. You need to be aware that resources found on the web and other electronic media are also covered by rules of plagiarism. If you are found to have committed plagiarism, a claim of lack of knowledge that the type of material or length required a specific citation method or permission will not excuse your behavior.

Plagiarism is a form of cheating. It is also theft (Kornblau, 2003). Not only does it falsely represent a student's knowledge, but it also fails to provide well-deserved credit to individuals who have worked hard to add to the body of knowledge. It is also stealing intellectual property. This theft includes using work found not only in books or journals but also information from presentations or workshops at conferences, digital video discs (DVDs) or other such media, and the internet (Kornblau, 2003).

Plagiarism can be the result of poor time management or lack of understanding about professional writing. However, neither of these reasons is sufficient excuse for this behavior. Drummond (1998) differentiates between active plagiarism and passive plagiarism. Active plagiarism is the purposeful act of using another person's work without giving credit, whereas passive plagiarism is the use of copying and pasting passages from a variety of sources with no credit given to the original sources. Students engaging in passive plagiarism incorrectly assume they have created original work through this patchwork approach. Every OT student is responsible for knowing what plagiarism is and for taking steps to prevent it. Plagiarism is also inconsistent with the core values of justice and truth addressed in Principles 4 through 6 of the AOTA *Occupational Therapy Code of Ethics*.

Lack of Respect for Resources

There are probably few experiences that are more frustrating to students than to spend time identifying articles needed for a project and then find that the articles have been ripped out of the identified journals (Reitz, 1997). It is also frustrating for students planning to print a paper in a computer lab to find that they cannot do so because someone failed to correctly logout the computer or incorrectly reconfigured the printer cables. Students need to respect shared learning resources and take responsibility for learning to use technology correctly. Vandalism and theft of materials, which are more extreme examples of failure to respect shared resources, are a breach of Principle 5A of the AOTA *Occupational Therapy Code of Ethics*. This principle states that "occupational therapy personnel shall familiarize themselves with and seek to understand and abide by applicable Association policies; local, state, and federal laws; and institutional rules" (AOTA, 2000, p. 615).

Faculty and Student Collaboration

Excellent research and program development can occur when students and faculty work together. To ensure that this relationship is positive, it is important to address a number of issues prior to the initiation of the project. These issues include "authorship, ownership of data, and subsequent use of data" (O'Rourke, 1989, p. 101). Students who work on a collaborative project with a faculty member and then write an article based on the project may be unaware of the need to share authorship or acknowledge the assistance of others. Depending upon the scope of the faculty member's contribution, it may be appropriate to share or possibly use a form of joint authorship with the faculty member acknowledged as primary author. O'Rourke (1989) indicates that the following contributions merit joint authorship: idea generator, designer, implementer, data processor, data analyzer, editor or writer, or graduate assistant (p. 102).

The *APA Publication Manual* (APA, 2001) provides the following guidance: "principal authorship and other publication credit [should] accurately reflect the relative scientific or professional contributions of the individuals involved, regardless of their relative status... minor contributions to the research or to the writing for publications [need to be]... appropriately acknowledged" (pp. 395-396). If a joint publication results primarily from a student's thesis or dissertation, it is customary for the student to be the first author. Assigning appropriate authorship is supported by Principle 7B, which states "occupational therapy personnel shall accurately represent their qualifications, views, contributions, and findings of colleagues" (AOTA, 2000, p. 615).

As a student you should be aware of any published policies or procedures in your program that pertain to student and faculty responsibilities associated with faculty projects. If you are planning to participate in a collaborative activity with a faculty member and your school does not have a policy, helpful resources can be found in the health education literature (Greenberg, Allen, & Noland, 1981) and the OT literature (Kyler-Hutchison, 1998). In addition, other OT educational programs may be willing to share their research and publication ethics policies.

Limited/Specialized Interest

Some faculty members strongly believe that future OT practitioners should be committed to all humans and their quest to maximize their human potential. Students who wish to be OT practitioners but only work with a certain subset of clients are often viewed with concern by these faculty. They may question the appropriateness of admitting students who wish to work only with children, clients with hand injuries, or clients with physical disabilities.

These concerns are based on a number of factors. When students make premature decisions about areas of specialization, they may close themselves to opportunities for learning and other future career possibilities. Student biases concern faculty, as they may indicate a lack of compassion for humanity as a whole, a lack of the ability to work with chronic patients, or a lack of desire to work with patients that are seen in some way as undesirable. With today's changing job market, there is no guarantee that future employment options will match the selected client group desired by the student. Students need to be competent and willing to work with any and all individuals, families, and communities in need of OT services.

The profession's practitioners must uphold their responsibility to address the above concerns, which are clearly supported by Principle 1A: "OT personnel shall provide services in fair and equitable manner. They shall recognize and appreciate the cultural components of economics, geography, race, ethnicity, religious and political factors, marital status, sexual orientation, and disability of all recipients of their services" (AOTA, 2000, p. 614).

Misguided Motivation to Become an Occupational Therapy Practitioner

In the past, potential practitioners were frequently attracted to the field by its creative, humanistic approach to health. Individuals who wished to make a difference in the health and welfare of society could do so by becoming either an OT or OTA. As the demand for OT services increased through the years, so did salaries. Some faculty members voiced concern regarding the commitment of students who were primarily attracted to the profession by job security and financial rewards. As the employment outlook becomes more expansive and lucrative, these concerns are re-emerging.

The following questions are examples of this concern. What happens now that the job market has shifted and salaries are increasing in medical model settings? Will individuals practicing in the community remain committed to their community-based clients? Will students view financial benefits as the primary factor in the decision making as to whom they will serve?

The need to pose and answer questions similar to those above is supported by Principles 1A, 1B, and 1C. In addition to these principles, one can argue that an individual selecting the profession for misguided reasons is not being truthful or honest to the ideals as articulated in the *Core Values and Attitudes of Occupational Therapy Practice* (AOTA, 1993).

One may argue, however, that the values of a profession change as both society and the profession itself change. What if students are only partially attracted to the profession due to high salaries? Is the concern raised above still appropriate? An emphasis on financial compensation may not be "wrong" as long as practitioners are competent and uphold the AOTA *Occupational Therapy Code of Ethics*. What do you think?

The above example shows that ethical decision making is often not clear at first. A situation that may initially appear to be problematic may not truly be so once more information is gathered. It is important to avoid jumping to conclusions when confronted with a possible ethical dilemma. It is equally important to avoid rashly accusing someone of wrongdoing in the "heat" of the moment. In addition, care needs to be taken to make sure that your actions are based not on "personal bias or prejudice," but on objective data before accusations are made or a complaint filed (AOTA, 2003, p. 29). In addition, prior to lodging a complaint, you should first be sure you have all the information available, address the issue with the person or persons involved, and have made a good faith effort to resolve the dilemma. The best way to approach a potential ethical issue is to systematically analyze the situation and follow one of the various models available to guide decision making.

PRACTICE DILEMMAS

Many of the problem behaviors described above would be considered unethical if exhibited in a practice setting. For example, lack of respect for resources in the clinical environment is unethical in the case of practitioners using either computers or copying machines for personal reasons. Arriving late for team meetings or engaging in side conversations during meetings, family conferences, supervisory conferences, or rounds is unethical since it impacts negatively on colleagues and the care of the client. Thus, this type of behavior is contrary to the concept of beneficence described earlier in this chapter. Individuals encountering peers engaging in unethical workplace behaviors such as these are obligated to take appropriate action. In the case of tardiness or talking in class or meetings, the appropriate action would be to confront the individual regarding his or her behavior and its impact on others, especially those we serve. As a rule, the first step in resolving a potential breach of ethics is to discuss your concerns with the individual(s) involved. In this way, you are modeling both professional and ethical conduct.

Practice dilemmas can involve issues of documentation, supervision, and billing. Documentation must be timely, accurate, and describe practice that is appropriate for the level of education and experience of the OT or OTA. This assertion is supported by Principle 4E, which states that "Occupational therapy practitioners shall protect service recipients by ensuring that duties assumed by or assigned to other OT personnel match credentials, qualifications, experience, and scope of practice" (AOTA, 2000, p. 615). It is also supported by Principles 4D and 5E.

One aspect of supervision is addressed in Principle 4E as stated above. In addition, Principles 4F and 5A state that OT practitioners shall comply with local, state, and federal laws. This means that the practitioner is responsible for being familiar with laws that relate to OT practice, including those associated with supervision. Since laws and institutional rules—especially those pertaining to supervision—can vary, it is recommended that students and practitioners be aware of all laws that relate to their geographic and specialty areas. State regulatory boards can be helpful in obtaining this information. All OT practitioners have an ethical obligation to know and understand state licensure, registration, or certification regulations.

All billing must be accurate and appropriate. It is the responsibility of practitioners to be aware of coding and billing regulations as well as charges. Without this knowledge, it is difficult to fulfill Principle 1B, which states:

> Occupational therapy practitioners shall strive to ensure that fees are fair and reasonable and commensurate with the service performed. When occupational therapy practitioners set fees, they shall set fees considering institutional, local, state, and federal requirements, and with due regard for the service recipient's ability to pay. (AOTA, 2000, p. 614)

ANALYZING ETHICAL DILEMMAS

There are several methods to use when analyzing an ethical situation (Aroskar, 1980; Hansen, Kamp, & Reitz, 1988; Morris, 2003; Reitz & Kyler, 1998; Trompetter, Hansen, & Kyler-Hutchison, 1998). These methods are similar in many ways. One method that embodies the essence of the various methods was developed by Hansen and Kyler-Hutchison and used by Kyler-Hutchison in her contribution to the text *Ethical and Legal Dilemmas in Occupational Therapy* (Bailey & Schwartzberg, 1995). This method includes finding the answers to the following 4 questions:

1. Who are the players in the dilemma?
2. What other facts or information are needed?
3. What actions may be taken?
4. What are the possible consequences of each action? (Kyler-Hutchison in Bailey & Schwartzberg, 1995, p. vi)

After answering these 4 questions, you should have a better understanding of the situation and be able to select a course of action you are comfortable with and are able to defend.

PROFESSIONAL BEHAVIORS

A variety of human resources are available to assist you in analyzing an ethical dilemma and following through with your decision. These resources include your faculty advisor, faculty members, program director, and state association president. Other individuals include state regulatory board members, Credentialing Services Staff at the NBCOT, the Chairperson or members of the AOTA's Commission on Standards and Ethics (SEC), the AOTA Ethics Officer, or the AOTA SEC Staff Liaison.

Various documents that provide guidance are also available and should be referred to if you are thinking of reporting a potential breach of ethics. One of these documents, the Enforcement Procedure for *Occupational Therapy Code of Ethics* (AOTA, 2002), is included in the *Reference Guide to the Occupational Therapy Code of Ethics* (Scott, 2003). Another document, *Disciplinary Action: Whose Responsibility?* (Hansen, 2003b), provides a useful chart that helps the student or practitioner determine the organization(s) to which a report should be directed.

Hansen (2003a) further details the ethical jurisdiction and roles of 3 primary organizations that process complaints regarding potential ethical violations. These organizations include the AOTA, the National Board for Certification in Occupational Therapy, Inc. (NBCOT), and State Regulatory Boards. Additional articles in the *Reference Guide to the Occupational Therapy Code of Ethics* (Scott, 2003) cover such important topics as payment for services, patient abandonment, discrimination, plagiarism, confidentiality, and documentation.

Additional literature exists that helps the student and practitioner to continue to study this important area of OT practice. Another AOTA publication, *Effective Documentation for Occupational Therapy* (Acquaviva, 1998), contains chapters that discuss fraud and ethical and legal issues surrounding OT documentation. The OT Search is an on-line bibliographic database that is accessible from the AOTA home page to individuals and institutions subscribing to this service. This database can assist the student in locating relevant articles pertaining to ethics. The student is encouraged to use the reference list following this chapter to further his or her understanding of OT ethics.

SOCIAL AND OCCUPATIONAL JUSTICE

Social justice emerged as a topic of discussion in the discipline with the work of Townsend (1993) and has led to a collaborative venture by Townsend and Wilcock to develop the construct of occupational justice (Wilcock & Townsend, 2000). The beliefs embodied in the construct of social justice is consistent with the values of the profession from its inception. A variation of social justice, occupational justice specifically focuses on the relationship between occupational opportunities and health and justice (Wilcock, 1998; Wilcock & Townsend, 2000). Occupational justice is "the promotion of social and economic change to increase individual, community, and political awareness, resources, and equitable opportunities for diverse occupational opportunities which enable people to meet their potential and experience well-being" (Wilcock, 1998, p. 257).

Social justice and its relationship to the well-being of communities was the topic of the University of Southern California, Department of Occupational Science and Occupational Therapy's (University of Southern California, 2002) *14th Annual Occupational Science Symposium, Occupational Science and the Making of Community.* Wilcock (1998) defined "an occupationally just society" as a society "that provided opportunity for people to develop their own potential, rather than be expected to fit into socioeconomically established roles" (p. 237). The World Federation of Occupational Therapists recently ratified a position paper on Community Based Rehabilitation that outlines the role of OT in "helping to overcome occupational deprivation and occupational apartheid leading to occupational justice" and is preparing a position paper on human rights (Sinclair, 2004).

Do you believe you have a duty to combat occupational and social injustice? Does the *Occupational Therapy Code of Ethics* support occupational justice? The concepts of social justice and occupational justice are being embraced by academia. Rybski and Arnold (2003) described a course developed and taught at St. Louis University entitled *Broadening the Concepts of Community and Occupation: Perspectives in a Global Society.* One of the course objectives was for students to "define occupational justice and compare and contrast it to social justice" (Rybski & Arnold, p. 2). The *Occupational Therapy Code of Ethics* is an example of the highest level of universal moral principles and includes "principles that apply to all OT personnel, regardless of race, gender, and creed. The spirit of the Code is not limited only to members of AOTA, but extends an obligation of respect and care toward all" (Morris, 2003, p. 22).

Does this obligation support your responsibility to combat social inequities and occupational injustice through practice, education, research, and advocacy to promote social participation for all individuals?

SUMMARY

A profession must uphold its duty to society and do all that is reasonable to protect the public from unethical practitioners. OTs and OTAs have a duty and responsibility to educate and assist students in developing and maintaining a high level of ethical practice by modeling such behavior. OT students must prepare to be fully competent, ethical practitioners. This preparation includes the development of a solid foundation in ethical behavior. This chapter has provided an introduction to ethics, terminology, the AOTA's *Occupational Therapy Code of Ethics*, a method to analyze ethical dilemmas, and thoughts regarding our duty to address issues of social and occupational injustice. It has also provided information regarding resources for further study and assistance with ethical concerns. Students are strongly encouraged to use these resources. Students and practitioners must consistently demonstrate the highest ethical standards in their behavior and all actions, which reflect directly on the OT profession. Failure to do so is a disservice to our patients, their families, and the society we serve.

ACKNOWLEDGMENTS

The author would like to express her appreciation for the assistance provided by the following individuals: members of the AOTA's SEC for review of content; Frederick D. Reitz, editing skills; as well as Elizabeth Frey and Gar Wing Tsang for locating resources.

LEARNING ASSIGNMENTS

1. Does your state or territory have a regulatory board? See if they have a Web site and find the code of ethics or ethics statement. Is it the same or different from the AOTA's *Occupational Therapy Code of Ethics*? Identify the similarities and differences.

2. Does your school and program have a Code of Ethics? An Honor Code? Are they the same or different from the AOTA's *Occupational Therapy Code of Ethics*? Identify the similarities and differences.

3. Identify 3 possible ethical dilemmas you have experienced as an OT student. Use the method described in this chapter to analyze one of the dilemmas.

4. Do you believe you have a duty to combat occupational and social injustice? Does the AOTA's *Occupational Therapy Code of Ethics* support occupational justice?

REFERENCES

Acquaviva, J. D. (1998). *Effective documentation for occupational therapy* (2nd ed.). Bethesda, MD: American Occupational Therapy Association.

American Psychological Association. (2001). *Publication manual of the American Psychological Association* (5th ed.). Washington, DC: Author.

American Occupational Therapy Association. (1993). Core values and attitudes of occupational therapy practice. *American Journal of Occupational Therapy, 47*, 1085-1086.

American Occupational Therapy Association. (2000). Occupational therapy code of ethics. *American Journal Occupational Therapy, 54*, 614-616.

American Occupational Therapy Association. (2003). Enforcement procedures for Occupational Therapy Code of Ethics. In J. B. Scott (Ed.), *Reference guide to the occupational therapy code of ethics* (pp. 29-35). Bethesda, MD: Author.

Aroskar, M. (1980). Anatomy of an ethical dilemma: The practice (Part II). *American Journal of Nursing, 80*, 661-663.

Bailey, D. M., & Schwartzberg, S. L. (1995). *Ethical and legal dilemmas in occupational therapy*. Philadelphia: F. A. Davis.

Beauchamp, T. L., & Childress, J. F. (2001). *Principles of biomedical ethics* (5th ed.). New York: Oxford University Press.

Drummond, L. (1998). ENGW 2323: Research & Argumentation Policies: Plagiarism. St Edward's University. Retrieved May 16, 2004, from http://stedwards.edu/hum/drummond/23pol.html

Greenberg, J., Allen, R., & Noland, M. (1981). Ethics and policy governing faculty and students. *Journal of the American College Health Association, 30*, 141-142.

Hansen, R. (2003a). Purpose of a professional code of ethics and an overview of the ethical jurisdiction of the AOTA, NBCOT, and SRBs. In J. B. Scott (Ed.), *Reference Guide to the OT Code of Ethics* (pp. 24-26). Bethesda, MD: American Occupational Therapy Association Press. (Excerpted from 1998 publication)

Hansen, R. (2003b). Disciplinary action: Whose responsibility? In J. B. Scott (Ed.), *Reference Guide to the Occupational Therapy Code of Ethics* (p. 23). Bethesda, MD: American Occupational Therapy Association Press. (Originally published 1994, revised, 1999, edited 2000)

Hansen, R. A., Kamp, L., & Reitz, S. (1988). Two practitioner's analyses of occupational therapy practice dilemmas. *American Journal of Occupational Therapy, 42*, 312-319.

Kasar, J., & Clark, E. N. (2000). *Developing professional behaviors*. Thorofare, NJ: SLACK Incorporated.

Kornblau, B. L. (2003). Commission on standards and ethics of the American Occupational Therapy Association advisory opinion on plagiarism. In J. B. Scott (Ed.), *Reference guide to the occupational therapy Code of Ethics* (pp. 52-54). Bethesda, MD: Author.

Kyler-Hutchison, P. (1998). Issues in ethics: Who's the author? Who's the owner? In AOTA, *Commission on Standards and Ethics, 1998 Reference guide to the occupational therapy Code of Ethics* (pp. 51-52). Bethesda, MD: American Occupational Therapy Association.

Kyler-Hutchison, P., & Mah, A. (2003). Unethical and illegal: What's the difference? In J. B. Scott (Ed.), *Reference guide to the occupational therapy Code of Ethics* (p. 81). Bethesda, MD: Author.

McCabe, D. L., Treviño, L. K., & Butterfield, K. B. (2001). Cheating in academic institutions: A decade of research. *Ethics & Behavior, 11*(3), 219-232.

Morris, J. (2003). Is it possible to be ethical? *OT Practice, 8*(4), 18-23.

Mosey, A. C. (1981). *Occupational therapy: Configuration of a profession*. New York: Raven Press.

O'Rourke, T. W. (1989). The student-professor relationship. In N. K. Iammarino, T. W. O'Rorke, R. M. Pigg, & A. D. Weinberg (Eds.), Ethical issues in research and publication. *Journal of School Health, 59*, 101-102.

Pigg, R. M. (1989). Integrity in the publication process. In N. K. Iammarino, T. W. O'Rorke, R. M., Pigg, & A. D. Weinberg (Eds.). Ethical issues in research and publication. *Journal of School Health, 59*, 103-104.

Reitz, S. M. (1997). Ethics for students. In K. Sladyk (Ed.), *OT primer: A guide to college success* (pp. 245-255). Thorofare, NJ: SLACK Incorporated.

Reitz, S. M., & Kyler, P. (1998). Ethical issues in documentation. In J. D. Acquaviva (Ed.), *Effective documentation for occupational therapy* (2nd ed., pp. 237-272). Bethesda, MD: American Occupational Therapy Association.

Rybski, D., & Arnold, M. J. (2003). Broadening the concepts of community and occupation: Perspectives in a global society. Paper presented October 17, 2003 at the Society for the Study of Occupation: USA Second Annual Research Conference, Park City, Utah.

Scott, J. B. (Ed.). (2003). *Reference guide to the occupational therapy Code of Ethics*. Bethesda, MD: American Occupational Therapy Association.

Sinclair, K. (2004). Message to the AOTA Representative Assembly from the WFOT President. Department of Rehabilitation Sciences, Hong Kong Polytechnic University.

State of Maryland, Title 10, Department of Health and Mental Hygiene. (1992). Board of Examiners of Psychologists, Code of Ethics and Professional Conduct, p. 2. [10.36.05]. Health Occupation Article.

Townsend, E. (1993). Muriel Driver Memorial Lecture: Occupational therapy's social vision. *Canadian Journal of Occupational Therapy*, 60(4), 174-183.

Trompetter, L., Hansen, R. A., & Kyler-Hutchison, P. (1998). Frameworks for ethical decision making-revised. In P. Kyler (Ed.), *Reference guide to the occupational therapy Code of Ethics* (p. 34). Bethesda, MD: American Occupational Therapy Association. (Originally published 1994, revised, 1998)

University of Southern California, Department of Occupational Science and Occupational Therapy. (2002). 14th Annual Occupational Science Symposium, Occupational Science and the Making of Community. Davidson Center, Los Angeles.

Wilcock, A. A. (1998). *An occupational perspective of health.* Thorofare, NJ: SLACK.

Wilcock, A. A., & Townsend, E. (2000). Occupational terminology interactive dialogue: Occupational justice. *Journal of Occupational Science, 7*(2), 84-86.

Key Concepts

- Teamwork: Successful team dynamics working to the patient's benefit.
- Team building: Members feel ministration, mastery, and maturation.

Essential Vocabulary

interdisciplinary: Several disciplines collaborate in decision-making.
intradisciplinary: Treatment within a discipline.
mastery: Feeling control over one's environment.
maturation: Goal renewal and improvement.
ministration: Feeling closeness with coworkers.
multidisciplinary: Several disciplines treat the person.
transdisciplinary: An integrated team collaborates and often shares treatments.

TEAMWORK AND TEAM BUILDING

Ellen Berger Rainville, MS, OTR, FAOTA; Tone Blechert, MA, COTA, ROH; Marianne Christiansen, MA, OTR; and Nancy Kari, MPH, OTR

When you ask people about what it is like being part of a great team, what is most striking is the meaningfulness of the experience. People talk about being part of something larger than themselves, of being connected, of being generative. It becomes quite clear that, for many, their experiences as part of truly great teams stand out as singular periods of life lived to the fullest. Some spend the rest of their lives looking for ways to recapture that spirit. (Senge, 1990, p. 13)

In recent years OTs have been included as members of teams—in education, in health care, on treatment units, in community settings, in management systems, etc.—the list is endless. The expectations inherent in these requests are as variable as the requests themselves. OTs who do not fully understand team dynamics may unintentionally respond to these expectations inappropriately and then feel unsuccessful in their team-related work activities. Because teamwork is such an important part of today's world, OTs need to be knowledgeable and competent in teamwork theory and practice in order to serve their consumers well.

Being an effective team member requires specialized knowledge and responsibility (Dunn et al., 1989). Team members must possess highly sensitive interpersonal communication skills (Navarra, Lipkowitz, & Navarra, 1990; Spencer, 1989), have knowledge and understanding of team development and dynamics (Blechert, Christiansen, & Kari, 1987; Gardner, 1988; Heming, 1988; Magrab, Elder, Kazuk, Pelosi, & Wiegerink, 1981), and demonstrate the ability to engage in collaborative work relationships (Grady, 1990; Guiffrida, 1991; Scheller, 1990). While team participation can be a challenging and sometimes even painful process (Dunn et al., 1989), its rewards include shared pride in goal achievement, increased confidence, and the satisfaction of high rapport (Gardner, 1988; Navarra et al., 1990; Scheller, 1990). The purpose of this chapter, therefore, will be to increase your knowledge and skill related to professional team process and function.

Becoming a respected and accepted member of the team is an important goal and a satisfying experience. There are many kinds of teams. We have all been on one type or another—sports, scouts, church or civic groups, charitable activities, and other activities. A team is defined as "a group of individuals who are committed to a shared purpose, to each other and to working together to achieve common goals" (Briggs, 1997, p. xxi). Effective teamwork can contribute to the welfare of one's patients, create high morale among staff members, and foster a collaborative and an educational climate in the work setting (Beggs, 1962).

The term *effectiveness* is a "buzz word" that has remained with us since the 1990s. Increased health care costs, productivity demands, and personnel shortages, coupled with maldistribution and attrition patterns, have produced problems in the effective delivery of OT services (AOTA, 1991). In geographic areas where there is an ample supply of both therapists and assistants, often only therapists are hired or, when assistants are hired, they are underutilized. The latter situation may result in job dis-satisfaction, decreased commitment and attrition for assistants. With increased demands for cost-effective services, every effort must be made to reduce this attrition. Intra- and interprofessional team building are possible solutions.

Some OT leaders feel that teamwork is "critically important to the vitality and expansion of the profession" (Blechert et al., 1987). An effective team is built on the character and competencies of its members. Team efforts are strengthened as members improve their professional and personal abilities. Satisfied contributing team members are helpful to patients and to each other. These individuals demonstrate a basic personal security. They are confident of their knowledge and abilities and comfortable and honest about their limitations. Much has been written about the team process. This chapter will provide an overview of some key information about this important aspect of service delivery. Once you have begun to serve on a team, if not before, you will wish to peruse some of the additional information available. Some ideas for obtaining further information about teams are provided for you at the end of this chapter.

Table 44-1

Groups Versus Teams

Groups	*Teams*
Members think they are grouped together for administrative purposes only. Individuals work independently; sometimes at cross purposes with others.	Members recognize their interdependence and understand both personal and team goals are best accomplished with mutual support. Time is not wasted struggling over "turf" or attempting personal gain at the expense of others.
Members tend to focus on themselves because they are not sufficiently involved in planning the unit's objectives. They approach their job simply as a hired hand.	Members feel a sense of ownership for their jobs and unit because they are committed to goals they helped establish.
Members are told what to do rather than being asked what the best approach would be. Suggestions are not encouraged.	Members contribute to the organization's success by applying their unique talent and knowledge to team objectives.
Members distrust the motives of colleagues because they do not understand the role of other members. Expressions of opinion or disagreement are considered divisive and nonsupportive.	Members work in a climate of trust and are encouraged to openly express ideas, opinions, disagreements, and feelings. Questions are welcomed.
Members are so cautious about what they say that real understanding is not possible. Game playing may occur and communication traps may be set to catch the unwary.	Members practice open and honest communication. They make an effort to understand each other's point of view.
Members may receive good training but are limited in applying it to the job by the supervisor or other group members.	Members are encouraged to develop skills and apply what they learn on the job. They receive the support of the team.
Members find themselves in conflict situations that they do not know how to resolve. Their supervisor may put off intervention until serious damage is done.	Members recognize conflict is a normal aspect of human interaction, but they view such situations as an opportunity for new ideas and creativity. They work to resolve conflict quickly and constructively.
Members may or may not participate in decisions affecting the team. Conformity often appears to be more important than positive results.	Members participate in decisions affecting the team, but understand that their leaders must make a final ruling whenever the team cannot decide or an emergency exists. Positive results, not conformity, are the goal.

WHAT IS A TEAM?

Katzenbach and Smith (1993) describe a "real" team as "a small group of people with complementary skills who are committed to a common purpose, performance goals and approaches for which they are held mutually accountable" (p. 45). Teams are different than work groups in that they are by nature collaborative. Teams share leadership, accountability, and success. Teams create specific goals and objectives that they discuss, work toward, and evaluate together. Work groups have a designated leader and they respond to goals and objectives determined by the organization. They run efficient meetings, deliver individual outcomes (products), have polite discussions, and meet because they are required to. Teams have fun and enjoy working together. In each organization, there are opportunities for teams or work groups. Remember that they are both important methods to get work done but that they are not the same.

Types of Teams

Table 44-1 illustrates important differences between groups and teams. As you can see, teams involve careful, intentional interactions aimed at facilitating achievement of the team's mission and goals. Service on a team offers opportunities for creative expression, for professional development and specialization, and for ongoing learning, along with great responsibility. Each team member shares responsibility for the actions of the group. For some, this is a supportive environment; for others, it can be intimidating. In any case, it can be a great adventure!

There are many types of teams. Teams are characterized by their purpose, such as educational teams, rehabilitation services teams, management teams, as well as by the ways in which they are organized and how their members interact. These interactions fall along a continuum from multidisciplinary to transdisciplinary as illustrated in Table 44-2.

Table 44-2

Team Interaction Continuum

Intradisciplinary

One or more members of one discipline provide treatment to the individual. Generally, other disciplines are not involved. If other disciplines are involved, communication is limited.

Multidisciplinary

A number of professionals conduct assessments and interventions independent from one another. Some formal communications occur between involved professionals. Resources and responsibilities are individually allocated between disciplines.

Interdisciplinary

Several disciplines agree to collaborate for decision making. Evaluation and intervention are still conducted independently, within defined areas of each profession's expertise. Formal communications, such as treatment planning meetings, do occur to exchange information, prioritize needs, and allocate resources and responsibilities.

Transdisciplinary

An interdisciplinary team whose members are committed to ongoing communication, collaboration, and share decision making for the patient's benefit. Evaluations and interventions are planned cooperatively. Programs are often the responsibility of a primary interventionist, but treatments are often shared. Ongoing training, support supervision, cooperation, and consultation among disciplines is important to this model.

QUALITIES OF EFFECTIVE TEAMS

Team members need to have effective communication, they must listen to each other, assert their own points of view, and negotiate constructively in order to have the best outcomes (Alpert et al., 1992; Henneman, Lee, & Cohen, 1995; Stewart, 1990). Teamwork is characterized by shared understandings, goals, values, visions, and responsibilities. These must occur in both word and deed (Brown, Thurman, & Pearl, 1993; Crepeau, 1991; Dunst, Trivette, & Deal, 1988; Lawlor & Mattingly, 1998; Stewart, 1990).

In the early 1960s, Levinson (1962) and his colleagues conducted an important study of workers at a new company. They found that the employees were engaged in a process of fulfilling mutual needs and expectations. A climate of successful reciprocity (a mutual giving and receiving or exchange) was built and the following contributing behaviors were observed (Blechert & Hansen, 1986; Levinson, 1962):

- Others are treated as individuals.
- Individual differences are appreciated.
- Relationships are established with those who are different.
- Flexibility is shown in stressful situations.
- Satisfaction is derived from a wide variety of sources.
- Strengths as well as limitations are accepted.
- Realistic self-concepts are exhibited.
- Activity and productivity are evident.

We have known for a rather long time that these behaviors and others are important to the success of teamwork and team building efforts. The mutual trust and respect that characterize successful team collaborations are evident when the team demonstrates the following:

- Equitable access to information
- Equal opportunity
- Fair representation
- Reliable interactions
- Open, positive attitudes
- Frequent kudos (Briggs, 1997; Hinojosa & Anderson, 1991; Kurtz, Dowrick, Levy, & Batshaw, 1996)
- Mutual recognition of competence and caring (Alpert et al., 1992; Henneman, Lee, & Cohen, 1995; Stewart, 1990)

Factors that inhibit successful teamwork include the following (Rosin, 1996):

- Problems with scheduling and time
- Differing values about team interaction, emanating either from the team members or from their organizations
- Unacknowledged or unresolved differences among team members
- Inadequate resources
- Inadequate communication
- Poor management

Among the qualities of a successful OT practitioner, several are worthy of discussion as they relate to effective teamwork. These are cooperation, flexibility, and creativity.

Cooperation

The old adage "united we stand, divided we fall…" is so true here. Team members work together to achieve common goals. In this effort, each individual must pay attention to the details that make cooperation possible. The OTs and OTAs on the team must be well informed about one another's activities.

Cooperation allows the opportunity to teach and learn, to give and receive, and to increase the competence of all involved. A respectful attitude toward the other members of one's team is extremely important. As people work together more closely, they will learn a great deal of information about each other. Team members must be discreet and avoid petty gossip. Cooperation is easiest if trust is maintained.

Flexibility

A successful team member sees change as positive. New or changing approaches and methods are met with an open and accepting mind. This openness to change encourages all team members to think creatively and express ideas freely.

Creativity

OT personnel pride themselves on their creative abilities. Certainly one would hope for an atmosphere that encourages creativity among staff members. Teamwork demands an environment that is permissive enough to allow new ideas to develop and yet structured enough to provide order and direction for all members. The organizational environment can facilitate or inhibit team functioning. Therefore, the purpose and philosophy of the work setting and each team member's understanding of his or her own duties and the duties of other departmental members is very important.

LEARNING

Understanding and collaborating with colleagues and consumers in order to improve quality of life and ability to function are expressed purposes of health care and educational teams. Together, team members explore the available sources of information from the literature, from the consumer's voice (interview or observation), from physical and psychosocial testing and evaluation, from ongoing attention to the process of therapy, etc. At each step of the process, team members' knowledge increases and they learn not just about their consumer but about each other and, if they are willing, themselves. Effective team leaders are teachers who facilitate (not instruct) learning for everyone on the team (Senge, 1990).

There are many management tools that support team members. One such tool is the job description, a list of the tasks that one is expected to perform at work. A written copy of one's job description as well as those of coworkers can increase team members' understanding of shared and individual responsibilities. Other tools, including mission statements, strategic plans, team building activities, even office design, influence the team's function. Every team develops its own culture, rituals, values, and practices, all of which are recognized, respected, and shared.

TEAM BUILDING

Napier and Gershenfeld (1983) defined team building as a process that facilitates the development of a group of people

with respect to their unique needs, their degree of readiness, and their past experience. They also point out the importance of team members having opportunities "to experience each other in a wide variety of situations" as well as through activities that "provide permission for a group to look at its own behavior and also to explore new ways of approaching problems in order to be more effective." Effective workplace team building is founded on the principle that teamwork meets specific needs of people in the areas of ministration, mastery, and maturation. When these needs are effectively met, both the individual and the team will grow and flourish. If they are not met, team dysfunction will occur (Blechert & Christiansen, 1986; Levinson, 1962).

Ministration

Ministration refers to our need to feel a sense of closeness with coworkers; to feel safe, guided and supported; and to experience acceptance, trust, and respect. For example, think about how it feels to be a new OTA student or employee unfamiliar with everything or so it seems. Team members who provide extra orientation, anticipate questions, and indicate a willingness to listen to the students fears and uncertainties help meet your ministration needs. When a team member tells you that it is okay to make a mistake and demonstrates an understanding that errors are an inherent part of the learning process, you feel a certain level of safety and support. Being able to "shadow" an experienced colleague, observing his or her actions, and listening to his or her reasoning is an incredible way to learn and to become a team member. Even after you have been working for some time, it is very helpful to collaborate with others by shadowing or cotreating with colleagues.

Some people may need a significant amount of support (ministration) in their work, whereas others may require very little. Some staff and students are uncomfortable telling their supervisor how much support they need in order to function effectively; however, a supervisor will often sense these needs in their behavior. It is important nonetheless for people to take responsibility and communicate any feelings of discomfort or lack of support. If the supervisor is unable to provide the support needed, he or she should be prepared to offer other sources of gratification. The team experience often helps to fill this gap. When students' and staff members' needs for ministration are met, they are likely to perceive the workplace as "caring."

Mastery

The need for mastery is concerned with the desire to explore, understand, and, to some extent, control one's self and one's environment (Levinson, 1962). Mastery involves increasing proficiency in job activities. This occurs through role exploration, practice experience, reflection, and performance review. The need for mastery can be met in a variety of ways, such as developing a high level of expertise and an enhanced role in a particular area of therapeutic intervention. Shadowing, mentoring, and other forms of collegial collaboration are also important. Also, taking advantage of opportunities to provide leadership to others through assuming supervisory and educational roles enhances mastery at many levels. Feedback on all professional activities should be actively sought from supervisors, peers, consumers, and other knowledgeable persons and these ideas should be incorporated into your practice.

A supervisor who is sensitive to the student or staff person's need for mastery will provide an appropriate measure of control early in the fieldwork or employment experience. This control may take the form of offering choices in assignments for instance. Supervisors usually appreciate a student or employee's interest in achieving independence; therefore, it is important to verbalize one's specific goals and needs. For the OTA, important competencies to be achieved must include more than those relevant to consumer care. For example, the ability to deal adequately with professionals from other departments, as well as other OT personnel, should be important goals.

Maturation

Maturation involves personal and professional goal renewal, risk taking for goal achievement, and the empowerment of others. For example, the OTA who seeks out activities and programs that maintain as well as expand his or her professional roles is demonstrating a mature desire to be a lifelong learner. Seeking new responsibilities involving risks, such as developing a new program, and becoming a mentor to another person are other ways that this need can be addressed. If maturation needs are met, a person unfolds; if they are not met, the person stagnates. Fieldwork provides reality-testing opportunities for a student as concepts learned in school are applied in a real situation. This reality testing takes the form of feedback from supervisors and patients as a result of one's efforts. Feedback provides a student with the sense of growth necessary for some maturation to take place.

DEVELOPMENTAL TEAM BUILDING

The developmental team chart shown in Table 44-3 presents a team building process organized according to stages of team development, characteristics of the particular stage, supervisor tasks, team member tasks, and communication issues. The levels of ministration, mastery, and maturation are also delineated. When using this chart it is important for the reader to consider the following (Blechert et al., 1987):

- Developmental information may be used to assess current team functioning.
- Developmental factors that may enhance group functioning are important team builders.
- The stages listed are not absolute and may overlap.
- Teams are unique and their experiences may not always parallel the chart.
- Teams evolve according to their experiences along the developmental continuum (Bull, 1976; Corey, 1981; Hagberg, 1984).

TEAM MEMBERSHIP

The purpose of a health care, educational, or rehabilitative team is to provide the best possible service to the consumer through the sharing of information and expertise and the coordination of services. A professional member usually heads the team, although it is possible for the consumer to serve as team leader. It is most common for a representative of the organization(s) with professional responsibility for the implementation of services to serve in that role. The members of the team may include any number of people who provide services or assistance for the consumer. For example, in home health care, the team might include the consumer, the physician, the nurse, social worker, certified nurse assistant, homemaker, spouse, and OT. In the public school, it might include the special education administrator, classroom teacher, parent, child, and OT. Involvement of the consumer at every level of team decision making and action is critical to outcome. It is important to assess for yourself how much teams value and respect the consumers of their care. Those who respect their consumers even to the level of seeing them as equal participants on the team are likely to have such respect for all team members. As stated earlier, such mutuality contributes to the success and satisfaction of a team. Table 44-4 provides brief definitions of the professionals with whom OTs commonly interact.

As we work with professionals from other disciplines, it is useful to ask them about their professional fields. Remember that your consumers are your colleagues as well as other professionals and their perspectives are invaluable to your understanding. You will learn a great deal about their knowledge and skills by understanding their education, philosophy, goals, values, etc. You will enhance your professional services by drawing on the expertise of others and you in turn will enhance theirs. Listen carefully to your colleagues as they express their opinions about the strengths and needs of individual consumers. Compare your perspectives and discuss openly where you agree, where you disagree, and where you might be able not only to compromise but also to learn more together. Be open to the perspectives of others. I think that you will find that you may have more similarities than differences and by respecting others you will find that they are better able to listen to and respect you. The type of collaborative teaching and learning that happens in effective teams is a remarkable experience.

Although the information on effective team building presented in this section can be applied to many professional team interactions, a critical focus is the intraprofessional relationship between OTs and OTAs. The relationship of teamwork to effective service delivery in OT has been identified as a major theme for our profession. If personnel within the same profession can work effectively as team players, it seems that teamwork that includes others will follow easily.

In summary, it is very helpful to understand the roles and responsibilities as well as the respective contributions of each team member. Teams that work well together are best able to accomplish such objectives as:

Table 44-3

Developmental Team Chart

Stage of Team Development	Characteristics	Supervisor's Tasks	Team Members' Issues	Communication
I. Initiation Stage Exploration and definition of member roles and responsibilities within the context of team and work settings.	Prior to and in the beginning phase of team formation, individuals may experience self-doubt, lack of trust, role ambiguity, and a degree of powerlessness in the work setting.	Promote atmosphere of acceptance and trust: state expectations openly, encourage discussion of members' expectations. Encourage commitment to learn building by helping members: identify skills, areas of strength and interest, increase self-esteem. Provide general definition and direction for newly formed team: define situation and resources available, define roles/responsibilities for members.	Learn and explore role expectations. Begin to share resources, identify own areas of expertise and interests.	Express anxieties and insecurities of new relationships. Verbalize support for team efforts. Demonstrate acceptance and begin to develop trust.
II. Transition Stage Adjustment and rearrangement of roles to create a team.	Team members experience increased anxieties, defensiveness, and struggles for control. Reclarification and adjustments of roles are evident. Group norms are forming. Relationship issues are important at this stage.	Provide encouragement. Manage conflict openly. Provide structures for team to make decisions, solve problems, and set priorities. Evaluate intervention strategies if needed. Reclarify roles, team goals.	Develop skills, gain confidence. Learn about the organizational structure. Commit self to teamwork.	Begin to identify and deal with conflicts openly. Verbalize group norms and values. Encourage team affiliation by engaging in community building activities.
III. Working Stage Tasks are identified and achieved.	Team members experience cohesion and productivity. Conflicts are dealt with openly and are effectively managed.	Refine leadership skills. Allow team members more autonomy and support development of their professional skills. Provide liaison functions with the external organization. Help team members find solutions to difficult problems; provide resources and support services. Assess and evaluate work done relative to the team's overall performance.	Participate in the planning, decision-making, and execution of tasks. Clarify personal goals. Ask for direction/support from supervisor. Participate in task evaluation. Develop sense of mastery.	Communicate support and challenge members through feedback. Discuss how methods of problem solving, decision making, and conflict management occur in the team.
IV. Interdependence Stage Team members are effective in their work; achieve interdependence in their working relationships.	Team members are mutually supportive, take pride in the team, value each other, and experience the team as interlocking roles.	Model collegial relationships. Become a mentor; empower others. Continue to develop personal and professional skills.	Reflect on self as a professional, reassess goals, offer peer evaluations. Form multiple points of view. Take risks; achieve greater competency.	Express valuing of team members and demonstrate support for each other's achievements.
Separation Team separation occurs at any stage; however, characteristics and tasks will be different depending on the maturity of the team.	Team members experience anxiety as they anticipate separation. There is an awareness of the successes and failures of the team.	Ensure opportunity for and assist members in summarizing, integrating, and interpreting the team experience. Provide a framework that will help members evaluate the team effort/individual roles. Allow time for members to resolve unfinished business and express feelings about the separation.	Summarize the team experience and the attainment of personal and professional goals. Evaluate personal and team performance. Define tasks for new members.	Express separation feelings. Avoid withdrawal/distancing of members. Give and receive feedback; discuss effect of current experiences on future teams.

Reprinted with permission from Blechert, T. E., Christiansen, M. F., & Kari, N. (1987). Intraprofessional team building. *American Journal of Occupational Therapy, 41,* 576-582.

Table 44-4

Professionals Who Often Serve on Teams With Occupational Therapy Personnel

Physician

A physician is a medical doctor who practices the science and art of preventing and curing disease and preserving health. In most states, physicians must prescribe medical treatments such as medication, surgery, and therapy. OT personnel work with physicians who have varying specialty backgrounds. These specialists may include physiatrist (physical medicine and rehabilitation), psychiatrist (mental illness), neurologist (nervous system disease), orthopedist (musculoskeletal), ophthalmologist (vision), pediatrician (children), gerontologist (elders), and many more.

Clinical Psychologist

The psychologist is not a medical doctor, although he or she may have a PhD. A clinical psychologist functions in 3 areas: diagnosis, psychotherapy, and research. The psychologist administers diagnostic tests and conducts interviews. Psychological tests are made up of a kind of standard situation in which varying reactions of different patients may be observed. Many people are reluctant to reveal their thoughts in an interview, but may show a characteristic way of thinking in response to tests. Psychotherapy may be performed with individual patients or in patient groups, and families may be involved. Psychologists have a background in statistics and research methods and are prepared to assist staff members who wish to do research by helping construct experimental procedures and interpret results.

Nurse

The nurse is concerned with the health of the consumer as well as his or her comfort and care if ill. This involves evaluating and addressing the patient's physical, spiritual, and emotional needs through established nursing procedures and techniques. Nurses are responsible for a variety of therapeutic measures prescribed and delegated by the physician (such as administering medications) and must be able to observe and evaluate patient symptoms, reactions, and progress. Education, support, and anticipatory guidance for the consumer are important aspects of nursing practice.

Social Worker

The role of the social worker is to act as a liaison between the consumer and the community in order to make the best use of the resources available. Social workers may work in public or private hospitals, clinics, community settings, schools, agencies, correctional institutions, and home health. Individuals may be referred to a social worker for help with financial problems, nursing home, or other specialized placement or to access other needed services and benefits. Social workers are also skilled in individual counseling and group work as well as community organization. They may provide both direct services and consultation related to psychosocial issues.

Speech and Language Pathologist

Speech pathologists are concerned with an individual's ability to communicate. This includes attention to his or her understanding of language as well as his or her expression of ideas. Speech pathologists are concerned also with auditory (hearing) ability and work closely with audiologists.

Physical Therapist

A PT provides treatment for patients with disabilities resulting from disease or injury. Various modalities are used in PT, including light therapy, which involves ultraviolet and infrared light; electrotherapy, which may involve diathermy and electrical stimulation; hydrotherapy, which includes equipment such as the Hubbard tank, whirlpool, and contrast baths; mechanical therapy, which involves massage, traction, and therapeutic exercise of various kinds; and thermotherapy, which involves heat such as paraffin baths and whirlpool. The purpose of the treatment may be to relieve pain, to increase function of a body part by improving muscle strength and joint ROM, to increase overall strength and endurance, or to improve mobility. Physical therapists assist people to be mobile with and without assistive devices. They are skilled in the use of wheelchairs, adaptive seating and positioning, walkers, crutches, canes, and other posture and mobility aides.

Therapeutic Recreation Specialist

A therapeutic recreation specialist uses play, leisure, exercise, and other activity to meet individual needs. For example, for some people, group recreation may encourage positive relationships with others, improve body image, allow an outlet for emotional release, aid circulation and other body functions, and provide enjoyment and relaxation. Some activities used in therapeutic recreation are swimming, music, games and conduct dancing, dramatics, special events, and outings. Leisure counseling is also provided.

Vocational Rehabilitation Counselor

A person may need assistance in selecting appropriate and meaningful work or changing careers as a result of his or her illness or injury. For instance, a truck driver who has had a heart attack may need to find a job with less physical demands and stressors. A high school student may need help with career planning and with adaptations for college classes or job training programs. The vocational rehabilitation counselor may administer standardized tests, interest inventories, and aptitude tests as well as personal interviews in order to develop individualized plans for training and job placement. The OT and OTA may work with the vocational counselor in evaluating work readiness, tolerance, coordination, and special skills.

(continued)

Table 44-4

Professionals Who Often Serve on Teams With Occupational Therapy Personnel (continued)

Nutritionist/Dietician

The function of the nutritionist is to advise about (for people living on their own) or actually manage (e.g., in the hospital setting) the preparation and serving of food for consumers. This includes understanding complex nutritional needs and planning and preparing special diets. The nutritionist considers the caloric value, nutrient content, attractiveness, taste, and texture of foods and drinks. OT personnel collaborate with nutrition staff in many ways, from the use of adaptive eating utensils and techniques, to the preparation of nutritious meals and snacks, to decisions about the texture of foods (so as to diminish risks such as swallowing problems or drooling).

Educator

The educator is concerned with the individual's learning. Educators are also known as teachers and have varied educational backgrounds. For example, some teachers are trained to work with children at certain ages and grade levels in schools; others are trained to work with young children and their families. Some educators have specialized knowledge in inclusion, reading, language, arts, music, etc. Their expertise and experience in creating environments and activities that promote learning and understanding is essential to the development of children and adults. OT personnel often collaborate with educators on such areas as curriculum design, activity analysis, environmental modification, and special educational or instructional strategies.

- Establishing a climate of mutual respect and effective working relationships.
- Appreciating the value of others' perspectives on assessment and intervention.
- Communicating effectively regarding the consumers needs, including scheduling.
- Cooperating in planning and providing cost-efficient, considerate services.
- Evaluating the outcomes of services and the consumer's satisfaction with care.

TEAM ROLES AND FUNCTIONS

Table 44-5 illustrates the interrelationships of group individual and situational characteristics on the team process. Team members play multiple roles on the team, often quite different from those specific to their discipline. As the team develops, personality, education, values, and experience interact to influence team members toward different roles. Skilled team leaders can use this phenomenon to benefit their team, and team members learn to rely on each other through the sharing of roles and responsibilities. Table 44-6 lists typical task, maintenance, and self-oriented (personal) roles of team members.

SUMMARY

There is a fable about a farmer whose children did not get along. He asked them to come together and to make a pile of sticks. He laid the sticks side by side and bound them together with string. He then challenged each child to pick up the bundle and break it. One by one they tried and failed. The farmer then untied the bundle and gave the children the sticks one at a time. They broke each one with ease. He said to them, "As long as you remain united, you are a match for anything, but differ and separate and you are undone."

Effective teamwork and team building are essential processes in the profession of occupational therapy. They contribute to quality service delivery and morale, and they can also have a significant influence on reducing OTA attrition. Teamwork qualities include cooperation, flexibility, and creativity. OT practitioners work with many different people to share information, coordinate schedules, and provide the most effective overall services. The basic needs of ministration, mastery, and maturation provide a theme that carries over into the developmental team chart, which presents a team building process organized according to specific developmental stages of teams. The identification of team characteristics, supervisor and member tasks, and communication issues provides a matrix that can serve as an important tool for improved team building.

LEARNING ACTIVITIES

1. Observe various teamwork activities in a health care, educational, or community service setting. List the characteristics that appear to contribute to or hinder effective teamwork. Interview team members about their experiences with the team.

2. Observe various teamwork activities in an athletic setting. List the characteristics that appear to contribute to or hinder effective teamwork. Interview team members about their experiences with the team. What are the similarities/differences with health care, educational, and community teams?

3. Participate in a self-assessment exercise with a peer. Identify the characteristics and experiences that each of you possesses that would contribute to teamwork and

Table 44-5

Team Dynamics

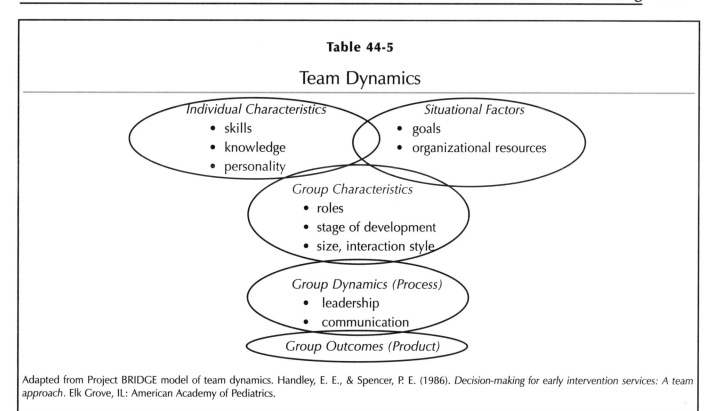

Adapted from Project BRIDGE model of team dynamics. Handley, E. E., & Spencer, P. E. (1986). *Decision-making for early intervention services: A team approach.* Elk Grove, IL: American Academy of Pediatrics.

Table 44-6

Roles of Team Members

Clarifier: Makes sure that the proposed plans are clear to everyone.
Compromiser: Makes accommodations to others, especially in conflict situations.
Consensus tester: Determines the team readiness to make decisions or take action.
Elaborator: Makes sure that proposed plans are fully evaluated.
Encourager: Praises others for their efforts and contributions.
Energizer: Motivates the team into action.
Gatekeeper: Makes certain that all team members have an opportunity to express their opinions.
Harmonizer: Mediates conflicts on the team.
Information gatherer: Collects information that is relevant to the issues.
Initiator: Brings issues to the attention of the team.
Observer: Provides constructive feedback on team dynamics and performance.
Standard setter: Helps the team establish guidelines for the activities.
Summarizer: Reviews all aspects of team issues and ideas.
Tension reliever: Uses humor or changes in routine to reduce or avoid negative interactions.

---

team-building relationships. Try to make some decisions together. Observe how accurate your predictions were.

4. Review the material on professional team members and identify the areas of their services that may overlap with those provided by OT personnel. Interview professionals and consumers about how they see their roles coinciding with those of OT personnel.

5. Study the chart found in Table 44-4 and list additional team member and supervisor tasks for each of the levels as they relate to a particular team problem you have experienced.

6. List and discuss additional communication issues for the stages of team development in terms of a specific personal team situation.

ACKNOWLEDGMENT

I would like to gratefully acknowledge the important influence that my friend and colleague Joanne Miller has had on my understanding of collaboration between OTs and OTAs.

REFERENCES

Alpert, H. B., Goldman, L. D., Kilroy, C. M., & Pike, A. W. (1992). 7 Gryzmish: Toward an understanding of collaboration. *Nursing Clinics of North America, 27*, 47-59.

American Occupational Therapy Association. (1991). Member data survey: Executive summary. *OT Week*, June 6, 1991.

Beggs, D. (Ed.). (1962). *Team coaching: Bold new venture* (pp. 44-47, 131, 456-465). Indiana University: United College Press.

Blechert, T. F., & Christiansen, M. E. (1986). Intraprofessional relationships and socialization: The maturation process. In S. E. Ryan (Ed.), *The certified occupational therapy assistant: Roles and responsibilities*. Thorofare, NJ: SLACK Incorporated.

Blechert, T., Christiansen, M., & Kari, N. (1987). Intraprofessional team building. *American Journal of Occupational Therapy, 41*(9), 576-582.

Briggs, M. H. (1997). *Building early intervention teams: Working together for children and families*. Gaithersburg, MD: Aspen.

Brown, W., Thurman, S. K., & Pearl, L. F. (1993). *Family centered early intervention with infants and toddlers: Innovative cross disciplinary approaches*. Baltimore, MD: Brookes.

Bull, N. (1976). *Teamwork: Working together in the human services*. New York: J. B. Lippincott.

Corey, G. (1981). *Theory and practice of group counseling*. Monterey, CA: Brooks/Cole.

Crepeau, E. B. (1991). Achieving intersubjective understanding: Examples from an occupational therapy treatment session. *American Journal of Occupational Therapy, 45*, 1016-1025.

Dunn, W., Campbell, P., Oetter, P., Hall, S., Berger, E., & Stickland, L. R. (1989). *Guidelines for occupational therapy services in early intervention and preschool settings*. Rockville, MD: American Occupational Therapy Association.

Dunst, C., Trivette, C., & Deal, A. (1988). *Enabling and empowering families: Principles and guidelines for practice*. Cambridge, MA: Brookline Books.

Gardner, H. G. (1988). *Helping others through teamwork*. Washington, DC: Child Welfare League of America.

Grady, A. P. (1990). Nationally speaking—Collaborative relationships: Opportunities for occupational therapy in the 1990s and beyond. *American Journal of Occupational Therapy, 44*(2), 105-108.

Guiffrida, C. (1991). Partnerships for change: Collaboration within and between professions. *Sensory Integration Special Interest Section Newsletter, 14*(4).

Hagberg, J. (1984). *Real power: Stages of personal power in organizations*. Minneapolis: Winston Press.

Heming, D. (1988). The titanic triumvirate: Teams, teamwork, and team building. *Canadian Journal of Occupational Therapy, 55*(1), 15-20.

Henneman, E. A., Lee, J. L., & cohen, J. J. (1995). Collaboration: A concept analysis. *Journal of Advanced Nursing, 21*, 103-109.

Hinojosa, J., & Anderson, J. (1991). Mother's perceptions of home treatment programs for their preschool children with cerebral palsy. *American Journal of Occupational Therapy, 45*, 273-279.

Katzenbach, J. R., & Smith, D. K. (1993). *The wisdom of teams: Creating the high-performance organization*. New York: Harper Business.

Kurtz, L. A., Dowrick, P. W., Levy, S. E., & Batshaw, M. L. (1996). *Handbook of developmental disabilities: Resources for interdisciplinary care*. Gaithersburg, MD: Aspen.

Lawlor, M. C., & Mattingly, C. F. (1998). The complexities embedded in family-centered care. *American Journal of Occupational Therapy, 52*, 259-267.

Levinson, H. (1962). *Men, management and mental stealth*. Cambridge: Harvard University Press.

Magrab, P., Elder, J., Kazuk, E., Pelosi, J., & Wiegerink, R. (1981). *Developing a community team*. Washington, DC: Georgetown University.

Napier, R. W., & Gershenfeld, M. K. (1983). *Making groups work*. Boston: Houghton Mifflin

Navarra, T., Lipkowitz, M. A., & Navarra, J. G. (1990). *Therapeutic communication: A guide to effective interpersonal skills for health care professionals*. Thorofare, NJ: SLACK Incorporated.

Rosin, P. Whitehead, A. D., Tuchman, L. I., Jesien, G. S., Regun. A. I., & Irwin, L. (1996). *Partnerships in family-centered care: A guide to collaborative early intervention*. Baltimore, MD: Paul Brookes.

Senge, P. M. (1990). *The fifth discipline: The art and practice of the learning organization*. London: Random House.

Scheller, M. D. (1990). *Building partnerships in health care*. Palo Alto, CA: Bull Publishing.

Spencer, P. (1989). Team dynamics relative to exemplary early services. In B. E. Hanft (Ed.), *Family centered care* (pp. 4-43-4-50). Rockville, MD: American Occupational Therapy Association.

Stewart, K. (1990). Collaborating with families: Reflections on empowerment. In B. E. Hanft (Ed.), *Family centered care*. Rockville, MD: American Occupational Therapy Association.

SUGGESTED READING

Katzenbach, J. R., & Smith, D. K. (1993). *The wisdom of teams: Creating the high-performance organization*. New York: Harper Business.

Senge, P. M. (1990). *The fifth discipline: The art and practice of the learning organization*. London: Random House.

Senge, P. M., et al (1994). *The fifth discipline fieldbook: Strategies and tools for building a learning organization*. City, ST: Publisher.

Wellins, R. S., Byham, W. C., & Wilson, J. M. (1991). *Empowered teams: Creating self-directed work groups that improve quality*. San Francisco: Jossey-Bass.

Key Concepts

- Effective management: Considers both internal and external factors when making decisions.
- Cost-containment measures: Have both positive and negative effects on OT.
- Laws: Past, current, and pending legislation impact the provision of OT services.
- Reimbursement: Varies based on the type of setting in which one practices.
- Quality of care: Can be enhanced through special accreditation agencies.
- Role of the manager: Performs multiple traditional roles as well as leadership roles.
- Leadership: In order to be effective, management and leadership qualities should not be mutually exclusive.

Essential Vocabulary

case mixed groups: A classification system developed for reimbursement of services provided at the acute rehabilitation level of care.

Commission on Accreditation of Rehabilitation Facilities (CARF): An independent body that accredits rehabilitation programs based on specific standards of care and criteria.

current procedural terminology (CPT) codes: A numerical coding system used to determine reimbursement rates.

diagnostic related group (DRG): A classification system developed for reimbursement of services provided at the acute care level of care.

Functional Independence Measure (FIM): A standardized functional assessment tool utilized in acute rehabilitation settings; a component of the IRF-PAI.

gross domestic product (GDP): The total value of all goods and services produced within a country.

Inpatient Rehabilitation Facilities-Patient Assessment Instrument (IRF-PAI): A patient assessment system used to classify patients for reimbursement of services provided at inpatient rehabilitation facilities.

Joint Commission on Accreditation of Healthcare Organizations (JCAHO): An independent body that accredits a variety of health care organizations based on specific standards of care and criteria.

Medicaid: A state run government health insurance program for lower income individuals.

Medicare: A federal government health insurance program for those over the age of 65 or for those with a disability who qualify for services.

national health care expenditures: The percentage of the GDP that is spent on the delivery of health care services.

prospective payment system (PPS): A process of financing that requires payment in advance for services rendered based on the classification system required at each level of care.

resource utilization group (RUG): A classification system developed for reimbursement of services provided at the subacute level of care.

MANAGEMENT ISSUES

Claudine Bogosian, MHA, OTR

INTRODUCTION

The purpose of this chapter is twofold. First, it will give the reader a global understanding of both the external and internal factors the OT manager faces. What are the external forces and variables that the manager deals with in today's health care environment? What are the internal factors and challenges that the manager must tackle? How does the manager effectively integrate both the internal and external factors to manage and lead a productive and efficiently run organization, department, or program?

Secondly, this chapter will briefly examine the traditional role and functions of the manager, as well as the qualities of effective leadership. Developing an understanding of both areas is imperative when you are in the workforce. The words *manager/management* and *leader/leadership* are often viewed as two separate entities. The manager must integrate these 2 entities for any health organization, OT department, or program to achieve its goals.

It is a fallacy to believe that this chapter is only important to those who aspire to manage a department or organization, develop a program, or for those who are interested in the "business" side of health care. Whether you aspire to any of the above or have a passion for focusing all your efforts on clinical skills, management in some form or another will have an impact on you and your workplace. It is essential to develop an appreciation of the various functions of a manager, as well as an understanding of the management process, as you, as an individual practitioner, are an integral part of the success of this process. Keep in mind that an effective manager asks many questions and he or she may or may not have the answers.

EXTERNAL CONSIDERATIONS

There are a variety of external factors that will have a direct or indirect affect on OT. What happens on Capitol Hill does impact a rural outpatient clinic in Minnesota as it does a major rehabilitation hospital in New York City. The level of funding and type of reimbursement systems for health services, whether through Medicare, Medicaid, managed health care plans, or traditional private insurance, will also have a direct impact on the health organization, OT department, and/or program. Now consider the influence of federal and local regulatory agencies, changes in demographics, technology, research, and costs/utilization, and the manager in today's health care environment faces a multitude of challenges (Spiegel & Hyman, 1994).

Therefore, it is essential to have an appreciation for the various types of external forces, particularly those of an economic and political basis, that will directly affect any health organization. It is imperative for the OT manager to have an understanding of the local, state, and federal political and economic environments in which he or she works, as well as have an understanding of a variety of other external considerations, as mentioned above, in order to make key decisions for the OT program that, in essence, will affect you, the OT practitioner.

The Economic Environment

The current "health" of the economy, as well as economic trends will have a direct impact on the delivery of health care and OT.

It is important for the OT manager to be aware of changes in the GDP, changes in inflation and interest rates, national debt, the federal budget, health care trends, and overall costs of the delivery of health care. All of these factors and trends, either seemingly directly or indirectly related to health care, will have a bearing on your organization's growth and survival in such a dynamic, ever-changing environment. An OT manager who spends time understanding the external environment and its potential impact on the organization is a manager who is keenly aware of how external forces will have an effect on his or her health care organization, and OT in particular.

Overall trends of the economy also need to be considered. Generally speaking, the economy is cyclical. It has a period of prosperous years, and then will have a period of down years. How significant is the national deficit during times of an economical downturn? Is it significant enough for cost containment efforts to be implemented? Will reimbursement rates from insurance companies be lowered? Will new mandates occur at the federal level and change the process of reimbursement from Medicare? Should the economy head for a tailspin, how will the manager foresee its impact on OT, and what changes will need to be made in order to remain viable? These are just a few sample questions the manager must consider when planning and making decisions for the department and/or program.

Quite obviously, it is of great value for the manager to have a solid understanding of the direct relationship between health care and the economy. The delivery of health care is quite costly for the United States government, and it is a system that places a great financial stress to the overall economy. In 1990, the percentage of the GDP for health expenditures was 12%. In 2001, it was just over 14% (CMS, 2002). The Office of the Actuary at the Centers for Medicare and Medicaid (CMS) projects the percentage to reach close to 18% by the year 2012, placing overall health expenditures at $3.1 trillion (CMS, 2002). It is noted that when there is a rapid rise in the GDP, it may be a reflection on the strain within the health care system. An example of this is government's and businesses' inability to finance health care costs that are rapidly increasing faster than our ability to finance them (Levit, 2003). The consequences of such a burden has been the introduction of a variety of cost containment measures, greater scrutiny of resource utilization, increased accountability, and a greater emphasis on outcomes and EBP.

Given this environment, the manager will be challenged to foresee how the current economic environment, as well as the health care sector of the economy, will impact OT. Therefore, the manager must look at the efficiency of processes and cost containment measures within the organization or program in which the OTA practices. A manager may look for involvement from the OTA by seeking creative solutions or ideas for program development. Perhaps committees may be formed to look at current practices and ways to improve quality of care, while reducing overall costs. OTAs may be asked to be participants in ongoing re-evaluation of current practices and programs; therefore, the OTA will be practicing in an ever-changing environment. The OTA has the ability to bring a unique "day-to-day" perspective to the manager, which will allow him or her to gain valuable insight and aid him or her in the planning and decision-making process.

Cost containment measures have a variety of ramifications to the profession of OT and OTAs. For example, there has been a shift toward using case managers who control resource utilization, a focus on decreasing lengths of stay in hospitals, increasing the prevalence of overlapping clients' treatments to increase the number of interventions per session, as well as reducing the number of professional staff compared to nonprofessional staff (Jacobs, 2003). The role of the OTA is evolving as well. Jacobs (2003) states, "to control costs, organizations are asking OTAs to take on more responsibilities" (p. 59). Cost containment measures need not be viewed as a negative. The result of many cost containment measures inherently creates the impetus to re-evaluate and improve a process that was status quo, redundant, and inefficient. In many instances, cost containment measures cut out waste and inefficiencies through creativity and development of new thought processes. The role of the manager is to facilitate this process and identify when excessive cost containment begins to affect the quality of care.

When considering the economy, it is also important to have an understanding of the pulse of society. What is currently of value to our society as a whole? In the early 1990s, both at the national and local level, the focus of debates across the country was on the consideration of taking steps toward a universal health care system. After 2001, it was homeland security and national defense. More recently, the national discussion has focused on a national prescription drug plan. Why is it important to understand what values society regards as a priority? It is important because perhaps what was once earmarked in the federal budget as the "health care dollar" may shift and become the "national defense dollar" based on what society and the government deems important. Again, this would then have a direct effect on the environment in which you are practicing OT. It is key to understand that money earmarked for one program generally tightens the budget of another.

Political Environment

The political environment of the times, at the federal, state, and local levels, is another area that the OT manager must consider. Consequences to the profession may occur from federal and/or state legislative action that is specific to and targeted directly toward OT. Or, as an example, it may be a change in political parties that causes proposals and discussions to be geared toward either expanding or redefining health care expenditures and programs, such as Medicare. Either way, it is important to note that legislation that is passed, whether related to health care or not, may have a significant impact on OT. For instance, at the federal level, enactment of the Balanced Budget Act of 1997 was the impetus for the drive toward further cost containment measures for Medicare. The change in reimbursement from a fee for service system to a prospective payment system (PPS), an area further discussed later in this chapter, for rehabilitation hospitals, skilled nursing facilities, and home health care is a specific example of this (Rovinsky, 1999). As a result, this law had a direct effect on the way OT services are delivered.

During the presidential campaign of 2000, all candidates pledged a commitment to a prescription drug plan for Medicare recipients that in some form came to fruition in late 2003. How does a prescription drug plan have any affect on OT? Perhaps it may have not have any effect at all, but time will tell. Nevertheless, the manager needs to be aware that it is considered additional spending of monies for the Medicare program, and perhaps, indirectly, reimbursement for OT may or may not be reduced. Again, one must remember that all sectors of health care are competing for the same health care dollar. A manager needs to be aware of this and will try to foresee and be proactive in the planning and decision-making process so as not to allow external factors to affect the quality of care the therapists are providing. The manager may ask him- or herself the following questions: Will this legislation have an effect on reimbursement of OT services? Will this legislation impact the scope of practice for the OT practitioner? How would this legislation affect the clients, consumers, and society we serve (Goodman-Lavey &

Dunbar, 2003)? The answers to these questions may impact OT as a profession, you as an OTA, and your workplace.

There are many other areas of consideration regarding the external environment. A manager's role is to continually ask him- or herself questions and think through hypothetical scenarios. Some examples are: Have there been any changes in the demographics in the community of which OT services are being delivered? Are their advances in technology that may allow for greater efficiency of services provided by the OTA? Are there any proposed changes in the scope of practice for other health care professionals that overlap with OT and would then have an impact on our profession and practice? What and who are in direct competition with our program and/or organization? Is there a niche in the community that the OT program can fulfill to stay ahead of the competition (Richmond, 2003)?

It is important to be aware of current local and state laws, licensure and certification laws, projected changes to these, and its potential impact on the service delivery of OT. In addition, it is also crucial for the manager to be aware of actions by insurance carriers, such as the possibility of excluding OT as a reimbursable service.

Special interest groups, at the local and federal level, also need to be monitored for any potential actions that may have an impact on OT. The OT manager cannot underestimate the power of lobbying and grassroots efforts by these groups.

Reimbursement

Another crucial area that a manager needs to follow closely is the reimbursement process for the services he or she provides. Developing a solid understanding of funding sources and reimbursement for OT services rendered is essential for every manager and practitioner alike. Rules and regulations are constantly changing, as cost containment becomes the utmost priority. The largest reimbursement source for OT is Medicare and Medicaid.

Medicare is considered a federally funded entitlement program that provides health services to its beneficiaries. The Medicare program is overseen by the Centers for Medicare and Medicaid Services within the United States Department of Health and Human Services. Medicare was established in 1965 as Title XVIII of the Social Security Act. Recipients include individuals over the age of 65, some less than 65 years of age with a disability, and those with end stage renal disease (CMS, 2003). It consists of the Hospital Insurance Program, Part A and the Supplementary Medical Insurance Program, Part B. The circumstances in which OT will be provided are as follows: It must be 1) prescribed by a doctor, 2) performed by an OT practitioner, 3) medically indicated for the treatment of the persons diagnosis (Thomas, 2003).

Medicaid, which is Title XIX of the Social Security Act, is administered at the state level for those with lower incomes. Although Medicaid derives some of its funding at the federal level, it is considered a state run program. Therefore, each state has its own eligibility requirements, range of available services, and reimbursement rates. It is important to note that Medicaid rules and regulations do vary between states (CMS, 2004a).

Other funding sources for OT services may be from private insurances or managed care plans. The reimbursement rate for OT will differ from the various plans, and it is important to note what the clients whom you are treating are eligible for. For example, does the plan cover OT services? Is there a set amount of visits? Does the plan cover durable medical equipment? There are a variety of other questions that need to be explored prior to your intervention. It is important to note that parameters such as extent and type of coverage, eligibility of services, reimbursement processes, and limitations vary from each insurance company and even vary among the variety of plans the insurance carrier offers (Thomas, 2003).

The types of payment systems for Medicare vary for each setting. Below is a brief overview of the most common payment systems. Keep in mind that this is an area that requires the practitioner to remain vigilant and mindful of the basic premise for payment based on the setting in which you practice. This is an area that is under constant scrutiny and rules and payment policies are ever changing, perhaps even at the time of this publication.

Acute care hospitals were the first to be reimbursed by a PPS. Since 1983, clients admitted to acute care hospitals are classified into a DRG. Clients are grouped based on factors including, but not limited to diagnosis, age, comorbidities, and status upon discharge (Logigian, 1989). Each DRG has a payment associated with it that the hospital will receive. Therefore, it is left to the hospital to determine the mix of services and diagnostic interventions reasonable and appropriate for the patient within the given predetermined payment rate. Historically, acute hospitals were paid retrospectively. The patient would be admitted, receive necessary services and diagnostic tests, and then would be discharged. The hospital then generated a bill and submitted it to Medicare. Medicare would then provide payment to the hospital, within reason, and certain limitations would apply. Now, Medicare determines what the average cost would be, based on the diagnosis and other factors, to receive care for each patient upon admission. Prospective payment systems were introduced to acute care hospitals as a cost containment measure.

Inpatient rehabilitation hospitals and units, referred to as inpatient rehabilitation facilities (IRFs), also use a PPS, which was implemented in 2000. The system is set up similarly to DRGs; however, IRFs use a different assessment system for determining payment. The IRF PPS utilizes information from a patient assessment instrument (IRF-PAI) to classify patients into case mix groups (CMGs) (CMS, 2004b). The FIM is a component of the IRF-PAI. It is a widely utilized functional assessment instrument in the acute rehabilitation setting, consisting of 18 functional items that are scored on a scale based on the level of assistance the patient requires to perform the 18 identified areas (University of Buffalo Foundation Activities (UBFA), Inc., 2002).

Skilled nursing facilities (SNFs) utilize a PPS system of payment as well through a different process. As similar with other settings, SNFs receive a set payment for each admission. However, a resident is evaluated using the Minimum Data Set (MDS). The MDS consists of protocols, guidelines, and assessments. Upon completion of the MDS based on the protocols, the patient is placed into a Resource Utilization Group (RUG). Each RUG category is based on the number of total minutes of therapy provided to the patient per week (CMS, 2004c).

The rehabilitation categories include the following:

- Ultra high: Treatment minimum of 720 minutes weekly. At least 2 disciplines, one discipline at least 5 days per week and one discipline 3 days per week.
- Very high: Treatment minimum of 500 minutes weekly. At least one discipline 5 days per week.
- High: Treatment minimum of 325 minutes weekly. At least one discipline 5 days per week.
- Medium: Treatment minimum of 150 minutes weekly. Five days across 3 disciplines.
- Low: Treatment minimum of 45 minutes weekly over at least 3 days (Murer, 2001).

Outpatient OT is covered under Medicare Part B. Medicare must certify the outpatient facility in order to be eligible for reimbursement. Once the patient has paid his or her yearly deductible, Medicare will reimburse the provider, in this case, the outpatient facility, 80% of the costs incurred. The system, which the outpatient facility is reimbursed, is called the Medicare Physician Fee Schedule (MPFS). Interventions that the OT practitioner performs are based on the Current Procedural Terminology (CPT) codes. It is important for one to be aware of the variety of CPT codes for appropriate and legal billing procedures. If not billed under the correct CPT code, your services will not be reimbursed (Thomas, 2003).

Home health agencies are also reimbursed through a PPS system. Reimbursement is received for each client based on the results of the Outcome and Assessment Information Set. The agency is then paid the corresponding rate for a 60-day time period (CMS, 2003). A client qualifies for OT services in the home if he or she is homebound and requires intermittent skilled nursing care, PT, or speech-language therapy. Once that criteria is met, an OT practitioner may provide services (CMS, 2002).

Reimbursement for OT, to an extent, does influence the scope of services that are provided. Therefore, it is important for the manager to be aware of changes, such as, for example, amendments to the original Balanced Budget Act of 1997, adjustments to the standard rates of reimbursement, or procedural and/or policy changes that are made by CMS and/or the legislative branch of the government. As a practitioner, it is essential to develop strong documentation skills to ensure that the treatment rendered will be reimbursed.

One may argue that the above external considerations are out of the individual manager's control. While this may be true, an effective manager will identify and consider all the external factors and trends of the time to effectively make decisions and implement changes in order for OT to remain viable and cutting edge. In addition, practitioners can promote favorable changes to these external factors by becoming involved with advocacy groups for the community that they serve, as well as involvement with state and national OT associations.

Regulatory Agencies

It is important to note that federal, state, and local laws and regulations will affect your practice, the OT department, and/or place of employment. It is important to become familiar with these agencies and how these regulations affect you and the OT department and/or program. For example, the focus of many regulatory agencies is on safe practices for the protection of clients and employees. The Department of Public Health requires that certain safety standards be met. Local agencies may require that specific regulations be met as they relate to fire safety and local emergency planning.

An example of a federal law that was passed that is not specific to OT but indirectly impacts an aspect of how we practice is the Health Insurance Portability and Accountability Act (HIPAA). HIPAA was signed into law on August 21, 1996. In summary, this law helps protect citizens by affording them new protections that improve "portability" and continuous health care coverage when, for example, one changes jobs, loses his or her health care coverage, or gets married (U.S. Department of Labor, 2004). A specific aspect of this law that was recently effective as of April 2003 was implementation of the HIPAA Privacy Rules. These new regulations affect all areas of the health care continuum, and OT departments and programs were also expected to be in compliance. There are many aspects of this rule, but in summary, it allows for additional protections for the safeguard and protection of medical information and records as it pertains to the client. In today's technologically driven society, this new rule, for example, allows for control mechanisms to be in place when information is transmitted via computer, limits medical information being disclosed to a third party without authorization, and allows for easier access to one's health information (U.S. Department of Health and Human Services, 2003. As an individual practitioner, it is imperative that one is aware of these regulations when discussing and/or transmitting confidential information regarding clients.

In addition, state licensure or certification laws specifically regulate OTAs. It is important for both the manager and the individual practitioner to be aware of the state laws and regulations to be sure all are in compliance. States may also require ongoing continuing education requirements. Since each state's requirements vary considerably, it is important to become familiar with the laws of the state in which you practice. It is also helpful to contact either the AOTA and/or the state OT association to help guide you through this process.

Accreditation

There are also agencies from which health care organizations choose to seek accreditation. The two most common organizations that directly impact OT are JCAHO and CARF. JCAHO accredits organizations across the health care spectrum, whereas CARF specifically accredits rehabilitation programs with specialty accreditation for spinal cord and brain injury programs. Should the health care facility choose to be certified from such agencies, there are specific outlined standards that should be achieved by the facility/program. The manager needs to have a solid understanding of these standards, as the basic framework and processes that are followed by the OT department are modeled after the agency's standards. For example, a specific JCAHO standard is "a patient receives education and training specific to the patient's needs and as appropriate to the care, treatment, and services provided" (JCAHO, 2004a).

Although accreditation from these types of agencies is voluntary, the majority of health organizations choose to seek their "seal of approval" as it provides for a slight edge against the competition, provides for a comparison against national standards, and allows for identification of strengths and weaknesses of the health care organization (JCAHO, 2004b).

INTERNAL CONSIDERATIONS

This section will give an overview of both the traditional role of the manager as well as the characteristics that set an effective and successful manager apart from an everyday manager.

Planning

Planning and/or strategic planning is a function of the manager that is a continual process. The ultimate end goal of a strategic plan is to run an efficient, viable, high quality OT department and/or program. As a result, the manager plans both on a short-term and long-term basis. This includes the development of goals and objectives for the OT department and/or program. In the short term, the focus of planning is on the day-to-day operations, including scheduling of clients and staff meetings, staffing plans, and program development. In the long term, the focus of planning is on assessing the external factors, mentioned in the previous section, and planning for its potential impact on OT. Development of policies and procedures are also completed. In addition, developing and/or redefining strategic goals and identifying the objectives to achieve those goals are part of the planning process for the manager (Liebler & McConnell, 2004; Rakich, Longest Jr., & Darr, 1992).

For example, if one of the strategic goals for the OT department is to provide high quality care in the most cost effective manner, then one needs to develop plans in order to achieve and maintain this goal. How is high quality maintained? Is it through staff training? Is it through reimbursement for continuing education classes? How do we keep costs to a minimum? The answer to these questions will be the framework for the objectives.

Planning for any structural changes to improve efficiency and quality of care must be carefully thought out as well. What are the benefits of the structural changes? Do they improve communication? Do they improve client satisfaction? Do they improve the practitioners' ability to carry out the necessary treatments? Do the benefits outweigh the budgetary impact it may have?

Planning is all encompassing for every aspect of the OT department, whether it is staffed with 5 therapists or 35 therapists. Very often, planning starts when a vision is conceptualized. Therefore, planning is the process of bringing the vision into reality. It is important to note that "visions" and "strategic plans" are not the same. Planning tends to be a step-by-step intended and deliberate process to reach a goal that is written on paper (Kouzes & Posner, 2002). Visions look beyond the strategic plan and require active involvement with the people of the organization. Visions will be discussed later in the chapter.

The participants in the planning process are not just executives and department heads. It can involve the practitioner as well. You may be called upon to offer your input and perspectives since you can offer a unique vantage point that can aid the manager in the planning process.

Decision Making

Decision making is another traditional role of the manager. The decision a manager makes affects all members of the OT staff. The manager is faced with making several decisions each day. He or she may be presented with several choices, and by understanding and analyzing all the considerations, alternatives, and ramifications, the manager tries to make the most informed and effective decision. Whether the perception is that the decision made was correct or incorrect, the manager is responsible for the final decision and subsequent consequences from that decision. Therefore, in order to make effective decisions, the manager must be able to take a step back and define and analyze the problem prior to developing possible solutions and alternatives (Drucker, 1986). Decisions are sometimes not popular with staff; however, the manager needs to make decisions that will be beneficial to the organization and OT on the whole and not what is best for individuals. Whenever possible, an effective manager will explain the rationale behind the decisions that are made.

Organizing

Organizing includes determining who reports to whom, such as what the organizational chart represents. Organizing also includes development of roles and responsibilities and outlining the processes that occur during the workday. For example, how will the OT treatment and workday be structured? What are the roles and responsibilities of staff members? What are the job descriptions, expectations, and responsibilities at each level (Liebler & McConnell, 2004; Rakich et al., 1992)?

Organizing may also include development of committees for program development or for short-term projects. Committees formed should always have goals and objectives, action plans associated with each objective with timeframes, as well as a general timeframe for the committee to be in existence. Committees usually disband once the objectives are met.

Directing

Directing involves the manager exerting his or her influence so as to guide others toward achieving their professional goals as well as achieving the global goals of the organization. Directing often incorporates the manager's use of his or her inherent authority and by making statements and commands to the staff that the manager expects to be followed (Perinchief, 2003). This role has evolved throughout the past decade from a more authority-like figure to one who is collaborative, mentoring, and empowering of others in order to achieve the objectives of the department. This area, linked closely with leadership, will be discussed in greater detail later in the chapter.

Staffing

Staffing includes development of the right staffing mix, such as the OT-to-OTA-to-OT aide ratio. It also involves interviewing and selecting potential employees. This area consists of ongoing performance appraisals of staff members, staff development, and staff retention efforts.

In addition, this is an area that includes outlining verbal and written action plans for staff. The OT manager works closely with the human resources personnel during the above-mentioned process (Liebler & McConnell, 2004; Rakich et al., 1992).

Controlling

Controlling involves assessment of the internal practices of the organization and/or department, identifying areas that require intervention, making changes, monitoring those changes, and making a final assessment as to the effectiveness of changes implemented. Generally, this process has undergone many name changes throughout the decades, from quality assurance to continuous quality improvement to performance improvement. Whatever the current term is, the process and goals remain the same. Many facilities have their own performance improvement department or a key staff member that will oversee this process for the entire organization (Liebler & McConnell, 2004; Rakich et al., 1992). In addition, areas of resource allocation/budgeting, information systems, and productivity for therapy personnel are examples of "control" or "control systems."

In summary, the above-mentioned "roles" of the manager are considered fluid. The manager may be performing one of these roles exclusively, but more often than not, the manager may be performing 2 or more simultaneously, or perhaps he or she may be "moving" between one role and another if circumstances deem it necessary. The traditional roles outlined have been around for decades. What has been changing is the approach the manager takes in performing these roles. For example, when making decisions, is the manager making them independently of others' opinions or is he or she considering the opinions of other staff members? If decisions are made while considering the opinions and input of staff, then the manager is aware of how to blend the traditional roles of the manager with qualities that make one an effective leader.

Is it Leadership or Management?

Is there a difference between leadership and management? In theory, perhaps there is. However, in order to be a successful manager, one needs to believe in and practice the qualities of a leader. Therefore, the leader should understand the roles of the manager, and the manager should possess the qualities of a leader. The two should not be exclusive of one another.

As mentioned in the introduction, as an OTA, it is important to have a solid understanding of management roles and issues whether you aspire to become a manager or not. If you are part of an OT staff, you will be part of and involved with a process of continually seeking ways to improve the quality of care of the clients you treat. Once you start practicing as an OTA, understanding and developing the below mentioned skills will provide a solid foundation for leadership development. It is okay not to aspire to the highest level in your organization, but perhaps you have an idea for a new program, community outreach service, or you are a senior therapist overseeing other OTAs. You will be faced with incorporating some components of the management roles or leadership qualities in some capacity or another. One does not need to be a manager to be a leader. Implementing the characteristics outlined will allow you to elicit behaviors required of others in order to achieve your goals.

Communication

Communication is the cornerstone to effective leadership/management. It is important for the manager to effectively communicate the strategic goals as well as to communicate the vision and roadmap for attaining the objectives. It is also vital to communicate in other areas, as well. In fact, there is not one area that is not important to communicate about. If you want your communication to be effective, it must be clear and simply stated. The only way to establish a connection with others and to be heard is to keep away from fancy jargon and abstract conversations. You will capture attention when others understand the points you are trying to convey. Communication must be truthful and honest. Whatever you communicate you must believe in and what you believe in you must live by example. An effective communicator also allows time for others to respond. Doing so allows others to participate in the process or otherwise you will be perceived as just "talking" (Maxwell, 1999). Communication regarding staffing, brainstorming ideas, policies and procedures, current treatment interventions, and staff development are just some examples that are essential to communicate about. It is also important for communication to occur regarding any possible changes that may impact the practitioner and the rationale for those changes. As OTAs, it is essential to be able to communicate your thoughts, ideas, and concerns to your supervisor and/or manager.

Trust

A manager must develop an environment that fosters trust. Trust and communication compliment each other well. The more open communication there is, the greater level of trust will develop. Trust develops with ongoing open communication, as well as teamwork. Understanding that all of us speak from our own unique perspective or paradigm is the first step to developing trust. Developing an understanding of others' perspectives will allow you to view the same idea, thought, or challenge differently. When that occurs, trust begins to develop. When we work in an environment of trust, it inherently allows for people to try out new strategies, take risks, and feel comfortable making mistakes (Goleman, Boyatzis, & McKee, 2002).

Active Listening

Active listening is beyond hearing what another person is saying. It is developing compassion and reinforcing that what another person is saying is significant. Reiterating what the person to whom you are listening is speaking about is one technique of allowing the person to know you understand what he or she is trying to convey. Maintaining good eye contact is another technique. Often active listening to coworkers and/or clients will allow you to find out information that you otherwise would have not known. Mastering active listening takes time to develop. When you are able to develop this skill, others will see you as approachable and will be willing to discuss their thoughts and ideas openly.

Vision

It is important for the manager to have a vision. Visions are beyond a tangible goal. As mentioned earlier, it is something beyond a goal or plan. Visions are what the manager sees for the future of the team, department, or organization. It creates a sense of unity, purpose, and motivation toward the stated vision. Not all managers are visionary. One needs to look beyond his or her current potential, challenges, and obstacles and see where the organization or department needs to be. Once the vision is developed, there must be a shared commitment from staff members to work toward the identified vision. Again, this is done through open communication, empowering others to feel that they are part of the team, and through motivation (Kouzes & Posner, 2002).

Influencing/Motivating

It is essential for the manager to develop skills that motivate and influence others toward the shared vision. This may occur in a variety of ways, such as empowering staff by allowing for involvement in the decision-making process, holding staff and managers equally accountable, allowing opportunities for opinions to be expressed, and providing positive feedback to staff. If you show you have tremendous confidence in a person, that in itself empowers them, which translates into motivating the individual (Maxwell, 1998). It is essential for the manager to possess these skills to allow for unity, productivity, and staff retention. Yes, it can be argued that motivation should occur from within: self-motivation. However, true leaders are motivational. They recognize that individuals are motivated by different factors. Understanding these factors is key to optimizing staff participation in the process of achieving goals and working toward the vision of the department and/or program (McCormack, Jaffe, & Goodman-Lavery, 2003).

SUMMARY

The role of the manager and the issues he or she faces are challenging and complex. This chapter gives the reader a brief overview of some of these challenges and briefly discusses how one can effectively meet these challenges. Developing a solid understanding of the impact of the external factors coupled with the internal considerations requires considerable skill and ability to balance both areas to create a viable, high quality, efficiently run OT program. It is necessary for all therapists, both the OT and OTA alike, to become involved with the management process as all the roles and functions of the manager will have a direct impact on the practitioner and his or her work environment. Involvement of everyone is key to the success of the OT program as well as to the high level of job satisfaction by the OT practitioner. The OTA can be involved in the process in a variety of ways, including, but not limited to, quality assurance projects, staff supervision, program development, and committee responsibilities.

LEARNING ACTIVITIES

1. Schedule a meeting with the director of an inpatient OT department or rehabilitation department at a local hospital. Inquire as to what service operation tasks they perform on a regular basis. Ask about JCAHO or CARF accreditation and what they had to do to prepare for the site visit by these organizations.

2. Meet with the clinical director of a local mental health clinic and the clinical director of a local substance abuse clinic. How do they differ in their clinical record-keeping procedures, and how might they differ with respect to confidentiality laws?

3. Design a fact sheet for other health care professionals that clearly indicates what services can be provided by an OT or OTA department.

REFERENCES

Centers for Medicare and Medicaid Services.(2002). National health care expenditures projections: 2002-2012. Retrieved February 13, 2004, from www.cms.hhs.gov/statistics/nhe/projections-2002/proj2002.pdf.

Centers for Medicare & Medicaid Services. (2003). Medicare information resource. Retrieved February 13, 2004, from http://www.cms.hhs.gov/medicare.

Centers for Medicare & Medicaid Services. (2004a). Welcome to Medicaid: Site for state & territorial government information. Retrieved April 26, 2004, from http://www.cms.hhs.gov/states.

Centers for Medicare & Medicaid Services. (2004b). Inpatient rehabilitation facility prospective payment system. Retrieved May 6, 2004, from http://www.cms.hhs.gov/providers/irfpps/default.asp.

Centers for Medicare & Medicaid Services. (2004c). Case mix prospective for skilled nursing facilities balanced budget act of 1997. Retrieved May 11, 2004, from http://www.cms.hhs.gov/providers/snfpps_overview.asp.

Drucker, P. F. (1986). *The practice of management.* New York: Harper & Row, Publishers, Inc.

Goleman, D., Boyatzis, R., & McKee, A. (2002). *Primal leadership: Learning to lead with emotional intelligence.* Boston, MA: Harvard Business School Press.

Goodman-Lavey, M., & Dunbar, S. (2003). Federal legislative advocacy. In G. L. McCormack, E. G. Jaffe, & M. Goodman-Lavey (Eds.), *The occupational therapy manager* (4th ed). Bethesda, MD: American Occupational Therapy Association.

Jacobs, K. (2003). Evolution of occupational therapy: the medical model and beyond. In G. L. McCormack, E. G. Jaffe & M. Goodman-Lavey (Eds.), *The occupational therapy manager* (4th ed). Bethesda, MD: American Occupational Therapy Association.

Joint Commission on Accreditation of Hospital Organizations. (2004a). *2004 CAMH—Comprehensive accreditation manual for hospitals.* Oakbrook Terrace, IL: Joint Commission Resources Inc.

Joint Commission on Accreditation of Healthcare Organizations. (2004b). Facts about joint commission in accreditation of healthcare organizations. Retrieved on May 1, 2004, from http://www.jcaho.com/about+us/index.htm.

Kouzes, J. M., & Posner, B. Z. (2002). *The leadership challenge.* San Francisco, CA: Jossey-Bass Publishing.

Levit, K. (2003). Forum on health care spending and medicaid: Trends in U.S. health care spending. Retrieved January 7, 2003, from http://www.kaisernetwork.org/health_cast/uploaded_files/ACF1E.pdf.

Liebler, J. G., & McConnell, C. R. (2004). *Management principles for health professionals* (4th ed.). Boston, MA: Jones & Bartlett Publishing.

Logigian, M. R. (1989). Cost accounting. In K. Jacobs & M. Logigian (Eds.), *Functions of a manager in occupational therapy.* Thorofare, NJ: SLACK incorporated.

Maxwell, J. C. (1998). *The 21 irrefutable laws of leadership: Becoming the person others will want to follow.* Nashville, TN: Thomas Nelson, Publishers, Inc.

Maxwell, J. C. (1999). *The 21 indispensable qualities of a leader: Follow them and people will follow you.* Nashville, TN: Thomas Nelson Publishers, Inc.

McCormack, G. L., Jaffe, E. G., & Goodman-Lavery, M. (2003). *The occupational therapy manager* (4th ed.). Bethesda, MD: American Occupational Therapy Association.

Murer, C. G. (2001). Trends and issues. Rehabilitation management: The Centers for interdisciplinary journal of rehabilitation. Retrieved May 19, 2004, from http://www.rehabpub.com/departments/112001/6.asp.

Perinchief, J. M. (2003). Documentation and management of occupational therapy services. In E. B. Crepeau, E. S. Cohen, & B. A. Boyt Schell (Eds.), *Williard and Spackman's occupational therapy* (10th ed.). Philadelphia: Lippincott, Williams and Wilkins.

Rakich, J. S., Longest, Jr., B. B., & Darr, K. (1992). *Managing health services organizations* (3rd ed.). Baltimore, MD: Health Professions Press, Inc.

Richmond, T. (2003). Marketing. In G. L. McCormack, E. G. Jaffe, & M. Goodman-Lavey (Eds.), *The occupational therapy manager* (4th ed.). Bethesda, MD: American Occupational Therapy Association.

Rovinsky, M. (1999). Provisions of the balanced budget act challenge integrated delivery systems care coordination patterns. Healthcare financial management. Retrieved April 30, 2004, from http://www.findarticles.com/cf_0/m3257/8_53/55471452/print.jhtml.

Spiegel, A. D., & Hyman, H. H. (1994). *Strategic health planning: Methods and techniques applied to marketing and management.* Norwood, NJ: Ablex Publishing Corporation.

Thomas, J. V. (2003). Reimbursement. In G. L. McCormack, E. G. Jaffe, & M. Goodman-Lavey (Eds.), *The occupational therapy manager* (4th ed.). Bethesda, MD: American Occupational Therapy Association.

University of Buffalo Foundation Activities, Inc (2002). *IRF-PAI training manual.* Buffalo, NY: Author.

U.S. Department of Health and Human Services. (2003). Why is the HIPAA privacy rule needed?. Retrieved July 21, 2004, from http://answers.hhs.gov/cgi-bin/hhs.cfg/php/enduser.

U.S. Department of Labor. (2004). Fact sheet: The health insurance portability and accountability act (HIPAA). Retrieved July 21, 2004, from http://www.dol.gov/ebsa/newsroom/fshipaa.html.

Key Concepts

- Continuing competence is a way of life. Health professionals must give priority to the continual development of knowledge and skills in order to provide up-to-date and effective care.
- Professional development is the personal responsibility of the OTA and is crucial to continuing competency.
- Learning relationships are the professional relationships that support, enhance, and prompt learning throughout the OTA's career.
- Self-assessment, establishing learning goals, selecting learning activities, participating in learning activities, and reassessing progress toward goals are crucial elements of the professional development process.
- Documentation of professional development and continuing competency is crucial.

Essential Vocabulary

clinical competence: Having the knowledge, performance skills, interpersonal abilities, critical reasoning skills, and ethical reasoning skills necessary to perform successfully as an OT practitioner.

continuing competence: The development and maintenance of competence in accordance with a specified standard within the OT practitioner's practice context and across time.

professional development: The process of assessing, planning, and engaging in learning relationships and activities for continuing competence within a practitioner's current practice area and/or to expand his or her competence into additional areas of practice to facilitate ongoing growth and development.

portfolio: A collection of evidence that demonstrates the practitioner's ongoing acquisition of the knowledge, skills, and attitudes necessary for fulfilling his or her professional roles.

PROFESSIONAL DEVELOPMENT

Anne Birge James, MS, OTR and Marijke Thamm Kehrhahn, PhD

This chapter describes the process of developing and maintaining clinical competence, the combination of complex knowledge and skills needed to provide effective client care. Clinical competence is developed and maintained through professional development, a lifelong process that begins during an OT practitioner's formal education and spans his or her entire career. During the OTA's coursework and fieldwork, professional development is heavily structured by the academic faculty and clinical supervisors. As OTAs move into clinical practice, however, they must assume primary responsibility for engaging in professional development to maintain clinical competence (Youngstrom, 1998). Fortunately, many resources exist to help the OTA in this crucial component of practice. This chapter will discuss the importance of continuing competence, describe the process of professional development, and provide valuable resources to assist OT practitioners in maintaining the competence needed for providing excellent client care.

COMPETENCE IN OCCUPATIONAL THERAPY PRACTICE

An OTA who has clinical competence possesses the knowledge, performance skills, interpersonal abilities, critical reasoning skills, and ethical reasoning skills necessary to perform successfully as an OT practitioner (AOTA, 1999). Several broad-based essentials of OT practice are inherent to the components of clinical competence, including the demonstration of professional behaviors (Fidler, 1996; Youngstrom, 1998), client-centered care (Moyers, 2003), and EBP (Case-Smith, 2004; Holm, 2000). Clinical competence must be assessed in a professional context (i.e., practitioners are expected to demonstrate competence in the roles that they assume with the client populations served [AOTA, 1999]).

Meeting the OT course requirements, successfully completing fieldwork, and passing the NBCOT certification examination are all methods of establishing initial competence. The profession of OT, however, is continually changing and evolving to meet the demands of the clients, the health care system,

and society (Hinojosa & Blount, 1998). Expansion of technology and information occurs rapidly, constantly altering and improving the theories and techniques used by OT practitioners. OTAs can expect that a significant portion of their professional knowledge is likely to be out of date within 5 years of graduation (Alsop, 2002). The following examples demonstrate just a few of the recent changes in OT practice:

- In 1977, there were 5 Special Interest Sections in the AOTA. In 2004, that number has increased to 11 with 4 subsections 2 specialty networks (AOTA, 2003b).
- It would have been unusual 15 years ago to have a client with a personal computer. Now, it is important for the OTA to be familiar with computers as it is an important ADL for many clients. Additionally, computers provide practitioners with an effective tool for providing home programs that include graphics (including video) capability, providing a level of detail not possible with handwritten programs.
- The World Wide Web was not widely available in 1994. OT practitioners did not require skills in accessing computer networks, either for patient care or for locating and accessing literature to support EBP. Now, the Internet offers a tremendous range of potential services for people with disabilities, including shopping, communication, education, and social support. OT practitioners have a responsibility to remain abreast of Internet-based information and services that may enhance the function of the clients they serve.
- Practice settings have changed dramatically over the past 20 years. In the early 1980s, most OT practitioners worked in institutionalized settings, such as hospitals and nursing homes. Today, many work in community settings, including schools, outpatient clinics, adult day care programs, and homes.
- Ten years ago, few OT practitioners were familiar with the term EBP. Today, practitioners are expected to engage in EBP, which requires skills in locating, accessing, interpreting, critiquing, and applying research evidence to clinical practice (Moyers, 2003; Tickle-Degnen, 1999).

The constantly changing face of OT practice means that OT practitioners must frequently update their knowledge and skills to maintain competence after graduation. Continuing competence incorporates the standards of clinical competence within a temporal context (i.e., the maintenance of clinical competence over time). Developing entry-level competence is typically a joint venture between academic and clinical educators and the student. The educators play a primary role in determining what should be learned and the student works hard to learn the knowledge and skills presented by the educator. The focus is on the basic skills needed to begin practicing as an OTA. Unlike entry-level competence, however, continuing competence cannot be broadly defined. It must be determined based on the needs of the individual OTA, the clients served, the practice setting, and available professional knowledge. Continuing competence, then, becomes the responsibility of the individual practitioner. Several AOTA documents describe the personal responsibility practitioners have for continuing competence (AOTA, 1993, 1998, 1999, 2000), suggesting that the OTA who does not maintain continuing competence has failed to meet the standards of professional practice.

Recently, there has been increased attention on the issue of continuing competence in OT. Questions have been raised regarding the adequacy of current approaches to continuing competence, which have primarily been through self-regulation and continuing education (Hinojosa et al., 2000a). Support for maintaining continuing competence has been variable and is often dependent on the practitioner's practice context and type of supervision (Lysaght, Altschuld, Grant, & Henderson, 2001). To address this issue, the NBCOT has reduced the certification renewal period to 3 years and has initiated continuing competence requirements, requiring OT practitioners to engage in "acceptable professional development activities" (NBCOT, 2003). Some of the professional development activities that are "acceptable" to NBCOT will be described later in this chapter. In 2002, the AOTA's Representative Assembly established the Commission on Continuing Competence and Professional Development (CCCPD) (AOTA, 2002). The focus of the CCCPD is to support continuing education that contains evidence-based content and to develop the Professional Development Tool (PDT) to facilitate practitioners' continuing competence (AOTA, 2002). The NBCOT's well-defined continuing competence requirements and the AOTA's PDT provide additional structure to a rich array of options available to OTAs for maintaining continuing competence.

PROFESSIONAL DEVELOPMENT

Professional development is the process by which health care professionals maintain continuing competence by building and maintaining a rich body of professional knowledge. In OT practice, professional development is now required to maintain certification and, in many states, to maintain licensure as an OTA. Professional development is the ongoing process of assessing one's professional abilities, planning development activities, and engaging in learning relationships and learning activities. Engagement in professional development builds competence within a practitioner's current practice area and/or expands his or her competence into additional areas of practice to facilitate ongoing growth and development (Burkhardt, Braveman, & Gentile, 2002; Hinojosa et al., 2000a).

Stages of Professional Development

Professional development is a continuous process; however, the activities and the focus of professional development vary at different career points. The stages of professional development that follow were selected because they tend to be career "breakpoints" (i.e., times when significant change occurs in one's professional life). Established relationships may come to an end and new ones formed. Responsibilities may change significantly, requiring new skills or knowledge. Van Maanen (1977) stated that breakpoints "require the individual to discover or reformulate certain everyday assumptions about [his or her] working life" (p. 322). Hinojosa et al. (2000b) suggest that "triggers"— "catalysts that help us step back and reflect on our competence to practice at an important juncture in our professional life" (p. CE-2)—can come from external sources (e.g., changes in reimbursement structures) or internal sources (e.g., the practitioner's desire to shift into a new practice area). In other words, these triggers signal increased opportunities for professional challenges that facilitate learning and professional growth. The learning focus for each professional development stage, key learning relationships, and activities associated with each stage are summarized in Table 46-1.

Educational Setting

The professional development process begins within the required coursework for OTAs. Clearly, the learning focus at this stage is on the knowledge and skills needed for competent practice with an emphasis on knowledge within the classroom setting. As described earlier, however, professional development requires an integration of knowledge and skills with professional behaviors. Educational programs are paying increased attention to professional behaviors and are making them a more explicit component of the curriculum by including them into course objectives and teaching students specific skills (Fidler, 1996; Raveh, 1995). Professional behaviors include abilities such as interpersonal and communication skills, management of time and resources, response to constructive feedback, problem solving, critical thinking, professionalism, responsibility, commitment to learning, and stress management (May et al., 1995). Students may be presented with new ways of assessing and enhancing these behaviors that conflict with previously held beliefs and habits.

Fieldwork

Fieldwork offers continued opportunities for students to develop knowledge, but the learning focus shifts from knowledge to skills and professional behaviors. Students do not learn as many new concepts, but they learn how to apply what they know in practical ways. They are frequently presented with situations that do not match their expectations, presenting conflicts that become learning opportunities. For example, a stu-

Phases of Professional Development

Phase of Socialization	Content Focus	Learning Relationships	Process Directed By	Learning Activities
Educational	General knowledge Professional behaviors (Basic skills)	College faculty (Clinical faculty)	College faculty Guidelines for accreditation	Lectures Case studies Reading Written assignments Lab exercises Role playing Observation Reflection
Fieldwork	Skills Professional behaviors Knowledge	Clinical instructor Clients (Other OT personnel) (Team members) (College faculty)	Clinical instructor (Student)	Hands-on experience Reflective dialogue Team meetings Reading/reviewing school notes
Entry-level practice	Knowledge and skills that are setting specific Professional behaviors with focus on independent self-management	Clients Supervisor Other OT personnel Team members OT practitioners outside the institution	OTA (self) - Supervisor collaboration Institutional needs	Hands-on experience Reflective dialogue Reading Online searches In-services Team meetings Conferences Workshops Professional memberships
Job changes	Shift in knowledge and skills to meet needs of new setting Refine professional behaviors in new relationships	Clients Supervisor Other OT personnel Treatment team members OT practitioners outside the institution (expanded since entry-level practice)	OTA (self)-directed with Supervisor input Institutional needs	Renewed focus on: Hands-on experience Reflective dialogue Reading In-services On-line searches Team meetings Conferences Workshops Revise professional memberships (establish new affiliations) Volunteer on committees
Specialization	Focus on knowledge and skills specific to content area Complexity of knowledge and ability to apply in varied situations is developed	Clients Supervisor Team members Specialists outside the institution Other OT personnel	OTA (self)-directed Expert input (may or may or may not be OT) Institutional needs	Hands-on experience Reflection Reading Writing Assist with research On-ine research Presentations Membership in specialty organizations Volunteer on committees Community service

dent with an idea about what spasticity will look and feel like based on a description from a book may find that his or her abstract mental model is very different from what he or she actually sees and feels when he or she first works with a client with spasticity.

Entry-Level Practice

Significant changes in the professional socialization process occur at the trigger point at which an OTA enters practice. The learning focus shifts to meet the demands of the employment setting. The new graduate will still be working on developing the skills and professional behaviors needed in clinical practice but will be presented with new challenges that may not have occurred during fieldwork. Managing his or her own caseload rather than sharing a caseload, meeting productivity demands, learning about available resources, and learning the "politics" of an institution are all examples of new challenges for the entry-level OTA.

Now that the practitioner is an OTA and no longer a student, the process of professional development is more self-directed. An OTA in an entry-level position should have ample opportunity for feedback and direction from the supervising OT, but the final decision about professional goals, learning relationships, and learning activities will be up the OTA.

Job Changes

The professional development process continues even when the OTA stays with a single employer. A job change, however, often "recharges" growth and development by providing the OTA with new learning relationships and an environment that presents more challenges to resolve. Enhancement of knowledge and skills often accelerates immediately following a job change as the OTA's learning focus shifts to refine and adapt the OTA's expertise to fit the needs of a different client group. A change in practice setting can put new demands on professional behaviors, too, such as critical thinking, problem-solving, and communication skills.

Specialization

Not all OT practitioners choose to specialize in one practice area. Many practitioners enjoy the challenge of variety and opt to work in settings that require a breadth of skills. They may opt for varied practice settings when changing jobs in order to keep their skills well-rounded. However, the process of professional socialization in a specialized area of practice can offer the OTA unique experiences and opportunities. When the OTA specializes, the learning focus shifts to developing a depth of knowledge (i.e., learning a lot about one practice area). Examples of specialty areas in OT practice include pediatric mental health, hand injuries, industrial rehabilitation, geriatrics, neurological rehabilitation, early intervention (birth-to-3 years), and community mental health. When entering a specialty field, the OTA's learning focus narrows, delving deep in the specialty content, and enhancing the complexity of the OTA's knowledge base.

Learning Relationships

Professional development literature in recent years has focused on the potential of relationships as sources of learning. Working as a professional offers many opportunities for developing the knowledge and skills of an OTA. One of the greatest sources of learning is the OTA's relationships with others—in the classroom, in fieldwork sites, on the job, in continuing education courses, and through professional associations. In all that has been written on mentoring, clinical supervision, peer coaching, and team learning, the common element is the interaction between people for the purpose of promoting continued development. The OTA will encounter many people in the health care field who have the capacity to help him or her learn and become a more proficient practitioner, such as teachers, fellow students, clients, supervisors, mentors, treatment team members, and colleagues. The number of people who can serve as learning guides expands as the OTA's career continues.

Sheckley and Keeton (1997) developed principles of professional development that highlight the importance of learning relationships. They pointed out that professionals who want to develop expertise must rely on a social network of fellow learners to challenge their thinking and share knowledge. Professional associates can promote reflection on experiences, add conceptual knowledge, develop applications of what has been learned to new situations, and assess the outcomes of interventions. They provide support, guidance, feedback, and input that further professional learning. In this section, we will look at the relationships that will be part of the OTA's developing career and how those relationships promote the development of continuing clinical competence. The relative influence of learning relationships at different stages of professional development is highlighted in Table 46-1.

Supervision

Supervision is an important component of the education, training, and socialization of an OTA. Loganbill, Hardy, and Delworth (1984) define supervision as "an intensive, interpersonally focused, one-to-one relationship in which one person is designated to facilitate the development of therapeutic competence in the other person" (p. 4). The 4 primary functions of the supervisor are to:

1. Ensure the welfare of the client.
2. Enhance the growth of the supervisee.
3. Promote the supervisee's transition from one developmental stage to the next.
4. Evaluate the supervisee's performance.

To facilitate growth, the supervisor must find ways to promote the developing OTA's reflection on his or her clinical experiences, conceptualization of working knowledge, and application of newly acquired knowledge and skills. In addition, the supervisor encourages self-assessment and facilitates the development of new techniques and skills based on what is being learned through practice.

Supervisors use specific techniques, each serving an important function in the promotion of overall development. Goal setting and goal clarification are techniques that allow both the supervisor and the supervisee to state expectations and set a learning and performance agenda. Goal setting is important because it clarifies what the supervisee is to achieve and how the supervisor will judge his or her performance. Observation gives the supervisor a chance to see the OTA in action and to note his or her performance strengths and growth needs in light of expectations, standards of practice, and job requirements. At times, supervisory observation will reveal opportunities for instruction or providing information, demonstration, and direction. Observation should also be coupled with feedback, "sharing knowledge of the results of an individual's performance with intent of changing that individual's behavior in a desirable direction" (Cohn, 2003, p. 911). Feedback is not judgmental of the person, but an assessment of the person's performance to clarify areas for specific improvement and provide examples of where to modify behavior.

Coaching is a process used by supervisors to help supervisees increase their sense of self-responsibility and ownership of their performance by promoting reflection and inquiry into their practices and professional activities. Good coaching from a supervisor will result in new awareness and new understanding that will ultimately have a positive effect on performance (MacLennan, 1995). Finally, evaluation is the systematic assessment of the OTA's performance to highlight areas of competence and specify areas that need improvement.

Perhaps the biggest challenge for both supervisor and supervisee is to work out a collaborative relationship that is inclusive of both the supervisor's style and the OTA's skills and needs. The OTA's collaborative behavior, maturity, level of expertise, and level of commitment will have an effect on how he or she is supervised and on his or her overall experience of supervision (Glickman, Gordon, & Ross-Gordon, 1995). On a first fieldwork assignment, the student OTA will find that the supervisor will take more of the responsibility for supervisory activities and will observe and evaluate the OTA's performance closely, being more directive and explicit. As the OTA develops clinical competence, he or she will be expected to take on more of the responsibility for the supervisory relationship. Fully developed professionals are quite autonomous and become more of a partner in the supervisory process. They bring questions, concerns, and clinical issues to their supervisors for feedback and bring successes to their supervisors' attention. Over time, the supervisor becomes less directive and more collaborative with the supervisee. The OTA's responsibility for growth increases as he or she develops into a full professional (Glickman et al., 1995).

Supervision is truly a collaborative activity. The OTA and his or her supervisor must work together in the interest of growth and development. Bordin (1994) suggested that the working alliance between the supervisor and the supervisee helps make the relationship work. The development of a working alliance means agreeing on goals, agreeing on the ways to work together to reach those goals, and creating a positive bond or relationship. A good supervisor-supervisee relationship requires care, commitment, communication, respect, truthfulness, and trust (Bennett, 1997). Too many professionals ultimately stall their careers because they become defensive and unwilling to accept the feedback and advice of others. All professionals experience some barriers to being supervised. Personal barriers such as resistance to change, previous negative experiences, or attitudinal barriers, such as "I already know what I am doing" or "You're just picking on me," can really get in the way of benefiting from supervision. Sometimes organizational barriers, such as time pressures or limited opportunities for interaction with a supervisor, can stifle the learning relationship. Process barriers such as conflict or ineffective communication between the supervisor and the supervisee can also limit the value of supervisory feedback (MacLennan, 1995). Supervisees should be willing to try suggestions and evaluate barriers in an effort to overcome them. The OTA can enhance his or her own learning by being open to supervision, seeing supervision as a learning relationship, asking questions, listening thoughtfully, and taking advantage of the expertise that his or her supervisor has to offer.

Mentoring

Mentoring relationships are extremely helpful in promoting professional growth and development. A mentor is a senior professional who is selected by the developing professional or assigned by an employer to foster professional orientation and growth. Mentors often do not have supervisory responsibility for the OTA, but fill the OTA's need for a role model and guide to how the system works and what is expected in the employing organization (MacLennan, 1995). A mentor may serve as an "inspirer," motivating and encouraging the new OTA to persist through difficult learning episodes; "investor," devoting significant time and energy to the long-term future of the OTA; and "supporter," providing a listening ear and a gentle push (Butterworth, 1992). Many health care professionals look back over their careers and remember various colleagues who served as mentors during those times when their assumptions and knowledge were challenged through problems they could not solve on their own.

Treatment Teams

The OT practitioner almost always works as part of a team of professionals who must work collaboratively to solve client-centered problems. Treatment teams provide collaborative opportunities for interprofessional learning, or learning among a group of professionals, often from different disciplines (Headrick, Wilcock, & Batalden, 1998). Sheckley and Keeton (1997) pointed out that adults learn best when they can tackle real problems, derive concepts from their experiences, and test those concepts in new situations. The treatment team is an effective vehicle for continued learning because it offers opportunities for knowledge sharing and problem solving in a practical, relevant context.

Interprofessional learning does not occur when professionals are focused on rivalries, professional boundaries, and proprietary knowledge. Fortunately, as Headrick et al. (1998) point out, most health care professionals have in common the personal desire to learn and the professional obligation to meet the needs of their patients or clients. The desire to learn and meet client needs often helps team members overcome the barriers to working and learning together.

Clients

There is no doubt that health care providers can and do learn from their clients. In the day-to-day work of the OTA, the information and feedback that clients give are a continuous source of knowledge and skill refinement. The process of assessing, identifying individual needs, and implementing individual treatment plans helps the OTA develop an understanding of how theoretical and procedural knowledge applies to real-life situations. Working directly with a client gives a multitude of opportunities to learn what works, what does not, and why. It helps the OTA develop the skills for individualization, adaptation, and evaluation that are critical to providing quality services. Some clients may agree to serve as formal research subjects, allowing the OTA to develop an extensive description and case study from which to inform and develop practice. Other clients are natural teachers, providing the OTA with challenges, questions, and insights that lead to a higher level understanding of individuals in need of OT, the conditions under which they live and work, and the value OT can have in supporting the client's goals. Almost any OT practitioner will be able to tell you stories about people he or she has served and how those people had a profound impact on his or her learning and growth as a professional.

Professional Relationships

Relationships with other OT practitioners will provide many opportunities for continued learning. For example, consider how much can be learned through conversations with fellow students. Some relationships developed in school will carry on into one's professional life, providing opportunities to share ideas, solve problems, give and get advice, and locate resources. Allen, Nelson, and Sheckley (1987) found that meeting with fellow professionals on a regular basis to discuss specific cases and general clinical issues was one of the 2 most highly valued and rewarding means of continuing professional development for psychologists. OTAs form relationships through work with fellow OT practitioners who offer ongoing opportunities for client- and content-focused dialogue that leads to continued competence.

Continued learning and professional development are cornerstones of almost all professional organizations. Professional organizations offer many opportunities for members to get together and learn from each other. It is in the best interest of your professional growth to join local, state, and national professional associations, such as AOTA, and to participate in them to form strong professional relationships. The potential number of learning relationships continues to grow through the OTA's career. The OTA should seek out and build relationships that will not only support the development of continue competence but provide opportunities to share knowledge with others.

Learning Activities

The NBCOT has described 30 professional development activities that they will accept as professional development units (PDU) needed for continued certification (NBCOT, 2003). A list of these activities and their corresponding PDU value and documentation requirements is available on the NBCOT Web site at www.nbcot.org/WebArticles/article-files/55-PDAChart.pdf. Some of the more commonly used activities will be described here. Professional development can be structured in both formal and informal ways to offer the OTA many, many options for reaching and maintaining competence.

A number of learning activities are initiated and developed by other people or organizations, including technical schools, colleges and universities, professional associations, independent professional development providers, and employers. Typically, the OT practitioner has little input into the content of these learning activities, so that careful selection is crucial for choosing learning activities that will progress the practitioner toward his or her specific learning goals. Externally-developed learning activities include:

- Continuing education classes. Similar to the classes that are taken in pursuit of a degree, continuing education classes are centered on a topic, meet a number of times, and are developed and led by one or more instructors. Many continuing education courses are offered online, which has opened up opportunities to OT practitioners by eliminating travel and time restrictions.

- Seminars. Professional seminars are generally more interactive than classes because the participants are more actively engaged in developing the learning goals and contributing what they know to the learning process. Seminars may meet a number of times, like classes, which provides the advantage of getting to know other OT practitioners and sharing expertise with them.

- Workshops. Workshops are one-time learning events focused on a topic of interest, usually work-related skills or knowledge. Workshops are designed and conducted by a workshop leader and are often advertised through workplaces and professional publications.

- In-service training. Many employers offer professional development opportunities in the workplace. These presentations, workshops, and classes are called in-service training. Health care agencies often use in-service training to update practitioners on agency policies and practices, as well as necessary health care information that is required for licensing or accreditation.

- Conferences. Conferences offer a large number of learning opportunities at one time in one location. At a conference, you can access current materials through vendor displays and demonstrations, attend workshops and presentations, and network with fellow OT practitioners. For example, AOTA sponsors a national conference and exposition annually that attracts thousands of OT practitioners. Conferences are a good way to find out about current issues and topics in your field. Many people find conferences fun and revitalizing.

- Publications. Magazines and journals offer OTAs another way to keep up to date. Reading articles and research on current practices and issues in OT gives practitioners a good sense of the current standards and expectations in the field, as well as a glimpse at what will be important in the future. There are many publications written specifically for OT practitioners. The *American Journal of Occupational Therapy* is an excellent resource that comes as one of many benefits for AOTA members. There are many other valuable journals. The Wilma L. West Library at the American Occupational Therapy Foundation (AOTF) has many resources and lists all available OT journals on its Web site (www.aotf.org). They will mail reprints of articles from any OT journal for a nominal fee. In order to receive PDUs for independent reading, practitioners must select recent, peer-reviewed articles or chapters and write a report describing ways in which the content could be used to enhance competency in their current roles (NBCOT, 2003).

- On-line resources. The World Wide Web can be a valuable and convenient resource for professional development because it provides access to specific Web sites, electronic conferences, some full-text articles, and interpersonal communication with other professionals. A brief search on the Internet can reveal hundreds of links to OT-specific and OT-related sites, including information on continuing education courses, job information, diagnostic and treatment information, and research reports.

As OTAs become socialized as OT practitioners, they will discover opportunities for self-directed learning (i.e., learning activities that are designed and pursued independently). Self-directed learning activities have tremendous educational potential and, if documented appropriately, they are another way for the OTA to obtain PDUs. Self-directed learning activities include:

- Case conferences. Meetings to review specific cases and solve therapeutic problems surrounding the cases provide opportunities to learn new information, see other practitioners in action, debate and resolve clinical issues, as well as develop clinical reasoning skills. While collaborative learning with other professionals can be an excellent vehicle for learning, in order to obtain PDUs for certification renewal, case conferences need to include collaboration with an advanced certified OT colleague (NBCOT, 2003).
- Mentoring. While working with a mentor can facilitate continued competence, the act of mentoring another professional (OT or other) also provides the mentor with an opportunity for professional development. As OTAs gain experience, they may wish to collaborate with another, less experienced practitioner as a mentor.
- Research. There are many forms of research that can yield new knowledge and skills. Conducting a literature review gives the researcher access to a tremendous amount of written information on a specific topic and requires that the researcher summarize and synthesize current knowledge. Participating in research on current practice promotes EBP, providing the practitioner with opportunities to learn about how and why new treatment methods are effective. Often, research is done collaboratively so that practitioners can share ideas and split up time-consuming tasks.

- Writing and speaking. Writing an article, giving a talk to consumer groups, presenting at a conference, or teaching a class all offer the opportunity for the OT practitioner to reflect on and synthesize knowledge and experience and to share a unique viewpoint with others in the field.
- Volunteer participation on committees, commissions, and organizations. Volunteering to serve on professional committees gives the OTA a unique window into the field, including current issues and concerns of the health care community and consumers. Committees or commissions can be at the institutional level, such as a hospital-based CVA support group; the regional level, such as a county commission on aging; or the national level, such as a certification policy task force. In this role, the OTA has the opportunity to contribute expertise to resolve issues or develop new ways of thinking, providing a very rewarding experience along with opportunity for growth.
- Professional memberships and meetings. Joining and actively participating in professional associations, at the local, state, or national level can bring OTAs in contact with a wide variety of learning relationships and provides opportunities to develop professional leadership skills. Professional organizations are run by volunteers who participate through activities such as organizing conferences, working with state licensure boards, lobbying state and federal legislators, or helping to produce a special interest newsletter.

Making a Professional Development Plan

Just as clients benefit from the implementation of well thought-out treatment plans, the OTA will benefit from devising a plan for professional development (Figure 46-1). Health care practitioners should learn to identify competence needs and specific activities for meeting those needs on a continual basis. Professional development plans should reflect the OTAs unique clinical abilities, goals, and visions for professional growth (Hinojosa, 2004) and should include documentation of the plan and the resulting change(s) in professional performance (Hinojosa et al., 2000a). The PDT, available online to AOTA members, provides a road map for the OT practitioner, describing each step of the professional development process and providing resources and worksheets (AOTA, 2003a).

Assessment

The first step in the professional development planning process is assessment, which occurs through reflection (AOTA, 2003a; Hinojosa et al., 2000a). OTAs can initiate reflection by asking themselves questions that assess both the practice environment and their own skills. For example: What is the current environment demanding of me as a professional? What are the trends in the near future? How am I prepared to meet the challenges of the future? What do I value in my practice and where would I like to go in the future? What knowledge and skills currently support clinical competence and what areas should I target for professional development?

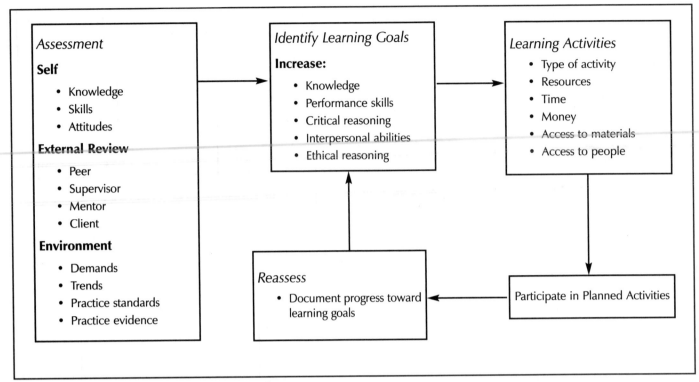

Figure 46-1. The professional development plan.

OT practitioners may also benefit from external evaluations. These may be initiated by the practitioner (e.g., OTAs may ask a peer, mentor, or client to provide feedback regarding specific aspects of their knowledge or skills) (AOTA, 2003a, Hinojosa et al., 2000a). More formal evaluations may also be used to inform the assessment process (e.g., employee performance evaluations or an institution's client satisfaction questionnaire).

Identifying Learning Goals

It is well established that learners who have identified learning goals perform better than those who do not have goals, in both academic (Utman, 1997) and professional contexts (VandeWalle, Brown, Cron, & Slocum, 1999). Learning goals are effective in at least 3 ways. First, goals help learners focus on crucial components of their learning needs, helping OTAs concentrate on those areas that are important for continued competence in their practice context. Second, articulating clear goals can help OTAs select the most appropriate and effective type of learning activity. For example, a learning goal that targets a psychomotor skill such as splinting is best achieved through hands-on learning activities rather than through reading. Third, learning goals provide target outcomes for reassessment and an effective way of reporting continued competence.

Documenting Professional Development

In clinical practice, the documentation of clients' progress toward well-defined goals is crucial. This is also true for professional development. Without effective and objective documentation of professional development, the OT practitioner has no evidence of continuing competence. Initial clinical competence

is easier to establish because it focuses on a single set of basic knowledge and skills; however, as practitioners gain experience and become focused in their roles, documenting competence through a written examination becomes impossible. Although there are a number of ways to document evidence of professional development, maintaining a professional portfolio is probably the most comprehensive.

A portfolio is a collection of evidence that demonstrates the practitioners' ongoing acquisition of the knowledge, skills, and attitudes necessary for fulfilling their professional roles (Alsop, 2002; Crist, Wilcox, & McCarron, 1998). Portfolios are recognized as an effective mechanism for documenting continuing competence by AOTA, which has included a portfolio template in its PDT (AOTA, 2003a) and is planning to use portfolio review as the process for establishing specialty certification for OT practitioners, a program under development at the time of this writing (Glantz & Moyers, 2003). Portfolios may contain an array of documents that demonstrate continuing competence, including certificates of learning, performance evaluations, self-assessments, goals, published and unpublished written works, professional awards, and testimonials from clients or colleagues. The process of developing a portfolio instantly engages the OT practitioner in the professional development process, so that the portfolio becomes both a means (i.e., learning activity) and an end (i.e., documentation) (Crist et al., 1998). While portfolio use is relatively new to OT practice, the relevant references included in this chapter provide excellent guidance to OTAs who need help getting started with their own portfolio (Alsop, 2001, 2002; Crist et al., 1998, AOTA, 2003b).

SUMMARY

This chapter described the process of professional development as it relates to developing and maintaining professional competence. The importance of continuing competence, the role of learning relationships, and the process and stages of professional development were all described.

Youngstrom (1998) described several traits and attitudes that can help the individual practitioner take responsibility for professional development and continuing competence. These include:

- Have an open attitude toward learning. Learning should be seen as a continuous process that is facilitated by questioning one's own practice and conferring with others. The OTA with an open attitude for learning will always strive to find a better way.

- Be a self-evaluator. The OTA who assesses his or her own performance and seeks out feedback will open up many learning opportunities. Even though learning occurs naturally through experience, "without time given to self-evaluation and reflection, the practitioner cannot accurately assess the level of competence or target areas for development" (Youngstrom, 1998, p. 720).

- Make a professional development plan and make the time to carry it out. Without a plan that includes specific activities and dates, it is too easy to let time slip away, allow professional development to slow, and to lose competence in the practice setting.

LEARNING ACTIVITIES

1. Work in pairs to conduct an Internet search for OT Web sites. Find 3 sites and write reviews of each site, including a description of the site, the types of information available, the resources available, and the usefulness or value for students and professionals.

2. Obtain information about conferences, seminars, and workshops for OT professionals. Assist the class in conducting an analysis of the various opportunities based on cost, convenience, content, relevance, and other features.

3. Conduct an investigation into the state and national continuing education requirements associated with certification and licensing. Conduct a class discussion about the meaning of continuing education requirements and help others see the variety of options for meeting them.

4. Choose a professional development plan. Develop your own plan for professional development for the coming year. Be sure to include the environmental assessment section and look carefully at the trends and demands of the field.

REFERENCES

Allen, G. J., Nelson, W. J., & Sheckley, B. G. (1987). Continuing education activities of Connecticut psychologists. *Professional Psychology: Research and Practice, 18*(1), 78-80.

Alsop, A. (2001). Competence unfurled: Developing portfolio practice. *Occupational Therapy International, 8,* 126-131.

Alsop, A. (2002). Portfolios: Portraits of our professional lives. *British Journal of Occupational Therapy, 65,* 201-206.

American Occupational Therapy Association. (1993). Occupational therapy roles. *American Journal of Occupational Therapy, 47,* 1087-1099.

American Occupational Therapy Association. (1998). Standards of practice for occupational therapy. *American Journal of Occupational Therapy, 52,* 866-869.

American Occupational Therapy Association. (1999). Standards for continuing competence. *American Journal of Occupational Therapy, 53,* 599-600.

American Occupational Therapy Association. (2000). Occupational therapy code of ethics. *American Journal of Occupational Therapy, 54,* 614-616.

American Occupational Therapy Association. (2002). The 2002 Representative Assembly summary of minutes. *American Journal of Occupational Therapy, 56,* 693-694.

American Occupational Therapy Association (2003a). Professional development tool. Retrieved April 30, 2004, from http://www.aota.org/pdt.

American Occupational Therapy Association. (2003b). SIS Contacts. Retrieved April 29, 2004, from http://www.aota.org/members/area3/links/link03.asp?PLACE=/members/area3/links/link03.asp

Bennett, T. (1997). *Clinical supervision marriage: A matrimonial metaphor for understanding the supervisor-teacher relationship.* Paper presented at the Annual Meeting of the Southwest Educational Research Association, Austin, TX, January 23-25, 1997.

Bordin, E. S. (1994). Theory and research on the therapeutic working alliance. New directions. In A. O. Horvath & L. S. Greenberg (Eds.), *The working alliance: Theory, research, and practice.* New York, NY: John Wiley & Sons.

Burkhardt, A., Braveman, B., & Gentile, P. (2002). Evaluating and documenting staff competence for accreditation reviews and staff development. Administration & Management Special Interest Section Quarterly, 18, 1-3, 6. Retrieved April, 28, 2004, from http://www.aota.org/members/area3/archs/amdec02.pdf.

Butterworth, T. (1992). Clinical supervision as an emerging idea in nursing. In T. Butterworth & J. Faugier (Eds.), *Clinical supervision and mentorship in nursing.* New York, NY: Chapman & Hall.

Case-Smith, J. (2004). Continuing competence and evidence-based practice. OT Practice ... Online, 8. Retrieved April 28, 2004 from http://www.aota.org//featured/area2/links/link16HAA.asp?PLACE=.

Cohn, E. S. (2003). Interdisciplinary communication and supervision of personnel. In E. B. Crepeau, E. S. Cohn, & B. A. B. Schell (eds.), *Willard & Spackman's occupational therapy* (10th ed., pp. 907-918). Philadelphia: Lippincott, Williams & Wilkins.

Crist, P., Wilcox, B. L., & McCarron, K. (1998). Transitional portfolios: Orchestrating our professional competence. *American Journal of Occupational Therapy, 52,* 729-736.

Fidler, G. S. (1996). Developing a repertoire of professional behaviors. *American Journal of Occupational Therapy, 50,* 583-587.

Glantz, C. H., & Moyers, P. A. (2003). New AOTA specialties board and programs established. OT Practice ... Online. Retrieved April 28, 2004, from http://www.aota.org//featured/area2/links/link16GP.asp?PLACE=.

Glickman, C. D., Gordon, S. P., & Ross-Gordon, J. M. (1995). *Supervision of instruction: A developmental approach.* Boston, MA: Allyn and Bacon.

Headrick, L. A., Wilcock, P. M., & Batalden, P. B. (1998). Interprofessional working and continuing medical education. *British Medical Journal, 316,* 771.

Hinojosa, J. (2004). Developing personal professional competencies. OT Practice ... Online, 9. Retrieved online April 28, 2004, from http://www.aota.org//featured/area2/links/link16HJ.asp?PLACE=.

Hinojosa, J., & Blount, M. L. E. (1998). Nationally speaking: Professional competence. *American Journal of Occupational Therapy, 52,* 699-701.

Hinojosa, J., Bowen, R., Case-Smith, J., Epstein, C. F., Moyers, P., & Schwope, C. (2000a). Self-initiated continuing competence. *OT Practice, 5*(23), CE-1-CE-7.

Hinojosa, J., Bowen, R., Case-Smith, J., Epstein, C. F., Moyers, P., & Schwope, C. (2000b). Standards for continuing competence for occupational therapy practitioners. *OT Practice, 5*(20), CE-1-CE-8.

Holm, M. B. (2000). Our mandate for a new millennium: Evidence-based practice, 2000, Eleanor Slagle Lecture. *American Journal of Occupational Therapy, 54,* 575-585.

Loganbill, C., Hardy, E., & Delworth, U. (1984). Supervision: A conceptual model. *The Counseling Psychologist, 10*(1), 3-41.

Lysaght, R. M., Altschuld, J. W., Grant, H. K., & Henderson, J. L. (2001). Variables affecting the competency maintenance behaviors of occupational therapists. *American Journal of Occupational Therapy, 55,* 28-35.

MacLennan, N. (1995). *Coaching and mentoring.* Brookfield, VT: Gower.

May, W. W., Morgan, B. J., Lemke, J. C., Karst, G. M., & Stone, H. L. (1995). Model for ability-bases assessment in physical therapy education. *Journal of Physical Therapy Education, 9,* 3-6.

Moyers, P. A. (2003). Five competencies for the future. OT Practice ...Online, 8. Retrieved April 28, 2004, from http://www.aota.org/featured/area2/links/link16GX. asp?PLACE=.

National Board for Certification in Occupational Therapy. (2003). NBCOT professional development activities chart. Retrieved May 3, 2004, from http://www.nbcot.org/WebArticles/articlefiles/55-PDAChart.pdf.

Raveh, M. (1995). Configuration of OT, professionalism and experiential learning—An integrated introductory course. *OT International, 2,* 65-78.

Sheckley, B. G., & Keeton, M. T. (1997). *Professional development: perspectives from research and practice.* Chicago, IL: CAEL.

Tickle-Degnen, L. (1999). Organizing, evaluating, and using evidence in occupational therapy practice. *American Journal of Occupational Therapy, 53,* 537-539.

Utman, C. H. (1997). Performance effects of motivational state: A meta-analysis. *Personality and Social Psychology Review, 1,* 170-182.

Van Maanan, J. (1977). *Organizational careers: Some new perspectives.* New York, NY: Wiley.

VandeWalle, D., Brown, S. P., Cron, W. L., & Slocum, J. W. (1999). The influence of goal orientation and self-regulation tactics on sales performance: A longitudinal field test. *Journal of Applied Psychology, 84,* 249-259.

Youngstrom, M. J. (1998). Evolving competence in the practitioner role. *American Journal of Occupational Therapy, 52,* 716-720.

HUMAN
DEVELOPMENTAL CHART

Neuromotor Development

Reflex Development

	Column 1	Column 2	Column 3	Column 4
Prenatal/Neonatal	Rooting Sucking Incurvation of spine Moro Extensor thrust ATNR STNR	Moro Asym. tonic m. Symm. tonic m. Tonic. labyr. Neon. neck r.	Plantar grasp Stepping Moro Placing Flexor withdrawal Extensor thrust Crossed extension	Palmar grasp Placing Traction Avoidance ATNR STNR
2 mo. 6 mo.	Laby. righting Landau Prot. extension	Neck/body r. Laby. r-su Landau Tilt – pr/su	Laby. r.-pr. Pos. supporting Laby. righting Prot. extension	
11 mo. 15 mo.	Tilting		Tilting/Hopping See-saw	
			Tilt – all 4s	

Voluntary Control

	Head/Trunk Control	Rolling/Crawling	Standing/Walking	Arm/Hand Function	Writing/Drawing
2 mo.	Lifts head when prone Head lag when pulled to sitting Falls forward in sitting position Back rounded				
3 mo.		Rolls back-to-side		Hands to midline Visual grasp Hands often open	
4 mo.	Had lag slight when pulled to sitting Lumbar curve only			Arms activate on sight of object Crude palm grasp Bilateral approach Holds 1 object	
5 mo.	Sits hyperflexed Head in line on pull-to-sit	Pivots in prone, arm propulsion movements			
6 mo.	Sits with support Begins to use supporting reactions	Automatic rolling Assumes 4-point crawling posture		Unilateral approach begins Circuitous arm motion	

Age	Sitting	Crawling	Standing / Walking	Prehension / Manipulation	Crayon / Drawing
7 mo.	Sits alone momentarily		Sustains weight on extended legs; Bounces		
8 mo.	No longer uses arms for support in sitting; Assumes sitting independently; Leans forward, re-erects	Belly crawling; Deliberate rolling		Holds 2 objects; Transfers object	
9 mo.		4-point crawl	Stands holding rail	Release beginning	
10 mo.	Sitting to prone		Pulls up to rail and lowers	Thumb and index tip prehension beginning	
11 mo.	Sits and pivots		Lifts foot at rail; Cruises		
12 mo. / 1 yr.			Walks with one hand held	Neat prehension; Places cube on cube; Casts object	Marks by banging or brushing
15 mo.	Seats self in small chair	Discards crawling	Assumes standing on own; Walks a few steps; Falls by collapse	Crude release (on contact with surface)	Marks rather than bangs
18 mo.			Heel-toe progression in walking; Walks sideways (17 m); Walks backwards (17 m)		Holds crayon butt end; Scribbles off page; Whole arm movements; One color
21 mo.			Squats in play; Down stairs hand held; Tries to stand on 6 cm Walking board; Kicks large ball	Towers 5 to 6 blocks	
24 mo. / 2 yrs.			Runs well; Walks with one foot on 6 cm walking board (27 cm)	Less handedness shift	Overhand grasp of crayon; Wrist action; Process rather than product
2½ yrs.			Jumps with both feet; Tries standing on one foot; Hops 1 to 3 steps on preferred foot; Attempts to step on walking board (33 m); Stands on 6 cm walking board with both feet (38 m)	Throws ball but with poor direction about 5 to 7 feet; Throws bean bag into 12 in hole from 3 ft	Holds crayon in fingers; Small marks; Imitates vertical/horizontal stroke

Age			
3 yrs.	Rides tricycle Alternates feet going up stairs Alternates feet part way on 6 cm walking board (38 m) Ascends small ladder alternating feet (38 m)	Towers 10 blocks 10 pellets into bottle, 30 sec. Catches large ball with stiff arms Throws ball without losing balance, 6 to 7 ft Handedness	Copies circle Imitates cross Encloses space Simple figures Beginning designs Names drawing
3½ yrs.	Stands on 1 foot, 2 seconds Jumps from 8 in. elevation Leaps off floor with feet together	Throws small ball	
4 yrs.	Propels and manipulates wagon Skips on 1 foot only Down stairs foot-to-step Balance on 1 foot, 4 to 8 seconds Walk 6 cm board part way before stepping off Crouch for broad jump of 8 to 10 in Hop on toes with both feet same time Carry cup of water without spilling Reciprocal arm motion in running pattern Ascends large ladder, alternating feet (47 m)	Throws ball overhand Beginning adult stance throwing Catches large ball arms flexed but rigid	Pencil held like adult, wrist flexed "Suns" Crude human figures Copies cross
4½ yrs.	Hops on 1 foot, 4 to 6 steps Alternates feet full length of 6 cm walking board (56 m) Descends small ladder		More detailed human figures

5 yrs.

Buildings and houses
Animals
Idea before starting
Copies triangle

Adult posture
distance throwing
Boys 24 feet
Girls 15 feet
Catches ball, hands more than arms, misses
Bounces large ball

Roller skates, ice skates, and rides small bicycle (5 or 6 yrs.)
Skips alternating feet
Stands indefinitely on 1 foot
Hop a distance of 16 ft
Walks long distance on tip toes
Walks length of 6 cm walking board in 6 to 9 sec. (60 m)
Running broad jump 28 to 35 in
Runs 11.5 ft per second
Descends large ladder

6 yrs.

Finger and wrist movement
Copies diamond

Reach, grasp, release, and body movement smooth
Catch ball, 1 hand
*Grip strength
Boys 11.3 lbs
Girls 3.2 lbs

Stand on each foot alternately with eyes closed
Walk a 4 cm walking board in 9 seconds with one error
Jump down from 12 in landing on toes only
Standing broad jump of 38 in.
Running broad jump of 40 to 45 in.
Hop 50 ft in 9 seconds

7 yrs.

*Grip strength
Boys 18.5 lbs
Girls 8.7 lbs

Motor performance continues to become more refined (running, jumping, balancing, etc.)
Strength increases
Learns to inhibit motor activity

8 yrs.

*Grip strength
Boys 26 lbs
Girls 14.4 lbs

Runs 5 yards per second
Standing broad jump of 45 in.

* Dynamometer norms for dominant hand (average/mean) (unpublished)
Scottish Rite Hospital for Crippled Children, Dallas, Texas.

3-dimensional geometric figures

Linear perspective

Distance throw
Boys 60 feet
Girls 35 feet

*Grip strength
Boys 45.2 lbs.
Girls 33.8 lbs.
Distance throw
Boys 95 feet
Girls 60 feet

*Grip strength
Boys 71.2 lbs
Girls 46.2 lbs

Boys distance throw
150 feet

Runs 6 yards per second
Standing broad jump of
60 in

Boys standing broad
jump 76 in.
Girls standing broad
jump 63 in.
Boys run 6 yd, 8 in
per second
Girls run 6 yd, 3 in
per second

Boys run 7 yd per
second
Boys standing broad
jump 90 in.

Daily Living Skills

*Social and Play
Development*

Individual – mothering
person most important

Body Scheme

*Sensorimotor
Development*

Other

Sensorimotor development
(0 to 2 yrs.):
Tactile functions
Vestibular functions
Kinesthetic functions
Auditory functions
Olfactory functions
Gustatory functions

Vision

Rudimentary fixation
Reflexive tracking for
brief periods
Sees light, dark, color,
and movement

Real convergence and
coordination

9 yrs.

10 yrs.

11 yrs.

14 yrs.

17 yrs.

Prenatal
Neonatal

2 mo.
6 mo.

11 mo.
15 mo.

2 mo.

Human Developmental Chart

Age	Visual / Perceptual	Sensorimotor	Social / Play	Self-Help
3 mo.	Accommodation more flexible and eye coordinate smoothly			
4 mo.	Size and shape consistency			
5 mo.				
6 mo.	Depth perception; Visual tracking 90 degrees; V and H planes; Color perception; Acuity; Discriminates strangers			
7 mo.			Stranger anxiety	
8 mo.				
9 mo.				
10 mo.				Holds bottle; Finger feeds
11 mo.				Drinks from cup (held)
12 mo.		Integration of body sides (1 to 4 yrs.): Gross motor planning; Form and space perception; Equilibrium response	Immediate family group important	Cooperates in dressing
1 yr.				
15 mo.				Grasps spoon and into dish
18 mos.		Postural flexibility; "Tummy," legs, feet, arms, hand, face parts	Solitary or onlooker play	Feeds self, spills; Takes off hat, socks, mittens; Unzips zippers; Toilet trained daytime
21 mos.				Handles cup well
24 mos.	Distinguishes vertical from horizontal lines	Strong tactile sense	Parallel play; Imitation	Hold small glass 1 hand; Helps in getting dressed; Pulls on socks; Pulls up pants; Removes shoes
2 yrs.				
2½ yrs.				Strings beads, snips with scissors, opens jar lid, turns door knob

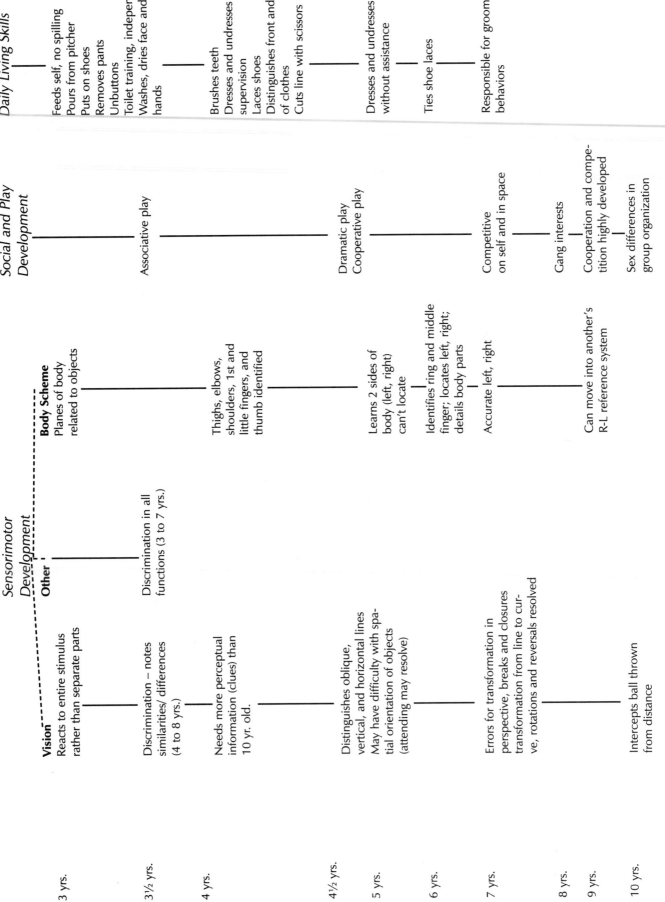

Daily Living Skills

3 yrs.
- Feeds self, no spilling
- Pours from pitcher
- Puts on shoes
- Removes pants
- Unbuttons
- Toilet training, independent
- Washes, dries face and hands

3½ yrs.
- Brushes teeth
- Dresses and undresses with supervision
- Laces shoes
- Distinguishes front and back of clothes
- Cuts line with scissors

7 yrs.
- Dresses and undresses without assistance

8 yrs.
- Ties shoe laces

- Responsible for grooming behaviors

Social and Play Development

3½ yrs.
- Associative play

- Dramatic play
- Cooperative play

- Competitive on self and in space

- Gang interests

- Cooperation and competition highly developed

- Sex differences in group organization

Sensorimotor Development

Body Scheme
- Planes of body related to objects

- Thighs, elbows, shoulders, 1st and little fingers, and thumb identified

- Learns 2 sides of body (left, right) can't locate

- Identifies ring and middle finger; locates left, right; details body parts

- Accurate left, right

- Can move into another's R-L reference system

Vision
- Reacts to entire stimulus rather than separate parts

Other
- Discrimination in all functions (3 to 7 yrs.)

- Discrimination – notes similarities/ differences (4 to 8 yrs.)

- Needs more perceptual information (clues) than 10 yr. old.

- Distinguishes oblique, vertical, and horizontal lines
- May have difficulty with spatial orientation of objects (attending may resolve)

- Errors for transformation in perspective, breaks and closures transformation from line to curve, rotations and reversals resolved

- Intercepts ball thrown from distance

3 yrs.
3½ yrs.
4 yrs.
4½ yrs.
5 yrs.
6 yrs.
7 yrs.
8 yrs.
9 yrs.
10 yrs.

BIBLIOGRAPHY

Ayers. (1962). Perceptual-motor training for children. Approaches to the treatment of patients with neuromuscular dysfunction. Third International Congress WPOT.

Barsch. (1967). *Achieving Perceptual-Motor Efficiency.*

Cratty. (1970). *Perceptual and Motor Development in Infancy and Early Childhood.*

Gesell. (1940). *The First Five Years.*

Espenschade & Eckert. (1967). *Motor Development.*

Llorens. (1970). *Human development: The promise of occupational therapy.* Rockville, MD: AOTA

McGraw. (1945). *The Neuromuscular Maturation of the Human Infant.*

Mussen, Conger, & Kagan. (1963). *Child Development and Personality.* 3rd ed.

Peiper. (1963). *Cerebral Function in Infancy and Childhood.*

Appendix compiled by Mary K. Cowan, MA, OTR, FAOTA.

STANDARDS OF PRACTICE FOR OCCUPATIONAL THERAPY

Linda Kohlman Thomson, MOT, OT(C), FAOTA,
Chairperson, Commission on Practice, AOTA

Permission was granted for the reproduction of this document by AOTA.

PREFACE

The Standards of Practice for OT are requirements for the OT practitioner (OTR and COTA) for the delivery of OT services that are client centered and interactive in nature (AOTA, 1995). The OTR supervises the COTA, and both work together in a collaborative manner to meet the needs of the client. However, the OTR is ultimately responsible and accountable for the delivery of OT services. This document identifies minimum standards for OT practice.

The minimum educational requirements for the OTR are described in the current Essentials and Guidelines of an Accredited Educational Program for the OT (AOTA, 1991a). The minimum educational requirements for the COTA are described in the current Essentials and Guidelines of an Accredited Educational Program for the OTA (AOTA, 1991b).

DEFINITIONS

- Assessment: Specific tools, instruments, or interactions used during the evaluation process. An assessment is a component part of the evaluation process (Hinojosa & Kramer, 1998).
- Client: A person, group, program, organization, or community for whom the OT practitioner is providing services (AOTA, 1995).
- Evaluation: The process of obtaining and interpreting data necessary for understanding the individual, system, or situation. This includes planning for and documenting the evaluation process, results, and recommendations, including the need for intervention and/or potential change in the intervention plan (Hinojosa & Kramer, 1998).
- OT practitioner: Any individual initially certified to practice as an OT or OTA or licensed or regulated by a state, district, commonwealth, or territory of the United States to practice as an OT or OTA (AOTA, 1997).
- Performance areas: Broad categories of human activity that are typically part of daily life. They are activities of daily living, work and productive activities, and play or leisure activities (AOTA, 1994c).
- Performance components: Elements of performance required for successful engagement in performance areas, including sensorimotor, cognitive, psychosocial, and psychological aspects (AOTA, 1994c).
- Performance contexts: Situations or factors that influence an individual's engagement in desired and/or required performance areas. Performance contexts consist of temporal aspects (chronological, developmental, life cycle, disability status) and environmental aspects (physical, social, political, cultural) (AOTA, 1994c).
- Screening: Obtaining and reviewing data relevant to a potential client to determine the need for further evaluation and intervention.
- Transition: Process involving actions coordinated to prepare for or facilitate change, such as from one functional level to another, from one life stage to another, from one program to another, or from one environment to another.

STANDARD I: PROFESSIONAL STANDING AND RESPONSIBILITY

1. An OT practitioner delivers OT services that reflect the philosophical base of OT (AOTA, 1979) and are consistent with the established principles and concepts of theory and practice.
2. An OT practitioner delivers OT services in accordance with AOTA's standards and policies. The nature and scope of OT services provided must be in accordance with laws and regulations.
3. An OT practitioner maintains current licensure, registration, or certification as required by laws or regulations.
4. An OT practitioner abides by AOTA's OT Code of Ethics (AOTA, 1994a).
5. An OT practitioner assures continued competency by establishing, maintaining, and updating professional performance, knowledge, and skills.

6. An OTR provides supervision for a COTA in a collaborative manner as defined by official AOTA documents and in accordance with laws or regulations.

7. A COTA seeks and follows supervision from a OTR in the delivery of OT services.

8. An OT practitioner is knowledgeable about AOTA's Standards of Practice for OT; the Philosophical Base of OT (AOTA, 1979); and other AOTA, state, and federal documents relevant to practice and service delivery.

9. An OT practitioner maintains current knowledge of legislative, political, social, cultural, and reimbursement issues that affect clients and the practice of OT.

10. An OTR is knowledgeable about research in the practitioner's areas of practice. An OTR applies timely research findings ethically and appropriately to evaluation and intervention processes and discusses applicable research findings with the COTA.

11. An OTR systematically assesses the efficiency and effectiveness of OT services and designs and implements processes to support quality service delivery.

12. A COTA collaborates with the OTR in assessing the efficiency and effectiveness of OT services and assists in designing and implementing processes to support quality service delivery.

Standard II: Referral

1. An OTR accepts and responds to referrals in accordance with AOTA's Statement of OT Referral (AOTA, 1994b) and in compliance with laws or regulations.

2. An OTR accepts and responds to referrals for evaluation or evaluation with intervention in performance areas, performance components, or performance contexts when clients may have a functional limitation or disability or may be at risk for a disability or may be a risk for a disabling condition.

3. An OTR refers clients to appropriate resources when the needs of the client can best be served by the expertise of other professionals or services.

4. An OT practitioner educates current and potential referral sources about the scope of OT services and the process of initiating OT services.

Standard III: Screening

1. An OTR screens independently or as a member of a team in accordance with laws and regulations. A COTA may contribute to the screening process under the supervision of an OTR.

2. An OTR selects screening methods appropriate to the client's performance context.

3. An OTR communicates screening results and recommendations to the appropriate person, group, or organization. A COTA may contribute to this process under the supervision of an OTR.

Standard IV: Evaluation

1. An OTR evaluates performance areas, performance components, and performance contexts. A COTA may contribute to the evaluation process under the supervision of an OTR.

2. An OT practitioner educates clients and appropriate others about the purposes and procedures of the OT evaluation.

3. An OTR selects assessments to evaluate the client's level of function related to performance areas, performance components, and performance contexts.

4. An OT practitioner follows defined protocols when standardized assessments are used.

5. An OTR analyzes, interprets, and summarizes assessment data to determine the client's current functional status and to develop an appropriate intervention plan. The COTA may contribute to this process under the supervision of an OTR.

6. An OTR completes and documents OT evaluation results within the time frames, formats, and standards established by practice settings, government agencies, external accreditation programs, and payers. A COTA may contribute to documentation of evaluation results under the supervision of an OTR and in accordance with laws or regulations.

7. An OTR communicates evaluation results, within the boundaries of client confidentiality, to the appropriate person, group, or organization. A COTA may contribute to this process under the supervision of an OTR.

8. An OTR recommends additional consultations when the results of the evaluation indicate that intervention by other professionals would be beneficial.

Standard V: Intervention Plan

1. An OTR develops and documents an intervention plan that is based on the results of the OT evaluation and the desires and expectations of the client and appropriate others about the outcome of service. A COTA may contribute to the intervention plan under the supervision of an OTR.

2. An OTR ensures that the intervention plan is documented within time frames, formats, and standards established by the practice settings, agencies, external accreditation programs, and payers.

3. An OTR includes in the intervention plan client-centered goals that are clear, measurable, behavioral, functional, contextually relevant, and appropriate to the client's needs, desires, and expected outcomes. A COTA may contribute to this process.

4. An OTR includes in the intervention plan the scope, frequency, duration of services, and the needs of the client.

5. An OTR reviews the intervention plan with the client and appropriate others. A COTA may contribute to this process.

STANDARD VI: INTERVENTION

1. An OTR implements the intervention plan through the use of specified purposeful activities or therapeutic methods that are meaningful to the client and are effective methods for enhancing occupational performance. A COTA may implement the intervention plan under the supervision of an OTR.

2. An OT practitioner informs clients and appropriate others regarding the relative benefits and risks of the intervention.

3. An OT practitioner maintains or seeks current information on resources relevant to the client's needs.

4. An OTR reevaluates during the intervention process and documents changes in the client's goals, performance, and needs. A COTA may contribute to the reevaluation process.

5. An OTR modifies the intervention process to reflect changes in client status, desires, and response to intervention. A COTA may identify the need for modifications and may contribute to the intervention modifications under the supervision of an OTR.

6. An OT practitioner documents the OT services provided within the time frames, formats, and standards established by the practice settings, agencies, external accreditation programs, and payers.

STANDARD VII: TRANSITION SERVICES

1. An OTR prepares a formal transition plan that is based on identified needs. A COTA may contribute to the preparation of a formal transition plan.

2. An OT practitioner facilitates the transition process in cooperation with the client, family members, significant others, team, and community resources and individuals, when appropriate.

STANDARD VIII: DISCONTINUATION

1. An OTR discontinues services when the client has achieved predetermined goals, has achieved maximum benefit from OT services, or does not desire to continue services. A COTA may recommend discontinuation of OT services to the supervising OTR.

2. An OTR prepares and implements a discontinuation plan that addresses appropriate follow-up resources. A COTA may contribute to the implementation of a discontinuation plan under the supervision of an OTR.

3. An OTR documents changes in the client's status between the initial evaluation and discontinuation of services. A COTA may contribute to the process under the supervision of an OTR.

4. An OTR documents recommendations for follow-up or reevaluation, when applicable.

REFERENCES

American Occupational Therapy Association. (1979). The philosophical base of OT. *American Journal of Occupational Therapy, 33,* 785.

American Occupational Therapy Association. (1991a). Essentials and guidelines of an accredited educational program for the OT. *American Journal of Occupational Therapy, 45,* 1077-1084.

American Occupational Therapy Association. (1991b). Essentials and guidelines of an accredited educational program for the OTA. *American Journal of Occupational Therapy, 45,* 1085-1092.

American Occupational Therapy Association. (1994a). OT code of ethics. *American Journal of Occupational Therapy, 48,* 1037-1038.

American Occupational Therapy Association. (1994b). Statement of OT referral. *American Journal of Occupational Therapy, 48,* 1034.

American Occupational Therapy Association. (1994c). Uniform terminology for OT (3rd ed.). *American Journal of Occupational Therapy, 49,* 1047-1054.

American Occupational Therapy Association. (1995). Concept paper: Service delivery in OT. *American Journal of Occupational Therapy, 49,* 1029-1031.

American Occupational Therapy Association. (1997). Bylaws. Article III, Section 1. Bethesda, MD: Author.

Hinojosa, J., & Kramer, P. (Eds.). (1998). *OT evaluation of clients: Obtaining and interpreting data.* Bethesda, MD: AOTA.

Adopted by the Representative Assembly 1998M15

Note: This document replaces the 1994 Standards of Practice for OT.

Occupational Therapy Code of Ethics—2000

Ruth Hansen, PhD, OTR, FAOTA,
Chairperson, Commission on Standards and Ethics (SEC), AOTA

Permission was granted for the reproduction of this document by AOTA.

PREAMBLE

The AOTA's *Code of Ethics* is a public statement of the common set of values and principles used to promote and maintain high standards of behavior in OT. The AOTA and its members are committed to furthering the ability of individuals, groups, and systems to function within their total environment. To this end, OT personnel (including all staff and personnel who work and assist in providing OT services, (e.g., aides, orderlies, secretaries, technicians) have a responsibility to provide services to recipients in any stage of health and illness who are individuals, research participants, institutions and businesses, other professionals and colleagues, students, and to the general public.

The OT Code of Ethics is a set of principles that applies to OT personnel at all levels. These principles to which OTs and OTAs aspire are part of a lifelong effort to act in an ethical manner. The various roles of practitioner (OT and OTA), educator, fieldwork educator, clinical supervisor, manager, administrator, consultant, fieldwork coordinator, faculty program director, researcher/scholar, private practice owner, entrepreneur, and student are assumed.

Any action in violation of the spirit and purpose of this Code shall be considered unethical. To ensure compliance with the Code, the Commission on Standards and Ethics (SEC) establishes and maintains the enforcement procedures. Acceptance of membership in the AOTA commits members to adherence to the Code of Ethics and its enforcement procedures. The Code of Ethics, Core Values and Attitudes of Occupational Therapy Practice (AOTA, 1993), and the Guidelines to the Occupational Therapy Code of Ethics (AOTA, 1998) are aspirational documents designed to be used together to guide OT personnel.

Principle 1. OT personnel shall demonstrate a concern for the well-being of the recipients of their services (beneficence).

OT personnel shall provide services in a fair and equitable manner. They shall recognize and appreciate the cultural components of economics, geography, race, ethnicity, religious and political factors, marital status, sexual orientation, and disability of all recipients of their services.

OT practitioners shall strive to ensure that fees are fair and reasonable and commensurate with services performed. When OT practitioners set fees, they shall set fees considering institutional, local, state, and federal requirements, and with due regard for the service recipient's ability to pay.

OT personnel shall make every effort to advocate for recipients to obtain needed services through available means.

Principle 2. OT personnel shall take reasonable precautions to avoid imposing or inflicting harm upon the recipient of services or to his or her property (nonmaleficence).

OT personnel shall maintain relationships that do not exploit the recipient of services sexually, physically, emotionally, financially, socially, or in any other manner.

OT practitioners shall avoid relationships or activities that interfere with professional judgment and objectivity.

Principle 3. OT personnel shall respect the recipient and/or their surrogate(s) as well as the recipient's rights (autonomy, privacy, confidentiality).

OT practitioners shall collaborate with service recipients or their surrogate(s) in setting goals and priorities throughout the intervention process.

OT practitioners shall fully inform the service recipients of the nature, risks, and potential outcomes of any interventions.

OT practitioners shall obtain informed consent from participants involved in research activities and indicate that they have fully informed and advised the participants of potential risks and outcomes. OT practitioners shall endeavor to ensure that the participant(s) comprehend these risks and outcomes.

OT personnel shall respect the individual's right to refuse professional services or involvement in research or educational activities.

OT personnel shall protect all privileged confidential forms of written, verbal, and electronic communication gained from educational, practice, research, and investigational activities unless otherwise mandated by local, state, or federal regulations.

Principle 4. OT personnel shall achieve and continually maintain high standards of competence (duties).

OT practitioners shall hold the appropriate national and state credentials for the services they provide.

OT practitioners shall use procedures that conform to the standards of practice and other appropriate AOTA documents relevant to practice.

OT practitioners shall take responsibility for maintaining and documenting competence by participating in professional development and educational activities.

OT practitioners shall critically examine and keep current with emerging knowledge relevant to their practice so they may perform their duties on the basis of accurate information.

OT practitioners shall protect service recipients by ensuring that duties assumed by or assigned to other OT personnel match credentials, qualifications, experience, and scope of practice.

OT practitioners shall provide appropriate supervision to individuals for whom the practitioners have supervisory responsibility in accordance with Association policies, local, state and federal laws, and institutional values.

OT practitioners shall refer to or consult with other service providers whenever such a referral or consultation would be helpful to the care of the recipient of service. The referral or consultation process should be done in collaboration with the recipient of service.

Principle 5. OT personnel shall comply with laws and Association policies guiding the profession of OT (justice).

OT personnel shall familiarize themselves with and seek to understand and abide by applicable Association policies; local, state, and federal laws; and institutional rules.

OT practitioners shall remain abreast of revisions in those laws and Association policies that apply to the profession of OT and shall inform employers, employees, and colleagues of those changes.

OT practitioners shall require those they supervise in OT-related activities to adhere to the *Code of Ethics*.

OT practitioners shall take reasonable steps to ensure employers are aware of OT's ethical obligations, as set forth in this Code of Ethics, and of the implications of those obligations for OT practice, education, and research.

OT practitioners shall record and report in an accurate and timely manner all information related to professional activities.

Principle 6. OT personnel shall provide accurate information about OT services (veracity).

OT personnel shall accurately represent their credentials, qualifications, education, experience, training, and competence. This is of particular importance for those to whom OT personnel provide their services or with whom OT practitioners have a professional relationship.

OT personnel shall disclose any professional, personal, financial, business, or volunteer affiliations that may pose a conflict of interest to those with whom they may establish a professional, contractual, or other working relationship.

OT personnel shall refrain from using or participating in the use of any form of communication that contains false, fraudulent, deceptive, or unfair statements or claims.

OT practitioners shall accept the responsibility for their professional actions which reduce the public's trust in OT services and those that perform those services.

Principle 7. OT personnel shall treat colleagues and other professionals with fairness, discretion, and integrity (fidelity).

OT personnel shall preserve, respect, and safeguard confidential information about colleagues and staff, unless otherwise mandated by national, state, or local laws.

OT practitioners shall accurately represent the qualifications, views, contributions, and findings of colleagues.

OT personnel shall take adequate measures to discourage, prevent, expose, and correct any breaches of the and report any breaches of the Code of Ethics to the appropriate authority.

OT personnel shall familiarize themselves with established policies and procedures for handling concerns about this Code of Ethics, including familiarity with national, state, local, district, and territorial procedures for handling ethics complaints. These include policies and procedures created by the AOTA, licensing and regulatory bodies, employers, agencies, certification boards, and other organizations who have jurisdiction over OT practice.

REFERENCES

American Occupational Therapy Association. (1993). Core values and attitudes of occupational therapy practice. *American Journal of Occupational Therapy, 47,* 1085-1086.

American Occupational Therapy Association. (1998). Guidelines to the occupational therapy code of ethics. *American Journal of Occupational Therapy, 52,* 881-884.

AUTHORS

The Commission on Standards and Ethics (SEC):

Barbara L. Kornblau, JD, OTR, FAOTA, Chairperson
Melba Arnold, MS, OTR/L
Nancy Nashiro, PhD, OTR, FAOTA
Diane Hill, COTA/L, AP
Deborah Y. Slater, MS, OTR/L
John Morris, PhD
Linda Withers, CNHA, FACHCA
Penny Kyler, MA, OTR/L, FAOTA, Staff Liaison

Adopted by the Representative Assembly 2000M15

Note: This document replaces the 1994 document, OT Code of Ethics (*American Journal of Occupational Therapy, 48,* 1037–1038).

Prepared 4/7/2000

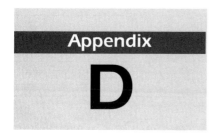

Karen Sladyk, PhD, OTR, FAOTA

INTERNET RESOURCES

Trying to keep an Internet resource list current is like trying to hold water in your hands; but these sites are good places to start. Each site has been reviewed for accurate contact and has been judged as stable. The reader is cautioned to evaluate Internet information with extreme care. Because Internet information is not peer reviewed and the author is often unknown, the worth of Internet material is often of no scientific value. Internet information is fast but students are cautioned that the Internet does not replace scholarly inquiry.

To evaluate a Web site, look for content accuracy first. Does the site publish information that you know is true from other reliable print forms such as journals? What seems to be the mission of the Web site? To sell you something? Fundraise for their cause? Both sales and fundraising are acceptable Internet tools but does that seem to be the main purpose of a national organization's Web site? Are author's names and peer-reviewed material available on the site?

Formats that are user friendly and assessable make a Web site easier to use but do not be mislead by slick Web sites that lack scientific content. Reliable sites usually have Web masters that can accurately blend content and ease of use. The bottom line: Be careful of Internet information and make sure you confirm all content with non-Internet resources.

SITES THAT PROVIDE LINKS TO OTHER OCCUPATIONAL THERAPY SITES

OT Seeker
www.otseeker.com

OT
www.occupationaltherapist.com

SITES OF INTEREST TO OCCUPATIONAL THERAPY ASSISTANTS

Administration on Aging
www.aoa.dhhs.gov

Advance for OT
http://occupational-therapy.advanceweb.com/

Alzheimer's Association
www.alz.org

American Association of Retired Persons
www.aarp.org

American Cancer Society
www.cancer.org

American Diabetes Association
www.diabetes.org

American Dietetic Association
www.eatright.org

American Occupational Therapy Association
www.aota.org

American Occupational Therapy Foundation
www.aotf.org

Arthritis Foundation
www.arthritis.org

CBS Healthwatch
www.cbsnews.com/sections/health/main204.shtml

Centers for Medicare and Medicaid Services
www.cms.hhs.gov

CINAHL
www.cinahl.com

CNN Health
www.cnn.com/health

Discovery Channel
www.discovery.com

Elderhostel
www.elderhostel.org

HealthFinder
www.healthfinder.gov

Health on the Net Foundation
www.hon.ch

HealthWeb
www.healthweb.org

Humor Matters
www.humormatters.com

ICIDH-2
www.who.int/icidh

Juvenile Diabetes Research Foundation International
www.jdrf.org

Leisure and Aging Center
http://web.indstate.edu/nrpa-las/links.html

Medicare
www.medicare.gov

Muscle charts of the human body
www.ptcentral.com/muscles

Muscular Dystrophy Association
www.mdausa.org

National Board for Certification in Occupational Therapy
www.nbcot.org

National Cancer Institute
www.nci.nih.gov

National Council on the Aging
www.ncoa.org

National Eye Institute
www.nei.nih.gov

National Institute of Arthritis and Musculoskeletal and Skin Diseases
www.niams.nih.gov

National Institute of Child Health & Human Development
www.nichd.nih.gov

National Institute of Diabetes & Digestive & Kidney Diseases
www.niddk.nih.gov

National Institutes of Health
www.nih.gov

National Institute of Mental Health
www.nimh.nih.gov

National Institute of Neurological Disorders and Stroke
www.ninds.nih.gov

National Institute on Aging
www.nia.nih.gov

National Institute on Alcohol Abuse and Alcoholism
www.niaaa.nih.gov

National Institute on Deafness and Other Communication Disorders
www.nidcd.nih.gov

National Institute on Drug Abuse
www.nida.nih.gov

National Library of Medicine
www.nlm.nih.gov

National Mental Health Association
www.nmha.org

National Osteoporosis Foundation
www.nof.org

National Parkinson Foundation
www.parkinson.org

National Rehabilitation Information Center
www.naric.com

National Stroke Association
www.stroke.org

Prevent Blindness America
www.preventblindness.org

Public Broadcasting System
www.pbs.org

Sensory Integration International
http://home.earthlink.net/~sensoryint

Social Security
www.ssa.gov

US Government guidelines on evidence-based practice
www.ahrq.gov

Veterans' Administration
www.va.gov

World Federation of Occupational Therapists
www.wfot.org

World Health Organization
www.who.int

INDEX

ABCD method, for goals and objectives, 502
abstinence, 304
abstract, of research article, 484
accommodation, 348
accreditation, 554-555
acetabulum, 292, 293
Achenbach Child Behavior Checklist, for ADHD, 186
ACS (Activity Card Sort), for Alzheimer's disease, 369, 374
action research, 486
active listening, in management, 557
activity(ies)
  of daily living. See ADLs (activities of daily living)
  definition of, 46
  demands of, 48
  director of. See activity director
  documentation of, 522-523
  motivation for, 522
  participation in, 523
  plan for, 518-523
  properties of, 54
  regulations on, 517-518
  in treatment plan, 502
  types of, 54
activity analysis, 52-64
  adaptation in, 55
  checklist for, 56, 59-63
  examples of, 56-59
  forms for, 56-59
  frame of reference for, 55
  grading in, 55-56
  history of, 53-54
  principles of, 54
  process and purpose of, 54-55
  skills for, 55
  time clock for, 309
Activity Card Sort (ACS), for Alzheimer's disease, 369, 374
activity configuration, for multiple sclerosis, 262
activity director, 516-527
  activities plan development by, 518-523
  definitions of, 517
  documentation duties of, 522-523
  job description for, 518
  in long-term care, 526
  program management by, 524-526
  regulations on, 517-518

staffing needs of, 524
activity groups, 385. See also crafts
  format for, 393-394
  task-oriented, 385-386
ADA (Americans with Disabilities Act of 1990), 429, 465
adaptation
  in activity analysis, 55
  in developmental theory, 36
  occupational, 78, 354, 400
adaptive equipment. See assistive technology
adaptive response, 138
Addams, Jane, 5
ADHD. See attention deficit hyperactivity disorder (ADHD)
ADLs (activities of daily living), 442-461
  in Alzheimer's disease, 370-371
  in arthritis, 283
  assistive technology for. See assistive technology
  in cognitive dysfunction, 452-453
  in decreased range of motion, 450
  definition of, 45, 443
  description of, 46
  documentation of, 453-458
  evaluation of, 444-445
  evidence-based treatment of, 459
  frameworks of reference for, 443
  in hemiplegia, 450, 452
  importance of, 443
  in incoordination, 448, 450-451
  measurement of, 443-444
  in multiple sclerosis, 264-265
  in muscle weakness, 447-449
  in Parkinson's disease, 340
  performance skills for, 446-452
  psychosocial issues in, 452-453
  in stroke, 324
  in total hip arthroplasty, 296
  in traumatic brain injury, 218
  treatment approaches for, 445-446
  in visual impairment, 356-357
  in wheelchairs, 452
adolescence
  depression in, 202-210
  developmental theories of, 41-42
adult education, wellness programs in, 430
adulthood, developmental theories of, 42-43
advanced-level practice, 510, 511
affect, flattened, 250

Age of Enlightenment, 3
age-related macular degeneration, 351, 352
aging, sensory loss with, 349-350
agitation, in traumatic brain injury, 218-219
agnosia, in Alzheimer's disease, 368
agoraphobia, 89, 276
AIMS (Alberta Infant Motor Scale), for cerebral palsy, 160
akinesia, in Parkinson's disease, 337, 338, 340
Alberta Infant Motor Scale (AIMS), for cerebral palsy, 160
alcohol abuse, 307-317
Alcoholics Anonymous, 306
Alert Program, for ADHD, 189
Allen, Claudia, 389
Allen Cognitive Level Test, 99-100
  for depression, 204
  for schizophrenia, 252, 253
alternative living environments, 442
Alzheimer's disease (DAT), 366-379
  ADLs in, 452
  assessment of, 369
  case study of, 100, 373-375, 378-379
  interventions for, 370-371
  progression of, 367-369
  treatment of, 371-373
American Occupational Therapy Association (AOTA)
  career mobility discussions in, 18
  Code of Ethics, 496, 499, 530-535, 587-588
  Commission on Continuing competence and Professional Development, 562
  documentation documents of, 499
  founding of, 8-10
  OT Roles paper, 408
  philosophy of, 30
  position on early intervention, 106-107
  principles of, 8-10
  Reference Manual of the Official Documents of the AOTA, 81
  report on philosophical base of OT, 28
  roster of honor of, 21-22
  Standards of Practice of, 583-585
  supervision guidelines of, 512-513
  uniform terminology system of, 45-46
Americans with Disabilities Act of 1990 (ADA), 429, 465
AMPS (Assessment of Motor and Process Skills), for TBI, 219
analysis of variance (ANOVA), 484

andragogy, 97
anonymity, in research, 495
ANOVA (analysis of variance), 484
anxiety disorders, 272-280, 337
APGAR scale, 37
aphasia, in Alzheimer's disease, 368
applied research, 486
apraxia, in Alzheimer's disease, 368
ARMD (age-related macular degeneration),
    351, 352
arousal deficits, in sensory integration dys-
    function, 141
arthritis, 282-290
    case studies of, 285-289
    energy conservation in, 284
    frame of reference for, 283
    interventions for, 283-284
    joint protection in, 284
    juvenile rheumatoid, 286-287
    osteoarthritis, 284-286
    rheumatoid, 287-289
arthrogryposis multiplex, splints for, 478
arthroplasty, hip, 292-303
artifacts, for qualitative research, 493
arts, vs. crafts, 400
Asperger's syndrome, 131, 205, 206
assessment, in OT process, 83
Assessment of Motor and Process Skills
    (AMPS), for TBI, 219
assets, patient, 501
assisted living, 430
assistive technology, 406-425
    for arthritis, 284
    characteristics of, 409, 411-413
    design of, 413
    effectiveness of, documentation of, 414
    fabricating, 414
    for hearing loss, 357
    for hemiplegia, 450, 452
    history of, 407
    for incoordination, 448, 450
    instruction for, 408
    for muscle weakness, 448
    for Parkinson's disease, 340
    personnel involvement with, 408
    precautions with, 409-410
    presentation to client, 414
    for range of motion limitation, 450
    for SCI, 234
    selection of, 408
    for total hip arthroplasty, 295
    for visual impairment, 356-357
asylums, history of, 3-7
ataxia
    in cerebral palsy, 159
    in multiple sclerosis, 261
athetosis, in cerebral palsy, 159
attention deficit hyperactivity disorder
    (ADHD), 184-200
    in adults, 197
    assessment of, 186-188
    case study of, 190-197
    diagnosis of, 185-186

eligibility for special education with, 187
evidence-based treatment of, 199, 477-478
interventions for, 189-190
symptoms of, 197
theory of, 186
attitudes, case studies of, 91-92
autism spectrum disorder, 122-137
    assessment of, 126-127
    case studies of, 127-129, 135-137
    evidence-based treatment of, 132
    historical perspective of, 123-124
    symptoms of, 124, 125
autocratic leadership, 392
autoimmune disease, multiple sclerosis as,
    258, 259
autonomic dysreflexia, in spinal cord injury,
    233
autonomy, 587
Award of Excellence, 21-22
axiology, 26
Ayres, A. Jean, sensory integration approach
    of, 124, 126, 139, 141-148
Azima, H., and Azima, F., 385

BADLs (basic activities of daily living), in
    SCI, 234, 236-239
BADS (Behavioral Assessment of Dysexecu-
    tive Syndrome), for TBI, 222
baking group, for oppositional defiant disor-
    der, 177
Bandura, Albert, 36-37
Barnett, Patty Lynn, 22
Bartel Index, for stroke, 319
Barton, George, 5-8
basic activities of daily living (BADLs), in
    SCI, 234, 236-239
basic research, 486
bathing
    in multiple sclerosis, 264-265
    after total hip arthroplasty, 295
bed mobility, in stroke, 321-323
Beery Developmental Test of Visual-Motor
    Integration (VMI)
    for autism spectrum disorders, 127
    for depression, 204
    for oppositional defiant disorder, 174
behavior, professional, 530-531, 534-535
Behavioral Assessment of Dysexecutive Syn-
    drome (BADS), for TBI, 222
behavioral frame of reference, 70-71
behavioral problems, in Alzheimer's disease,
    371
belonging, 433
beneficence, 529-530, 587
Benne, Kenneth, 392-393
biomechanical frame of reference, 68
    for spinal cord injury, 235
    for total hip arthroplasty, 294
    for work injury, 464
Black, Teri, 22
Blechert, Toné Frank, 21
blindness, 351
The Bloomingdale (hospital), 4

Bobath neurodevelopmental treatment frame
    of reference, 68-69, 157
body functions, definition of, 48
body structures, definition of, 48
bolsters, 411-412
bony prominence, 416
BOTMP (Bruininks-Oseretsy Test of Motor
    Proficiency)
    for ADHD, 187
    for autism spectrum disorders, 127
bradykinesia, in Parkinson's disease, 336, 337,
    338
brain attack. See stroke
brain injury, traumatic. See traumatic brain
    injury (TBI)
Brigance Diagnostic Inventory of Early
    Childhood Development
    for autism spectrum disorders, 127
    for cerebral palsy, 161
Brittell, Terry, 21
Brown, Ilenna, 21
Brown-Sequard lesion, 232
Bruininks-Oseretsy Test of Motor Proficiency
    (BOTMP)
    for ADHD, 187
    for autism spectrum disorders, 127
Burke, Janice, 10-11
Byers, Sue, 22

calf board, for wheelchair, 411
Canadian Model of Occupational Perfor-
    mance (CMOP), 77-78
    for anxiety disorders, 274
    for multiple sclerosis, 262
Canadian Occupational Performance
    Measure (COPM)
    for anxiety disorders, 274, 275
    for schizophrenia, 252
cardiovascular disease risks, case study of, 88
career opportunities, 513-514
    activity director, 518
    for professional development, 564
CARF (Commission on Accreditation of
    Rehabilitation Facilities), 550, 554-555
carpal tunnel syndrome, repair of, splints
    after, 418
CARS (Childhood Autism Rating Scale),
    128
case mixed groups (CSGs), 550, 553
case studies
    agoraphobia, 89
    Alzheimer's disease, 100, 373-375, 378-
        379
    anxiety disorders, 273-280
    arthritis, 285-289
    attention deficit hyperactivity disorder,
        190-197
    autism, 127-129, 135-137
    cardiovascular disease risks, 88
    cerebral palsy, 111, 161-164, 169-171
    conferences on, 567
    cooking deficits, 90-91
    depression, 202-210, 504-505

diabetic neuropathy, 49-50
impact of change, 93
juvenile rheumatoid arthritis, 286-287
learning, 100
life skills, 435-437
low vision, 358-359
multiple sclerosis, 261-267, 269-270
occupational therapy process, 49-50
oppositional defiant disorder, 173-182
osteoarthritis, 285-286
Parkinson's disease, 338-343, 345-347
reclusive person, 92
research designs using, 491, 494
retinopathy of prematurity (retrolental
        fibroplasia), 107-111, 114-120
return to work, 462-469
rheumatoid arthritis, 90, 288-289
schizophrenia, 251-257
self-abuse, 131-132
sensory integration dysfunction, 139-154
severe disruptions, 93
shoulder sling, 92
spinal cord injury, 235, 240-242
splints, 89-90, 92
stroke, 320-328, 330-332, 505, 507
substance abuse, 307-317
superstitions, 91
supervision, 514
total hip arthroplasty, 294-303
traditions, 91
traumatic brain injury, 216-223, 226-229
underweight, 88
visual impairment, 107-111, 358-359
work injury, 465-468
The Casino, 6
cataract, 351, 352
catatonia, 251
catheterization, urinary, in SCI, 230
CCCPD (Commission on Continuing
        Competence and Professional Develop-
        ment), 562
center vision, 348
ceramics, 402
cerebral palsy (CP), 156-171
    assessment of, 160-161
    case studies of, 111, 161-164, 169-171
    etiology of, 157
    evidence-based treatment of, 166
    frames of reference for, 157
    prevalence of, 157
    signs of, 158
cerebrovascular accident. See stroke
certification, renewal period for, 562
certified occupational therapy assistants
        (COTAs), 15, 583-585
chair, for multiple sclerosis, 467
challenge, 434
change, impact of, case studies of, 93
cheating, 532
chewing difficulties, in Parkinson's disease,
        337
Chicago School of Civics and Philanthropy, 7

Childhood Autism Rating Scale (CARS),
        128
children and childhood
    attention deficit hyperactivity disorder in,
        184-200
    autism spectrum disorder in, 122-137
    cerebral palsy in, 156-171
    development of, chart for, 574-580
    developmental theories of, 40-41
    juvenile rheumatoid arthritis in, 286-287
    oppositional defiant disorder in, 172-182
    sensory integration dysfunction in, 138-
        154
    visual impairment in, 104-120
Choctaw-Chickasaw Sanitarium, 9
Chomsky, Noam, 40
Circle of Courage model, 433-434
client factors, 48, 566
client-centered models, 77-78
climate, 88-89
clinical competence, 560
clinical dementia rating, 366
Clinical Observations of Motor Performance
        (COMPS), for sensory integration dys-
        function, 141
clinical reasoning process, 406, 479
closed head injury, 213
CMOP. See Canadian Model of Occupational
        Performance (CMOP)
coaching, supervision of, 565
Code of Federal Regulations, on human sub-
        ject rights, 494-495
Coffey, Margaret S., 22
Cognitive Behavioral Model, for anxiety dis-
        orders, 273, 274
cognitive development, 34
Cognitive Disabilities Model, for schizophre-
        nia, 251
cognitive dysfunction
    ADLs in, 452
    in Alzheimer's disease, 367-369, 371
    in multiple sclerosis, 260, 261
cognitive function, assessment of, in stroke,
        320
cognitive rehabilitation, 75-76
cognitive theory, of Piaget, 36, 38, 40-41
cognitive-behavioral frame of reference, 72-
        74, 99-100
cohesiveness, in group dynamics, 391
cohorts, in research, 484
Cole, Marli, 393-394
collaborative approach
    activity director in, 525
    to ADL deficits, 445
    vs. cheating, 532
    faculty-student, 533
    in professional development, 565
    to work injury, 465
Commission on Accreditation of Rehabilita-
        tion Facilities (CARF), 550, 554-555
commitment, 434
Committee on Occupational Therapy Assis-
        tants, 15

communication
    in group intervention, 385
    in management, 556
    in Parkinson's disease, 340-341
    of research findings, 479
    in SCI, 236-239
    with sensory loss, 357
    skills for, 47
    in teaching, 98
    therapeutic, 392
community, re-entry into, 212
community redesign, 430
compensatory strategies, for ADL deficits, 445
competence, 560, 561-562
Comprehensive Occupational Therapy Evalu-
        ation Scale (COTE)
    for anxiety disorders, 274-275
    for TBI, 219
Comprehensive Trail Making Test (CTMT),
        for TBI, 221
COMPS (Clinical Observations of Motor Per-
        formance), for sensory integration dys-
        function, 141
compulsion, 272
computer crafts, 402
conceptual practice model, 77
conduct, rules of, 28-30
conferences, 566
confidentiality, 531, 587
    in documentation, 499
    in research, 495
confusion, in traumatic brain injury, 218-221
Conners' Parent Rating Scale or Conners'
        Teacher Rating Scale, for ADHD, 186
consensual validation, 382
Consolation House, 5-6, 8
constipation, in Parkinson's disease, 337
consultation, 429, 430, 517
content, in group, 382
context, 44, 47
continuing competence, 560
continuous reading, 348
control, 434
controlling, 556
cooking, 401
    deficits of
        case study of, 90-91
        in multiple sclerosis, 265-266
    in depression, 206
    in visual impairment, 356
cooperation, in teamwork, 541-542
cooperative group, 387
coordination, deficits of, ADLs in, 448, 450,
        451
coping, life skills for, 432-440
COPM (Canadian Occupational Performance
        Measure)
    for multiple sclerosis, 262
    for schizophrenia, 252
correlational research designs, 490-491
cost containment, 552
cost-effectiveness, of OTAs, 513

COTAs (certified occupational therapy assistants), 15, 583-585
COTE (Comprehensive Occupational Therapy Evaluation Scale)
  for anxiety disorders, 274-275
  for TBI, 219
coup and contrecoup effect, 214
Cowan stabilizing pillow, 409, 410, 413
Cox, Betty, 21
CP. See cerebral palsy (CP)
CPT (Current Procedural Terminology) codes, 550, 554
  crafts, 398-404
  vs. arts, 400
  ceramics, 402
  computer, 402
  cooking, 401
  for depression, 205-206
  fiber, 402
  found materials, 403
  framework of reference for, 400
  indications for, 400
  kits for, 400-401
  leatherwork, 401
  metal, 402
  mosaics, 402
  needle, 401-402
  theoretical basis of, 399-400
  usage of, 399
  woodworking, 401
Crampton, Marion W., 15, 16
creative activities, 516, 519
creativity, in teamwork, 542
CSGs (case mixed groups), 550, 553
CTMT (Comprehensive Trail Making Test), for TBI, 221
cultural considerations, 90-92, 98
cumulative trauma disorders, 462
Current Procedural Terminology (CPT) codes, 550, 554
customs, case study of, 90-91
CVA. See stroke

Daily Living Interview, 204
DAT. See Alzheimer's disease (DAT)
data analysis, in research, 493
data collection, for research, 492-493
databases, of evidence-based results, 475
dating, policies on, 531-532
De Gangi-Berk Test of Sensory Integration (TSI)
  for autism spectrum disorders, 127
  for sensory integration dysfunction, 141
death and dying, stages of, 43
decision making
  in Life Skills Program, 435
  in management, 555
declarative memory, 369
decoupage, 403
decubitus ulcers, in SCI, 234
deductive reasoning, 487
delusions, 250

dementia
  of the Alzheimer's type. See Alzheimer's disease
  in Parkinson's disease, 337
democratic community activities, 516, 519
democratic group leadership, 392
depression, 202-210
  case study of, 504-505
  in oppositional defiant disorder, 175
  in Parkinson's disease, 337
  in visual impairment, 354
descriptive research designs, 490
detoxification, 304
development
  human, 34-43, 391-392
    chart for, 574-581
    evaluation of, 37
    prenatal, 37
    stages of, 38-43
    theories of, 35-37
  professional, 560-570
development groups, for life skills, 434-435
developmental groups, Mosey model for, 386-387, 392
developmental team building, 543, 544
developmental/spatiotemporal model, crafts and, 399
diabetic neuropathy, 49-50
diabetic retinopathy, 352
Diagnostic and Statistical Manual of Mental Disorders-IV
  on attention deficit hyperactivity disorder, 185
  on autism, 123
  on substance abuse, 305
diagnostic related groups (DRGs), 550, 553
diffuse axonal injury, 213, 214
dilemmas, 534
diplopia, 258, 260
directing, 555-556
directive groups (Kaplan), 387-388
discharge planning, 502. See also specific disorders
discontinuation, of treatment program, 84, 585
disorganized schizophrenia, 251
disorganized speech, 250
disruptions, severe, case study of, 93
distractibility, 184
Dix, Dorthea Lynde, 4
Doane, Joseph C., 10
documentation, 498-508
  of activity program, 522-523
  of ADL performance and progress, 453-458
  AOTA documents on, 499
  of assistive technology efficacy, 414
  of autism services, 129
  components of, 500
  confidentiality in, 499
  examples of, 504-507
  for Medicare, 500
  of professional development, 568

of progress, 503-504
of treatment plans, 500-503
Donahue, Mary, 387
dopamine deficiency, Parkinson's disease in, 336
double-blind studies, 490
dressing
  in hemiplegia, 450
  in incoordination, 448
  in muscle weakness, 448, 449
  in range of motion limitation, 450
  in visual impairment, 356
  in wheelchair, 452
DRGs (diagnostic related groups), 550, 553
drug abuse, 304-317
DSM-IV. See Diagnostic and Statistical Manual of Mental Disorders-IV
Dunton, William Rush, Jr., 6-9, 385
duty, 530, 588
dynamic interactional frame of reference, 76-77
dynamic splints, 418
dysarthria, in Parkinson's disease, 340-341
dysphagia, in Parkinson's disease, 337
dyspraxia, 138
Early Intervention Program for Infants and Toddlers with Disabilities, 107
EBP. See evidence-based practice
eccentric viewing techniques, 348
economic environment, 89-90, 551-552
Eddy, Thomas, 4
EDPA (Erhardt Developmental Prehension Assessment), for cerebral palsy, 161
education. See also learning
  for activity director, 518, 525
  continuing, 566
  lack of commitment to, 532
  for occupational therapy, 15, 18-19
  for professional development, 562
Education for All Handicapped Children Act of 1975, 19
Education of the Handicapped Act (EHA) of 1975
  for ADHD, 187
  for visual impairment, 107
educational activities, 516, 519
EDVA (Erhardt Developmental Vision Assessment), for cerebral palsy, 161
effectiveness, of teams, 539, 541-542
EFRT (Executive Function Route Finding Task), for TBI, 221
egocentric-cooperative group, 387
EHA (Education of the Handicapped Act) of 1975, 107, 187
elderly persons
  Alzheimer's disease in, 366-379
  developmental theories of, 42-43
  functional status of, evidence-based studies of, 478
  identification for, 357-358
  osteoarthritis in, 284-286
  Parkinson's disease in, 338-343, 345-347
  rheumatoid arthritis in, 287-289

sensory dysfunction in, 348-364
stroke in, 318-332
substance abuse in, 307-317
total hip arthroplasty in, 292-303
Eleanor Clarke Slagle Award, 22
Ellis, Lady, 4
Ellis, Sir William Charles, 4
embryology, 37
empirical research, 486-487
employment, injury during, 462-469
empowerment activities, 519
endurance, decreased, in multiple sclerosis, 261
energy conservation, in arthritis, 284
entry-level practice, 510, 511, 564
environmental considerations, 88-90
    in ADL deficits, 445
    in Alzheimer's disease, 372-373
    in multiple sclerosis, 259
    in muscle weakness, 448
episodic memory, 369
epistemology, 26
equipment
    for activity program, 525
    adaptive. See assistive technology
ergonomics, 430, 466-467
Erhardt Developmental Prehension Assessment (EDPA), for cerebral palsy, 161
Erhardt Developmental Vision Assessment (EDVA), for cerebral palsy, 161
Erikson, Erik, 35-36, 38-42
ethics, 29-30, 528-537
    code of, 496, 499, 530-535, 587-588
    definition of, 529
    dilemmas in, 534
    guidelines for, 496, 499
    justice, 535
    language of, 529-530
    professional behavior and, 530-531, 534-535
    in research, 496
    resources for, 534-535
    student behavior problems and, 531-534
    vs. unethical behavior, 531
ethnic factors, 90-92
ethnographic studies, 494
evaluation. See also activity analysis
    in occupational therapy process, 48, 81, 83
    standards for, 584
Evaluation of Sensory Processing, for sensory integration dysfunction, 141
Everhardt, Kathleen Melin, 22
evidence-based practice, 472-482. See also specific disorders
    communication of findings in, 479
    definition of, 384, 473
    examination of evidence in, 475-480
    framing question in, 474-475
    reasons for, 473-474
    steps for, 474-479
Executive Function Route Finding Task (EFRT), for TBI, 221

exercise
    for arthritis, 283
    for fracture rehabilitation, 310
    for Parkinson's disease, 340
    progressive resistive, 334
    for stroke, 324-327
experiential learning, in groups, 384-385, 390
experimental research designs, 490
external environment, 88-89

facilitation techniques, for stroke, 318
fatigue, in multiple sclerosis, 260, 261
FBP (Functional Behavior Profile), for Alzheimer's disease, 369, 374
FCE (Functional Capacity Evaluation), for work injury, 462, 464
feedback
    in group intervention, 390
    on professional behavior, 530-531
feeding
    in hemiplegia, 450
    in incoordination, 448
    in muscle weakness, 448
    in Parkinson's disease, 337
    in range of motion limitation, 450
    in visual impairment, 356
    in wheelchair, 452
festination, in Parkinson's disease, 337
fiber crafts, 402
fidelity, 530, 588
Fidler, Gail, task-oriented group model of, 385-386
Fidler, Jay, 386
fieldwork, 562, 564
FIM (Functional Independence Measure), 319-320, 443-444, 484
financial aspects, of activity program, 525-526
fingers, splints for. See splints and splinting
Five-Stage Group, 388
flaccidity, 318, 323
flattened affect, 250
flexibility, in teamwork, 542
food preparation. See cooking
force, effect of, 416
Forte, Barbara, 22
found materials, for crafts, 403
Fowler, Thomas, 4
fractures, of upper extremity, with substance abuse, 307-317
frames of reference, 66-77
    for activity analysis, 55
    for Alzheimer's disease, 370-371
    for anxiety disorders, 273
    for arthritis, 283
    for autism spectrum disorders, 124, 126
    for cerebral palsy, 157, 160
    cognitive/perceptual, 75-77
    for crafts, 400
    definition of, 67
    for depression, 203-204
    vs. models, 77
    for Parkinson's disease, 338
    pediatric, 74-75

for physical function, 68-69
for psychosocial function, 69-74
for schizophrenia, 251
sensory integration as, 139
for spinal cord injury, 235
for stroke, 319
for traumatic brain injury, 216
for visual impairment, 106, 353-354
for work injury, 464-465
framework
    for activity analysis, 55
    for OT practice, 45-50
free play, for oppositional defiant disorder, 175
Freud, Sigmund, 35, 38-41, 385
FSI (Functional Status Index), 445
Functional Behavior Profile (FBP), for Alzheimer's disease, 369, 374
Functional Capacity Evaluation (FCE), for work injury, 462, 464
functional impact, of oppositional defiant disorder, 175
Functional Independence Measure (FIM), 319-320, 443-444, 484
functional performance, measurement of, 325
functional position, of hand, 416, 418-419
Functional Status Index (FSI), 445
function/dysfunction continua, 66, 68-77

gait, in Parkinson's disease, 337
games, 403
Gardner, Howard, 41
GCP (gross domestic product), 550, 552
generosity, 434
Gilbert, Martha, 9
Glasgow Coma Scale, 214, 216
glaucoma, 351, 352
goals
    for professional development, 568
    setting of, 435-438
    treatment, 99
    in treatment plan, 501-502
graded activities and work tasks, 462
grading, in activity analysis, 52, 55-56
grief, 43
grip strength
    in multiple sclerosis, 263
    splint design and, 418
grooming
    in hemiplegia, 452
    in incoordination, 448
    in multiple sclerosis, 264-265
    in muscle weakness, 448
    in range of motion limitation, 450
    in visual impairment, 356
    in wheelchair, 452
grooming group, for depression, 205-206
gross domestic product (GDP), 550, 552
group(s), vs. teams, 540
group dynamics, 385
    roles in, 392-393
    stages of, 391-392
group intervention, 382-396
    activity groups, 385-386, 393-394

advantages of, 383-384
Allen's cognitive approach, 389
development of, 385
evidence-based strategies for, 395
experiental learning and, 384-385
Fidler's task-oriented model of, 385-386
group development in, 391-392
group norms in, 390-391
Kaplan's directive approach, 387-388
King's sensory integration approach, 389
leadership styles for, 392
membership roles in, 392-393
Mosey's developmental model of, 386-387, 392
process of, 389-390
Ross' integrative approach, 388-389
group support
for anxiety disorders, 276-277
for spinal cord injury, 241
habit(s), 47
habit training, 7
half-lapboard, 406, 411
hallucinations, 250
hand
function and functional position of, 416, 418-419, 574-578
splints for. *See* splints and splinting
strength of, evidence-based studies of, 476
handwriting
in ADHD, 187
in Parkinson's disease, 338, 340
in visual impairment, 357
hardiness, 434
Hawaii Early Learning Profile (HELP)
for autism spectrum disorders, 127
for cerebral palsy, 161
Hawkins, Diane S., 22
head injury. *See* traumatic brain injury (TBI)
Head Start Act of 1964, 107
Health Insurance Portability and Accountability Act (HIPAA), 554
health insurance reimbursement, documentation for, 500
health promotion, 428-431
hearing loss, with aging, 350, 357-358
HELP (Hawaii Early Learning Profile)
for autism spectrum disorders, 127
for cerebral palsy, 161
hemianopia, 318
hemiparesis, 318
hemiplegia
ADLs in, 450, 452
in stroke, 320
Henry Phipps Clinic, 7, 8
"here and now," 382
heterotopic ossification, in SCI, 234
Hierarchy of Needs (Maslow), 487
hip, total arthroplasty of, 292-303
HIPAA (Health Insurance Portability and Accountability Act), 554
history, of occupational therapy, 2-10
holism, 26, 27-28
home health agencies, reimbursement of, 554

home management
in hemiplegia, 452
in incoordination, 450, 451
in muscle weakness, 448
in range of motion limitation, 450
in visual impairment, 356
in wheelchair, 452
Home Observation for Measurement of the Environment, 37
homunculus, 214
hope, 430
Hull House, Chicago, 5, 7, 8
human development. *See* development
human subject rights, in research, 494-496
hyperactivity, in ADHD. *See* attention deficit hyperactivity disorder (ADHD)
hyperthermia, in SCI, 233
hypertonia, in cerebral palsy, 159
hypotension, orthostatic, in SCI, 233
hypothermia, in SCI, 233
hypotonia, in cerebral palsy, 159

IADLs (instrumental activities of daily living)
definition of, 443
description of, 46
evaluation of, 444-445
measurement of, 443-444
in SCI, 236-239
IDEA (Individuals with Disability Education Act) of 1997, 107, 187
identification, for elderly persons, 357-358
IEP (Individualized Education Plan), for cerebral palsy, 163-164
IFSP (Individualized Family Service Plan), 114-120, 161-162
illusions, 250
implementation, in OT process, 84
impulsivity, 184
inattention, in ADHD. *See* attention deficit hyperactivity disorder (ADHD)
incoordination
ADLs in, 448, 450, 451
in Parkinson's disease, 336
independence, 433-434
individuality
in activity plans, 521
in occupations, 86-94
Individualized Education Plan (IEP), for cerebral palsy, 163-164
Individualized Family Service Plan (IFSP)
for cerebral palsy, 161-162
for visual impairment, 114-120
Individuals with Disability Education Act (IDEA) of 1997, 107, 187
inductive reasoning, 487
infants, development of
chart for, 574-575, 578-579
theories of, 37-40
infarction, 318
informed consent, in research, 495
inpatient rehabilitation facilities (IPFs), 550, 553
insane people, moral treatment of, 3-7

institutional review board, 495
instrument(s), for evaluation and research, 489. *See also* specific instruments
instrumental activities of daily living. *See* IADLs
integrative group intervention (Ross), 388-389
intelligence, multiple, 41
interdisciplinary model, for traumatic brain injury, 216
interdisciplinary teams, 541
interdisciplinary treatment plan, 172
intermediate-level practice, 510, 511
internal environment, 89
Internet resources, 591-592
evidence-based data on, 475
for professional development, 567
intervention, 48-49. *See also* specific disorders
definition of, 383
group. *See* group intervention
process of, 80-85
standards for, 584-585
interviews
for ADL evaluation, 445
for research, 493
intradisciplinary teams, 541
IPFs (inpatient rehabilitation facilities), 550, 553

JCAHO (Joint Commission on Accreditation of Healthcare Organizations), 554-555
Jewish Sanitarium and Hospital for Chronic Diseases, 10
job injury, 462-469
Johnson, Susan Cox, 8
Joint Commission on Accreditation of Healthcare Organizations (JCAHO), 554-555
joint protection, in arthritis, 284
Jones, Robin, 22
journals, with research studies, 475
JRA (juvenile rheumatoid arthritis), 286-287
justice, 535, 588
juvenile parkinsonism, 336
juvenile rheumatoid arthritis, 286-287

Kabat proprioceptive neuromuscular facilitation frame of reference, 69
Kanner, Leo, 123
Kaplan, Kathy, directive group of, 387-388
Kelley, Florence, 5
KELS (Kohlman Evaluation of Living Skills), 219, 445
Kidner, Thomas B., 8
Kielhofner, Gary, 10-11
King, Lorna Jean, 389
Kitchen Task Assessment (KTA), for Alzheimer's disease, 369
kits, for crafts, 400-401
Klein-Bell ADL Scale, 445
knitting device, 412
Kohlman Evaluation of Living Skills (KELS), 219, 445

Kransee, Margaret, 7
KTA (Kitchen Task Assessment), for Alzheimer's disease, 369

laissez-faire leadership, 392
language, development of, 40
lapboards, for wheelchair, 411
Larson, Barbara, 21-22
lassitude, 258, 260
Lathrop, Julia, 5
Lazarus Project, 526
leadership. See also management issues
    in group intervention, 392
    vs. management, 556
learning, 96-101
    case studies of, 100
    with cognitive disability, 99-100, 399
    experiential, in groups, 384-385, 390
    in groups, 384-385, 390
    interpersonal, 390
    Mosey's teaching-learning process for, 98-99
    in professional development, 564-567
    in teams, 542
    theories of, 97-98, 100
leatherwork, 401
legal blindness, 351
legal hold, 172
leisure activities, 516, 519
    assessment of, 83
    in multiple sclerosis, 266
    in SCI, 236-239
levodopa/carbidopa, for Parkinson's disease, 338
Lewin, Kurt, 384, 385, 392
life skills, 432-440
    case study of, 435-437
    development groups for, 434-435
    evidence-based strategies for, 439
    hardiness, 434
    resilience, 433-434
lifestyle, redesign of, 428, 429
lifestyle/adaptive performance model, crafts and, 399
listening, in management, 557
long-term care, activity director for, 516-527
long-term memory, 368-369
loose associations, 250
LOTCA (Lowenstein Occupational Therapy Cognitive Assessment), for TBI, 220
low vision, 350-352, 358-359
Lowenstein Occupational Therapy Cognitive Assessment (LOTCA), for TBI, 220
Luther, Martin, 3

McDonald Play Activity Inventory-Revised (MPAI-R), for oppositional defiant disorder, 174
McKee, Nelda, 10
macular degeneration, 351, 352
maintenance activities, 519
make-up board, 412
management issues, 550-558

accreditation, 554-555
economic environment, 551-552
internal considerations, 555-557
political environment, 552-553
regulations, 552-554
reimbursement, 553-554
Manhattan State Hospital, 7
Marcia, James, 42
Maslow's Hierarchy of Needs, 487
mastery, 433, 542-543
maturation, in teamwork, 543
mature group, 387
Maudsley, Henry, 123
MBPC (Memory and Behavior Problem Checklist), for Alzheimer's disease, 369
MDS (Minimum Data Set), 553-554
mean, in research, 484
median, in research, 484
Medicaid, reimbursement by, 553
Medicare
    documentation for, 500
    politics of, 552-553
    reimbursement by, 553-554
    Resident Assessment System of, 522
MEDLS (Milwaukee Evaluation of Daily Living Skills), 445
Memory and Behavior Problem Checklist (MBPC), for Alzheimer's disease, 369
memory deficits, Alzheimer's disease in, 366-369
memory notebook, for traumatic brain injury, 218, 219
mental illness. See also specific disorders
    historic treatment of, 3-7
mental retardation, with autism, 130-131
mentoring, 565, 567
meta-analysis, 484
metacognition, 212
metal crafts, 402
metaphysics, 26
Meyer, Adolph, 6, 7, 8, 27-20, 385
micrographia, in Parkinson's disease, 338, 340
middle childhood, 172
Miller Assessment for Preschoolers, for sensory integration dysfunction, 141
Milwaukee Evaluation of Daily Living Skills (MEDLS), 445
mind-body interaction, 9
Minimum Data Set (MDS), 553-554
ministration, in teamwork, 542
mobile arm support (MAS), 442
mobility, bed, in stroke, 321-323
model(s)
    of ADHD, 186
    client-centered, 77-78
    crafts and, 399-400
    definition of, 67
    description of, 77
    of group intervention, 385-389
    of human occupation, 78
    occupational adaptation, 78, 354, 400
    occupational science, 78
    of resilience, 433-434

of sensory integration, 140
Model of Human Occupation (MOHO), 11, 78
    for arthritis, 283
    for crafts, 400
    for visual impairment, 354
    for work injury, 464
MOHO. See Model of Human Occupation (MOHO)
moral treatment, 3-7
mosaics, 402
Mosey, Anne Cronin, 69-70
    developmental group model of, 386-387, 392
    on ethics, 529
    teaching-learning process of, 98-99
motivation
    for activity participation, 522
    in management, 557
    for OT practice, 533-534
motor skills
    acquisition of, as frame of reference, 74
    deficits of, in sensory integration dysfunction, 141
    development of, 574-578
movement disorders
    in Alzheimer's disease, 368
    in multiple sclerosis, 260, 261
    Parkinson's disease as, 334-347
MPAI-R (McDonald Play Activity Inventory-Revised), for oppositional defiant disorder, 174
MS. See multiple sclerosis (MS)
multidisciplinary teams, 541
multiple sclerosis (MS), 258-270
    case study of, 261-267, 269-270
    clinical signs and symptoms of, 259-260
    epidemiology of, 259
    etiology of, 259
    medical treatment of, 260
    motor vehicle violations in, 476-477
    occupational impact of, 261
    patterns of, 260
    referrals in, 260
    workplace modifications for, 467-468
Multiple Sclerosis Society, 259
muscle weakness, ADLs in, 447-448
myelin sheath, 258, 259

Narcotics Anonymous, 306
narrative notes, 503
National Board for Certification of Occupational Therapists (NBCOT), 566-567
national health care expenditures, 550
National Society for the Promotion of Occupational Therapy, 6, 8
National Wellness Association, 429
NBCOT (National Board for Certification of Occupational Therapists), 566-567
needle crafts, 401-402
neglect, unilateral, 318
neural plasticity, 212

neurodevelopmental treatment frame of reference, 68-69, 157
neurofunctional approach, as frame of reference, 77
Neuromotor Behavior Model
    for anxiety disorders, 273
    crafts and, 398
    for schizophrenia, 251
Newton, Isabelle, 8
nonexperimental research designs, 490-491
nonmaleficence, 529-530, 587
normative ethics, 528
norms, group, 390-391
NPI Interest Checklist, for anxiety disorders, 276
nystagmus, 258, 260

OA (osteoarthritis), 284-286
obesity, case study of, 88
O'Brock, Irene, 9-10
observation
    for ADL evaluation, 445
    for research, 493
    of sensory integration dysfunction, 141-142
Observed Tasks of Daily Living (OTDL), for TBI, 222
obsession, 272
occupation
    areas of, 44
    deficiency of, 87
    definition of, 28, 46
    performance of, 46-47
        in MS, 261, 266
        in SCI, 236-239
        in visual impairment, 106
    sensory integration and, 140
    types of, 87
Occupational Adaptation model, 78, 354, 400
occupational behavior, 8, 11, 173-174
occupational nurse, 5
occupational performance areas, 484
occupational rehabilitation, 462
Occupational Safety and Health Administration (OSHA), 465
occupational science, 11, 78
occupational therapy
    before 1960, 15
    case studies of. See case studies
    definition of, 46, 54, 87
    developmental milestones of, 19-21
    distrust in, 18
    domain of, 45-48
    early training needs in, 15
    evolution of, 27-30
    history of, 2-10
    as learning process, 9-10
    origin of term, 6-7
    personal qualities for, 10
    philosophy of, 8, 24-30
    process of, 48-50, 80-85
    questionnaire for, 308, 313-315
    recent practice changes in, 561-562
    short courses in, 15

terminology of, 45-48, 77, 583
occupational therapy assistants (OTAs)
    as activity directors, 516-527
    developmental milestones of, 19-21
    distrust of, 18
    education for, 15, 18-19
    history of, 14-18
    occupational therapist interactions with, 146
    practice settings for, 19
    roster of honor of, 21-22
    supervision of, 510-515, 564-565
    utilization of, 513
Occupational Therapy Practice Framework: Domain and Process, 45-50, 106
    on activity analysis, 57
    on ADLs, 443
    on assessment, 83
    on documentation, 499
    on intervention, 383
Omnibus Budget Reconciliation Act of 1987, Nursing Home Reform Amendments of, 517-518
ontogeny, 382
open head injury, 213
open seclusion, 172
ophthalmologist, 348
oppositional defiant disorder, 172-182
optometrist, 348
organizational skills, 184
organizing, 555
orientation stage, of group development, 391
Orthoplast, for splint fabrication, 421
orthostatic hypotension, in SCI, 233
OSHA (Occupational Safety and Health Administration), 465
OTAs. See occupational therapy assistants (OTAs)
OTDL (Observed Tasks of Daily Living), for TBI, 222
outcomes
    in occupational therapy process, 49
    in treatment plan, 502

palmar arches, 416, 418
panic, 272
parallel group, 387
paraplegia, 232, 452
Parkinson's disease (PD), 334-347
    case study of, 338-343, 345-347
    causes of, 336
    evidence-based treatment of, 343
    frame of reference for, 338
    juvenile, 336
    medical management of, 338
    signs and symptoms of, 335-338
    surgical management of, 338
pauciarticular JRA, 282, 286
Pavlov, Ivan, 36
PD. See Parkinson's disease (PD)
PDMS-2 (Peabody Developmental Motor Scales-2)
    for ADHD, 187
    for autism spectrum disorders, 127

pedagogy, 97
pediatric patients. See also children and childhood; infants
    frames of reference for, 74-75
PEOP model. See Person-Environment Occupation-Performance (PEOP) model
performance patterns, crafts and, 400
performance skills, 47
    for ADLs, 446-452
    crafts and, 400
    for visual impairment, 106
peripheral vision, 348
Person-Environment-Occupation Performance (PEOP) model, 77-78
    for ADHD, 186
    for anxiety disorders, 273, 274
    for multiple sclerosis, 262
    for schizophrenia, 251
pervasive developmental disorders (PPDs), 122. See also autism spectrum disorder
phenomenological studies, 494
Philadelphia Geriatric Center Instrumental Activities of Daily Living, for stroke, 319
philosophy, of occupational therapy, 24-30
phobias, 272
physical activities, 516, 519
physical development, 34
physical function, frames of reference for, 68-69
Piaget, Jean, 36, 38, 40-41
Pierce, Franklin (president), 4
pillow, Cowan, 409, 410, 413
pill-rolling, in Parkinson's disease, 336
Pinel, Phillipe, 3-4
pinch strength, in multiple sclerosis, 263
plagiarism, 532-533
planning, in OT process, 83-84, 555
play
    for autism spectrum disorders, 126
    development of, 578-580
    for oppositional defiant disorder, 175
PNF (proprioceptive neuromuscular facilitation), 69, 338
policy and procedure manual, for activities, 523
political environment, 552-553
polyarticular JRA, 282, 286
Polyform, for splint fabrication, 421
polysubstance abuse, 306
portfolios, of professional development, 560, 568
positioning, in stroke, 321-322
post traumatic stress disorder, 172, 272
postural instability, in Parkinson's disease, 336, 337, 340
PPSs (prospective payment systems), 553-554
practice settings, for OTAs, 19
praxis deficits, in sensory integration dysfunction, 141
PRE (progressive resistive exercise), 334
prehension, 418
prenatal development, 37
presbyopia, 350

pressure injuries, in SCI, 234
printing, 403
privacy, 587
problem list, in treatment plan, 501
procedural memory, 369
process, definition of, 382
productive activities, 516, 519
professional behavior, 530-531, 534-535
professional development, 560-570
    competence, 560, 561-562
    educational setting for, 562, 564
    at entry-level, 564
    fieldwork in, 562
    job changes in, 564
    learning relationships and activities in, 564-567
    plan for, 567-568
    specialization in, 564
    stages of, 562, 563
progress, documenting, 503-504
progress notes, 503
Progressive Era, 5-6
progressive resistive exercises (PRE), 334
project group, 387
projection, as defense mechanism, 382
projective media, 385
proprioceptive neuromuscular facilitation (PNF), 69, 338
prospective memory, 369
prospective payment systems (PPSs), 553-554
psychiatric occupational therapy, vs. holism, 28
psychoanalytic theory, in group intervention, 385-386
psychodynamic frame of reference, 71-72
psychomotor agitation, 202
psychosexual developmental stages (Freud), 35, 38-41
psychosis, 250
psychosocial developmental theory (Erikson), 35-36, 38-42
psychosocial function, frames of reference for, 69-74
psychosocial issues, ADLs and, 452
PTSD (post traumatic stress disorder), 172, 272
puberty, 41-42
public relations, in activity planning, 521
publications, for professional development, 566-567
purposeful work and leisure, 9
putty, therapeutic, 402

quadriplegia, 232
Quakers, mental illness treatment facilities of, 4
qualitative research, 491-494
quality of life, 24, 29
quantitative research, 488-491
quasi-experimental research designs, 490
question, in research, 488
questionnaires
    for activity interest, 520

for occupational therapy, 308, 313-315

RA (rheumatoid arthritis), 90, 287-289
Rancho Levels of Cognitive Functioning-Revised (RLA), for TBI, 214-224
randomized clinical trials (RCTs), 484
range, in research, 484
range of motion (ROM)
    decreased, ADLs in, 450
    in fracture rehabilitation, 310
    in juvenile rheumatoid arthritis, 287
    in Parkinson's disease, 340
    restriction of, in spinal cord injury, 233
    in rheumatoid arthritis, 288
    with splint, 420
    in stroke, exercises for, 321
RCTs (randomized clinical trials), 484
reading
    continuous, 348
    spot, 348
    with visual impairment, 357
reasonable accommodations, 184, 462
reasoning
    clinical, 406, 479
    in research, 487
reclusive lifestyle, case study of, 92
records. See documentation
recovery, from substance abuse, 304
recreation groups, for depression, 205-206
reference, frames of. See frames of reference
referral, 81-82, 584
reflexes
    development of, 574
    infant, 37
regulations, 552-554
    on activities, 517-518
    on human research subject rights, 494-495
    supervision and, 512
    on work injury, 464-465
rehabilitation
    cognitive, 75-76
    as frame of reference, 69
        for ADL deficits, 445
        for crafts, 400
        for multiple sclerosis, 262
        for spinal cord injury, 235
        for total hip arthroplasty, 294
        for visual impairment, 353-354
    occupational, 462
    in stroke, 320
    in visual impairment, 353
    in work injury, 464
Reilly, Mary, 10-11, 27-28
    on play experiences, 126, 157, 160
reimbursement, 553-554
relapse, in multiple sclerosis, 258, 259
reliability, in research, 484
remission, in multiple sclerosis, 258, 259
reports. See documentation
research, 484-496. See also evidence-based practice
    action, 486
    applications of, 485-486

applied, 486
basic, 486
definition of, 485
empirical, 486-487
ethics in, 496
faculty-student collaboration in, 533
human subject rights in, 494-496
problem definition in, 487-488
for professional development, 567
qualitative, 491-494
quantitative, 488-491
question in, 488
reasoning in, 487
theoretical, 486-487
Resident Assessment System, 522
residential treatment facility, 172
resilience, 433-434
Resource Utilization Group (RUG), 554
resources, lack of respect for, 533
respiratory impairment, in SCI, 233
responsibility, for service delivery, 583-584
retinopathy
    diabetic, 352
    of prematurity (retrolental fibroplasia), 107-111, 114-120
return-to-work process, 462-469
rheumatoid arthritis, 287-289
    case study of, 90
    juvenile, 286-287
rigidity, in Parkinson's disease, 336-338, 340
RLA (Rancho Levels of Cognitive Functioning -Revised), for TBI, 214-224
Robeson, Harriet, 9
Robinson, Col. Ruth A., 15, 16
Rochester, New York State Hospital, 7
role acquisition frame of reference, 69-70
role dysfunction, 202
ROM. See range of motion (ROM)
room check program, in depression, 206
Ross, Mildred, integrative group of, 388-389
Routine Task Inventory-2 (RTI-2)
    for schizophrenia, 253
    for TBI, 219
RUG (Resource Utilization Group), 554
Ryan, Sally E., 21

safety, of assistive equipment, 409, 412
Saki-Chydenius, Sisko, survey of, 387
sampling, in research, 489-492
sanction, 528
Sands, Ida, 9
San-Splint, for splint fabrication, 421
scapegoat, in group dynamics, 391
scapular mobilization exercises, for stroke, 324-327
Schindler, Victoria, 386, 387
schizophrenia, 250-257
Schwagmeyer, Mildred, 15, 17
SCI. See spinal cord injury (SCI)
scotoma, 348
screening, for OT services, 81, 83
    in cerebral palsy, 160
    standards for, 584

self-abuse, in autism, 131-132
self-care training, in depression, 205-206
self-catheterization, urinary, in SCI, 230
self-instruction interventions, for Alzheimer's disease, 372-373
self-regulation deficits, in sensory integration dysfunction, 141
Seltser, Charlotte Gale, 21
semantic memory, 369
seminars, 566
sensorimotor development, 578-580
sensory defensiveness, 122, 138
sensory dysfunction, 348-364
    hearing loss, 350, 357-358
    in multiple sclerosis, 260, 261
    in SCI, 233-234
    in SID, 138-154, 474
    visual. See visual impairment
sensory integration
    for ADHD, 189
    for autism spectrum disorders, 124, 126
    for cerebral palsy, 157
    definition of, 139
    dysfunction of (SID), 138-154, 474
    as frame of reference, 74-75
    model of, 140
    as theory, 139
Sensory Integration and Praxis Tests (SIPT)
    for autism spectrum disorders, 124, 126
    for sensory integration dysfunction, 141
Sensory Integration Inventory of Individuals with Developmental Disabilities (SII-DD)
    for autism spectrum disorders, 127
    for cerebral palsy, 160
sensory modulation, deficits of, in SID, 141
Sensory Profile
    for ADHD, 186
    for sensory integration dysfunction, 141
sensory stimulation, for traumatic brain injury, 217
service competency, 292
service management, 84
sewing, 401-402
sexual relationships, policies on, 531-532
Shannon, Phillip, 10-11
Sheats, Paul, 392-393
Sheppard and Enoch Pratt Asylum, 6
shock, spinal, in SCI, 234
short courses, for occupational therapy, 15
short-term memory, 368
shoulder
    subluxation of, 318, 323-324
    work-related injury of, 465-466
SID (sensory integration dysfunction), 138-154, 474
sight, problems with. See visual impairment
SII-DD (Sensory Integration Inventory of Individuals with Developmental Disabilities)
    for autism spectrum disorders, 127
    for cerebral palsy, 160
single-subject study designs, 491

SIPT (Sensory Integration and Praxis Tests)
    for autism spectrum disorders, 124, 126
    for sensory integration dysfunction, 141
skilled nursing facilities (SNFs), 553-554
skills
    for activity analysis, 55
    life, 432-440
    performance. See performance skills
skin
    pressure injuries of, in SCI, 234
    problems with, in Parkinson's disease, 337
Skinner, B.F., 36
Slagle, Eleanor Clarke, 5, 7, 8, 54, 385
    award named for, 22
sleep disturbance, in Parkinson's disease, 337
slings
    custom-made, 92
    for hemiplegia in stroke, 324, 327
SNFs (skilled nursing facilities), 553-554
SOAP notes, 503
sobriety, 304, 306
social access activities, 516, 519
social microcosm concept, 389
social-emotional development, 34
socialization
    in Alzheimer's disease, 375
    in professional development, 563
Society of Friends, mental illness treatment facilities of, 4
sociocultural considerations, 90-92
somatic complaints, 202
Spackman, Clare, 9
spasticity
    in cerebral palsy, 159
    in multiple sclerosis, 260
    in SCI, 234
specialization, 533
    vs. holism, 28
    for professional development, 564
specific needs, for assistive technology, 406
speech, disorganized, 250
spinal cord injury (SCI), 230-249
    ADLs in, 452
    case study of, 235, 240-242
    complications of, 233-234
    definition of, 232
    etiology of, 232
    evaluation of, 234
    initial treatment of, 233
    interventions for, vs. level, 236-240
    levels of, 232-233, 236-240
    prevalence of, 232
    prognosis for, 233-234
    splints for, 418
spinal shock, in SCI, 234
spirituality, 430, 516, 519
splints and splinting, 416-426
    for arthrogryposis multiplex, 478
    assessment of, 420
    custom-made, 89-90, 92
    environmental effects on, 89
    evidence-based strategies for, 425
    fabrication of, 420-425

    history of, 417
    prefabricated, 418
    principles of, 418-420
    purpose of, 417-418
    types of, 418
spot reading, 348
staffing, 556
standard deviation, 484
standards
    case studies of, 91-92
    of practice, 81, 583-585
    study of (axiology), 26
    supervision and, 512
static splints, 418
stress
    case study of, 93
    hardiness and, 434
    management of, for anxiety disorders, 276-277
stroke, 318-332
    assessment in, 319-320
    case study of, 320-328, 330-332, 505, 507
    definition of, 319
    epidemiology of, 319
    evidence-based treatment of, 474-475
    frames of reference for, 319
    functional impact of, 320
    treatment of, 320, 329
    visual impairment in, 351-353
substance abuse, 304-317
substance dependence, 304
substantia nigra, degeneration of, in Parkinson's disease, 336
suctioning, in SCI, 233
suncatchers, 403
superstitions, case study of, 91
supervision, 510-515
    in professional development, 564-565
    in teamwork, 544
support groups
    for anxiety disorders, 276-277
    for spinal cord injury, 241
supportive activities, 518-519
swallowing difficulties, in Parkinson's disease, 337

tactile discrimination deficits, in sensory integration dysfunction, 141
task, of group, 382
task groups, 175, 385-386
TBI. See traumatic brain injury (TBI)
TCA (Toglia Categorization Assessment), for TBI, 222
TEA (Test of Everyday Attention), for TBI, 220
Teacher Questionnaire of Sensorimotor Behavior, for ADHD, 186
teaching. See also learning
    Mosey's process for, 98-99
teams, 531-548
    building of, 542-543
    definition of, 539, 540
    dynamics of, 547

effective, 539, 541-542
functions of, 546, 547
vs. groups, 540
learning in, 542
membership in, 543-546
professional development in, 565
roles in, 546, 547
tenodesis, 230, 242
Test of Everyday Attention (TEA), for TBI, 220
Test of Functional Executive Abilities (TOFEA), for TBI, 221
Test of Playfulness, for ADHD, 187
Test of Sensory Function in Infants, for SID, 141
Test of Visual Motor Skills-Revised (TVMS-R), for autism spectrum disorders, 127
Test of Visual Perceptual Skills-Revised (TVPS-R), for autism spectrum disorders, 127
tetraplegia, 232, 452
T-groups, 384
THA. See total hip arthroplasty (THA)
theoretical research, 486-487
theory(ies)
    definition of, 67
    developmental, 35-42
    of learning, 97-98, 100
    neurodevelopmental treatment, 68-69, 157
    sensory integration, 139
therapeutic communication, 392
therapeutic potential, 52
therapy putty, 402
thermoplastic materials, 416, 420-422
thinking, steps of, 98
third-party payer, 498, 500
thrombosis, 292
TIME (Toddler and Infant Motor Evaluation)
    for autism spectrum disorders, 127
    for cerebral palsy, 160
time clock, for activity analysis, 309
toddler(s), developmental theories of, 38-40
Toddler and Infant Motor Evaluation (TIME)
    for autism spectrum disorders, 127
    for cerebral palsy, 160
TOFEA (Test of Functional Executive Abilities), for TBI, 221
Toglia Categorization Assessment (TCA), for TBI, 222
Toglia dynamic interactional frame of reference, 76-77
toilet training, 39
toileting, after total hip arthroplasty, 295
total hip arthroplasty (THA), 292-303
    assessment in, 294-296
    case study of, 294-303
    frames of reference for, 294
    indications for, 293
    precautions after, 295, 298

procedure for, 293-294
    statistics on, 293
    treatment of, 295, 297, 299-301, 303
Touch Inventory for Elementary School-Aged Children, for ADHD, 186
Tracy, Susan, 5, 8, 53-54
traditions, case studies of, 91
transdisciplinary teams, 541
transfers
    in hemiplegia, 452
    in incoordination, 450
    in muscle weakness, 448
    in range of motion limitation, 450
    in stroke, bed-to-chair, 321
    in wheelchair, 452
transition plan, 585
traumatic brain injury (TBI), 212-229
    case study of, 216-223, 226-229
    categories of, 213
    epidemiology of, 213
    evaluation in, 216
    frames of reference for, 216
    interdisciplinary approach to, 216
    neuroanatomy of, 213-214
    recovery from, 214-216
Traumatic Brain Injury Act of 1996, 213
treatment plan, documenting, 500-503
tremor, in Parkinson's disease, 336, 338
Trendelenburg gait, 292
trial use, of assistive technology, 406, 413
trust, in management, 556-557
trustworthiness, of research results, 493-494
truth, 26
TSI (De Gangi-Berk Test of Sensory Integration)
    for autism spectrum disorders, 127
    for sensory integration dysfunction, 141
Tuke, William, 4, 53
TVMS-R (Test of Visual Motor Skills-Revised), for autism spectrum disorders, 127
TVPS-R (Test of Visual Perceptual Skills-Revised), for autism spectrum disorders, 127
twelve-step programs, for substance abuse, 306

ulcers, decubitus, in SCI, 234
ULOS (upper limb orthotic system), 442
underweight, case study of, 88
Uniform Terminology, 45-46
unilateral neglect, 318
upper limb orthotic system (ULOS), 442
urinary problems, in Parkinson's disease, 337

vaccinations, for infants, 37
values
    case studies of, 91-92
    clarification of, 437
    study of (axiology), 26
variables, in research, 488-489

variance, 484
veracity, 530, 588
vestibular processing deficits, 141
vision
    center, 348
    development of, 578-580
    in management, 557
    peripheral, 348
visual acuity, 348, 350
visual field deficits, 318
visual impairment, 104-120, 348-364
    with aging, 349-350
    AOTA policy on, 106-107
    assessment of, in stroke, 320
    case study of, 107-111, 358-359
    causes of, 352-353
    evidence-based treatment of, 113
    frames of reference for, 106, 353-354
    functional impact of, 105-106, 351-352
    interventions for, 353-357
    low vision, 350-352, 358-359
    resources for, 355
    terminology of, 105
    types of, 350-351
visual motor integration, 202
visual perceptual deficits, 318
VMI (Beery Developmental Test of Visual-Motor Integration)
    for autism spectrum disorders, 127
    for depression, 204
    for oppositional defiant disorder, 174
volunteers, in activity programs, 524

Wade, Beatrice, 9
Watson, John B., 36
weakness, ADLs in, 447-448
wellness, 428-431
wheelchair
    ADLs and, 452
    assistive equipment for, 411
    for stroke, 324, 327
Wiemer, Ruth Brunyate, 15, 17-18
Wilbarger Protocol, in autism, 128
woodworking, 401
work injury, 462-469
workers' compensation, 241, 465
workshops, 566
World Wide Web. See Internet
wrist, splints for. See splints and splinting
writing. See also handwriting
    creative, 402

Yalom, I.D., 389-392
Yerxa, Elizabeth, 10-11, 78
York Retreat, 4, 53

Zarit Burden Interview, for Alzheimer's disease, 369, 374

WAIT

...There's More!

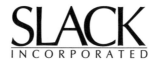